SECOND EDITION

Occupational Therapy
in Community-Based Practice Settings

Marjorie E. Scaffa, PhD, OTR/L, FAOTA
Professor and Chair
Department of Occupational Therapy
University of South Alabama
Mobile, Alabama

S. Maggie Reitz, PhD, OTR/L, FAOTA
Professor and Chair
Department of Occupational Therapy and
Occupational Science
Towson University
Towson, Maryland

F.A. Davis Company • Philadelphia

F. A. Davis Company
1915 Arch Street
Philadelphia, PA 19103
www.fadavis.com

Printed in the United States of America

Last digit indicates print number: 10 9 8 7 6 5 4 3 2 1

Senior Acquisitions Editor: Christa Fratantoro
Manager of Content Development: George Lang
Developmental Editor: Peg Waltner
Art and Design Manager: Carolyn O'Brien

As new scientific information becomes available through basic and clinical research, recommended treatments and drug therapies undergo changes. The author(s) and publisher have done everything possible to make this book accurate, up to date, and in accord with accepted standards at the time of publication. The author(s), editors, and publisher are not responsible for errors or omissions or for consequences from application of the book, and make no warranty, expressed or implied, in regard to the contents of the book. Any practice described in this book should be applied by the reader in accordance with professional standards of care used in regard to the unique circumstances that may apply in each situation. The reader is advised always to check product information (package inserts) for changes and new information regarding dose and contraindications before administering any drug. Caution is especially urged when using new or infrequently ordered drugs.

Library of Congress Cataloging-in-Publication Data

Scaffa, Marjorie E.
  Occupational therapy in community-based practice settings / Marjorie E. Scaffa, S. Maggie Reitz. — 2nd ed.
    p. ; cm.
  Includes bibliographical references and index.
  ISBN 978-0-8036-2580-8 (pbk. : alk. paper)
  I. Reitz, S. Maggie. II. Title.
  [DNLM: 1. Occupational Therapy—methods. 2. Community Health Services. WB 555]
  RM735
  615.8'515—dc23   2013011686

For all those special people
who see what others ignore,
embrace what others fear,
and create new paths that others can follow.

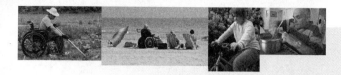

This text is dedicated to the memory of Dr. Gary Kielhofner (1949–2010), scholar, teacher, mentor, and friend. His extraordinary contributions to occupational therapy education, research, and practice are unparalleled.

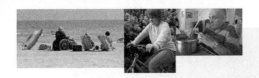

Introduction to the Foreword

This is the foreword that appeared in the first edition of this text. It is particularly meaningful to me as it was written by Dr. Gary Kielhofner, who was my occupational therapy professor and mentor. Dr. Kielhofner died in September 2010 after a short battle with cancer, but his legacy lives on in the many students he taught and professionals he mentored. For these reasons, we have chosen to retain this foreword and dedicate the second edition of this text to Dr. Gary Kielhofner.

—MARJORIE E. SCAFFA, PhD, OTR, FAOTA

Foreword

Twenty-five years ago I collaborated on my first publication with one of my mentors, Florence Cromwell. The paper described preparation of occupational therapy students to work in community settings (Cromwell & Kielhofner, 1976). I had the good fortune of working with a mentor who appreciated that much of the future of occupational therapy would be in community practice. A quarter century ago, this was still a new idea.

In the intervening period a number of changes in health care, health demographics, and funding of health services have made community-based practice not only common but the most promising direction for the future of practice in occupational therapy.

It gives me great satisfaction to see that one of my former students has gone on to edit the first comprehensive volume in community practice. It is even more gratifying to note the scope and quality of chapters that make up this ambitious volume. Community practice means much more than physical placement in a community setting. Importantly, it represents a different paradigm of care than that seen in traditional hospital and rehabilitation settings. The therapist working in the community most likely works in an organization whose traditional medically defined settings. Moreover, the voices and viewpoints of those served will often carry much more weight than in a traditional setting. Therapists who wish to be effective in community practice must be prepared to take on new roles, to take unusual risks, and to envision service in creative ways. Thus, although community practice is not as anomalous as it was 25 years ago, it still represents new territory for most of occupational therapy.

Marjorie Scaffa and her colleagues have assembled a remarkable set of resources for the occupational therapist in community practice. The scope and depth of the chapters make this at once an authoritative work on community practice and an invaluable collection of resources.

—GARY KIELHOFNER, DrPH, OTR

Cromwell, F.S., & Kielhofner, G. (1976). An educational strategy for occupational therapy community service. American Journal of Occupational Therapy, 30, 629-633.

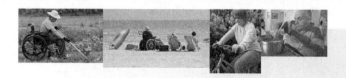

This book is the culmination of one aspect of the professional journey of Marjorie Scaffa that started when she was an undergraduate major in psychology with a minor in health education and continued on in an entry-level master's program to become an occupational therapist. During her years as an occupational therapy student at Virginia Commonwealth University, she was introduced to the Model of Human Occupation by Dr. Kielhofner and became increasingly excited about the potential for practice in nonmedical settings. When given the opportunity to choose a topic for a paper, Marjorie wrote about occupational therapy's role in community health, and the seeds of what would later become this book were sown.

As a practicing occupational therapist, she gained experience in a variety of settings but was most energized and excited by home health practice. Providing services in the home enabled her to become part of the person's daily life context in which the client participated in self-care, work, and leisure. Marjorie was impressed by how much more meaningful occupations were to individuals and their families in real-life environments.

Through our practice and further education, we both came to believe firmly that if occupation could restore function and enhance the quality of life for individuals with disabilities and their families, then it could also be used to prevent injuries and promote health in communities. Thus began our quests for doctorates in health education. We quickly realized that much of what we had learned in occupational therapy would be useful in community-based prevention and health promotion, but that we needed to become acculturated to the mind-set and conceptual frameworks of health educators, which were quite different from those of occupational therapy practitioners. We were exposed to planning, implementing, and evaluating preventive interventions directed at groups and populations rather than rehabilitative interventions directed at individuals.

Through time we were able to assimilate both of our professional identities as occupational therapists and health educators, which enabled us to envision this Second Edition. It is clearly and straightforwardly an occupational therapy text with an appreciation of the importance of community as a context for health.

We hope that you find the Second Edition of the book to be a useful and more developed discussion of the issues related to present-day community practice in occupational therapy and descriptions of a variety of settings in which this practice currently occurs. The book has grown from 18 chapters in the original edition to 29 chapters in this Second Edition, with sections devoted to each of the six areas of the American Occupational Therapy Association's Centennial Vision. Chapters have been added on community mental health services for children and youth as well as on forensic transition services. The number of chapters on productive aging has increased from one to five, with chapters being added on driving and community mobility, low-vision services, fall prevention, and aging in place. Chapters related to work have increased from one to three, with new chapters on ergonomics and welfare to work programs being the enhancements to this edition. The ability to add chapters on Lifestyle Redesign, technology in community-based practice, as well as chapters on health promotion in faith-based organizations, primary care settings, and academic communities together with the other additional chapters exemplifies how the profession's contributions to community health and well-being have significantly expanded since the first edition of this book.

The book remains designed as a textbook for entry-level occupational therapy students, but it also proves useful to practitioners wishing to facilitate a transition from medical model practice to community-based practice. We are grateful for the opportunity to participate in and contribute to the profession's expanding role in prevention, health promotion, and community health.

—MARJORIE E. SCAFFA
    S. MAGGIE REITZ

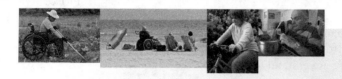

Abigail Baxter, PhD
Professor
Department of Leadership and Teacher Education
University of South Alabama
Mobile, Alabama

Mary Frances Baxter, OT, PhD, FAOTA
Associate Professor
School of Occupational Therapy
Texas Woman's University
Houston, Texas

Mary Becker-Omvig, MS, OTR/L
Program Manager
Howard County Office on Aging
Columbia, Maryland

Shirley A. Blanchard, PhD, ABDA, OTR/L, FAOTA
Associate Professor
Department of Occupational Therapy
Creighton University
Omaha, Nebraska

Peter Bowman, OTD, MHS, OTR/L, OT(C), Dip COT
Assistant Professor
Division of Occupational Therapy
Medical University of South Carolina
Charleston, South Carolina

Carol A. Brownson, MSPH
Program Director
Advancing Chronic Care through Excellence
in Systems & Support (ACCESS)
George Warren Brown School of Social Work
Washington University in St. Louis
St. Louis, Missouri

Kimberly Mansfield Caldeira, MS
Associate Director
Center on Young Adult Health and Development
University of Maryland School of Public Health
College Park, Maryland

Erin Guillory Caraway, MS OTR
Occupational Therapist
Physical Medicine Department
Lake Charles Memorial Health System
Lake Charles, Louisiana

Roxanne Castaneda, MS, OTR/L
Public Health Advisor
Center for Mental Health Service
Community Support Programs
Substance Abuse Mental Health Services
Administration
Rockville, Maryland

S. Blaise Chromiak, MD
Family Practice Physician
Mobile, Alabama

Camille Dieterle, OTD, OTR/L
Director
USC Occupational Therapy Faculty Practice
Assistant Professor of Clinical Occupational Therapy
Division of Occupational Science and Occupational
Therapy
University of Southern California
Los Angeles, California

Joy D. Doll, OTD, OTR/L
Assistant Professor
Director
Post-Professional OTD Program
Department of Occupational Therapy
Creighton University
Omaha, Nebraska

David Ensminger, PhD
Assistant Professor
Teaching and Learning Program
School of Education
Loyola University Chicago
Chicago, Illinois

Rebecca I. Estes, PhD, OTR/L, CAPS
Associate Professor
Occupational Therapy Department
Nova Southeastern University
Fort Lauderdale, Florida

Wendy M. Holmes, PhD, OTR/L
Associate Professor
School of Occupational Therapy
Brenau University
Gainesville, Georgia

Sonia Lawson, PhD, OTR/L
Associate Professor
Department of Occupational Therapy &
Occupational Science
Towson University
Towson, Maryland

Paula Lowrey, MOT, OTR/L, CAPS
Occupational Therapist
Independent Contractor
Home Health
Fort Lauderdale, Florida

M. Beth Merryman, PhD, OTR/L, FAOTA
Professor
Department of Occupational Therapy &
Occupational Science
Towson University
Towson, Maryland

Emily Wilson Mowrey, MS, OTR/L
Occupational Therapist
Westerville, Ohio

Penelope A. Moyers, EdD, OTR, FAOTA
Dean
Henrietta Schmoll School of Health
St. Catherine University
Saint Paul, Minnesota

Peggy Strecker Neufield, PhD, OTR/L, FAOTA
Community Consultant and Advocate
St. Louis NORC Research and Community Liaison
St. Louis, Missouri

Susan M. Nochajski, PhD, OTR/L
*Clinical Associate Professor and Occupational Therapy
  Program Director*
Department of Rehabilitation Science
University at Buffalo
State University of New York
Buffalo, New York

Shannon Norris, OTR/L
Private Practice Owner
Kids Kount
Daphne, Alabama

Laurette Olson, PhD, OTR/L, FAOTA
Professor
Graduate Program in Occupational Therapy
Mercy College
Dobbs Ferry, New York

Michael A. Pizzi, PhD, OTR/L, FAOTA
Assistant Professor
Department of Occupational Therapy
Long Island University
Brooklyn, New York

Ruth Ramsey, EdD, OTR/L
Associate Professor and Chair
Department of Occupational Therapy
Dominican University of California
San Rafael, California

Lauren Ashley Riels, MS, OTR/L
Occupational Therapist
Advanced Medical Personnel Services
Hattiesburg, Mississippi

Courtney Sasse, MA EdL, MS, OTR/L
Assistant Professor
Department of Occupational Therapy
University of South Alabama
Mobile, Alabama

Janie B. Scott, MA, OT/L, FAOTA
Occupational Therapy and Aging in Place Consultant
Columbia, Maryland

Theresa Marie Smith, PhD, OTR/L, CLVT
Assistant Professor
Department of Occupational Therapy & Occupational Science
Towson University
Towson, Maryland

Wendy B. Stav, PhD, OTR/L, SCDCM, FAOTA
Chair and Professor
Occupational Therapy Department
Nova Southeastern University
Fort Lauderdale, Florida

Virginia C. Stoffel, PhD, OT, BCMH, FAOTA
Associate Professor
Graduate Program Coordinator
Department of Occupational Science & Technology
University of Wisconsin-Milwaukee
Milwaukee, Wisconsin

President
American Occupational Therapy Association
Bethesda, Maryland

Lynn M. Swedberg, MS, OT
Consultant, Occupational Therapist
Outreach Therapy Consultants, Inc.
Spokane, Washington

Shun TAKEHARA, OTR
Assistant Professor
Department of Occupational Therapy
Yamagata Prefectural University of Health Sciences
Yamagata City, Japan

Nancy Van Slyke, EdD, OTR/L, FAOTA
Associate Professor (Retired)
Department of Occupational Therapy
University of South Alabama
Mobile, Alabama

Donna A. Wooster, PhD, OTR/L
Associate Professor
Department of Occupational Therapy
University of South Alabama
Mobile, Alabama

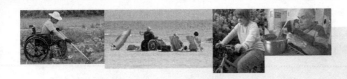

Reviewers

Mariana D'Amico, EdD, OTR/L, BCP
Assistant Professor
Medical College of Georgia
Augusta, Georgia

Carolyn R. Dorfman, PhD, OTR/L
Assistant Professor
The College of St. Scholastica
Duluth, Minnesota

Karen P. Funk, OTD, OTR
Clinical Associate Professor, Program Chair
University of Texas at El Paso
El Paso, Texas

Susan Leech, EdD, OT
Assistant Professor
University of Texas at El Paso
El Paso, Texas

Catherine McNeil, MS, OTR/L
Assistant Professor
Worcester State College
Worcester, Massachusetts

Jennifer J. Saylor, MEd, OT/L
Program Director, Fieldwork Coordinator
New Hampshire Community Technical College
Claremont, New Hampshire

Stacy Smallfield, DrOT, OTR/L
Assistant Professor
The University of South Dakota
Vermillion, South Dakota

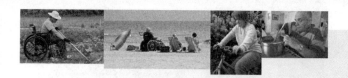

Acknowledgments

The Second Edition of this text would not have been possible without the encouragement and assistance of many people who share our enthusiasm for community practice. We would first like to acknowledge our universities, the University of South Alabama and Towson University, for funding graduate assistants and other forms of support. Several exceptional occupational therapy students and graduates were valuable contributors to the organization and production of this book, including Courtney Sasse from the University of South Alabama and Marie Chandler, Stacey Harcum, Hollie Hatt, and Stacey Greenberg from Towson University.

We are also indebted to the fine staff at F.A. Davis Company, especially Christa Fratantoro, Senior Acquisitions Editor, for her encouragement and unwavering faith in our work, and Peg Waltner, freelance developmental editor, for her exceptional guidance and assistance throughout the project.

And last, but certainly not least, we would like to acknowledge the support of family and friends. We are fortunate to have understanding, caring, and thoughtful people in our lives, as we could not have completed this textbook without their assistance. However, our spouses, Blaise Chromiak and Fred Reitz, deserve the South Alabama Jaguar and Towson Tiger share of our gratitude and love for their patience as this project unfolded, evolved, and finally came to fruition.

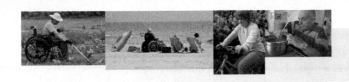

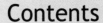

Contents

Chapter 4   Legislation and Policy Issues *51*

SECTION II   Community-Based Program Development *61*

Chapter 5   Program Planning and Needs Assessment *61*

SECTION VI Mental Health *271*

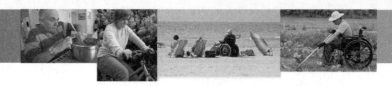

Basic Principles and Relevant Issues

Chapter 1

Community-Based Practice: Occupation in Context

Marjorie E. Scaffa, PhD, OTR/L, FAOTA

We know what we are, but we know not what we may be.

—Shakespeare

Learning Objectives

This chapter is designed to enable the reader to:

- Describe the history of community-based practice in occupational therapy.
- Describe the variety of roles for occupational therapy practitioners in community-based practice.
- Describe the characteristics of effective community-based practitioners.
- Describe the history of paradigm shifts in occupational therapy.
- Identify key characteristics of a community practice paradigm for occupational therapy.

Key Terms

Client-centered approach
Community
Community-based practice
Community-centered initiative/intervention
Community health promotion
Community-level intervention
Dynamical systems approach

Ecological approach
Health
Paradigm
Paradigm shift
Strengths-based
    occupational therapy

Introduction

In 2017, the profession of occupational therapy and the American Occupational Therapy Association (AOTA) will turn 100 years of age. In order to set a course for the future and to celebrate the profession's history, the AOTA developed a Centennial Vision that reads: "We envision that occupational therapy is a powerful, widely recognized, science-driven, and evidence-based profession with a globally connected and diverse workforce meeting society's occupational needs" (Baum, 2006, p. 610).

A community practice paradigm is entirely consistent with this vision. For example, expanding community-based occupational therapy services and population-based interventions could make occupational therapy more visible, thereby enhancing understanding and recognition of the profession. The improved awareness of occupational therapy also may increase consumer demand for services. If occupational therapy practitioners are working in more varied settings and providing needed services, then more opportunities to influence policies and take on leadership roles may result. Practicing in the community increases involvement with other professionals and assists in building alliances that also may expand the profession's power base. In addition, community practice enables the development of a variety of new roles for occupational therapy practitioners. Finally, because community practice occurs in environments where people work, play, go to school, and participate in activities of daily living, the profession is more likely to be aware of and meet society's occupational needs.

The AOTA Centennial Vision outlines six broad practice areas, including children and youth; productive aging; mental health; rehabilitation, work, and industry; disabilities and participation; and health and wellness (Baum, 2006, p. 611). Community-based services exist and can be developed within each of these practice areas, for example, ergonomic consultation, driver evaluation and training, hippotherapy, welfare-to-work programs, aging-in-place services, aquatic therapy, and violence prevention programs (Johansson, 2000; Scaffa, 2001). Occupational therapy as a profession has the opportunity to respond to and help resolve the social and health problems of the 21st century, including poverty, homelessness, addiction, depression, joblessness, chronic disease and disability, unintentional injury, violence and abuse, and social discrimination and stigma. Meeting the occupational needs of society will require not only the provision of occupational therapy services to individuals and families in community-based settings, but also the provision of occupational therapy services to organizations, communities, and populations.

An overview of community-based practice for occupational therapy is provided in this chapter. Also included are a review of the historical perspectives of community-based practice, an identification of the various roles associated with community-based practice, and a description of the characteristics necessary for effective community-based occupational therapy practice. The major paradigm shifts in occupational therapy, highlighting the impact of systems theory, are presented. Concluding the chapter is a discussion of the community practice paradigm as a client-centered approach to practice.

Historical Perspectives of Community-Based Practice

Community-based practice is not a new concept in occupational therapy (Table 1-1). Two founders of the profession, George Barton and Eleanor Clarke Slagle, developed community-based programs in the early 1900s. Barton, who was disabled by tuberculosis and a foot amputation, established Consolation House in New York in 1914. The program used occupations to enable convalescents to return to productive living (Punwar, 1994; Sabonis-Chafee, 1989). Eleanor Clarke Slagle was hired in 1915 to develop a program to provide persons with mental or physical disabilities an opportunity to work and become self-sufficient. The project was funded by philanthropic contributions and was located at Hull House, a settlement house in Chicago. In its first year of operation, the program served 77 persons who developed manual skills and received wages for their work. The goods produced in the workshop included baskets, needlework, rugs, simple cabinets, and toys (Reed & Sanderson, 1999).

Banyai (1938) wrote about the care individuals with tuberculosis were receiving while residing in sanitariums. While acknowledging the importance of occupational therapy intervention in the institution, she emphasized the need to follow the patient into the community. The ultimate goal was to restore the

Table 1-1	Historical Timeline of Community Practice in Occupational Therapy
Date	**Event**
1914	George Barton establishes Consolation House in New York.
1915	Eleanor Clarke Slagle establishes the work program at Hull House in Chicago.
1937	Humphreys advocates community treatment for persons with developmental disability.
1938	Banyai advocates following tuberculosis patients into the community after discharge from sanitariums.
1940	The AOTA reports on roundtable discussions held at national conference on the role of occupational therapy in community health.
1968	Bockhoven suggests that occupational therapy take responsibility for community occupational development.
1969–1973	In the United States, West, Reilly, and Mosey describe the need for occupational therapy services in the community.
1972	Llorens describes a community-based program in San Francisco for pregnant teenagers.
1972	Finn argues that the profession move beyond the role of therapist to "health agent."
1973	Hasselkus and Kiernat describe an independent living program for the elderly.
1974	The AOTA Task Force on Target Populations expands the role of the profession to include health promotion and disability prevention.
1977	Laukaran describes the major obstacles to community-based practice.
1982	Kirchman, Reichenback, and Giambalvo describe a prevention program for the well elderly.
1997	Well-elderly study published in the *Journal of the American Medical Association*.
2006	ACOTE accreditation standards revised with increased emphasis on health promotion and population-based services.
2006	AOTA adopts the 2017 Centennial Vision.

individual to a satisfactory level of social and economic functioning. Banyai (1938) believed that this required the occupational therapist to work with the person in the community after discharge from the institution.

The professional literature of the 1960s suggests that the field was on the verge of expanding its services outside of traditional medical settings (Laukaran, 1977). West (1969) asserted that "the traditional role of the occupational therapist, that of the reintegration of social function, is not a hospital service but rather a function that can be best filled in the community" (p. 231). Reilly (1971) advocated that the future growth of the profession was predicated on the transition of occupational therapy services from the hospital to the community. The focus of occupational therapy, in her view, should be to develop experiences and programs in the individual's community environment that enhance adaptive

competencies. This broader perspective requires the professional to provide therapeutic programming in the individual's milieu, including home, workplace, and community.

In spite of these early admonitions to focus on broader health needs and services outside of institutional settings, the move to community-based practice was short-lived and very limited in scope. In the 1970s and 1980s, examples of outreach into the community included an independent living project for the elderly (Hasselkus & Kiernat, 1973), a project in San Francisco for pregnant teenage girls (Llorens, 1972), and prevention services for the well elderly (Kirchman, Reichenback, & Giambalvo, 1982). According to Laukaran (1977), three major obstacles to community-based practice existed at that time. These barriers were practical constraints, historical factors within the discipline, and gaps in knowledge and theory related to community-based practice. The practical constraints were related to the limited number of opportunities for community-based practice at that time and the public perception of occupational therapy as a medical discipline. Historically, occupational therapy practitioners' professional identities had been associated with work in medical institutions. In addition, professional education programs emphasized preparation for practice in medical rather than community-based settings. Laukaran (1977) noted that some theoretical frameworks of that era (e.g., occupational behavior, biopsychosocial, and developmental models) were compatible with community-based practice. However, these early models were inadequate in providing guidelines and rationales for services in community settings.

Some of these same obstacles exist today, albeit in different forms. Opportunities for utilizing occupational therapy expertise in community settings are limitless but typically not designated as occupational therapy positions. For the profession to move into these settings, practitioners must seek out positions that although not labeled "occupational therapy" could benefit from the unique contributions of the discipline. The perception of occupational therapy as strictly a medical discipline continues to exist both outside and within the profession. The identity of "medical professional" is an alluring one, as in the past it denoted an aura of legitimacy. Many occupational therapy practitioners today are reluctant to "let go" of this restrictive image in favor of a more broadly defined role. In addition, professional preparation programs are slow to shift focus. However, many educators concur that the future of the profession will largely be determined by its ability to expand the scope of practice into community-based settings (Holmes & Scaffa, 2009a). Many more theoretical frameworks exist today than existed in the 1960s. These newly emerging models, based on the work of previous theorists, are readily applicable to community-based practice. Some of these theories and models are described in detail later in Chapter 3.

Interestingly, one of the boldest predictions and strongest support for the validity of occupational therapy services in the community came from a physician in 1968. Bockhoven (1968) suggested a new role for occupational therapists, described as "taking responsibility for community occupational development, alongside the businessman, city planner and the economist ... to support growth of respect for human individuality in occupation"

(p. 25). The AOTA (1974) Task Force on Target Populations redefined occupational therapy as "the science of using occupation as a health determinant" (p. 158). This definition advanced the notion that occupational therapy was not limited to the seriously or chronically ill but also could remediate mild to moderate impairments and contribute to health promotion and disability prevention.

Finn (1972), in the 1971 Eleanor Clarke Slagle Lecture, states: "In order for a profession to maintain its relevancy it must be responsive to the trends of the times ... Occupational therapists are being asked to move beyond the role of therapist to that of health agent. This expansion in role identity will require a reinterpretation of current knowledge, the addition of new knowledge and skills, and the revision of the educational process" (p. 59).

These words are still true today. The expanded role of health agent requires practitioners to move into the community and provide a continuum of services; these include health promotion and disability prevention in addition to the intervention services typically provided by the profession. Health agent is more than "therapist." Other roles, such as consultant, advocate, community organizer, program developer, and case manager, are also included.

Definitions of Terms

To conceptualize and operationalize community-based practice in occupational therapy, definitions of some terms have been adopted for the purposes of this textbook. These terms include health, community, community-based rehabilitation, community-based practice, community health promotion, community-level intervention, and community-centered initiatives/interventions.

Health

Health is defined as the ability to: "realize aspirations, to satisfy needs, and to change or cope with the environment. Health is, therefore, seen as a resource for everyday life ... a positive concept emphasizing social and personal resources, as well as physical capacities. . . . The fundamental conditions and resources for health are peace, shelter, education, food, income, a stable ecosystem, sustainable resources, social justice and equity" (World Health Organization, 1986, p. 1).

Community

"Community" means different things to different people. No single definition appears to capture the richness and diversity of the term, but combining the following definitions provides a broad and comprehensive perspective. Community refers to "non-institutional aggregations of people linked together for common goals or other purposes" (Green & Raeburn, 1990, p. 41). It is the "space where people think for themselves, dream their dreams, and come together to create and celebrate their common humanity" (O'Connell, 1988, p. 31). **Community** is "a social unit in which there is a transaction of common life among the people making up the unit" (Green & Anderson, 1982, p. 26). This social unit has its own norms and through the regulation of resources organizes both the environment and individual and group behavior.

The community or neighborhood setting is a vital part of growing up, raising families, and meeting the many challenges and stresses of modern life (Warren & Warren, 1979). According to Nisbit (1972), people do not come together in community relationships merely to be together; they come together to do something that cannot easily be done in isolation.

Community-Based Practice

Community-based practice is more comprehensive than community-based rehabilitation. Community-based practice includes a broad range of health-related services: prevention and health promotion, acute and chronic medical care, habilitation and rehabilitation, and direct and indirect service provision, all of which are provided in community settings. "Community" in this framework "means more than a geographic location for practice, but includes an orientation to collective health, social priorities, and different modes of service provision" (Kniepmann, 1997, p. 540). Community models are responsive to individual and family health needs in homes, workplaces, and community agencies. In this way, interventions are contextually embedded. The goal in community-based practice is for the client and the practitioner to become integral parts of the community. Some hospitals and rehabilitation centers provide field trips in the community for patients or clients and health fairs for community members, but these activities are not considered community-based services. They are more appropriately referred to as "community outreach" (Robnett, 1997).

Community Health Promotion

Community health promotion can be defined as "any combination of educational and social supports for people taking greater control of, and improving their own or the health of a geographically defined area" (Green & Ottoson, 1999, p. 729). Educational programs may be directed at individuals, families, groups, or communities through schools, work sites, organizations, and/or mass media. Social approaches focus on organizational, legal, political, and economic changes that support health and well-being. "Organized community effort is the key to community health. There are some things the individual can do entirely alone, but many health benefits can be obtained only through united community effort" (Green & Anderson, 1982, p. 4).

Community-Level Intervention

Community-level interventions "attempt to modify the socio-cultural, political, economic and environmental context of the community to achieve health goals" (Scaffa & Brownson, 2005, p. 485). These are population-based approaches to health and do not focus on individual health behavior change. Community-level interventions are directed at impacting systems that affect health in communities. Often initiated by health care and government agencies, they typically involve community organization strategies. Decisions are often based on the source of funding, and planning is done by a "lead" agency. The professional serves as an expert in a leadership capacity.

Community-Centered Initiatives/Interventions

Community-centered initiatives/interventions are often generated by leaders and members of the community and typically utilize existing community resources. Community coalitions form to identify common concerns and needs and to design approaches to solve community problems. Community-centered interventions follow the principles of client-centered practice, where the client is the entire community. In this way, community-centered initiatives promote community participation, exchange of information, and community autonomy. The role of the professional is as a consultant, facilitator, and mentor in the community. Occupational therapists can participate in community-centered initiatives by "identifying occupational risk factors, engaging in problem-solving and proposing and implementing solutions" that meet the community's unique occupational needs (Scaffa & Brownson, 2005, p. 485).

Trends and Roles in Community-Based Practice

The AOTA 2010 Workforce Study (AOTA, 2010) indicated that 2.0% of occupational therapy practitioners work in community settings including adult day care, independent living centers, assisted living facilities, senior centers, and supervised housing among others. In addition, 2.3% work in settings characterized as "other" including driving programs, supported employment, sheltered workshops, and industrial rehabilitation/work programs, all of which are community-based. A total of 4.8% of occupational therapy practitioners work in early intervention programs. These data reveal that approximately 9.1% of occupational therapy practitioners work in community settings. This does not include the 2.9% of occupational therapy practitioners who work in community-based mental health programs and the 5.8% who work in home health.

Median annual compensation for occupational therapists working full-time in community settings ranged from $59,000 to $71,350, depending on the number of years of experience. The overall median annual compensation for occupational therapists working in community settings was $68,000, while for occupational therapists working full-time across all settings it was $64,722. This demonstrates that the common perception that occupational therapists in community settings earn less than their counterparts in more traditional settings is a myth (AOTA, 2010).

Occupational therapy practitioners have a significant role to play in supporting individuals in their homes and workplaces, facilitating their independence, and promoting their integration into the community (Stalker, Jones, & Ritchie, 1996). More than 30 years ago, West (1967) described her vision of the changing responsibility of occupational therapists to the community. This vision acknowledged the newly emerging focus on prevention and health promotion in medicine and the impact this new focus would have on practice settings, roles, and responsibilities. West (1967) predicted that, as a result of the change in focus, practice would move into new settings, "namely, the communities in which our potential patients live, work and play" (p. 312). She described four emerging roles that at the time were adding new dimensions to the traditional role of the clinically based occupational therapist. These new roles included evaluator, consultant, supervisor, and researcher.

Other roles that community-based practitioners may fulfill include program planners and evaluators, staff trainers, community health advisors, policy makers, and primary care providers. Practitioners in the community may function as community health advocates, consultants, case managers, entrepreneurs, supervisors, and program managers. Descriptions of these roles follow in the next section. It is important for community-based practitioners in these roles to develop networks for support and collaboration with other occupational therapy practitioners, health and social service professionals, and community leaders.

Role Descriptions

Community Health Advocate

As a community health advocate, practitioners identify the social, physical, emotional, medical, educational, and occupational needs of community members for optimal functioning and advocate for services to meet those needs. In addition, practitioners act as advocates and lobbyists by providing input and shaping legislation and government policies, thereby affecting local and national physical and mental health issues and changing environmental conditions to promote health.

Consultant

Occupational therapy practitioners in the role of consultant provide information and expert advice regarding program development and evaluation, supervisory models, organizational issues, and/or clinical concerns. Consultation is "an interactive process of helping others solve existing or potential problems by identifying and analyzing issues, developing strategies to address problems and preventing future problems from occurring" (Epstein & Jaffe, 2003, p. 260). Consultation services are most often utilized when new programs are being developed or undergoing significant change and may be short-term or long-term, depending on the needs of the program. Within the community, occupational therapy practitioners can act as consultants to a variety of groups, such as Scouts or Boys & Girls Clubs, adult education programs, adult day care, transitional living programs, independent living centers, community development and housing agencies, health departments, military bases and organizations, and work site safety and health programs.

Case Manager

As a case manager, a practitioner coordinates the provision of services; advises the consumer, family, or caregiver; evaluates financial resources; and advocates for needed services. Case management requires a professional who has ample clinical experience, understands reimbursement mechanisms, and has good organizational skills. Frequently, the qualifications and duties of case managers are dictated by state regulations. Occupational therapy practitioners are most often designated as case managers in mental health and children and youth practice areas.

While the primary role of case managers is to ensure access to community services and resources, they may also assist in the development of independent living skills (e.g., money management, social interaction, and cognitive skills such as decision making and problem solving). Occupational therapists are qualified by their education and training to serve as case managers and/or to supervise others in case management positions.

Private Practice Owner/Entrepreneur

An occupational therapy entrepreneur is "an individual who organizes a business venture, manages its operation, and assumes the risks associated with the business" (Vaughn & Sladyk, 2011, p. 167). The entrepreneur may own a private practice, provide services on a contractual basis, and/or function as a consultant. In order for entrepreneurs to be successful, they must be able to assess and respond to the unique needs of their communities. Changing demographics, including the significant growth of the aging population, will provide a variety of opportunities for occupational therapy entrepreneurs. In order to be successful, entrepreneurs must have a wide range of skills including financial management, marketing, leadership, and organizational and team-building skills (Vaughn & Sladyk, 2011).

A broad overview of entrepreneurship is provided in Chapter 8.

Supervisor

Supervisors typically manage and are responsible for all the activities of their team members. A supervisor sets up work schedules, delegates tasks, recruits and trains employees, and conducts performance appraisals. In occupational therapy practice, supervision is designed to "ensure the safe and effective delivery of occupational therapy services and foster professional competence and development" (AOTA, 2009, p. 797). The role of an occupational therapy supervisor varies from facility to facility but generally includes training and evaluating staff and fieldwork students, developing and reviewing intervention plans and progress updates, solving problems as needed, and contributing to budget and program development. Supervisors typically do not have final budgetary or personnel authority but assume responsibility for the day-to-day operations of the program.

Program Managers

Program managers are responsible for the overall design, development, function, and evaluation of a program; budgeting; and staff hiring and supervision. Many occupational therapists have served as program managers in community settings (Fazio, 2008). Program managers conduct needs assessments, SWOT (strengths, weaknesses, opportunities, threats) analyses, strategic planning, and program development functions. Occupational therapists not in positions officially designated as program manager may be asked to expand existing programs or develop new programs to meet client needs. Program managers in community-based settings tend to "use a more interactive approach that promotes open communication, feedback and collaboration than managers in more traditional, institutionally-driven medical settings" (Scaffa, Doll, Estes, & Holmes, 2011, p. 320).

Characteristics of Effective Community-Based Occupational Therapy Practitioners

According to Learnard, "occupational therapy in community health is both an art and a science"

(Robnett, 1997, p. 30). In addition to the typical occupational therapy focus on enhancing function through task analysis and modification of important life tasks and the environment, occupational therapists in community-based practice need a variety of other skills and attributes. According to Robnett (1997), Learnard believes effective community-based therapists exemplify the following characteristics:

- Sense of positive hopefulness
- Understanding of individuals in their specific personal circumstances
- Creativity to envision a variety of possibilities
- Ability to set aside one's cultural, personal, and professional biases and respect individual choices rather than passing judgment

Holmes and Scaffa (2009b) studied twenty-three occupational therapists working in emerging practice areas and attempted to identify the competencies needed to work in new or underdeveloped practice settings. The competencies were identified through the use of the Delphi technique of forecasting, whereby respondents have multiple opportunities to identify, rate, and rank the characteristics they deem essential for emerging practice. The competencies and characteristics were classified into five categories used in the AOTA Standards for Continuing Competence (AOTA, 1999), which included:

1. knowledge required for multiple roles,
2. critical reasoning necessary for decision making in those roles,
3. interpersonal abilities to establish effective relationships with others,
4. performance skills and proficiencies for practice, and
5. ethical reasoning for responsible decision making.

A sixth category—traits, qualities, and characteristics—was added based on the Delphi panel responses. The competencies and characteristics identified by the Delphi panel are listed in Box 1-1 (Holmes & Scaffa, 2009b).

In addition, the following attributes and skills are recommended for those contemplating practice in community settings:

- Comfort with indirect service provision
- Grant-writing skills
- Networking skills
- Organizational skills
- Professional autonomy
- Program planning and evaluation skills
- Public relations skills

Paradigm Shifts in Occupational Therapy

A **paradigm** is a conceptual framework that allows explanation and investigation of phenomena. Kuhn (1970) defined a paradigm as "universally recognized scientific achievements that for a time provide model problems and solutions to a community of practitioners" (p. viii). Paradigms have two essential characteristics. They are (a) sufficiently unprecedented scientific achievements that draw a large number of constituents from competing areas of inquiry, and (b) adequately open-ended enough to allow for the exploration of solutions to a variety of problems. A paradigm is a worldview that characterizes a particular group or discipline that has common interests. It is a "consensus-determined matrix of the most fundamental beliefs or assumptions of a field" (Kielhofner, 1983, p. 6). A profession or discipline-specific paradigm determines

- how professionals view their phenomenon of interest;
- what puzzles, problems, or questions practitioners will seek out in their work;
- what solutions will emerge; and
- what goals will be set for the direction of the profession.

A paradigm is the "cultural core of the discipline" and "provides professional identity" (Kielhofner, 1997, p. 17).

Kuhn (1970) asserted that change within a discipline or profession does not occur gradually. Rather, it occurs very dramatically. When a discipline abandons one view of the world for another, it has undergone a revolution, a drastic conceptual restructuring, called a **paradigm shift.** Often, there is much resistance to paradigm shifts and to those initiating them. Paradigm shifts dramatically change the existing rules, create new trends, and trigger innovations. Paradigm shifts occur in four stages: preparadigm, paradigm, crisis, and return to paradigm.

Box 1-1 Competencies and Characteristics Needed for Emerging Practice Areas

Listed in order of importance ratings

Knowledge Competencies*

Occupation-based practice for evaluation and intervention
Philosophy of occupational therapy
Occupational therapy models and frames of reference applied to intervention
Principles of client-centered practice
Occupational therapy practice framework: domain and process
Core values of occupational therapy
Program development
Potential occupational therapy role and contribution in the practice area
Community systems
Public health principles and practice models

Performance Skills Competencies

Envision occupational therapy roles and service possibilities
Implement client-centered practices
Assess, evaluate, and provide intervention for occupational issues
Work collaboratively with others
Identify and access available resources
Search, analyze, and synthesize evidence-based research for emerging practice
Seek opportunities to demonstrate and use skills to meet clients' needs
Select, administer, and interpret evaluation results for variety of practice areas
Conduct comprehensive task and activity analyses
Provide consultation to groups and individuals

Critical Reasoning Competencies*

Reason holistically
Translate theory to practice
Solve problems
Use clinical reasoning for client services

Think outside of the box
Use good judgment—know when to seek assistance
Think abstractly
Complete a SWOT analysis

Ethical Reasoning Competencies*

Self-assessment of strengths and needs for ongoing professional development
Principles of social justice
Principles of occupational justice

Interpersonal Abilities Competencies*

Listen actively
Communicate occupational therapy concepts to a variety of audiences
Establish relationships with stakeholders and community leaders
Network effectively with other professionals
Demonstrate cultural competence
Establish and maintain relationships with professionals
Seek mentors within and outside of the occupational therapy profession
Understand and use language and terms of other professions
Negotiate effectively
Ask for feedback, advice, and assistance from colleagues and friends

Traits, Qualities, and Characteristics

Self-starter, self-directed
Adaptable to new situations
Able to step outside of the medical model
Self-confident
Persevering, determined, and persistent
Flexible
Tolerant of ambiguity
An independent worker
Creative
Able to challenge the status quo

Category headings* from "Standards for Continuing Competence" by the American Occupational Therapy Association, 1999, *American Journal of Occupational Therapy, 53,* 559–560.
Data from: Holmes & Scaffa (2009). An exploratory study of competencies for emerging practice in occupational therapy. *Journal of Allied Health, 38* (2), 81–90.

Kielhofner conducted an historical examination of paradigm shifts in occupational therapy (Fig. 1.1). According to Kielhofner (1983), the pre-paradigm stage in occupational therapy traces its roots to the moral treatment movement with its humanistic focus. Moral treatment proponents advocated that the treatment of persons with mental illness should emphasize

a daily routine of occupations in a family-like atmosphere (Neidstadt & Crepeau, 1998). Participation in occupations was believed to normalize disorganized habits and behaviors (Kielhofner, 1997). During the 18th and 19th centuries, the moral treatment philosophy was competing with a pathology-oriented approach in the treatment of the mentally ill.

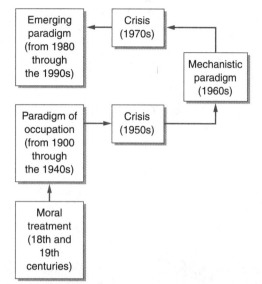

Fig. 1•1 Paradigm Shifts in Occupational Therapy. *(From Kielhofner, G. [1997, p. 48]. Conceptual foundations of occupational therapy [2nd ed.]. Philadelphia, PA: F.A. Davis. With permission.)*

During the first four decades of the 20th century, a remarkable degree of consensus emerged among practitioners and in the literature regarding "occupation" as the central phenomenon of interest. Although the paradigm of occupation originated in the mental health arena, it was easily applicable to physical disabilities. Occupation referred to the balance of work, play, self-care, and rest. Occupational therapists of the time viewed the individual holistically, composed of both mind and body, participating in daily tasks in interactions with his or her environments. Occupations were graded according to the individual's capabilities. Persons progressed from simple activities that stimulated the senses to more demanding occupations requiring concentration and skill (Kielhofner, 1997).

The first paradigm crisis is evident in the professional literature of the late 1940s and early 1950s, when increasing pressure from medicine to be more scientific led to the questioning of the paradigm of occupation. The literature began to favor kinesiological, neurophysiological, and psychoanalytic approaches to occupational therapy practice. The depression of the 1930s caused much job insecurity, compelling occupational therapy to develop a closer relationship with medicine. The American Medical Association began accrediting occupational therapy educational programs. Occupational therapy practice began to align itself more closely with the medical model and adopted the medical paradigm of reductionism with few modifications (Kielhofner, 1983).

The reductionist, or mechanistic, paradigm of the 1960s asserted that by focusing on the inner mechanisms of disease and disability (i.e., neurophysiology, anatomy, kinesiology, and psychoanalysis), occupational therapy could actually alter function and thereby gain professional respect as a scientific discipline. The early paradigm of occupation had a holistic appreciation of the occupational nature of human life. The new paradigm provided a more in-depth view and shifted professional thinking from the gestalt to a reductionist focus on parts. The medical model, or reductionist paradigm, was not simply added to the paradigm of occupation; the former replaced the latter and, as a result, the focus of occupational therapy practice changed dramatically in the 1960s and 1970s. Practitioners dropped "occupations" from therapy in favor of exercise, talk groups, specialized treatment techniques, and modalities (Kielhofner, 1983).

The reductionist, or mechanistic, paradigm was not, and is not, altogether negative. New assistive devices and technology, new techniques (e.g., sensory integration and neurodevelopmental treatment), and greater respect from the medical community emerged from this approach. The major loss was the profession's commitment to the occupational nature of human beings and the importance of occupation as a therapeutic medium. Without this common theme of early practice, the specialty areas within the field began to drift apart, leading to a second paradigm crisis.

This second paradigm crisis, which occurred in the 1970s, was precipitated by the recognition that reductionism was an inadequate framework for understanding the complexities of human occupational behavior. Awareness grew that the problems of the chronically disabled could not be solved by technology alone. In addition, occupational therapists expressed dissatisfaction over a loss of professional identity, a fragmented ideology, and a lack of professional unity (Kielhofner, 1983, 1997).

According to Kielhofner (2004), a new paradigm is emerging that recommits itself to the core construct of occupation and attempts to regain the profession's identity and holistic orientation. The emerging paradigm is characterized by a synthesis of useful concepts from the mechanistic paradigm with contemporary knowledge of occupation from many disciplines. In addition, the emerging paradigm utilizes a systems perspective. An underlying assumption of "systems theory is that no system (e.g., cell, person, or organization) can be fully explained by examining the component parts of which it is made" (Kielhofner, 2004, p. 66). A systems viewpoint emphasizes that occupational performance results from the dynamic interaction between the person, the environmental context, and the occupations in which the person engages. In addition, it allows for a more complex perspective on factors that impact occupational performance and therefore a broader range of potential solutions to occupational performance problems. The purpose of occupational therapy in this perspective is to provide "opportunities and environmental resources that support the emergence of new patterns of performance and participation in everyday life" (Kielhofner, 2004, p. 66).

Community Practice Paradigm

Community health care is more than just a decentralization of services through outreach into the community. It includes a focus on community health in addition to individual health. Functioning effectively in the community will require a range of new roles for the practitioner and a unique set of knowledge, skills, and attitudes (Wiemer & West, 1970). A main difference between the model of community health espoused by Wiemer and West (1970) and the model that is currently being proposed is that Wiemer and West believed that community health was merely an extension of the medical model into community-based settings. The current belief is that community health requires a paradigm different from that of the medical model, a reductionist perspective, that is, a shift to a new way of thinking. This new paradigm is, however, consistent with the early foundations of occupational therapy and represents a return to the early principles of the profession.

Though it is easy to critique the limitations of medical models of health care delivery, it is far more difficult to describe the essential components of a new, more community-oriented paradigm. Clearly,

the role of the professional and the therapeutic relationship between provider and "patient" is different in the two paradigms (Table 1-2). In addition, some basic terminology from the medical model, such as "patient," is clearly inappropriate in community settings. Occupational therapy practitioners must make a conscious effort to modify their use of terminology from patient to *client,* from treatment to *intervention,* and from reimbursement to *funding.* Use of medical language can limit one's perspective, unnecessarily narrow professional focus, and decrease the ability to perceive options.

In the transition from a medical model paradigm to community practice, professionals need to relinquish responsibility, power, and control to the recipient of services, client, or community member. The client is the expert regarding his or her situation, needs, and desires. Therefore, the client is the person who makes the decisions regarding the services utilized. For community practice to be successful, planning must be coordinated with and through a variety of agencies, organizations, and individuals in the community. The impact of culture also must be recognized, appreciated, and incorporated into service delivery. Ultimately, the professional reports to the client who is both the recipient and evaluator of the services provided.

In the community, professionals function as facilitators whose role is to build and reinforce capacity and develop leadership in others. This requires humility, the ability to share successes with

Table 1-2 Contrasting Paradigms	
Medical Model	**Community Model**
Professional is responsible	Community member is responsible
Professional has power	Community member has power
Professional makes decisions	Community member makes decisions
Professional is the "expert"	Community member is the "expert"
Professional answers to the agency	Professional answers to the consumer
Planning is fragmented	Planning is coordinated
Culture is denied	Culture is appreciated

others, and patience. Successful practice in the community requires more time than in the typical clinical setting, as consensus must be developed and resources identified and obtained to support individuals in maintaining a satisfying lifestyle in the community of their choice.

Assessment of individuals in community settings may include the traditional components of occupational therapy evaluation, such as areas of occupation, performance patterns, performance skills, and client factors (AOTA, 2008). However, this type of evaluation is usually insufficient in the community setting. Client factors are often the primary focus in the medical model. In community practice, the performance areas of activities of daily living, instrumental activities of daily living, rest/sleep, work, education, play/leisure, social participation, and contexts/environment take on much more significance. If the focus of intervention is not the individual but rather on a collection of individuals—for example, a family, a community, or some subpopulation of a community such as members of a senior center—then assessment must be much broader in scope. Assessment in community settings requires attention to the population to be served and the context in which the services will be delivered (Box 1-2). Intervention planning utilizes the information generated from the comprehensive assessment, and potential programs of services are identified with input from the intended service recipients and community organizations. Community institutions, such as schools, churches, mosques, temples, social organizations, health care providers, and political entities, are all part of the context of service and therefore are integral components of assessment and intervention. The process of program development in community settings is described in detail in Chapter 6 and program evaluation in Chapter 7.

Characteristics of the Community Practice Paradigm

A well-developed community practice paradigm can enhance the likelihood of achieving the Centennial Vision. The following are some preliminary suggestions on the nature of the community practice paradigm. The emerging community practice paradigm has the following characteristics. It is:

- Client-centered
- Occupation-based

Box 1-2	Assessment of Population and Context

I. Assessment of the population:
  A. General demographics (age, gender, diagnoses, etc.)
  B. Current and anticipated living and working environments and role expectations
  C. Current performance in areas of activities of daily living, instrumental activities of daily living, work, education, sleep/rest, play/leisure, and social participation
  D. General performance component assets and deficits
  E. Significance of these factors with respect to community members' goals and needs
II. Assessment of the context:
  A. General characteristics of the agency/program (mission, goals, etc.)
  B. Characteristics of the physical environment
  C. Characteristics of the social environment/milieu (norms, emotional and cultural climate, etc.)
  D. Availability of resources (space, materials, staff, etc.)
  E. Significance of these factors with respect to community members' goals and needs

---

- Supported with evidence
- Based on dynamic systems theory
- Ecologically sound, and
- Strengths-based

Client-Centered

The community practice paradigm requires a **client-centered approach** that "promotes participation, exchange of information, client decision-making, and respect for choice" and "focuses on the issues which are most important to the person and his or her family" (Law, 1998, preface). The collaborative process is designed to enable the client to identify occupational performance problems, engage in problem solving, and propose solutions that meet his or her unique individual needs and circumstances. The occupational therapist is a facilitator, educator, and mentor in the process (Law, 1998). A client-centered model has three key elements. It:

- Considers the values, goals, roles, activities, and tasks of the person, group, or community
- Involves the client as an active participant in the entire process of needs assessment,

intervention planning, implementation, and evaluation
- Establishes a partnership between the client and practitioner that enables the client to assume responsibility for the process and the outcome of services (Baum, Bass-Haugen, & Christiansen, 2005).

Use of the term "client" in the community practice paradigm may refer to an individual, a family, an organization, or an entire community (AOTA, 2008). Regardless of the type of client identified, the principles of client-centered practice are still relevant.

Occupation-Based

A community practice paradigm in occupational therapy should be occupation-based and supported with evidence. The focus on occupation is what makes the profession unique, and evidence of effectiveness is what makes occupational therapy services valuable. Occupation-based practice is defined as an "intervention in which the occupational therapy practitioner and client collaboratively select and design activities that have specific relevance or meaning to the client and support the client's interests, need, health, and participation in daily life" (AOTA, 2008, p. 672). Characteristics of occupation-based practice are listed in Box 1-3.

Supported With Evidence

Demonstrating the effectiveness and efficiency of occupational therapy services through research enhances the profession's credibility. Scientific evidence provides data for decision making regarding the importance and changeability of risk factors and the appropriateness of specific interventions. Evidence-based decision making is the "process of coming to a conclusion or making a judgment that combines clinical expertise, patient concerns, and evidence gathered from scientific literature to arrive at best practice recommendations" (Abreu & Chang, 2011, p. 331). According to Holm (2000), evidence-based practitioners:

- Examine what they do by asking questions
- Take the time to find the best evidence to guide their practice
- Appraise the evidence carefully
- Use the evidence to "do the right things right"
- Evaluate the impact of their evidence-based practices

Box 1-3	Characteristics of Occupation-Based Practice

- Occupation is infused throughout the evaluation and intervention process.
- Occupational history taking, occupational performance assessment, and the development of an occupational profile are essential elements of client evaluation.
- Occupational performance patterns including roles, habits, routines, and rituals are assessed and incorporated into the therapeutic process.
- Therapeutic goals are based on the client's occupational needs and values.
- Participation in occupation is used as an intervention modality and is a desired outcome of therapy.
- Activity selection, analysis, and modification take into consideration the client's desired and meaningful occupations.
- Environmental and contextual impacts on occupational performance and participation are considered and addressed.

Data from "Occupational Therapy Practice Framework: Domain & Process" (2nd ed.) by the American Occupational Therapy Association, 2008, *American Journal of Occupational Therapy, 62* (6), 625–683.

Based on Dynamic Systems Theory

Communities function as systems; therefore, a dynamic systems perspective is extremely useful in conceptualizing community practice. According to Capra (1982, p. 43), systems theory "looks at the world in terms of the inter-relatedness and interdependence of all phenomenon, and in this framework an integrated whole whose properties cannot be reduced to those of its parts is called a system." Dynamic systems are characterized by complete interconnectedness. This means that all variables are interrelated and that a change in one variable impacts all other variables that are part of the system. In addition, dynamic systems are nested; every system is part of another larger system with the same dynamic principles operating at each level. Subsystems settle into preferred, although not predictable, patterns called attractor states. Attractor states are temporary with various strengths. The development of dynamic systems is in part dependent on initial states. Minor differences in the beginning can become huge effects with dramatic consequences in the long term. Dynamic systems are constantly developing and changing through interactions with their environment and through internal reorganization (De Bot, Lowie, & Verspoor, 2007). Relationships among variables in dynamic systems are governed by heterarchy. "Heterarchy" refers to "the relation of elements to one another when they are unranked, or when they possess the potential for being ranked in a number of different ways, depending on systemic requirements" (Crumley, 2005, p. 39).

Throughout history (Green & Anderson, 1982, p. 22), "people have organized themselves into families, institutions, communities, and societies to exercise more control over the environment and over the behavior of each other. Rules of behavior become community norms that are transmitted from one generation to another as culture. Culture defines acceptable social organization (family interaction patterns, roles and responsibilities of institutions and leaders, and the functions of government) as well as individual behavior. The influence of all these cultural, economic, organizational, and institutional forces on the environment, on individual behavior, and on health may be referred to as the social history of health."

A **dynamical systems approach** recognizes the complexity of the social history of health and provides a framework for assessment and intervention at various levels of systems, including individual, interpersonal, organizational, community, and public policy levels. The focus of intervention in community practice might be the individual recipient of service. However, just as frequently, if not more frequently, the focus of intervention is the family or the community as a whole. Individuals are embedded in a number of systems that must be addressed even when the focus of intervention is at the individual level. For example, an individual's level of self-fulfillment and independence in the community may well be more a function of environmental, institutional, and social barriers than the individual's disability itself. Therefore, intervention may focus on several levels of systems simultaneously. According to dynamic systems theory, if one component of a system changes, "a chain reaction of adaptations and adjustments is created in other parts of the system" (Scaffa & Brownson, 2005, p. 482). Interventions to improve health and well-being are most effective when multiple components of a dynamic system are targeted. This creates a synergistic effect that resonates throughout all aspects of a community.

Ecologically Sound

An **ecological approach** considers the client embedded in and interacting with a variety of environments and contexts. This perspective requires the occupational therapy practitioner to consider both the client's capabilities and constraints and the environmental enablers and barriers. Client capabilities may include psychological, physiological, cognitive, neurobehavioral, and spiritual assets. Environmental enablers may include cultural and social, policy, socioeconomic, and built and natural environmental resources (Baum, Bass-Haugen, & Christiansen, 2005). Client constraints may include poor health status, occupational risk factors, and occupational performance limitations. Environmental barriers may include poverty, lack of natural and built environmental resources, economic recession, high unemployment rates, inadequate public transportation, and lack of access to social and occupational participation. Recognizing the interdependence between the client and the social and physical environment is critical to effective community practice.

Strengths-Based

Finally, a community paradigm for occupational therapy is **strengths-based,** meaning that the focus is on what the client can do—his or her assets, talents, resources, and capabilities—and not simply the client's deficits or functional limitations. A strength is the ability to consistently perform in a high-quality manner in a particular activity. A talent is a naturally occurring pattern of thought, feeling, or behavior that can be used productively. A strengths-based approach to intervention assesses the client's inherent strengths and talents and then incorporates these into the therapeutic process to facilitate occupational engagement and empowerment. A strengths-based model avoids the use of stigmatizing labels; reduces the sense of victimization; and fosters hope, growth, and self-efficacy. The development of strengths can be conceptualized as a three-step process:

1. identifying strengths and talents,
2. incorporating these strengths and talents into the client's view of himself or herself, and
3. changing behavior.

Behavior change may include acquiring knowledge to enhance strengths and talents, sharing one's talents with others, and creating and implementing strategies to maximize one's strengths and utilize them more consistently. A focus on the development of strengths increases life satisfaction and productivity (Hodges & Clifton, 2004).

The basic underlying tenets of the emerging community practice paradigm can be summarized as follows:

* Occupational therapy is best provided "in vivo" where people play, work, go to school, participate in social interactions, and engage in activities of daily living (Scaffa, 2001).
* Participation in occupation that structures everyday life is health promoting and enhances quality of life (AOTA, 2008).
* Occupational risk factors—for example, occupational deprivation, occupational alienation, and occupational imbalance—predispose individuals, families, groups, and communities to illness, disability, and dysfunction (AOTA, 2008; Wilcock, 2006).
* The physical, social, cultural, and temporal environments influence occupational choice, priorities, and organization, as well as quality and satisfaction with occupational performance (AOTA, 2008).
* Habits, routines, roles, and rituals are performance patterns that impact occupational participation (AOTA, 2008).
* Engagement in occupation contributes to self-identity and self-efficacy (AOTA, 2008).
* People have the right to fully participate in their communities and engage in occupations of their choice that provide purpose and meaning in their lives (AOTA, 2008).
* Health and health behaviors are influenced by a variety of factors: personal, social, economic, and ecological (USDHHS, 2011).
* Social isolation, low educational attainment, poverty, violence, pollution, crime, and discrimination are all threats to individual and community health and well-being (Scaffa & Brownson, 2005).
* The reduction of occupational risk factors and the enhancement of occupational resilience factors can improve the health and well-being of individuals, families, and communities. (Scaffa & Brownson, 2005).

The occupational therapy profession must reinterpret and expand its knowledge base to support community-based initiatives as well as think creatively and develop new models of practice appropriate for community-based settings. As occupational therapy services in the community increase and as practitioners become more comfortable with indirect service provision and designing interventions for populations, the paradigm of community practice will evolve.

Conclusion

It is time to start living out of our imagination, not out of our memory alone.

Over 25 years ago, Dasler (1984) stated that occupational therapists, regardless of their area of practice, should focus their attention on creating and filling more positions in community-based settings than in the traditional clinic environment. She believed that practitioners should adapt their roles and skills to fit with the "outside" community environment. Dasler (1984) referred to this as the "deinstitutionalization of the occupational therapist" (p. 31). Fidler (2000) echoed this sentiment when she stated, "as a profession, our single focus on and identity as a therapy, as a remedial rehabilitation service, has, I believe, significantly hampered our development. This narrow identity has, over many years, hindered our discovery and validation of the rich and broad dimensions of occupation" (p. 99).

For the future, Fidler (2000) envisioned an "occupationalist" who, in addition to rehabilitation services, provides health promotion services and programs of prevention, lifestyle counseling, and learning enhancement, and participates in organizational, institutional, and community planning and design. If occupational therapy practitioners continue to resist the move into community-based settings, where their services are most needed, in favor of hospital and clinic environments, then the future of the profession will surely be unnecessarily limited.

In 1972, Finn suggested a number of issues that need to be addressed as the profession moves from an emphasis on medical and clinical services to health promotion and community-based services. An updated interpretation of these issues follows. Occupational therapy practitioners need to:

- Gain knowledge about community organizations and institutions and how they operate.
- Acquire a thorough understanding of the unique services they can offer in community settings and be able to communicate these services clearly.
- Develop strategies to translate knowledge into actual programs that are responsive to community needs.
- Prepare to take risks when faced with challenges in unfamiliar environments.
- Learn to relate to and communicate effectively with non-medical personnel and avoid the use of professional jargon.
- Offer services to a community rather than waiting for services to be solicited.
- Develop the role of health agent while maintaining professional identity, and appreciate the opportunities for personal and professional growth in the experience.

Occupational therapy philosophy and services are very compatible with community-based service provision. However, the paradigm of direct-service provision to individuals in clinical settings is inadequate for these emerging areas of practice in the community. The old paradigms are insufficient for identifying relevant issues and solving the problems associated with community practice. Learning from other disciplines, which have had a community focus for all or most of their existence (e.g., sociology, social psychology, public health, and community health education), can be a powerful tool in facilitating occupational therapy's expansion into the community.

Now is the time for occupational therapy practitioners to move ahead with confidence. If the profession fails to assume the dynamic, new roles that are emerging in the community, other professionals will surely replace it. All occupational therapy practitioners, educators, and students are critical links in this monumental paradigm shift in the profession. With vision and creativity, the profession's potential contribution to the community and society is limitless.

Learning Activities

1. Interview an occupational therapist in community practice regarding the skills, abilities, and characteristics a person needs to be successful in providing community-based services. Assess your own readiness to practice in community settings. What do you need to learn to be able to make this transition?

2. In pairs or small groups, write a brief article for *OT Practice* describing the benefits for clients and practitioners of providing community-based services and the barriers to developing occupation-based community programs.

3. Read the local newspaper for a week and identify at least two community health problems that could be addressed by occupational therapists. Describe the populations and communities affected and the environmental and contextual characteristics that contribute to the health problems. Who would you contact in order to investigate volunteer or paid employment opportunities to help solve one or both of the health problems?

REFERENCES

Abreu, B. C. & Chang, P-F. J. (2011). Evidence-based practice. In K. Jacobs & G. McCormack (Eds.), *The occupational therapy manager, 5th edition* (pp. 331–347). Bethesda, MD: AOTA Press.

Agency for Healthcare Research and Quality. (2008). *2007 National Healthcare Quality Report.* Rockville, MD: US Department of Health and Human Services. AHRQ Pub. No. 08-0040.

American Occupational Therapy Association. (1974). Task force on target populations: Report of the task force on target populations, report I. *American Journal of Occupational Therapy, 28,* 158–163.

American Occupational Therapy Association. (1999). Standards for continuing competence. *American Journal of Occupational Therapy, 53,* 559–560.

American Occupational Therapy Association. (2008). Occupational therapy practice framework: Domain & process (2nd ed.). *American Journal of Occupational Therapy, 62* (6), 625–683.

American Occupational Therapy Association. (2009). Guidelines for supervision, roles, and responsibilities during the delivery of occupational therapy services. *American Journal of Occupational Therapy, 63* (6), 797–803.

American Occupational Therapy Association. (2010). *2010 Occupational Therapy Compensation and Workforce Study.* Retrieved from http://nxtbook.com/nxtbooks/aota/2010salarysurvey/index.php#/0

Banyai, A. L. (1938). Modern trends in the treatment of tuberculosis. *Occupational Therapy in Rehabilitation, 17,* 245–254.

Barker, J. A. (1992). *Future edge.* New York, NY: William Morrow.

Baum, C., Bass-Haugen, J. & Christiansen, C. (2005). Person-environment-occupation-performance: A model for planning interventions for individuals and organizations. In C. H. Christiansen, C. M. Baum & J. Bass-Haugen, *Occupational therapy: Performance, participation and well-being* (pp. 373–385). Thorofare, NJ: SLACK.

Baum, M. C. (2006). Presidential address, 2006 Centennial challenges, Millennium opportunities. *American Journal of Occupational Therapy, 60*(6), 609–616.

Bockhoven, J. S. (1968). Challenge of the new clinical approaches. *American Journal of Occupational Therapy, 22,* 23–25.

Capra, F. (1982). *The turning point.* New York, NY: Bantam.

Crumley, C. L. (2005). Remember how to organize: Heterarchy across disciplines. In C.S. Beekman & W.W. Baden (Eds.), *Nonlinear models for archaeology and anthropology* (pp. 35–50). Burlington, VT: Ashgate Publishing Company.

Dasler, P. J. (1984). Deinstitutionalizing the occupational therapist. *Occupational Therapy in Health Care, 1*(1), 31–40.

De Bot, K., Lowie, W. & Verspoor, M. (2007). A dynamic systems theory approach to second language acquisition. *Bilingualism: Language and Cognition, 10*(1), 7–21.

Epstein, C. F. & Jaffe, E. G. (2003). Consultation: Collaborative interventions for change. In G. McCormack, E. G. Jaffe & M. Goodman-Levy (Eds.), *The occupational therapy manager* (4th ed., pp. 259–286). Bethesda, MD: AOTA Press.

Fazio, L. (2008). *Developing occupation-entered programs for the community.* Upper Saddle River, NJ: Pearson-Prentice-Hill.

Fidler, G. S. (2000). Beyond the therapy model: Building our future. *American Journal of Occupational Therapy, 54*(1), 99–101.

Finn, G. L. (1972). The occupational therapist in prevention programs. *American Journal of Occupational Therapy, 26,* 59–66.

Green, L. W., & Anderson, C. L. (1982). *Community health* (4th ed.). St. Louis, MO: Mosby.

Green, L. W., & Ottoson, J. M. (1999). *Community and population health* (8th ed.). Boston: McGraw-Hill.

Green, L. W., & Raeburn, J. (1990). Contemporary developments in health promotion, definitions and challenges. In N. Bracht (Ed.), *Health promotion at the community level* (pp. 29–44). Newbury Park, CA: Sage.

Hodges, T. D., & Clifton, D. O. (2004). Strengths-based development in practice. In P. A. Linley & S. Joseph, *Positive Psychology in Practice.* Hoboken, NJ: John Wiley & Sons.

Holm, M. B. (2000). Our mandate for the new millennium: Evidence-based practice. *American Journal of Occupational Therapy, 54*(6), 575–585.

Holmes, W. M., & Scaffa, M. E. (2009a). The nature of emerging practice in occupational therapy: A pilot study. *Occupational Therapy in Health Care, 23*(3), 189–206.

Holmes, W. M., & Scaffa, M. E. (2009b). An exploratory study of competencies for emerging practice in occupational therapy. *Journal of Allied Health, 38*(2), 81–90.

Howe, M., & Dippy, K. (1968). The role of occupational therapy in community mental health. *American Journal of Occupational Therapy, 22,* 521–524.

Johansson, C. (2000). Top ten emerging practice areas. *OT Practice, 5*(3), 7–8.

Karan, O. C., & Greenspan, S. (1995). *Community rehabilitation services for people with disabilities.* Boston, MA: Butterworth-Heinemann.

Kielhofner, G. (1983). *Health through occupation: Theory and practice in occupational therapy.* Philadelphia: F.A. Davis.

Kielhofner, G. (1997). *Conceptual foundations of occupational therapy, 2nd edition.* Philadelphia, PA: F.A. Davis.

Kielhofner, G. (2004). *Conceptual foundations of occupational therapy, 3rd edition.* Philadelphia: F.A. Davis.

Kneipmann, K. (1997). Prevention of disability and maintenance of health. In C. Christianson & C. Baum, *Occupational therapy: Enabling function and wellbeing* (pp. 531–555). Thorofare, NJ: SLACK.

Kuhn, T. S. (1970). *The structure of scientific revolutions* (2nd ed.). Chicago: University of Chicago Press.

Laukaran, V. H. (1977). Toward a model of occupational therapy for community health. *American Journal of Occupational Therapy, 31*(2), 71–74.

Law, M. (Ed.). (1998). *Client-centered occupational therapy.* Thorofare, NJ: SLACK.

Neidstadt, M. E., & Crepeau, E. B. (1998). *Willard and Spackman's occupational therapy, 9th edition.* Philadelphia: Lippincott.

Nisbit, R. (1972). *Quest for community.* New York, NY: Oxford.

O'Connell, M. (1988). *The gift of hospitality: Opening the doors of community life to people with disabilities.* Evanston, IL: Center for Urban Affairs and Policy Research, Northwestern University.

Punwar, A. J. (1994). *Occupational therapy: Principles and practice* (2nd ed.). Baltimore: Williams and Wilkins.

Reed, K. L., & Sanderson, S. N. (1999). *Concepts of occupational therapy* (4th ed.). Philadelphia: Lippincott.

Reilly, M. (1971). The modernization of occupational therapy. *American Journal of Occupational Therapy, 25,* 243–246.

Robnett, R. (1997). Paradigms of community practice. *OT Practice, 2*(5), 30–35.

Sabonis-Chafee, B. (1989). *Occupational therapy: Introductory concepts.* St. Louis, MO: Mosby.

Scaffa, M. E. (2001). *Occupational therapy in community-based practice settings.* Philadelphia: F.A. Davis.

Scaffa. M. E. & Brownson, C. (2005). Occupational therapy interventions: Community health approaches. In C.

Christiansen & C. Baum, *Occupational therapy: Performance, participation and well-being.* Thorofare, NJ: SLACK.

Scaffa, M.E., Doll, J., Estes, R. & Holmes, W. (2011). Managing programs in emerging practice areas. In K. Jacobs & G. McCormack (Eds.), *The occupational therapy manager, 5th edition* (pp. 311–327). Bethesda, MD: AOTA Press.

Stalker, K., Jones, C., & Ritchie, P. (1996). All change? The role and tasks of community occupational therapists in Scotland. *British Journal of Occupational Therapy, 59*(3), 104–108.

U.S. Department of Health and Human Services. (2011). *Healthy People 2020.* Retrieved from http://healthypeople.gov/2020/default.aspx

Vaughn, L. & Sladyk, K. (2011). Entrepreneurship. In K. Jacobs & G. McCormack (Eds.), *The occupational therapy manager, 5th edition* (pp. 167–178). Bethesda, MD: AOTA Press.

Warren, R., & Warren, D. (1979). *The neighborhood organizer's handbook.* Notre Dame, IN: University of Notre Dame.

Watanabe, S. G. (1967). The developing role of occupational therapy in psychiatric home service. *American Journal of Occupational Therapy, 21,* 353–356.

West, W. A. (1967). The occupational therapist's changing responsibility to the community. *American Journal of Occupational Therapy, 21,* 312–316.

West, W. A. (1969). The growing importance of prevention. *American Journal of Occupational Therapy, 23,* 226–231.

Wiemer, R. B., & West, W. A. (1970). Occupational therapy in community health care. *American Journal of Occupational Therapy, 24,* 323–328.

Wilcock, A. A. (2006). *An occupational perspective of health.* Thorofare, NJ: SLACK.

World Federation of Occupational Therapists. (2004). *Perspective.* Retrieved from http://wfot.org/office_files/CBRposition%20Final%20CM2004%281%29.pdf

World Health Organization. (1986). *Ottawa Charter for Health Promotion.* Retrieved from http://euro.who.int/__data/assets/pdf_file/0004/129532/Ottawa_Charter.pdf

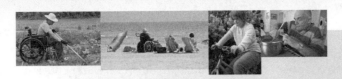

Chapter 2

Public Health, Community Health, and Occupational Therapy

Marjorie E. Scaffa, PhD, OTR/L, FAOTA, and Courtney S. Sasse, MA EdL, MS, OTR/L

If you do not know where you are going, you are likely to end up someplace else.

—Lao Tsu

Learning Objectives

This chapter is designed to enable the reader to:

- Describe the basic constructs associated with community and public health, prevention, and health promotion.
- Identify the determinants of health in a community.
- Discuss strategies for primary, secondary, and tertiary prevention.
- Describe the contributions occupational therapy can make to achieve the goals of *Healthy People 2020*.
- Discuss occupational therapy's role within the context of health promotion, community, and public health.

Key Terms

Community
Community health
Community health interventions
Determinants of health
Epidemiology
Health disparities
Health promotion

Incidence
Prevalence
Preventive occupation
Primary prevention
Public health
Secondary prevention
Tertiary prevention

Introduction

The profession's participation in public and community health efforts is affirmed in the *Occupational Therapy Framework: Domain and Process* (American Occupational Therapy Association [AOTA], 2008). In this document, health promotion and disability prevention are described as intervention approaches, and examples of the application of these approaches are provided focusing on performance skills, performance patterns, contexts, activity demands, and client factors. In addition, health management and maintenance are identified within the domain of occupational therapy as instrumental activities of daily living. Health and wellness, participation, prevention, quality of life, and occupational justice are

just a few of the outcomes that can result from the application of occupational therapy to public health problems.

Although having a sound knowledge base in occupational therapy is likely, the reader may be less familiar with the areas of public health and community health. The underlying constructs and principles of public health and community health as a foundation for providing occupational therapy from a population perspective are presented in this chapter. Key public and community health constructs such as health promotion, prevention, risk factors, and epidemiology are discussed in this chapter. Roles that may be assumed by occupational therapy practitioners and measures that may be implemented to improve the health of the community also are described.

Public Health

Public health is concerned with optimizing the health status of populations. Detels and Breslow (1997, p. 3) stated that public health is "the process of mobilizing local, state, national, and international resources to ensure the conditions in which people can be healthy." To achieve these healthy conditions, four public health strategies are used: promoting health and preventing disease, improving medical care, promoting health-enhancing behaviors, and controlling the environment (Detels & Breslow, 1997). These authors also identified three principles of public health that must be considered before any action can be taken to alleviate health concerns:

- The specific problems affecting the community's health must be assessed.
- Any strategies implemented must be based on scientific knowledge and available resources.
- The level of social and political commitment that currently exists must be determined.

A comprehensive definition of public health was put forth by Winslow in 1920: "Public health is the science and art of preventing disease, prolonging life, and promoting physical health and efficiency through organized community efforts for the sanitation of the environment, the control of communicable infections, the education of the individual in principles of personal hygiene, the organization of medical and nursing service for the early diagnosis and preventive treatment of disease, and the development of the social machinery which will ensure to every individual in the community a standard of living adequate for the maintenance of health" (p. 30).

Public health is often defined in terms of its aims and goals rather than being grounded in a specific body of knowledge (Detels, Holland, McEwen, & Omenn, 1997; Fee, 1997). Winslow's broad definition accurately implies that many disciplines contribute to the field of public health, including epidemiology, the biological and clinical sciences, biostatistics, nursing, health education, sanitation, industrial hygiene, sociology, psychology, economics, law, and engineering. However, the fundamental scientific basis of public health is **epidemiology,** the study of the distribution, frequencies, and determinants of disease, injury, and disability in human populations (MacMahon & Trichopoulos, 1996).

Epidemiologists use health statistics, including measures of incidence and prevalence, to estimate disease, injury, and disability in a variety of population groups; analyze health trends; plan and evaluate public health initiatives; and make informed health policy decisions. **Incidence** refers to the number of new cases of disease, injury, or disability within a specified time frame, typically a year. **Prevalence** refers to the total number of cases of disease, injury, or disability in a community, city, state, or nation existing at one point in time (Pickett & Hanlon, 1990).

According to Pickett and Hanlon (1990), preventive interventions attempt to reduce the incidence rate of a disease or an injury, and early detection procedures and rapid treatment attempt to reduce the duration of illness. Either strategy would result in a decreased prevalence rate. Combining the two strategies of prevention and early detection is the most effective approach to reducing overall prevalence.

Public health practitioners also are very interested in risk factors, both modifiable and nonmodifiable, that compromise health. Risk factors are those precursors that increase an individual's or population's vulnerability to developing a disease or disability or sustaining an injury (Scaffa, 1998). Often when people hear or use the term "risk factor," they are thinking of a physical condition that contributes to a disease. For example, high cholesterol, hypertension, and obesity are risk factors that can contribute to cardiovascular disease. However, risk factors are not just physical, behavioral, or genetic. They can also be social, economic, political, and environmental. Some risk factors are considered causal because the health problem cannot occur in the absence of the risk factor. Other risk factors are considered contributory because they interact with other risk factors leading to the development, exacerbation, or maintenance of disease, injury, or disability (Scaffa, 1998).

In addition to risk factors, public health professionals attempt to increase resiliency or protective factors that contribute to improved health and well-being. Resiliency factors are those precursors that appear to increase an individual's or population's resistance to developing a disease or disability or sustaining an injury (Scaffa, 1998). Resiliency factors may include the individual's genetic composition, personality, and health behavior patterns and social factors such as peer and family relationships and environmental and institutional supports for health. Public health interventions attempt to modify all types of risk factors and strengthen resiliency or protective factors to enhance the overall health and well-being of populations.

Prevention

Prevention refers to "anticipatory action taken to reduce the possibility of an event or condition from occurring or developing, or to minimize the damage that may result from the event or condition if it does occur" (Pickett & Hanlon, 1990, p. 81). When applying the term to public health, prevention refers to reducing the likelihood of the occurrence of disease/disability or inhibiting its progression to enhance optimal health and quality of life. Specifically, there are three levels of prevention: primary, secondary, and tertiary. Each level focuses on preventing health problems at a particular point along the continuum of the illness/injury process.

Primary prevention focuses on healthy individuals who potentially could be at risk for a particular health problem. The goal is to prevent the health problem from occurring by taking steps to maintain one's current healthy status and reduce susceptibility. For example, an already healthy person could continue to eat nutritious foods in the proper quantities and exercise regularly. Doing so could potentially avert obesity, diabetes, or cardiovascular disease. Another primary prevention strategy is to always wear a seat belt while in a motor vehicle, possibly avoiding injury if a crash occurred.

Secondary prevention focuses on the detection and treatment of disease early in its preclinical or clinical stages. The goal is to slow the progression, attempt to cure or control it as soon as possible, and prevent complications and disability. Arresting or reversing communicability also is a focus because early treatment of an infectious disease will limit exposure to others. An example of secondary prevention is an individual with hypertension exercising and maintaining an optimal weight so he or she can achieve normal blood pressure readings and thus reduce the risk of myocardial infarction (MI) and cerebrovascular accident (CVA).

Tertiary prevention, the third level, refers to measures used in the advanced stages of disease to limit disability and other complications. Tertiary prevention is implemented when a person is already ill or impaired, and the initial damage has already occurred. The goal is to restore as much functionality as possible, rehabilitate the individual, and attempt to prevent further damage. This level of prevention is the most familiar to occupational therapy practitioners. For example, occupational therapists routinely teach joint protection techniques to individuals with rheumatoid arthritis to prevent deformity and to enhance their ability to complete desired occupations with less pain. Energy conservation techniques are taught to individuals with cardiac conditions to prevent overexertion during the performance of occupations.

Health Promotion

Health promotion, a key public health strategy, is defined as any planned combination of educational, political, regulatory, environmental, and organizational supports for actions and conditions of living conducive to the health of individuals, groups, or communities (American Hospital Association, 1985; Green & Kreuter, 1991). More simply, it is "the process of enabling people to increase control over, and to improve, their health" (World Health Organization [WHO], 1986, para. 3). Health promotion encompasses strategies impacting all societal levels, including individuals, groups, organizations, communities, and government policy makers. A key purpose of health promotion is the prevention of disease and injury in individuals and populations.

Community Health

Typically, when people use the terms "community" and "health," they assume others define the words in the same manner. In reality, definitions can vary widely. To avoid misunderstandings, these two words are defined here for this discussion. **Community** refers to "noninstitutional aggregations of people linked together for common goals or other purposes" (Green & Raeburn, 1990, p. 41). Inherent is the idea that a community does not have to be composed of individuals within a particular geographical region. Communities may be "religious, professional, cultural, political, recreational, and a myriad of others based on groups of people with common bonds" (Rhynders & Scaffa, 2010, p. 209). Communities are dynamic entities that evolve with the changing characteristics of their members. **Community health** refers to the physical, emotional, social, and spiritual well-being of a group of people who are linked together in some way, possibly through geographical proximity or shared interests.

A community-based approach can be optimal when providing prevention and health care services to individuals. Social support, the ability to reach many consumers, targeted interventions that meet specific community needs, active community involvement, community-driven priorities, and the potential for a systems approach where problems can be addressed at multiple levels are included. A systems-oriented approach allows all involved to see the big picture and better understand relationships, connections, and dependencies. Because consequences and interactions are integral components, employing a systems view is helpful when trying to prioritize community needs and determine solutions to problems.

Community health interventions can be defined as "any combination of educational, social, and environmental supports for behavior conducive to health" (Green & Anderson, 1982, p. 3). Also, according to Green and Anderson (1982, pp. 3–4): "Educational interventions may be directed at high-risk individuals, families, or groups or at whole communities through mass media, schools, worksites, and organizations. Social interventions may include economic, political, legal and organizational changes designed to support actions conducive to health. Environmental supports include the structure and distribution of physical, chemical and biological resources, and facilities and substances required for people to protect their health. The health behavior of a community includes the actions of the people whose health is in question and the actions of community decision makers, professionals, peers, teachers, employers, parents and others who may influence health behaviors, resources or services in the community."

Community health interventions can be described on a continuum from community-based to community-level to community-centered (Scaffa & Brownson, 2005). Community-based interventions are health services provided in community settings targeted at individuals and families in order to improve health and facilitate health behavior change. Community-level interventions seek to modify the norms and behaviors of a population and improve health through sociocultural, political, economic, and environmental changes. Community-centered interventions are population-based approaches that are initiated and driven by the community itself using existing resources and seeking external support as needed. The goal of community health promotion is that every member of the community experiences a level of well-being and vitality, enabling him or her to choose, participate in, and enjoy the activities of the community (Scaffa & Brownson, 2005).

National Health Goals and Objectives for the United States

In 1979, the Surgeon General's office, in the U.S. Department of Health, Education, and Welfare (now the U.S. Department of Health and Human Services [USDHHS]), published a document titled *Healthy People*. This document was designed to identify national health goals and discuss health promotion and disease prevention in the United States so increasingly scarce healthcare resources could be used most efficiently and effectively. The concept underlying *Healthy People* came from Canada's *LaLonde Report*, a document published in 1974 describing the health status of Canadians. The authors of this framework proposed that all morbidity and mortality can be attributed to four primary elements:

- inadequacies in the existing health care system,
- behavioral factors or unhealthy lifestyles,
- environmental hazards,
- human biological factors (LaLonde, 1974).

The *Healthy People* document (U.S. Department of Health, Education, and Welfare, 1979) emphasized the importance of lifestyle changes in reducing morbidity and mortality rates. Five major health goals for the nation were identified and categorized according to life span; that is, one major goal was identified for each age group (i.e., infants, children, adolescents and young adults, adults, and older adults). Goals, several subgoals, and other problems experienced by each age group also were presented.

A new document, *Healthy People 2000*, was released in 1990. With this document, the focus became the improvement in quality of life and people's sense of well-being rather than solely the reduction of mortality rates. The new health goals for the United States were to:

- Increase the span of healthy life.
- Reduce health disparities.
- Achieve access to preventive health services for all (USDHHS, 1990).

In *Healthy People 2000*, 22 priority areas were identified for the focus of the nation's health promotion and disease prevention efforts. These areas were listed under the same three broad categories used in the 1979 document (i.e., health promotion, health protection, and preventive health services) with the addition of another category, surveillance and data systems. The purpose of adding this last category was to improve data collection methods. Additionally, social and environmental factors were emphasized as it became obvious that focusing on individual behaviors was insufficient.

Ten years later, due to advances in preventive therapies, vaccines and pharmaceuticals, assistive technologies, and computerized systems, the context in which *Healthy People 2010* was developed differed from that in which *Healthy People 2000* was framed (USDHHS, 1998). *Healthy People 2010*, released in January 2000, had two comprehensive goals: to increase the quality and years of healthy life and to eliminate health disparities. Progress toward these goals was measured by 467 objectives organized into 28 focus areas. "Healthy People in Healthy Communities" was the underlying premise of *Healthy People 2010* as individual health is dependent, to some degree, on the physical and social environments that exist in the community. Likewise, community health is affected by the collective attitudes and behaviors of community members. *Healthy People 2010* provided a framework for interdisciplinary collaboration in prevention and health promotion activities.

Healthy People 2020, released in November 2010, represents the fourth decade of goals and objectives that can be used to provide structure for prevention, health promotion, and well-being across a variety of population groups. The overarching goals outlined in *Healthy People 2020* are to:

- "Attain high-quality, longer lives free of preventable disease, disability, injury, and premature death.
- Achieve health equity, eliminate disparities, and improve the health of all groups.
- Create social and physical environments that promote good health for all.
- Promote quality of life, healthy development, and healthy behaviors across all life stages" (USDHHS, 2011a, para. 5).

According to *Healthy People 2020*, the range of factors that influence health status, or the **determinants of health**, fall into five broad categories: policy making, social factors, health services, individual behavior, and biology and genetics. Individual and population health are influenced by the interrelationships among these factors. Interventions that target multiple determinants of health are likely to be more effective than programs that address single factors.

A major focus of the *Healthy People 2020* initiative is to eliminate health disparities and achieve health equity. The term **health disparities** refers to "a particular type of health difference that is closely linked with social, economic, and/or environmental disadvantage. Health disparities adversely affect groups of people who have systematically experienced greater obstacles to health based on their racial or ethnic group; religion; socioeconomic status; gender; age; mental health; cognitive, sensory, or physical disability; sexual orientation or gender identity; geographic location; or other characteristics historically linked to discrimination or exclusion" (USDHHS, 2011b, para. 6).

Achieving health equity will require a coordinated and concerted effort to address the complex social, economic, educational, and environmental factors that produce health disparities, as well as to increase access to health care.

Three new features have been added to *Healthy People 2020* to support the vision of the initiative, "a society in which all people live long, healthy lives" (USDHHS, 2010a, p. 1). These include:

- an increased emphasis on achieving health equity through a determinants of health approach
- an interactive Web site that enables users to tailor information to their needs as the main vehicle for dissemination
- a collection of evidence-based resources to facilitate implementation

The long-range goals, topic areas, and measures of progress included in *Healthy People 2020* provide an action-oriented foundation for occupational therapy practitioners to consider in all phases of evaluation and intervention. There are 42 topic areas identified in the *Healthy People 2020* document (Box 2-1). These topical areas are sets of health objectives that have been grouped to bring attention and focus to the needs of certain populations or needs specific to each condition. Health objectives are assigned to particular federal agencies to develop, track, monitor, maintain, and periodically report to the public the status of each.

A significant number of the health objectives for the nation outlined in *Healthy People 2020* address the needs of persons with disabilities specifically. Box 2-2 contains examples of these objectives, many of which are directly relevant for occupational therapy intervention.

Ultimately, the goal of *Healthy People 2020* is to provide data and tools to enable practitioners and communities across the nation to easily integrate services and intervention efforts. In order to meet public health goals, a framework for implementation is included in *Healthy People 2020:* MAP-IT, or Mobilize, Assess, Plan, Implement, and Track (USDHHS, 2010b). The MAP-IT guide, available online, includes information on conducting a community needs assessment, a brief overview of *Healthy People 2020*, and tools for assessing and tracking progress.

Throughout the decade, the *Healthy People 2020* initiative will assess the general health status of the population, health-related quality of life, determinants of health, and health disparities. Health-related quality of life measures are particularly relevant for occupational therapists as they include physical,

---

Box 2-1 *Healthy People 2020* Focus Areas

Access to health services	Heart disease and stroke
Adolescent health	HIV
Arthritis, osteoporosis, and chronic back conditions	Immunization and infectious diseases
Blood disorders and blood safety	Injury and violence prevention
Cancer	Lesbian, gay, bisexual, and transgender health
Chronic kidney disease	Maternal, infant, and child health
Dementias, including Alzheimer's disease	Medical product safety
Diabetes	Mental health and mental disorders
Disability and disability health	Nutrition and weight status
Early and middle childhood	Occupational safety and health
Educational and community-based programs	Older adults
Environmental health	Oral health
Family planning	Physical activity
Food safety	Preparedness
Genomics	Public health infrastructure
Global health	Respiratory diseases
Health care–associated infections	Sexually transmitted diseases
Health communication and health information technology	Sleep health
Health-related quality of life and well-being	Social determinants of health
Hearing and other sensory or communication disorders	Substance abuse
	Tobacco use
	Vision

Data from: Healthy People 2020 by the U.S. Department of Health and Human Services, Office of Disease Prevention and Health Promotion, 2010, ODPHP Publication No. B0132. Retrieved from http://healthypeople.gov

Box 2-2   Selected Objectives Addressing the Needs of People with Disabilities

The overall goal in this focus area is to promote the health and well-being of people with disabilities. Objectives designed to address this goal include:
- DH-1: Include in the core of *Healthy People 2020* population data systems a standardized set of questions that identify "people with disabilities."
- DH-2: Increase the number of Tribes, States, and the District of Columbia that have public health surveillance and health promotion programs for people with disabilities and caregivers.
- DH-3: Increase the proportion of U.S. master of public health (M.P.H.) programs that offer graduate-level courses in disability and health.
- DH-4: Reduce the proportion of people with disabilities who report delays in receiving primary and periodic preventive care due to specific barriers.
- DH-7: Reduce the proportion of older adults with disabilities who use inappropriate medications.
- DH-8: Reduce the proportion of people with disabilities who report physical or program barriers to local health and wellness programs.
- DH-9: Reduce the proportion of people with disabilities who encounter barriers to participating in home, school, work, or community activities.
- DH-10: Reduce the proportion of people with disabilities who report barriers to obtaining the assistive devices, service animals, technology services, and accessible technologies that they need.
- DH-11: Increase the proportion of newly constructed and retrofitted U.S. homes and residential buildings that have visitable features.
- DH-13: Increase the proportion of people with disabilities who participate in social, spiritual, recreational, community, and civic activities to the degree that they wish.
- DH-14: Increase the proportion of children and youth with disabilities who spend at least 80% of their time in regular education programs.
- DH-16: Increase employment among people with disabilities.
- DH-17: Increase the proportion of adults with disabilities who report sufficient social and emotional support.
- DH-18: Reduce the proportion of people with disabilities who report serious psychological distress.
- DH-19: Reduce the proportion of people with disabilities who experience nonfatal unintentional injuries that require medical care.
- DH-20: Increase the proportion of children with disabilities, birth through age 2 years, who receive early intervention services in home or community-based settings.

Data from: Healthy People 2020 by the U.S. Department of Health and Human Services, Office of Disease Prevention and Health Promotion, 2010, ODPHP Publication No. B0132.

mental, and social aspects of quality of life, well-being and life satisfaction, and participation in common activities. Participation measures reflect how community members, regardless of functional limitations, participate in education, work, social, civic, and leisure activities (USDHHS, 2010c).

A Global Perspective

In 2005, the WHO established the Commission on Social Determinants of Health (CSDH) to develop strategies on reducing health inequities. Health inequities exist both within and between countries, with a 40-year life expectancy difference between the richest and poorest countries. The CSDH concluded that health inequities are not inevitable; instead they are due mainly to policy failures, and inequities in daily living conditions, access to power, and participation in society.

The CSDH proposed three comprehensive goals: to improve daily living conditions; address the inequitable distribution of power, money, and other resources; and measure and understand the problem and evaluate the outcomes of intervention (WHO, 2008). Nine key themes with implementation strategies were identified, including:

- early child development
- globalization
- health systems
- employment conditions
- social exclusion
- women and gender equity

- urbanization
- priority public health conditions
- measurement and evidence

At the 2011 World Conference on Social Determinants of Health in Brazil sponsored by the WHO, heads of governments and government representatives reaffirmed the belief that "health inequities within and between countries are politically, socially and economically unacceptable, as well as unfair and largely avoidable, and that the promotion of health equity is essential to sustainable development and to a better quality of life and well-being for all, which in turn can contribute to peace and security" (WHO, 2011, para. 4). The participants pledged to collectively take global action on the social determinants of health in order to create vibrant, inclusive, and healthy communities.

Improving Health and Well-Being Through Occupation

Wilcock (1998, p. 110) defines health from an occupational perspective as "the absence of illness, but not necessarily disability; a balance of physical, mental and social wellbeing attained through socially valued and individually meaningful occupation; enhancement of capacities and opportunity to strive for individual potential; community cohesion and opportunity; and social integration, support and justice, all within and as part of a sustainable ecology."

Seligman (2011) proposes that well-being consists of five elements: positive emotion, engagement, positive relationships, meaning, and accomplishment. This perspective suggests that occupation is a fundamental process for achieving health and well-being by facilitating engagement, meaning, and accomplishment. According to Wilcock (2005), the "occupations that will have the most obvious effects on wellbeing are those that are socially sanctioned and valued and that enable people freedom to effectively use physical and mental capacities in combination with social activity" (p. 153).

A variety of risk factors to health can result from less than optimal use, choice, opportunity, or balance in occupation. Risk factors for occupational dysfunction include occupational imbalance, occupational deprivation, and occupational alienation (Wilcock, 1998) as well as occupational delay, occupational interruption, and occupational disparities (Bass-Haugen, Henderson, Larson, & Matuska, 2005). These risk factors are described in Box 2-3.

Occupational therapy practice is based on the premise that participation in meaningful occupations can improve occupational performance and overall health and well-being. Therefore, **preventive occupation** can be characterized as the application of occupational science in the prevention of disease and disability and the promotion of health and well-being of individuals and communities through

Box 2-3 Occupational Risk Factors

- **Occupational alienation:** a lack of satisfaction in one's occupations. Tasks that are perceived as stressful, meaningless, or boring may result in an experience of occupational alienation (Wilcock, 1998).
- **Occupational delay:** occupational development that does not follow the typical schedule for the acquisition of occupational skills and is associated with occupational performance deficits (Bass-Haugen, Henderson, Larson, & Matuska, 2005)
- **Occupational deprivation:** circumstances or limitations that prevent a person from acquiring, using, or enjoying an occupation. Conditions that lead to occupational deprivation may include poor health, disability, lack of transportation, isolation, homelessness, etc. (Wilcock, 1998)
- **Occupational disparities:** inequalities or differences in occupational patterns among populations, often the result of occupational injustice (Bass-Haugen, Henderson, Larson, & Matuska, 2005)
- **Occupational imbalance:** occupational patterns that fail to meet an individual's physical or psychosocial needs, thereby resulting in decreased health and well-being (Wilcock, 1998)
- **Occupational interruption:** a temporary interference with occupational performance or participation as a result of a change in personal, social, or environmental factors (Bass-Haugen, Henderson, Larson, & Matuska, 2005)

meaningful engagement in occupations. An excellent example of the power of preventive occupation was demonstrated in a comprehensive research project commonly referred to as the "Well Elderly Study" conducted at the University of Southern California (Clark, Azen, Zemke, Jackson, Carlson, Mandel, Hay, Josephson, Cherry, Hessel, Palmer, & Lipson, 1997). This randomized, controlled trial, involving 361 men and women aged 60 years or older living independently in the community, was designed to evaluate the effectiveness of a preventive occupational therapy program. The main outcome measures of interest were "physical and social function, self-rated health, life satisfaction and depressive symptoms" (Clark et al., 1997, p. 1321). Older adults receiving occupational therapy services demonstrated improved vitality, physical and social functioning, life satisfaction, and general mental health. A six-month follow-up assessment indicated that 90% of the therapeutic gains had been maintained (Clark, Azen, Carlson, Mendale, LaBree, Hay, et al., 2001).

Practitioner Roles in Health Promotion and Community Health

The AOTA supports and promotes the involvement of occupational therapy professionals in the design and implementation of health promotion and prevention services (Scaffa, Van Slyke, & Brownson, 2008). Health promotion services may address the needs of individuals, families, groups, organizations, communities, and populations. The goals of occupational therapy in health promotion and prevention are to:

- Prevent or reduce the incidence of illness or disease, accidents, injuries, and disabilities in the population
- Reduce health disparities among racial and ethnic minorities and other underserved populations
- Enhance mental health, resiliency, and quality of life
- Prevent secondary conditions and improve the overall health and well-being of people with chronic conditions or disabilities and their caregivers and

- Promote healthy living practices, social participation, *occupational justice,* and healthy communities, with respect for cross-cultural issues and concerns (Scaffa et al., 2008, p. 695).

Occupational therapy practitioners may assume any combination of these three major roles in health promotion and disease/disability prevention:

1. Promoting healthy lifestyles for all clients and their families regardless of disability status. Lifestyle risk factors, such as tobacco use, unhealthy diet, physical inactivity, and substance abuse, are often overlooked among persons with disabilities. Standard health promotion programs and services may be inappropriate for persons with disabilities. Occupational therapy practitioners are capable of adapting these programs to meet the special needs of individuals living with disabling conditions.
2. Incorporating occupation in existing health promotion efforts developed by experts in areas such as health education, nutrition, and exercise. For example, in working with a person with a lower-extremity amputation due to diabetes, the occupational therapy practitioner may focus on the occupation of meal preparation using foods and preparation methods recommended in the nutritionist's health promotion program. This enables the achievement of the goal of functional independence in the kitchen while reinforcing the importance of proper nutrition for the prevention of further disability.
3. Developing and implementing occupation-based health promotion programs, targeting a variety of constituencies and levels of society, including individuals (both with and without disabilities), groups, organizations, communities, and governmental policies.

A variety of examples of occupation-focused health promotion interventions are listed in Box 2-4.

Conclusion

Philosophically, occupational therapy and public health are quite compatible and even complementary. Occupational therapy practitioners can learn

Box 2-4   Occupation-Based Health Promotion Interventions

Occupation-focused health promotion interventions at each level may include but are not limited to:

Individual-level interventions
- Adaptation of physical activities/exercises for persons with disabilities
- Education of caregivers about proper body mechanics for lifting to prevent back injuries
- Driving evaluation and training for persons with physical or cognitive impairments

Group-level interventions
- Repetitive strain injury education and prevention and management programs for workers
- Parenting skills training for adolescent mothers
- Education of day-care providers regarding normal growth and development, handling behavioral problems, and identifying children at risk for developmental delay

Organizational-level interventions
- Consultation with industrial managers regarding the benefits of ergonomic workspace design and worksite injury prevention strategies
- Disability awareness training for service-industry personnel such as those who work for airlines, hotels, restaurants, etc.

Community-level interventions
- Modification of community recreational facilities to increase accessibility for persons with disabilities
- Consultation with contractors, architects, and city planners regarding accessibility and universal design

Governmental-policy interventions
- Promotion of full inclusion of children with disabilities in schools and day-care programs
- Lobbying for public funds to support programs to improve the quality of life for at-risk populations

much from collaboration with public health, health promotion, and health education professionals in terms of primary and secondary prevention strategies and community health initiatives. Public health programs can benefit from the unique contribution of occupation and an occupational science perspective that occupational therapy practitioners can provide. The focus of *Healthy People 2020* on quality of life, satisfying relationships, and functional capacity to work and play invites the participation and inclusion of the occupational therapy profession in public health, health promotion, prevention, and community health initiatives.

In order for occupational therapists and other health care professionals to effectively participate in individual and population-based health promotion and prevention efforts, educational programs need to facilitate the development of competencies for this area of practice. The Association for Prevention Teaching and Research (APTR) has developed a curriculum framework for health professions education that focuses on interprofessional collaboration and serves as the educational underpinning for *Healthy People 2020* objectives related to the training of health professionals. The *Clinical Prevention and Population Health Curriculum Framework* consists of four components: evidence-based practice, clinical preventive services and health promotion, health systems and health policy, and population health and community aspects of practice (APTR, 2009). Adoption of this framework by occupational therapy educational programs could enhance the knowledge and skills of students needed for future health promotion practice.

Changes in demographics, including the rapid growth in the number of elderly who are at risk for injuries, illnesses, and disabilities, provide an opportunity for occupational therapy practitioners to expand their role in health promotion and disease/disability prevention. As in all areas of practice, health promotion interventions should be based on clear evidence. Although occupational therapy practitioners have the basic competencies to design and implement occupation-based health promotion interventions, continuing education to acquire specialized knowledge and skills is recommended for this practice area (Scaffa et al., 2008).

Learning Activities

1. Interview several individuals of various ages to ascertain their ideas, definitions, and perspectives on health and well-being. How are their perspectives on health and well-being different and how are they similar? Ask them to describe their current state of health and how participation in everyday activities (occupations) impacts their well-being.
2. Select a population in a specific geographic area and search for newspaper and magazine articles on the health needs of this population. Identify potential occupational risk factors for this population and occupational therapy interventions to address these risk factors.
3. Compare your occupational therapy educational program to the *Clinical Prevention and Population Health Curriculum Framework* (APTR, 2009) to determine content areas that need to be enhanced for effective participation in health promotion services.

REFERENCES

American Hospital Association. (1985). *Health promotion for older adults: Planning for action.* Chicago, IL: Center for Health Promotion.

American Occupational Therapy Association. (2008). Occupational therapy practice framework: Domain and process (2nd ed.). *American Journal of Occupational Therapy, 62*(6), 625–683.

Association for Prevention Teaching and Research. (2009). *Clinical prevention and population health curriculum framework.* Retrieved from http://aptrweb.org/about/pdfs/Revised_CPPH_Framework_2009.pdf

Bass-Haugen, J., Henderson, M. L., Larson, B. A., & Matuska, K. (2005). Occupational issues of concern in populations. In C. H. Christiansen, C. M. Baum, & J. Bass-Haugen (Eds.), *Occupational therapy: Performance, participation and well-being* (3rd ed.). Thorofare, NJ: SLACK.

Clark, F., Azen, S. P., Zemke, R., Jackson, J., Carlson, M., Mandel, D., Hay, J., Josephson, K., Cherry, B., Hessel, C., Palmer, J., & Lipson, L. (1997). Occupational therapy for independent living older adults: A randomized controlled trial. *Journal of the American Medical Association, 278,* 1321–1326.

Clark, F., Azen, S. P., Carlson, M., Mandel, D., LaBree, L., Hay, J., et al. (2001). Embedding health-promoting changes into the daily lives of independent-living older adults: Long-term follow-up of occupational therapy intervention. *Journal of Gerontology: Psychological Sciences, 56,* 60–63.

Detels, R., & Breslow, L. (1997). Current scope and concerns in public health. In R. Detels, W. W. Holland, J. McEwen, & G. S. Omenn (Eds.), *Oxford textbook of public health.* New York: Oxford University Press.

Detels, R., Holland, W. W., McEwen, J., & Omenn, G. S. (1997). *Oxford textbook of public health.* New York: Oxford University Press.

Fee, E. (1997). The origins and development of public health in the United States. In R. Detels, W. W. Holland, J. McEwen, and G. S. Omenn (Eds.), *Oxford textbook of public health* (pp. 35–54). New York: Oxford University Press.

Green, L. W., & Anderson, C. L. (1982). *Community health.* St. Louis, MO: Mosby.

Green, L. W., & Kreuter, M. W. (1991). *Health promotion planning: An educational and environmental approach* (2nd ed.). Mountainview, CA: Mayfield.

Green, L. W., & Raeburn, J. (1990). Contemporary developments in health promotion, definitions and challenges. In N. Bracht (Ed.), *Health promotion at the community level.* Newbury Park, CA: Sage.

LaLonde, M. (1974). *A new perspective on the health of Canadians: A working document.* Ottawa: Ministry of National Health and Welfare.

MacMahon, B., & Trichopoulos, D. (1996). *Epidemiology principles and methods.* Boston: Little, Brown.

Pickett, G., & Hanlon, J. J. (1990). *Public health: Administration and practice.* St. Louis, MO: Times Mirror/Mosby.

Rhynders, P. A., & Scaffa, M. E. (2010). Enhancing community health through community partnerships. In M. Scaffa, S. M. Reitz, & M. Pizzi, *Occupational therapy in the promotion of health and wellness* (pp. 208–224). Philadelphia: F.A. Davis.

Scaffa, M. E. (1998). Adolescents and alcohol use. In A. Henderson, S. Champlin, & W. Evashwick (Eds.), *Promoting teen health: Linking schools, health organizations and community.* Thousand Oaks, CA: Sage.

Scaffa, M. E., & Brownson, C. (2005). Occupational therapy interventions: Community health approaches. In C. H. Christiansen, C. M. Baum, & J. Bass-Haugen (Eds.), *Occupational therapy: Performance, participation and well-being* (3rd ed., pp. 477–488). Thorofare, NJ: SLACK.

Scaffa, M. E., Van Slyke, N., & Brownson, C. A. (2008). Occupational therapy in the promotion of health and the prevention of disease and disability. *American Journal of Occupational Therapy, 62*(6), 694–703.

Seligman, M. (2011). *Flourish: A visionary new understanding of happiness and well-being.* New York, NY: Free Press.

U.S. Department of Health and Human Services. (1990). *Healthy People 2000: National health promotion and disease prevention objectives* (Publication No. 017-001-00474-0). Washington, DC: U.S. Government Printing Office.

U.S. Department of Health and Human Services. (1998). *Healthy People 2010 objectives: Draft for public comment.* Washington, DC: U.S. Department of Health and Human Services.

U.S. Department of Health and Human Services. (2000). *Healthy People 2010* (2nd ed.). Washington, DC: U.S. Government Printing Office.

U.S. Department of Health and Human Services. (2010a). *Healthy People 2020* (ODPHP Publication No. B0132). Retrieved from http://healthypeople.gov

U.S. Department of Health and Human Services. (2010b). Implementing Healthy People 2020. *Healthy People 2020.* Retrieved from http://healthypeople.gov/2020/ implementing/default.aspx

U.S. Department of Health and Human Services. (2010c). Health-Related Quality of Life and Well-Being. *Healthy People 2020.* Retrieved from http://healthypeople.gov/ 2020/about/QoLWBabout.aspx

U.S. Department of Health and Human Services. (2011a). About Healthy People. *Healthy People 2020.* Retrieved from http://healthypeople.gov/2020/about/default.aspx

U.S. Department of Health and Human Services. (2011b). Disparities. *Healthy People 2020.* Retrieved from http:// healthypeople.gov/2020/about/DisparitiesAbout.aspx

U.S. Department of Health, Education, and Welfare. (1979). *Healthy People: Surgeon General's report on health promotion/disease prevention* (Publication No. 79-55071). Washington, DC: U.S. Government Printing Office.

Wilcock, A. A. (1998). *An occupational perspective of health.* Thorofare, NJ: SLACK.

Wilcock, A. A. (2005). Relationship of occupations to health and well-being. In C. H. Christiansen, C. M. Baum, & J. Bass-Haugen (Eds.), *Occupational therapy: Performance, participation and well-being* (3rd ed.). Thorofare, NJ: SLACK.

Winslow, C-E. A. (1920). The untilled fields of public health. *Science, 51,* 23–33.

World Health Organization. (1986). *The Ottawa Charter for Health Promotion.* Retrieved from http://who.int/health-promotion/conferences/previous/ottawa/en/

World Health Organization. (2008). *Commission on Social Determinants of Health: Report by the Secretariat.* Retrieved from http://apps.who.int/gb/ebwha/pdf_files/EB124/ B124_9-en.pdf

World Health Organization. (2011). *Rio Political Declaration on Social Determinants of Health.* Retrieved from http://who.int/sdhconference/ declaration/Rio_political_declaration.pdf

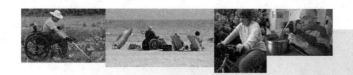

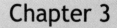

Chapter 3

Theoretical Frameworks for Community-Based Practice

S. Maggie Reitz, PhD, OTR/L, FAOTA, Marjorie E. Scaffa, PhD, OTR/L, FAOTA, and M. Beth Merryman, PhD, OTR/L, FAOTA

We envision that occupational therapy is a powerful, widely recognized, science-driven, and evidence-based profession with a globally connected and diverse workforce meeting society's occupational needs.

—Centennial Vision of the American Occupational Therapy Association [AOTA], 2007, p. 614)

Learning Objectives

This chapter is designed to enable the reader to:

- Appreciate the need for occupational therapists to be knowledgeable and competent in the use of theory in community-based practice.
- Identify and define terms related to theory and the relationships among these terms.
- Define the term "community organization," and describe strategies for organizing communities to meet health needs.
- Describe the general characteristics and principles of theories from related disciplines that could be used in community-based practice.

Key Terms

Community assets
Community organization
Concept
Conceptual model of practice
Construct
Human agency
Model

Outcome expectations
Paradigm
Principle
Reciprocal determinism
Self-efficacy
Theory

Introduction

In preparation for its 100th anniversary in 2017, the American Occupational Therapy Association (AOTA) developed its Centennial Vision, which highlights the importance of evidence-based practice. The utilization of theory is the first step in a profession's quest to be both science-driven and evidence-based. A well-developed theoretical foundation for community-based practice is essential for a variety of reasons. Theories and models provide the foundation and context for basic and applied research, program design, implementation, and evaluation. A brief review of terminology is provided to help establish a common basis for understanding the theoretical discussion. This review is followed by a description of a few select theoretical frameworks from public health, health education, and occupational therapy that can be applied to community-based practice. Theoretical frameworks such as these and others can be used to assist communities in their efforts to improve residents' occupational performance, health, participation, and quality of life. These four outcomes are consistent with those of occupational therapy, as detailed in the AOTA *Practice Framework*: *Domain and Processes* (AOTA, 2008).

In the current climate of rapid change and the need to justify and substantiate the role of occupational therapy, knowledge of theory is essential. Established and evolving theoretical models are well suited to support occupational therapy's role in health care institutions and in the community. However, before models can be fully implemented, it is important to understand the terminology used in the application of theory.

Review of Terminology

The following terms will be defined and described: concept, construct, principle, model, theory, paradigm, and conceptual model of practice. These terms are presented in sequence beginning with the basic building blocks of theory and then moving on to terms that describe higher levels of conceptualization.

Concepts and Constructs

Some authors and theorists simply use the term "concept," while others use both "concept" and "construct" in order to differentiate between types of ideas. A **concept** "describes some regularity or relationship within a group of facts" (Payton, 1988, p. 12). The term "construct" may be used to represent a specific type of concept. When this distinction is made, the term "concept" is employed to describe tangible physical objects such as a table or ball, while the term **construct** is used to refer to intangible ideas (Miller & Schwartz, 2004), such as health or quality of life. Occupational therapy uses a variety of constructs, for example, competence, mastery, achievement, adaptation, self-efficacy, and emotional regulation. It is essential that these and other constructs are examined, defined, and explained in terms of their potential contribution to occupational therapy community-based practice outcomes.

Principle

A **principle** describes the relationship between two or more concepts, two or more constructs, or a combination of constructs and concepts. Some writers use the term "postulate" interchangeably with the term "principle." Related principles can then be organized into theories (Miller & Schwartz, 2004; Payton, 1988). Examples of principles from Nelson's Conceptual Framework of Therapeutic Occupation (Nelson, 1997, p. 13) include:

- "Occupation influences the world around the person."
- "The person can affect his or her own future occupational forms."
- "A person can literally change his or her own nature by engaging in occupation."

These same principles can be adapted for use in the community as follows:

- Occupation influences the world around people and their community.
- The community can affect its own future occupational forms.
- A community can literally change its own nature through occupational engagement.

Model

A **model** can be defined as a semantic or diagrammatic representation of concepts and/or constructs and their interrelationships. This representation allows for operationalization, experimental assessment, and application of a theory (Parcel, 1984). Models can be viewed as a subclass of theories (McKenzie, Neiger, & Thackeray, 2009). However, not all theories possess corresponding models, and not all models are founded on specific, well-defined theories.

Theory

A **theory** "is a systematic way of understanding events or situations" that describes the relationships between the constructs, concepts, and principles on which it is built (National Cancer Institute [NCI], 2005, p. 4). Humans use theory to link an event or behavior to antecedent factors whether or not those factors are directly observable (Miller & Schwartz, 2004). A well-constructed theory satisfies four basic criteria:

- Fit,
- Understanding,
- Generality, and
- Control.

For a theory to have a good *fit,* it must reflect the everyday reality of the phenomenon it is designed to represent. *Understanding* refers to the need for the theory to be rational, be logical, and make sense both to the researcher/theorist and to the individuals who were studied. *Generality* means that a well-developed theory is comprehensive and includes sufficient variation to provide applicability to a diversity of contexts. Lastly, it should allow for a degree of *control* over the phenomenon in question (Strauss & Corbin, 1990).

Paradigm

A paradigm guides the thinking and development of new knowledge for the use of a discipline. The term is used by theorists in a variety of disciplines to describe both the overall vision of the discipline and the practical knowledge employed in daily activities of the discipline. A **paradigm,** according to Kuhn, is a "collective vision...a set of perspectives, ideas, and values that constitute a unique perspective shared by members of the discipline" (Kielhofner, 2004, p. 16). Kielhofner (2009) expands on this idea by identifying three elements of a paradigm:

- core constructs, which are broad ideas about the need, selection, and rationale of interventions,
- focal viewpoint, which provides a common lens to view practice possibilities, and
- values and priorities of the profession.

Conceptual Model of Practice

A **conceptual model of practice** "presents and organizes theory used by therapists in their work.... Each model explains an area of functioning and specifies the interventions pertaining to particular kinds of problems in that area" (Kielhofner, 2004, p. 20). The elements of a well-developed conceptual practice model are displayed in Box 3-1. Ideally these parts work together to support the continued development of best practice. Examples of conceptual models of practice identified by Kielhofner (2009) include the biomechanical model, cognitive model, functional group model, intentional relationship model, model of human occupation, motor control model, and sensory integration model.

Box 3-1 Conceptual Practice Model Components

- Theory specific to phenomena seen in practice
- Resources for practice (e.g., equipment, assessments)
- Research and evidence on utility of theory

Developed from "The Kind of Knowledge Needed to Support Practice?" by G. Kielhofner, 2009, in G. Kielhofner (Ed.), *Conceptual Foundations of Occupational Therapy Practice* (pp. 8–14). Philadelphia, PA: F.A. Davis.

Theories Related to Community-Based Practice

There are many theoretical supports available to occupational therapy practitioners as they engage in community-based occupational therapy practice. These supports include the academic discipline of occupational science as well as occupational therapy conceptual practice models. Theories and models from health education, health psychology, public health, and communication studies, as well as theories directly related to community organization, can also be helpful guides for community-based practice.

Community Organization Approaches

Community organization has been defined as "the process by which community groups are helped to identify common problems or goals, mobilize resources, and in other ways develop and implement strategies for reaching goals they have set" (Minkler & Wallerstein, 2005, p. 26). The goals of community organization include solving current community problems, building permanent organizational and community capacity for ongoing problem solving, and empowering individuals and neighborhoods to act collectively in their own best interest (Rubin & Rubin, 2005). Before initiating a community organization effort, familiarity with the community, as well as the language of community development and the values and assumptions of community organization, is important. Terms associated with community organization are listed and defined in Box 3-2 (McKenzie et al., 2009).

Box 3-2 Terms Associated With Community Organization	
Citizen Participation:	The bottom-up, grassroots mobilization of citizens for the purpose of undertaking activities to improve the condition of something in the community.
Community Capacity:	"The characteristics of communities that affect their ability to identify, mobilize, and address social and public health problems" (Goodman, Speers, McLeroy, Fawcett, Kegler, Parker, & Wallenstein, 1999, p. 259).
Community Development:	"A process designed to create conditions for economic and social progress for the whole community with its active participation and the fullest possible reliance on the community's initiative" (United Nations, 1955, p. 6).
Empowered Community:	"One in which individuals and organizations apply their skills and resources in collective efforts to meet their respective needs" (Israel, Checkoway, Schulz, & Zimmerman, 1994).
Grassroots Participation:	"Bottom-up efforts of people taking collective actions on their own behalf, and they involve the use of a sophisticated blend of confrontation and cooperation in order to achieve their ends" (Perlman, 1978, p. 65).
Macro Practice:	The methods of professional change that deal with issues beyond the individual, family, and small group level.
Social Capital:	"Relationships and structures within a community that promote cooperation for mutual benefit" (Minkler & Wallerstein, 2005, p. 35).
Participation and Relevance:	"Community organizing that 'starts where the people are' and engages community members as equals" (Minkler & Wallerstein, 2005, p.35).

From McKenzie, J. F., Neiger, B. L., & Thackeray, R., *Planning, Implementing, and Evaluating Health Promotion Programs: A Primer* (5th ed., p. 239). Copyright © 2009 by Pearson Benjamin Cummings. Reprinted with permission.

Ross (1967) describes several important principles underlying community organization. These include:

- Communities can develop strategies to respond to their specific needs and problems.
- Individuals have the ability to change and want to change.
- Community members should be involved in the change-making process.
- Changes that are internally motivated have more meaning and are more lasting than changes imposed from the outside.
- A "holistic" approach to change is more effective than a "fragmented" approach.
- Democracy requires the "cooperative participation and action" of community members and the requisite skills that make this possible.
- Communities may need assistance to effectively organize to meet their needs.

The majority of theoretical approaches to community organization are need- or problem-based, and involve identification and remediation of deficits in a community. However, Kretzmann and McKnight (2005) propose a strengths-based approach that involves identifying and mobilizing all of the existing and potential, but often unrecognized, assets in a community. **Community assets** include personal attributes and skills, relationships among people, local associations, and informal networks. Connecting community assets and strengths creates a synergy and multiplies their power and efficacy.

The models used in community organizing have been classified into different systems. One frequently cited classification method, developed by Rothman (Minkler & Wallerstein, 2005), separates the models into three categories:

1. locality development, which is heavily process-dominated;
2. social planning, which is heavily task-oriented; and
3. social action, which incorporates task and process.

Community organizing strategies take many forms but typically involve consensus, collaboration, and advocacy. Examples of effective strategies include developing critical awareness, creating community identity, building relationships, mapping community assets, organizing coalitions, identifying community successes, and leveraging resources and investments from outside the community, as well as leadership development, and political and legislative action (Mathie & Cunningham, 2003; Minkler & Wallerstein, 2005).

McKenzie et al. (2009, p. 242) provide a generic approach to community organization that combines the three types of models, with social planning being the most heavily used (Fig. 3.1). The steps, described by McKenzie et al. (2009), can serve as useful guides for occupational therapy practitioners who are new

to working with the community as the point of service. These steps provide the basic road map of tasks that are required to enter and organize a community. However, they do not provide sufficient guidance to develop and evaluate an intervention. These principles, combined with one or more of the other theoretical models discussed later in this chapter, provide an excellent framework for the development of an empowered community. Community organizing involves "transforming individual and collective values to build support for social justice and social equity" (Rubin & Rubin, 2005, p. 189) and as such is a useful tool for occupational therapy practitioners advocating occupational justice.

Selected Health Education and Public Health Models and Theories

Since the 1950s, the fields of health education, public health, and health psychology have been developing and employing models to explain why people do or do not engage in health behaviors. Many theories have been referred to in the health education and public health literature, but one of the most frequently cited is social cognitive theory (Bandura, 1977). This theory, as well as four additional models, will be described briefly, including: the health belief model (Rosenstock, Strecher, & Becker, 1994), Prochaska and DiClemente's transtheoretical model of health behavior change (1983, 1992), the PRECEDE-PROCEED framework (Green & Kreuter, 1991, 2005) and the Diffusion of Innovation model (Rogers, 2003). The health belief model (HBM) is a model of the precursors of health behavior, while the transtheoretical model of health behavior change explains the stages people experience as they seek to change their health behavior (McKenzie et al., 2009). The PRECEDE-PROCEED framework is a program planning and evaluation tool, while Diffusion of Innovation is a health communications approach.

Social Cognitive Theory

Bandura (2004) described the core determinants of health behaviors, the mechanisms through which these core determinants work, and the application

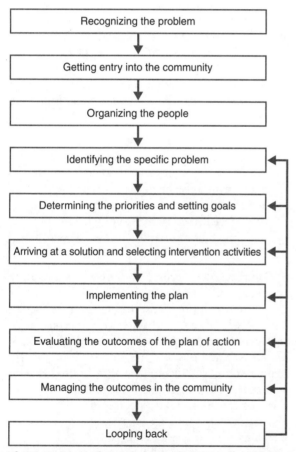

Fig. 3•1 Steps of Community Organization. *(From McKenzie, James F., Neiger, Brad, L., and Thackery, Rosemary, Planning, Implementing, and Evaluating Health Promotion Programs: A Primer [5th ed., p. 242]. Copyright ©2009 by Allyn & Bacon.)*

of social cognitive theory (SCT) to prevention and health promotion practices. The core determinants of health behaviors include: knowledge of the health risks and benefits of various behaviors, perceived self-efficacy, outcome expectations, self-determined health goals and strategies, and perceived facilitators and impediments to health behavior change. In addition, the SCT relies on the postulate of **reciprocal determinism,** which is present when there is a continuous reciprocal, interdependent interaction of the person, the person's behavior, and the environment. The relative contribution of each of these factors in the determination of an outcome differs according to the setting and the behavior in question (Bandura, 1977).

Knowledge of the health effects of various behaviors is a necessary, but not sufficient, precondition for change. Other factors also are involved. The individual's perception that he or she will be able to successfully perform a specific behavior, or perceived self-efficacy, plays a central role in motivation for change (Bandura, 2004). **Self-efficacy** is the belief in one's own competence and power to execute an action that will achieve the desired outcome. These efficacy beliefs have a profound impact on goal setting and aspirations. According to Bandura (2004, p. 145), "the stronger the perceived self-efficacy, the higher the goals people set for themselves and the firmer their commitment to them."

Self-efficacy, whether or not an individual believes in his or her ability to perform a given behavior, is derived from personal performance attainments, vicarious experiences, verbal persuasion, and emotional arousal. Successful accomplishment of a behavior enhances one's expectation for future endeavors. The more similar the current task to tasks performed successfully in the past, the greater the efficacy expectations will be. Observations of others who are perceived as similar to oneself, engaging in activities and achieving the desired outcome can also increase one's expectations for accomplishment. According to SCT, verbal encouragement, receipt of permission to attempt a specific behavior, and a perceived physiological and emotional state that is conducive to successful execution of the task will also enhance an individual's confidence and self-efficacy relative to that behavior.

Health behavior change also is mediated by expectancies. According to Bandura (1977), **outcome expectations** are the individual's belief that a given behavior will lead to specific outcomes. There are three types of outcome expectations: physical outcomes, the pleasurable and/or aversive effects of the health behavior; social outcomes, the social approval and/or disapproval the behavior evokes; and self-evaluative outcomes, the degree of satisfaction and/or self-worth the person derives from his or her health behavior and/or health status (Bandura, 2004).

Finally, health behavior is affected by personal values and goals, as well as perceived facilitators and barriers. **Human agency,** or the ability to intentionally create and influence one's future, enables goal setting, behavior change, and environmental adaptation (Bandura, 2006). Barriers, obstacles, and impediments to health behavior and health behavior change may be personal, social, economic, and environmental. Persons with high levels of self-efficacy are more likely to perceive obstacles as surmountable, while persons with low levels of self-efficacy will quickly become discouraged in the face of adversity (Bandura, 2004). Behavior change, in the SCT paradigm, can be achieved in the following ways:

- directly, by reinforcement of particular behaviors;
- indirectly, through social modeling or observing someone else being reinforced for the behavior; and
- through self-management or by having the individual monitor and self-reward (Parcel & Baranowski, 1981).

Bandura (2004) recommends the use of a stepwise approach to the development of health behavior interventions, tailoring the strategies to the particular level of self-efficacy and outcome expectations of the client. For example, persons with high levels of self-efficacy and positive outcome expectations will require minimal guidance to achieve health behavior change. However, persons who have doubts about their self-efficacy and the outcomes of their behaviors will need more guidance, support, and modeling. Persons with low levels of self-efficacy and negative outcome expectations will require considerable structure and personal guidance, as well as the incorporation of the occupational therapy principle of "the just right challenge" in order to build confidence through experiences of behavioral success.

In general, the SCT provides a unique perspective for community-based practice. The constructs of self-efficacy, outcome expectations, behavioral capability, modeling, reciprocal determinism, and self-control appear to be particularly relevant for the development of occupational therapy interventions.

Health Belief Model

The health belief model describes the relationships between a person's beliefs about health and his or her health-specific behaviors. The beliefs that mediate health behavior are, according to the model, perceived susceptibility, severity, benefits, and barriers. In addition to the beliefs just mentioned, cues to action are viewed as necessary triggers of behavior.

- *Perceived susceptibility* is the individual's subjective impression of the risk of a disease, illness, or trauma.
- *Perceived severity* refers to the convictions a person holds regarding the degree of seriousness of a given health problem.
- *Perceived benefits* are the beliefs a person has regarding the availability and effectiveness of a variety of possible actions in reducing the threat of illness or trauma.
- *Perceived barriers* are the costs or negative aspects associated with engaging in a specific health or preventive behavior.
- *Cues to action* are defined as instigating events that stimulate the initiation of behavior. These cues may be internal, such as perceptions of pain, or external, such as feedback from a health care provider (Rosenstock, 1974) or the media.

According to the model, in order for a person to take action to avoid illness or trauma, the positive forces need to outweigh the negative forces. If an individual believes the following, that:

- he or she is personally susceptible to the disease, illness, or trauma;
- occurrence of the health problem is severe enough to negatively impact his or her life;
- taking specific actions would have beneficial effects;
- barriers to such action do not overwhelm the benefits;

- the individual is exposed to cues for action,
- then it is likely that the health behavior will occur (Rosenstock, 1974).

The HBM has been used with a variety of populations and a diversity of health topics, including:

- Breast self-examination (Champion, 1985) and mammogram screening (Wang, Liang, Schwartz, Lee, Kreling, & Mandelblatt, 2008),
- Contraceptive behavior (Herold, 1983; Hester & Macrina, 1985),
- Diabetes self-management regimen (Becker & Janz, 1985; Bereolos, 2007),
- Health habits of college students (Deshpande, Basil, & Basil, 2009; Juniper, Oman, Hamm, & Kerby, 2004),
- Medication compliance among psychiatric outpatients (Kelly, Mamon, & Scott, 1987), and
- Osteoporosis prevention (Johnson, McLeod, Kennedy, & McLeod, 2008).

Perceived threat, which encompasses perceived susceptibility, has been suggested to be an important first cognitive step in the health-action link described by this model. Figure 3.2 presents an adapted schematic representation of the updated HBM as applied to the goal of increasing physical activity.

Within occupational therapy, the HBM has been used to support a program evaluation of CarFit®, a community-based program directed at educating older drivers about proper positioning while driving. CarFit was jointly developed by AOTA, AARP, and the American Automobile Association to enhance driving safety among older adults. Results from this study indicated that this type of community-based program can result in self-reported behavior change and the dissemination of educational content beyond the original participants (Stav, 2010).

Transtheoretical Model of Health Behavior Change

The transtheoretical model of health behavior change (TMHBC), also referred to as the Stages of Change Model, is a complex model consisting of stages (precontemplation, contemplation, preparation, action, maintenance, and relapse/re-cycling) and processes of change (Prochaska, Norcross, & DiClemente, 1994). The stages are depicted in

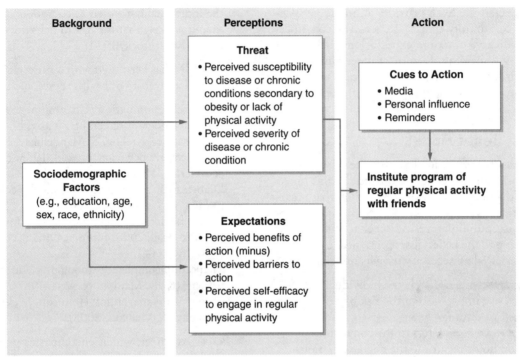

Fig. 3•2 Adapted from The Revised Health Belief Model as a Framework to Investigate Compliance with Required Physical Activity. *(From Rosenstock, I. M., Strecher, V. J., and Becker, M. H. [1994]. The health belief model and HIV risk behavior change. In R. J. DiClemente and J. L. Peterson [Eds.], Preventing AIDS: Theories and methods for behavioral interventions [p. 11]. New York: Plenum.)*

Figure 3.3 and the processes are described in Table 3-1.

The precontemplation stage refers to the individual's inability to identify that she has a problem, and, as a result, she has no intention of changing her behavior. In the contemplation stage, the individual can identify and acknowledge a problem behavior and is motivated to remedy it. The preparation stage is characterized by planning for change, acquiring needed resources to facilitate the behavior change, and making declarations about intentions to change to family and friends. The action stage involves overtly changing one's behavior and modifying the environment to facilitate and maintain the change. The maintenance stage requires long-term commitment to sustain the behavior change and to incorporate it into one's lifestyle permanently (Prochaska, Norcross, & DiClemente, 1994).

Relapse is included as many health behavior changes, such as smoking, follow a pattern of initiation,

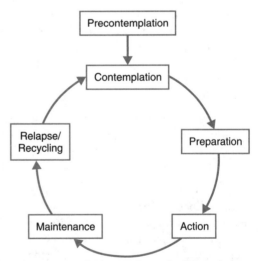

Fig. 3•3 Stages of Change from the Transtheoretical Model. *(Data from: Prochaska, Norcross, & DiClemente (1994).)*

Table 3-1	Processes Associated With the Transtheoretical Model
Process	**Description**
Consciousness-raising	Increasing one's level of awareness of the problem and its consequences, providing information that can be useful in the behavior change process
Social liberation	Alternatives to the behavior that the environment provides that free the person from having to make an individual decision
Emotional arousal	Similar to consciousness-raising, but works on a deeper feeling level in order to experience and express emotions about the problem and behavior change, as well as to understand one's resistance to change
Self-reevaluation	A thoughtful and emotional reappraisal of the problem that enables people to see when and how their behavior conflicts with their goals and values
Commitment (or self-liberation)	Accepting responsibility for the changes needed and announcing one's decision to change, which increases accountability for taking action
Countering	Substituting healthy responses and behaviors for unhealthy ones, for example, going for a walk instead of eating a piece of cake
Environment control	Restructuring the physical and social environment to maximize potential for effective behavior change; avoiding stimuli that elicit unhealthy behaviors
Rewards	Behaviors that are reinforced are repeated and maintained. Finding rewards for behavior change that are personally meaningful is critical for success.
Helping relationships	Soliciting, accepting, and receiving support and other types of assistance from significant others in one's life including friends, family, colleagues, clergy, and health-care professionals

Data from: Prochaska, Norcross, & DiClemente (1994). *Changing for Good: A Revolutionary Six-Stage Program for Overcoming Bad Habits and Moving Your Life Positively Forward.* New York, NY: Avon Books.

relapse, and re-initiation of change. It is important not to interpret relapse as a failure but to acknowledge it as a natural element in the long-term process of health behavior change. Following a relapse, an individual typically will re-enter the change process at the contemplation, preparation, or action stages. The National Cancer Institute (NCI, 2005) identified this model's circular nature as a strength, whereby an individual can enter the cycle at any point and repeated attempts to change behavior or "re-cycle" are possible.

The broad change processes listed in Table 3-1 should not be confused with techniques. There are potentially hundreds of techniques associated with the processes of change. Research indicates that:

- many methods for implementing change processes can be effective

- individuals who believe they have the autonomy and power to change their lives are the most likely to initiate and maintain a change, and
- tailoring the techniques employed to the individual's preferences and needs enhances the probability of successful long-term behavior change (Prochaska, Norcross, & DiClemente, 1994).

There has been limited use of this model within the occupational therapy literature. One exception is the work of Stoffel and Moyer (2004), in which they identify motivational strategies, based on the transtheoretical model, as one of four effective methods occupational therapy practitioners can use to assist persons with substance use disorders to eliminate use of risky substances. Hammond, Young, and Kidao (2004) conducted a study on the effectiveness of a pragmatic occupational therapy program that was developed over a period of years for clients with rheumatoid arthritis. From this experience, the researchers came to realize that the program may have been more effective had it been theory-based and matched to the client's readiness for change, an important construct of the transtheoretical model.

PRECEDE-PROCEED Planning Model

The PRECEDE model, developed by Green, Kreuter, Deeds, and Partridge (1980) with financial support from the National Institutes of Health, is a planning model for health education based on principles, both theoretical and applied, from epidemiology, education, administration, and the social/behavioral sciences. In the PRECEDE-PROCEED framework, the acronym PRECEDE stands for predisposing, reinforcing, and enabling causes in educational diagnosis and evaluation (Green, Kreuter, Deeds, & Partridge, 1980). A set of steps called PROCEED (policy, regulatory, and organizational constructs in educational and environmental development) were later superimposed on the original model (Green & Kreuter, 1991). The framework has since been revised in order to accommodate the evolving nature and broadening ecological perspective of health promotion. The complete PRECEDE-PROCEED framework is illustrated in Figure 3.4.

The PRECEDE portion of the framework is readily applicable across a variety of settings, providing structure and organization to health education program planning and evaluation. Application of this approach occurs in several phases and involves the diagnoses of variables in four domains: social, epidemiological, educational and ecological, and administrative and policy (Green & Kreuter,

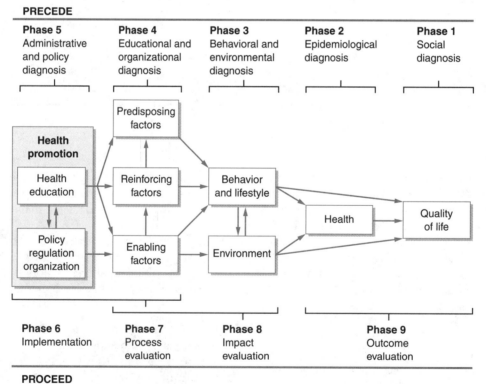

Fig. 3·4 The PRECEDE-PROCEED Model. *(From Health Promotion Planning: An Educational and Ecological Approach [4th ed., p. 17], by Lawrence W. Green and Marshall W. Kreuter. Copyright © 2005 by McGraw Hill.)*

2005). The approach is unique in that it begins with the desired final outcome and works backward, taking into account factors that must precede a certain result.

Phase 1, *social assessment,* is an analysis of the social problems that exist in a community, which is a necessary step in assessing the quality of life of the target population. The purpose of this phase is to ascertain the relationship between a given health problem and the social problems and priorities of the population. Phase 2, *epidemiological, behavioral, and environmental assessment,* is an evaluation of the health problems associated with the community's quality of life. It includes a review of vital indicators such as morbidity, mortality, fertility, and disability rates along with behavioral and environmental indicators (Green & Kreuter, 2005).

In phase 3, *educational and ecological assessment,* resources and barriers are differentiated by three categories of influence: predisposing, enabling, and reinforcing factors. *Predisposing factors* provide the motivation or rationale for the behavior(s); for example, knowledge, attitudes, values, and beliefs. *Reinforcing factors* supply the reward, incentive, or punishment of a behavior that contributes to its maintenance or extinction. *Enabling factors* include personal skills and assets as well as community resources and barriers. Predisposing and enabling factors are antecedent to the health behavior and allow for the behavior to occur. Each group of factors is analyzed in terms of importance and changeability, and priorities are established for the intervention. Based on the nature of the targets for intervention, educational methodologies are selected (Green & Kreuter, 2005).

The final phase (phase 4) of the process is *administrative and policy assessment, and intervention alignment,* which includes: reviewing budgetary implications; identifying and allocating other types of resources, including time; defining the nature of any cooperative agreements; and assessing the availability of and gaps in policies and regulations. Gaps in and barriers to the implementation of the health promotion program need to be addressed at this stage, prior to program implementation. This step and the steps proceeding are essential for the development of an ethical, evidence-based program. Neglect of this important step can doom an otherwise viable intervention to failure. After this phase is completed, the PROCEED portion of the model is activated.

The PROCEED phase follows the four phases of the PRECEDE portion and includes the implementation of the program (i.e., phase 5) as well as three phases of evaluation. The goal of the PROCEED portion is to monitor the program processes in order to make adjustments as needed to ensure quality as program implementation continues. The three types of evaluation include *process* (phase 6), *impact* (phase 7), and *outcome* (phase 8) evaluations (Green & Kreuter, 2005).

The PRECEDE-PROCEED planning framework has been used to develop a wide variety of community and population health programs, with over 950 applications of the use of the framework being published (Green & Kreuter, 2005). While this planning framework has not been used widely in occupational therapy, it has been used by an interdisciplinary team with members from a variety of health professions and disciplines, among them occupational therapy, to conduct a systematic literature review. The team used the PRECEDE portion of the PRECEDE-PROCEED framework to systematically investigate the literature and report risk and protective factors related to driving safety among older adults (Classen, Awadzi, & Mkanta, 2008).

Diffusion of Innovations Model

The diffusion of innovations model developed by Rogers (2003) is a very useful adjunct to specific occupation or health theories (Reitz, Scaffa, Campbell, & Rhynders, 2010). Whereas specific health or occupation theories inform the development of an effective structure and content for the program, the diffusion of innovations model provides a guide on how to most efficiently communicate the availability of the intervention and the adoption of new behaviors. The factors that influence the speed of behavior adoption appear in Table 3-2, together with questions to address in order to maximize success in communicating the message. In the AOTA's backpack awareness program, developed by Jacobs (Yamkovenko, 2010), the answer to each of these questions would be yes. The innovation (e.g., limiting weight and using both padded shoulder straps), once tried, is more comfortable and will impact the

Table 3-2	Key Attributes Affecting the Speed and Extent of an Innovations Diffusion
Attribute	**Key Question**
Relative advantage	Is the innovation better than what it will replace?
Compatibility	Does the innovation fit with the intended audience?
Complexity	Is the innovation easy to use?
Trialability	Can the innovation be tried before making a decision to adopt?
Observability	Are the results of the innovation observable and easily measurable?

From *Theory at a glance* (2nd ed., p. 28), by National Cancer Institute, 2005, Bethesda, MD: National Institutes of Health.

daily lives of the intended participants; the innovation is easy to use and easy to try, and it is easy to see other influential people adopting the innovation.

According to Rogers, people vary in their readiness to adopt new behaviors (NCI, 2005; Rogers, 2003). Rogers found that people, following a normal distribution, would fall in one of five categories of adopters: innovators, early adopters, early majority adopters, late majority adopters, or laggards. Most people fall into the early majority adopters or late majority adopters categories. Fewer individuals are classified as early adopters or laggards. The rarest categories are those on either end of the distribution, the innovators (i.e., those first to adopt) and the laggards (i.e., the last to adopt). Early adopters are often seen as trendsetters; once a trend becomes popular, people who often lag in trying new things may eventually adopt the innovation.

Whereas there is tremendous potential to use this theory to disseminate occupational therapy health promotion strategies (Reitz et al., 2010), there is little to no evidence in the literature. However, the theory has been used to develop recommendations for increasing the compatibility of reported research evidence for use by occupational therapists (Sudsawad, 2005) and to explore adherence to intervention guidelines for low back pain by physical therapists (Harting, Rutten, Rutten, & Kremers, 2009).

Selected Occupational Therapy Models

Descriptions of models found in the occupational therapy professional literature and application in community-based practice follows. This description is not meant to be an exhaustive account of relevant approaches but rather a sampling to illustrate how models within occupational therapy relate to community-based practice. Of the many occupational therapy models available to assist in community health program planning, three have been selected for analysis in this chapter. However, various other models also are potentially useful in community-based practice. It is hoped that readers will explore other models and conduct an independent analysis to determine the most appropriate model to address the health needs of their unique community. The three models discussed in this chapter were selected due to their applicability for use either individually or in conjunction with models and approaches from other disciplines presented earlier in this chapter. The models described include:

- model of human occupation (MOHO),
- ecology of human performance (EHP), and
- person-environment-occupation model (PEO).

Model of Human Occupation

The model of human occupation (MOHO) was developed by Kielhofner and Burke (1980) to provide a link between practice and Reilly's theory of occupational behavior (Scott, Miller, & Walker, 2004). In 1980, a four-part article describing the MOHO was published in the *American Journal of Occupational Therapy*. Kielhofner either authored or coauthored each of these articles and has been the catalyst for the model's further development. However, "scholars and clinicians worldwide now contribute to its development and application" (Kielhofner, 1997, p. 187). Originally the human system was portrayed as interacting with the environment via a cycle of input, throughput, output, and feedback (Kielhofner & Burke, 1980). The traditional application of this model views the individual as receiving input from the environment as well as being the site of the throughput process. *Throughput* is a process composed of three subsystems:

1. Volitional,
2. Habituation, and
3. Performance capacity.

This process was originally portrayed as being hierarchical in nature, where the higher subsystems "command lower ones and...lower ones constrain the higher" (Kielhofner, 1985, p. 504). Later the model was described as a heterarchy, where each of the subsystems works in unison to perform occupational behaviors "according to the demands of the situations in which they are performing, not according to a preordained or fixed structure" (Kielhofner, 1995, p. 34). A heterarchical process seems better suited to community-based practice.

The output of the system is occupational behavior (Kielhofner, 1997), or purposeful interaction with the environment. This interaction, which is termed *feedback,* produces additional information to the individual regarding his or her performance. A thorough understanding of the role of the three heterarchical subsystems of throughput is necessary before applying or adapting this model to community-based practice. These subsystems, when working in unison, serve to organize the individual's response to the environment.

Through the years, the description of the components of the environment has been modified to reflect both the continued development of the model and the influence of other theorists. In the current language of the MOHO (Kielhofner, 1997), the environment consists of physical aspects (i.e., objects and spaces) as well as social aspects (i.e., occupational forms and groups). The environment both "affords" and "presses" the individual (Kielhofner, 1997), meaning it simultaneously facilitates and constrains the human system.

The throughput subsystems play important roles. The *performance capacity subsystem* involves the "interplay of the musculoskeletal, neurological, perceptual, and cognitive phenomena" (Kielhofner, 1997, p. 194), which allows the individual to meet the demands of both the environment and the remaining two subsystems. The primary function of this subsystem is to produce "the actions required to accomplish occupation" (Kielhofner, 1997, p. 194).

The *habituation subsystem* functions to maintain the organism by providing "everyday patterns of behaviors without ongoing conscious choices" (Kielhofner & Burke, 1985, p. 24). This maintenance is done through the development and refinement of habits and internalized roles (e.g., worker, student, mother, and spouse). Habits and internalized roles provide humans with a sense of order and predictability. In addition, they allow humans to be energy and time efficient.

The *volitional subsystem,* the third component of the throughput process, motivates the individual to "enact" a behavior. This subsystem, which originally was viewed as the subsystem that governed the other subsystems, is composed of three "structural components: personal causation, values, and interests" (Kielhofner & Burke, 1980, p. 576). Kielhofner and Burke (1985) defined "personal causation" as "a collection of beliefs and expectations which a person holds about his or her effectiveness in the environment" (p. 15). These beliefs include "belief in skill, belief in efficacy of skill, expectancy of success/failure, and internal/external control" (Kielhofner & Burke, 1985, p. 16). In addition, Kielhofner and Burke view values as "images of what is good, right and/or important" (p. 17), whereas interests concern the self-knowledge of activities or occupations that provide pleasure to the individual. This self-knowledge includes the ability to recognize patterns of enjoyed activities and an understanding of which activities evoke more potency of interest than others.

Two related constructs that explain how the human system changes within, and in response to, the environment over time also are important to consider when applying this model in the community. These constructs are the trajectory of change and adaptive and maladaptive cycles. The *trajectory of change* is the self-transformation of the system over time. An *adaptive cycle* supports the individual in satisfying internal demands as well as the demands of the environment (Kielhofner & Burke, 1980). Kielhofner described a *maladaptive cycle* as failing "to meet one or both" of the internal or environmental demands just mentioned (1980, p. 737). It is possible, however, to reverse a maladaptive cycle and encourage the development of an adaptive cycle.

The MOHO has been applied to intervention with individuals with a variety of disorders. This model also has potential use for well individuals in an occupational therapy community-based program. In addition, it is believed that it can be used in community-based health promotion programming where the recipient of services is the community rather than an individual or family. Figure 3.5 illustrates a simplified adaptation of the MOHO for use as a community empowerment model (Reitz, 1990).

The following fictional example illustrates the possible use of the adapted MOHO, depicted in Figure 3.5, to community-based practice. In this scenario, an occupational therapy practitioner employed by a school system has been asked by the Parent-Teacher-Student Association (PTSA) to assist with the development of a violence (i.e., perpetrators from outside the school community) and bullying (i.e., perpetrators from within the school community) prevention program in the county's only high school. In this example, the community's volitional subsystem has already motivated the community to make the decision to seek assistance. Thus, the community is already exhibiting "community causation" by identifying the problem and believing it has the power to take steps to accomplish the goal of improving school and student safety.

The actual steps the community or PTSA decides to take will be greatly influenced by the community's cultural norms (e.g., values and interests) as well as the habits and roles of its members. The practitioner can assist the community in identifying values and interests that will influence decision making relative to changes in the structure of the school and community habits. The community may need to collectively determine the relative priorities of potentially conflicting values. For example, the community will need to weigh the value it places on personal freedom against the value it places on student safety and comfort when deciding whether to require students to wear identification or to install security cameras.

In addressing the habituation level of this model, the practitioner identifies potentially dangerous habits (e.g., propping open exterior doors on balmy days) and roles (e.g., identification of disengaged students with no apparent role in the school community). In addition, the community's skills and skill constituents would be identified. This analysis would then be used to facilitate the community's current skills to maximize habit and role performance as well as identify necessary skills requiring development in order to achieve the goals of the program.

Ecology of Human Performance

The ecology of human performance (EHP) model was developed by the faculty at the University of Kansas to address their concerns regarding the "lack of consideration for the complexities of context" in both evaluation and intervention (Dunn, Brown, & McGuigan, 1994, p. 595). Figure 3.6 depicts the major components of this conceptual model of practice—the person and his or her skills, abilities, tasks, and performance range.

A human's skills and abilities, in combination with a perception of his or her context, support the selection and performance of specific tasks, defined in the model as "objective sets of behaviors necessary to accomplish a goal" (Dunn et al., 1994, p. 599).

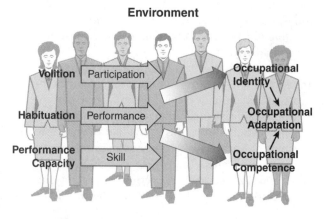

Fig. 3•5 The Model of Human Occupation as a Framework for Use in Community-Based Practice. *(Adapted from* Model of Human Occupation: Theory and Application *(3rd ed., p. 121), by G. Kielhofner, 2002, Baltimore, MD: Lippincott Williams & Wilkins. Copyright 2002 by Lippincott Williams & Wilkins.)*

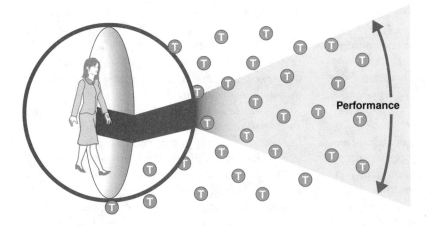

Fig. 3•6 The Major Components of the EHP. *(From Dunn, W., Brown, C., and McGuigan, A. [1994]. The ecology of human performance: A framework for considering the effect of context.* American Journal of Occupational Therapy, 48, *p. 600.)*

Each individual's performance range depends on both past experience and current resources. Limited resources, possibly due to a temporary state of affairs or a more permanent situation, may impact a human's performance range even if he or she has a variety of skills and abilities. For example, a competent parent of a toddler may find his or her parenting repertoire (i.e., performance range) significantly hindered by a change of context brought about by the cramped confines of an airplane seat. If the same competent parent were sentenced to serve a 10-year prison term, the change in resources for parenting would obviously be of longer duration. However, in this scenario, even though the parent had a variety of skills and abilities, he or she would not have access to resources to support a broad performance range.

The EHP model provides "five alternatives for therapeutic intervention" (Dunn et al., 1994, p. 603). The first of these five levels is identified as the *establish/restore* level. This level includes interventions that seek to restore function via the development and improvement of skills and abilities. Another level of intervention is that of *adapt*. At this level, the therapist adapts "the contextual features and task demands to support performance in context" (p. 604). Yet another intervention level is the *alter* level where the therapist changes the actual context rather than adapting the current one. An example of such an intervention would be moving an individual who uses a walker to a street-level apartment so the individual would not be forced to climb stairs. The *prevent* level of intervention seeks to "prevent the occurrence or evolution of maladaptive performance in context" (p. 604). The last level of intervention in the EHP is the *create* level. This level has great potential for community-based practice since its goal is to create "circumstances that promote more adaptable or complex performance in context" (p. 604). Policy initiatives, program development, community development, and community empowerment are all activities at this level of intervention.

When using the EHP model, regardless of the level of intervention chosen, intervention should always be guided by the culture of the individual or the community. Tasks that an individual or community selects to pursue are determined by its skills and abilities, as well as personal choices, priorities, and values that are often guided by both life experience and cultural values. For example, a child's choice to play soccer may at first be influenced by his or her family's cultural background, which highly values the sport. Continued interest may be influenced by natural aptitude and early skill development, coupled with pride for a grandfather's past achievements as a semiprofessional player overseas.

These five levels of intervention can be readily adapted to facilitate the development of community-based health promotion activities. An intervention at the *prevent* level may, for example, include the development of an interdisciplinary program to educate seniors with diabetes in healthy eating habits and cooking techniques to avoid complications of an uncontrolled disease process (Lutz, 1998). Forming a daily walking group at a senior center to promote exercise, leisure skills, and a healthy lifestyle is an example of a *create* level intervention. As stated earlier, the fifth level, *create*, appears to be particularly well suited for community-based program development since it "does not assume a disability is present" and it focuses on "providing enriched contextual and task experiences that will enhance performance" (Dunn et al., 1994, p. 606).

An example of a community that may request assistance from an occupational therapy practitioner might be a homeless shelter (i.e., a community of individuals). In this example, the community has acted based on concern for the healthy development of its children. The community has already taken the first two necessary steps by recognizing the problem and inviting the occupational therapy practitioner into the community. The practitioner can use the EHP model to define the scope of the problem from an occupation-based perspective and then work with the community to determine priorities and set goals. Interventions are then selected from the model's five intervention levels. The occupational therapy practitioner and the community then jointly implement the agreed-upon activities and evaluate the outcomes. The community then takes responsibility for continued monitoring, consulting the occupational therapy practitioner for assistance in program evaluation or expansion as desired.

Person-Environment-Occupation Model

The person-environment-occupation (PEO) model was initially conceptualized by Law and colleagues (1996) to operationalize client-centered practice across settings and populations. The model expands the awareness of the relationship between a person and his/her environment present in ecological models in order to recognize the transactive relationship among the three constructs—person, environment, and occupation (Strong & Rebeiro-Gruhl, 2011). In addition to explicitly identifying the person as the focus of intervention, this model also identifies the environment as a modality. Four aspects of the environment that have an influence on occupational performance are detailed in the model. These are external to the person and include cultural, institutional (including political and economic), social, and physical aspects (Law, Cooper, Strong, Stewart,

Rigby, & Letts, 1996). In the PEO model, activities, tasks, and occupations are differentiated by describing them as nested within one another, with activities being the smallest unit and occupations being the largest unit. An occupation is a group of tasks in which an individual engages across a period of time or his or her life span. Occupational performance is understood as a "dynamic, ever-changing experience of a person engaged in purposeful activities, tasks, and occupations within an environment" (Stewart, Letts, Law, Cooper, Strong, & Rigby, 2003, p. 229). The major assumption of the PEO model is that the greater the "fit" among the three key areas—person, environment, and occupation, in terms of matching the strengths and capacities of the person and the supports and demands of the environment and occupation—the better the person's or community's occupational performance.

One of the strengths of this model is its applicability across settings. For example, the proponents of this model assume that an intervention can occur at the person, program, or system level. This lends it to use in community practice, where a consultative approach or broader than person level intervention is the norm. Another strength is its relative simplicity and lack of jargon, lending to ease of use in interdisciplinary settings, such as community agencies. Because the roots of this model lie in an ecological framework, others in community health practice may be familiar with its basic tenets, such as the influence of the environment on engagement and participation. Those who work in the community are faced very directly with the effects of the environment in people's everyday lives, so this model is easily understood and applied in such settings.

Examples of Research Using the PEO Model

The PEO model was used to structure community-based research in which occupational engagement and time use relative to recovery were examined from the perspective of people with serious mental illness living in the community. A specific research question addressed participants' views of environmental supports and barriers to recovery, using the PEO to guide questions on a semi-structured interview about the physical, social, cultural, and institutional aspects of the environment (Merryman,

Magaha, Mullins, Pollock, & Waters, 2003). Findings from this population revealed that the social aspects of the environment were the most critical to support recovery. These primarily included the support of family and friends. The aspects of the environment that most served as a barrier to recovery were predictable: social and financial (Merryman & Sheffield, 2011).

The PEO model was used to structure other community-based research using participatory action methods (McIntyre, 2008) in designing sessions for a Photovoice project with fifth and sixth graders in a Youth Empowerment Program (Wilson, Dashio, Martin, Wallerstein, Wang, & Minkler, 2007). The grant used positive youth development (Damon, 2004) as the overarching framework, and employed the PEO in the design and implementation of intervention sessions. Sessions were designed by occupational therapy graduate students using the model's principles in decisions regarding the amount of structure, support, enrichment, and adaptation of approach, task, and environment. An example of a session in which participants selected photographs and generated quotes reflecting their responses to directions to take nine photos each of their daily life, their environment, and things they liked to do or wanted to share about what they liked, is presented in Table 3-3.

Although the positive youth development model was the primary driver of the program, the PEO model encouraged researchers to use specific strategies to enhance occupational performance and opportunities for skill development and competence to aid efficacy.

Conclusion

Community-based practice often involves a team approach wherein the membership of the team does not conform to the familiar, traditional, hospital-based interdisciplinary team. Public health experts, health educators, community developers and organizers, and politicians are all examples of potential community-based team members who may work together on a community initiative. Many of these professionals share a common language that is represented in the models from other disciplines presented in this chapter. It is hoped that exposure to these models will facilitate interdisciplinary work in the community by practitioners. For occupational therapy to reach its potential in the community, its practitioners must possess the knowledge and skill to join together with a varied group of stakeholders, gatekeepers, community members, and other health professionals to creatively and cost effectively

Table 3-3 Photovoice Storyboard Captions Using PEO to Reflect Themes of Self-Efficacy		
P = Daily Life	**E = My Environment**	**O = Things I Like to do**
"This one I chose because my CDs are my most important possession because if you're bored and your friends are punished, you can just sit back, get some popcorn, and watch a movie."	"The playground. It's fun to be playing on the playground because you can let out all your feelings there."	"This is my brother and he is posing with earphones in his ears. He's in my room and I took this picture he encourages me to do things like sing and don't let nobody tell me I can't do anything."
"I took this picture because every day I come home I have to do homework and do all my chores. I think this picture is very important because without homework you will have very low grades. This picture makes me feel very successful."	"I took a picture of the grass because me, my neighbor, and my mom helped it grow by planting seeds and watering it everyday. When I first moved in it was dirt. The picture made me feel good because I helped it grow."	"My best friend, (participant), is in the picture. She is smiling. I took the picture because she is one of my best friends. I think that it is nice of me to encourage her to be a wonderful student. The picture makes me feel great to have a friend to take care of me."

Data from Day, Y., DeHart, R., Grant, A., Kwebetchou, N., Lowther, S., & Weisburger, M. (2010) under the direction of Dr. Beth Merryman, *Photovoice: Engagement through action research with fifth graders in a Youth Empowerment Program.* Unpublished graduate project.

facilitate the achievement of the health goals of diverse communities.

As in all areas of occupational therapy practice, outcomes research is needed to evaluate the efficacy of interventions. This is particularly true in community-based practice. The profession can draw on the expertise of individuals conducting research on community empowerment initiatives in the fields of public health and health education. One such resource is a description of a "research model developed to study community organization influence on local public health care policy" (Brown, 1984, p. 205). Both the research methodology and the study's results are helpful to the potential researcher in this area. For example, one of the study's findings was that the group that used "political leverage" was more successful than those that used factual, educational testimony at public hearings. Another finding was that lobbying and the presence of "other groups and leaders" help encourage support within the community (Brown, 1984, p. 229). Political activism and the generation of research evidence supporting the efficacy of occupational therapy interventions in community-based practice will increase the likelihood that occupational therapy contributions will be valued in the public health arena.

Learning Activities

1. Review recent issues of *OT Practice* for articles about community-based programs. Read the articles and determine whether the programs were theory-based. If a theory was not mentioned, reflect on the description of the program and identify possible theories and constructs from those theories that could be used to support the implementation or evaluation of the program.

2. Concerned about a recent fatal bike crash, an occupational therapy student joins with a health education student to design a program to increase bicycle helmet usage on their college campus. Identify and describe how they could use constructs from one or more theories in the program development and evaluation plan.

3. After graduation you have contracted to work with a health educator to develop a falls prevention program on a cruise ship that caters to older adults. Identify and describe how you

would use constructs from one or more theories in your program. Draw a sketch of the theory and the corresponding constructs.

REFERENCES

American Occupational Therapy Association. (2007). AOTA's *Centennial Vision* and Executive Summary. *American Journal of Occupational Therapy, 61*(6), 613–614.

American Occupational Therapy Association. (2008). Occupational therapy practice framework: Domain and processes. *American Journal of Occupational Therapy, 62*(6), 625–683.

Bandura, A. (2006). Toward a psychology of human agency. *Perspectives on Psychological Science, 1*(2), 164–180.

Bandura, A. (2004). Health promotion by social cognitive means. *Health Education & Behavior, 31*(2), 143–164.

Bandura, A. (1977). *Social learning theory.* Upper Saddle River, NJ: Prentice Hall.

Becker, M., & Janz, N. (1985). The health belief model applied to understanding diabetes regimen compliance. *Diabetes Educator, 11*, 41–47.

Bereolos, N. M. (2007). *The role of acculturation in the health belief model for Mexican-Americans with type II diabetes* [Abstract]. Denton, TX. Retrieved from UNT Digital Library http://digital.library.unt.edu/ark:/67531/metadc4001/

Brown, E. R. (1984). Community organization influences on local public health policy: A general research comparative study. *Health Education Quarterly, 10*(3/4), 205–233.

Champion, V. (1985). Use of the health belief model in determining frequency of breast self-examination. *Research in Nursing and Health, 8*, 373–379.

Classen, S., Awadzi, K. D., & Mkanta, W. W. (2008). Person-vehicle-environment interactions predicting crash-related injury among older drivers. *American Journal of Occupational Therapy, 62*, 580–587.

Damon, W. (2004). What is positive youth development? *The ANNALS of the American Academy of Political and Social Science, 591*, 13–24.

Day, Y., DeHart, R., Grant, A., Kwebetchou, N., Lowther, S., & Weisburger, M. (2010). *Photovoice: Engagement through action research with fifth graders in a Youth Empowerment Program.* Unpublished manuscript, Department of Occupational Therapy & Occupational Science, Towson University, Towson, MD.

Deshpande, S., Basil, M. D., & Basil, D. Z. (2009). Factors influencing healthy eating habits among college students: An application of the health belief model. *Health Marketing Quarterly, 26*(2), 145–164.

Dunn, W., Brown, C., & McGuigan, A. (1994). The ecology of human performance: A framework for considering the effect of context. *American Journal of Occupational Therapy, 48*, 595–607.

Goodman, R. M., Speers, M. A., McLerooy, K., Fawcett, S., Kegler, M., Parker, E., ... Wallerstein, N. (1999). Identifying and defining dimensions of community capacity to provide a basis for measurement. *Health Education Quarterly, 25*(3), 258–278.

Green, L. W., & Kreuter, M. W. (1991). *Health promotion planning: An educational and environmental approach* (2nd ed.). Mountainview, CA: Mayfield.

Green, L. W., & Kreuter, M. W. (2005). *Health promotion planning: An educational and ecological approach* (4th ed.). New York: McGraw Hill.

Green, L. W., Kreuter, M. W., Deeds, S. G., & Partridge, K. B. (1980). *Health education planning: A diagnostic approach.* Palo Alto, CA: Mayfield.

Hammond, A., Young, A., & Kidao, R. (2004). A randomized controlled trial of occupational therapy for people with early rheumatoid arthritis. *Annals of the Rheumatic Diseases, 63,* 23–30.

Harting, J., Rutten, G. M., Rutten, S. T., & Kremers, S. P. (2009). A qualitative application of the diffusion of innovations theory to examine determinants of guideline adherence among physical therapists. *Physical Therapy, 89*(3), 221–232.

Herold, E. (1983). The health belief model: Can it help us understand contraceptive use among adolescents? *Journal of School Health, 53,* 19–21.

Hester, N., & Macrina, D. (1985). The health belief model and the contraceptive behavior of college women: Implications for health education. *Journal of American College Health, 33,* 245–252.

Israel, B. A., Checkoway, B., Schulz, A., & Zimmerman, M. (1994). Health education and community empowerment: Conceptualizing and measuring perceptions of individual, organizational, and community control. *Health Education Quarterly, 21*(2), 149–170.

Johnson, C. S., McLeod, W., Kennedy, L., & McLeod, K. (2008). Osteoporosis health beliefs among younger and older men and women. *Health Education and Behavior, 35*(5), 721–733.

Juniper, K. C., Oman, R. F., Hamm, R. M., & Kerby, D. S. (2004). The relationships among construct in the health belief model and the transtheoretical model among African-American college women for physical activity. *America Journal of Health Promotion, 18*(5), 354–357.

Kelly, G., Mamon, J., & Scott, J. (1987). Utility of the health belief model in examining medication compliance among psychiatric outpatients. *Social Science Medicine, 25,* 1205–1211.

Kielhofner, G. (1980). A model of human occupation, part 3: Benign and vicious cycles. *American Journal of Occupational Therapy, 34*(11*),* 731–737.

Kielhofner, G. (Ed.). (1985). *A model of human occupation: Theory and application.* Baltimore: Williams and Wilkins.

Kielhofner, G. (Ed.). (1995). *A model of human occupation: Theory and application* (2nd ed.). Baltimore: Williams and Wilkins.

Kielhofner, G. (1997). *Conceptual foundations of occupational therapy* (2nd ed.). Philadelphia: F.A. Davis.

Kielhofner, G. (2002). *A model of human occupation: Theory and application* (3rd ed.). Baltimore: Lippincott Williams & Wilkins.

Kielhofner, G. (2004). *Conceptual foundations of occupational therapy* (3rd ed.). Philadelphia: F.A. Davis.

Kielhofner, G. (2009). *Conceptual foundations of occupational therapy* (4th ed.). Philadelphia: F.A. Davis.

Kielhofner, G., & Burke, J. (1980). A model of human occupation, part 1: Conceptual framework and content. *American Journal of Occupational Therapy, 34,* 572–581.

Kielhofner, G., & Burke, J. (1985). Components and determinants of human occupation. In G. Kielhofner (Ed.), *A model of human occupation: Theory and application* (pp. 12–36). Baltimore: Williams and Wilkins.

Kretzmann, J. P., & McKnight, J. L. (2005). *Discovering community power: A guide to mobilizing local assets and your organization's capacity.* Evanston, IL: Asset- Based Community Development Institute in cooperation with the Kellogg Foundation.

Law, M., Cooper, B., Strong, S., Stewart, D., Rigby, P., & Letts, L. (1996). The Person-Environment-Occupation model: A transitive approach to occupational performance. *Canadian Journal of Occupational Therapy, 63*(1), 9–23.

Lutz, C. (1998). Interdisciplinary prevention in rural communities: Outcome evaluation of the *Strides for Life* walking program for older adults. Gerontology graduate research project. Unpublished master's project, Towson University, Towson, MD.

Mathie, A., & Cunningham, G. (2003). From clients to citizens: Asset-based community development as a strategy for community-driven development. *Development in Practice, 13*(5), 474–486.

McIntyre, A. (2008). *Participatory action research.* Thousand Oaks, CA: Sage.

McKenzie, J. F., Neiger, B. L., & Thackeray, R. (2009). *Planning, implementing, and evaluating health promotion programs: A primer* (5th ed.). San Francisco, CA: Pearson Benjamin Cummings.

Merryman, M. B., Magaha, C., Mullins, R., Pollock, F., & Waters, E. (2003). *Environmental questionnaire.* Unpublished manuscript, Department of Occupational Therapy & Occupational Science, Towson University, Towson, MD.

Merryman, M. B., & Sheffield, C. (2011). *Occupational engagement and recovery experiences of community living adults with serious mental illness.* Unpublished manuscript.

Miller, R. J., & Schwartz, K. (2004). What is theory, and why does it matter? In K. F. Walker & F. M. Ludwig (Eds.), *Perspectives on theory for the practice of occupational therapy* (3rd ed., pp. 1–26). Austin, TX: PRO-ED.

Minkler, M., & Wallerstein, N. (2005). Improving health through community organization and community building: A health education perspective. In M. Minkler, *Community organizing and community building for health* (2nd ed., pp. 26–50). Rutgers, NJ: The State University of New Jersey.

National Cancer Institute. (2005). *Theory at a glance* (2nd ed.). Bethesda, MD: National Institutes of Health. Retrieved from http://cancer.gov/theory.pdf

Nelson, D. L. (1997). Why the profession of occupational therapy will flourish in the 21st century. *American Journal of Occupational Therapy, 51*(1), 11–24.

Parcel, G. S. (1984). Theoretical models for application in school health education research. Special combined issue of *Journal of School Health, 54,* and *Health Education, 15,* 39–49.

Parcel, G. S., & Baranowski, T. (1981). Social learning theory and health education. *Health Education, 12,* 14–18.

Payton, O. D. (1988). *Research: The validation of clinical practice* (2nd ed.). Philadelphia: F.A. Davis.

Perlman, J. (1978). Grassroots participation from neighborhood to nation. In S. Langton (Ed.), *Citizen participation in America* (pp. 65–79). Lexington, MA: Lexington Books.

Prochaska, J. O., & DiClemente, C. C. (1983). Stages and processes of self-change of smoking: Toward an integrative model of change. *Journal of Counseling and Clinical Psychology, 51*(3), 390–395.

Prochaska, J. O., & DiClemente, C. C. (1992). Stages of change in the modification of behavior problems. In M. Hersen, R. M. Eisler, & P. M. Miller (Eds.), *Progress in behavior modification* (pp. 184–214). Sycamore, IL: Sycamore Press.

Prochaska, J. O., Norcross, J. C., & DiClemente, C. C. (1994). *Changing for good: A revolutionary six-stage program for overcoming bad habits and moving your life positively forward.* New York: Avon Books.

Reitz, S. M. (1990, Fall). Community development model: An application of the model of human occupation. Unpublished paper for Health 688—p, Community Health Issues for Minority Populations, University of Maryland, College Park.

Reitz, S. M., Scaffa, M. E., Campbell, R. M., & Rhynders, P. A. (2010). Health behavior frameworks for health promotion practice. In M. E. Scaffa, S. M. Reitz, & M. A. Pizzi (Eds.), *Occupational therapy in the promotion of health and wellness* (pp. 46–69). Philadelphia: F.A. Davis.

Rogers, E. M. (2003). *Diffusion of innovations* (5th ed.). New York: Free Press.

Rosenstock, I. (1974). Historical origins of the health belief model. In M. Becker (Ed.), *The health belief model and personal behavior.* Thorofare, NJ: SLACK.

Rosenstock, I. M., Strecher, V. J., & Becker, M. H. (1994). The health belief model and HIV risk behavior change. In R. J. DiClemente and J. L. Peterson (Eds.), *Preventing AIDS: Theories and methods for behavioral interventions* (pp. 5–24). New York: Plenum.

Ross, M. G. (1967). *Community organization: Theory, principles and practice.* New York, NY: Harper and Row.

Rubin, H. J., & Rubin, I. S. (2005). The practice of community organizing. In M. Weil (Ed.), *The handbook of community practice* (pp. 189–203). Thousand Oaks, CA: Sage.

Scott, P., Miller, R. J., & Walker, K. F. (2004). Gary Kielhofner. In K. F. Walker & F. M. Ludwig (Eds.), *Perspectives on theory for the practice of occupational therapy* (3rd ed., pp. 267–325). Austin, TX: PRO-ED.

Stav, W. (2010). CarFit: An evaluation of behavior change and impact. *British Journal of Occupational Therapy, 73*(12), 589–597.

Stewart, D., Letts, L., Law, M., Cooper, B., Strong, S., & Rigby, P. J. (2003). The Person-Environment-Occupation model. In E. B. Crepeau, E. S. Cohn, & B. A. Boyt Schell (Eds.), *Willard & Spackman's occupational therapy* (10th ed., pp. 227–233). Philadelphia: Lippincott Williams and Wilkins.

Stoffel, V. C., & Moyers, P. A. (2004). An evidence-based and occupational perspective of interventions for persons with substance-use disorders. *American Journal of Occupational Therapy, 58,* 570–586.

Strauss, A., & Corbin, J. (1990). *Basics of qualitative research: Grounded theory procedures and techniques.* London, U.K.: Sage.

Strong, S., & Rebeiro-Gruhl, K. (2011). Person-environment-occupation model. In C. Brown & V. Stoffel (Eds.), *Occupational therapy in mental health: A vision for participation* (pp. 31–44). Philadelphia: F.A. Davis.

Sudsawad, P. (2005). Concepts in Clinical Scholarship—A conceptual framework to increase usability of outcome research for evidence-based practice. *American Journal of Occupational Therapy, 59,* 351–355.

United Nations. (1955). *Social progress through community development.* New York: United Nations.

Wang, J. H., Liang, W., Schwartz, M. D., Lee, M. M., Kreling, B., & Mandelblatt, J. S. (2008). Development and evaluation of a culturally tailored educational video: Changing breast cancer-related behaviors in Chinese women. *Health Education & Behavior, 35*(6), 806–820.

Wilson, N., Dasho, S., Martin, A., Wallerstein, N., Wang, C., & Minkler, M. (2007). Engaging youth adolescents in social action through Photovoice: The youth empowerment strategies (YES!) project. *Journal of Early Adolescence, 27,* 241–261.

Yamkovenko, S. (2010). Backpack awareness day for people of all ages. Retrieved from http://aota.org/News/Consumer/Backpack-Day.aspx

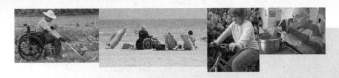

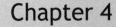

Chapter 4

Legislation and Policy Issues

M. Beth Merryman, PhD, OTR/L, FAOTA, and Nancy Van Slyke, EdD, OTR/L, FAOTA

Legislation that affects the lives of people with disabilities should be of more than just a passing interest to those who are involved with the disability community. Not only does legislation articulate who is to receive the services, but it also articulates what and how services are to be delivered.

—Fifield & Fifield, 1995, p. 38

Learning Objectives

This chapter is designed to enable the reader to:

- Discuss the need for a basic understanding of federal legislation pertinent to community-based practice.
- Compare and contrast legislation supporting reimbursement for services with those providing support and funding for programs.
- Identify specific legislation that focuses on issues related to each of the following categories: education and development, medical rehabilitation, consumer rights, and environmental issues.
- Compare and contrast federal and state policy environments and potential methods of influence for community practice.

Key Terms

Americans with Disabilities Act (ADA) of 1990
Civil rights referenced legislation
Consumer referenced legislation
Educational and developmental referenced legislation
Environment referenced legislation

Individuals with Disabilities Education Act (IDEA)
Medical rehabilitation referenced legislation
Protection and care referenced legislation
Social Security Act of 1935
Technology Related Assistance Act of 1988

Introduction

Occupational therapists practicing in the medical model have expected payment from, and therefore have been influenced by, the medical insurance providers, including programs offered by federal, state, and private sources. Although this reimbursement for services will continue to influence the practice of occupational therapy within the medical model, the current shift from the fee-for-service delivery model to community-based practice will require practitioners to broaden their perspectives to include knowledge of legislation that impacts community service programs. According to Baum

and Law (1998), occupational therapists must understand the mechanisms of service delivery for social programs, including the legislative policies and funding (i.e., provision of money for a specified purpose) resources that support them.

Globally, health and social policies have shifted away from institutional care and towards supporting inclusion and community participation. For example, the World Health Organization adopted the *International Classification of Functioning, Disability and Health (ICF)* (2001) to replace the *International Classification of Impairments, Disabilities and Handicaps (ICIDH)*, supporting a shift from a biomedical to a social paradigm. This occurred in recognition of the role of the environment in determining a person's health and disability status (Stewart & Law, 2003). In 2004, the World Federation of Occupational Therapists approved a position paper on community-based rehabilitation that supports full community participation by people with disabilities worldwide (Kronenberg, Algado, & Pollard, 2005). In the United States, it has been recognized that many people with serious mental illness live productive lives in the community. Mental health policy has shifted to support recovery by putting the person at the center of care decisions. Examples include the *Surgeon General's Report on Mental Health* (1999) and the *President's New Freedom Commission/Initiative* (2001; 2003), in which it is recommended that the entire mental health delivery system be transformed to support consumer recovery.

Historically, special-interest groups have influenced legislation and policies, resulting in the development of the majority of community services and programs currently available for special populations. Changing views of health and the environment have also influenced policy and funding decisions (Stewart & Law, 2003). The influence of federal legislation and regulation on the increased availability of community programs for persons with disabilities has been part of the impetus for the interest and shift in occupational therapy practice from the medical model to a variety of other environments within the community (Jacobs, 1996).

In this chapter, the legislation and policies that might influence community-based practice are presented. The legislation described is not intended to be all-inclusive. It should be emphasized that policy is constantly changing and practitioners must be alert to both existing and pending legislation that impacts the practice setting as well as the client population served. The basic themes described are an amalgamation of those described in publications by Fifield and Fifield (1995) and Reed (1992). An extensive outline of the relevant legislation is provided in Box 4-1.

Box 4-1 Outline of Major Legislation Influencing Community Practice

Protection and care referenced legislation/policy

- Social Security Act
  - Aid to the permanently and totally disabled
  - Supplemental security income program
- Maternal and Child Health and Mental Retardation Planning Amendments (P.L. 88-156)
- Mental Retardation and Community Mental Health Center Construction Act (P.L. 88-164)
- National Institute of Mental Health Community Support Program
- Omnibus Reconciliation Act of 1981 (P.L. 97-35)
- Reauthorization of P.L. 102-321 ADAMHA Re-Organization Act Substance Abuse Prevention and Treatment Services Block Grant

Educational and developmental legislation for persons with disabilities

- Education
  - National Defense Education Act (P.L. 85-864)
  - Maternal and Child Health and Mental Retardation Planning Amendments (P.L. 88-156)
  - Mental Retardation and Community Mental Health Center Construction Act (P.L. 88-164)
  - Education for All Handicapped Children Act (P.L. 94-142)
    - Part H Amendment to P.L. 94-142
- Developmental referenced legislation/policy
  - Developmental Disabilities Act of 1970 (P.L. 91-517)
  - 1973 Amendments to the Rehabilitation Act (P.L. 93-112)
  - Education for All Handicapped Children Act of 1975 (P.L. 94-142)
  - Part H of P.L. 94-142, Early Intervention Provisions

Box 4-1 Outline of Major Legislation Influencing Community Practice—cont'd

Legislation establishing reimbursement and funding for rehabilitation programs
- Rehabilitation Act of 1973 (P.L. 93-112)
- Subsequent Amendments to the Rehabilitation Act
  - 1965: P.L. 89-97 created Medicare and Medicaid
  - 1972: P.L. 92-223 established intermediate-care facilities for persons with mental retardation
  - 1972: P.L. 92-603 established supplemental security income to persons on standardized assistance programs
  - 1986: P.L. 99-506 clarified supportive employment
- Mental Retardation Facilities and Community Mental Health Center Construction Act of 1963 (P.L. 88-164)

Civil rights referenced legislation
- Civil Rights Act of 1964 (P.L. 88-352) and 1988 Civil Rights Restoration Act
- Architectural Barriers Act of 1968 (P.L. 90-480)
- Amendments to Developmental Disabilities Act
- Section 504 of the Rehabilitation Act of 1973 (P.L. 93-112)
- Education for All Handicapped Children Act (P.L. 94-142)
- Americans with Disabilities Act of 1990 (P.L. 101-336)

Environment referenced legislation
- Architectural Barriers Act of 1986 (P.L. 90-480)
- Independent Living Provisions of the 1973 Vocational Rehabilitation Act (P.L. 93-112)
- Education for All Handicapped Children Act (P.L. 94-142)
- Technology Related Assistance Act of 1988 (P.L. 100-407)
- Technology Assistance Act of 2004 (P.L. 108-364)

Consumer referenced legislation
- Developmental Disabilities Act of 1970
- 1977 Rehabilitation Act Amendments
- Education for All Handicapped Children Act (P.L. 94-142)
- Technology Related Assistance Act of 1988 (P.L. 100-407)
- Americans with Disabilities Act of 1990 (P.L. 101-336)

Sources: Reed, K. L. (1992). History of federal legislation for persons with disabilities. *American Journal of Occupational Therapy, 46,* 397–408.
Fifield, B., & Fifield, M. (1995). The influence of legislation on services to people with disabilities. In O. C. Karan and S. Greenspan (Eds). *Community rehabilitation services for people with disabilities* (pp. 38–70). Boston: Butterworth-Heinemann.
National Collaborative on Workforce and Disability for Youth. (2008). *Disability Legislation* Retrieved from http://ncwd-youth.info/resources_&_Publications?disability_Legislation/all_legislation.shtml

Legislation and Disabilities

To facilitate the shift in practice to the community model and promote the role of occupational therapy effectively, the practitioner must have a basic understanding of the historical background of legislation that affects the lives of people with disabilities. Although most practitioners are generally aware of legislation affecting reimbursement for services, this knowledge has been traditionally based on the location of service provision (e.g., inpatient hospital, outpatient rehabilitation facility, public school). According to Brownson (1998), current legislation and funding mechanisms have moved beyond the medical management of the client to addressing other societal and environmental factors that affect health.

Fifield and Fifield (1995, p. 38) state that "legislation not only articulates who is to receive services, but it also articulates what and how services are to be delivered and reflects the values, philosophies, and concerns of society." According to these authors, much of the early legislation provided compensation programs for military and work injuries, which later led to the emergence of rehabilitation and education legislation that provided funding for services rather than compensation for injury. Fifield and Fifield (1995) state that a majority of the current federal programs for persons with disabilities has evolved from legislation that was initiated under the administration of President John F. Kennedy. Although the work of the President's Panel on Mental Retardation of 1962 focused on mental retardation, it outlined legislative needs and programs that applied to almost all disabilities. These needs included prevention, education, public resources, research, coordination of services, and consumer participation. Subsequently, legislation has been developed in almost all of these areas. Fifield and Fifield (1995) categorized the legislation that emerged into five social concerns or themes:

(1) protection and care,
(2) development and opportunities,
(3) civil rights,
(4) environmental issues, and
(5) consumer responsiveness.

Protection and Care Referenced Legislation

Protection and care referenced legislation is intended to provide for the safety of those constituencies covered by the legislation. The focus of this type of legislation is on guardianship or protection of the citizenry. Legislation related to protection and care was initially introduced with the **Social Security Act of 1935.** This act was designed as a federally financed program that would be managed by the state to provide relief and assistance to indigent dependent children, elderly adults, and the blind. The Social Security Act originally provided old-age assistance (Title I) and aid to families with dependent children (Title IV). In addition, the act provided programs for the blind (Title VI), established state and public health authorities (Title X), and authorized grants to states for maternal and child health and crippled children services (Title V). The Social Security Act has been amended numerous times (1956, 1972, and 1980) to allow workers with disabilities to receive pensions before reaching retirement, to provide income maintenance for those who are permanently and totally disabled, and to provide income maintenance and health benefits (Medicaid and Medicare) to families and individuals with disabilities living in non-institutional and community-based settings (Fifield & Fifield, 1995; Reed, 1992).

Educational and Developmental Referenced Legislation

Educational and developmental referenced legislation is intended to provide for the instructional and training needs of those constituencies covered by the legislation. The focus of this type of legislation is on increasing the productivity and enriching the lives of people with disabilities. Because public education was primarily considered the responsibility of the state, the early education laws for children with disabilities came from the individual state legislatures. The first significant federal support for public education for people with disabilities was provided through the National Defense Education Act in 1957. Amended versions of the National Defense Education Act (Public Law 85-864 and Public Law 85-926) provided funds for mental retardation research and authorized the first federally supported programs to train teachers of children who were mentally retarded (Fifield & Fifield, 1995). Additional public policies, such as the Mental Retardation Facilities and Community Mental Health Center Construction Act of 1963 (Public Law 88-164) and the Developmental Disabilities Act of 1970 (Public Law 91-517), have attempted to better meet the needs of at-risk populations and individuals with developmental disabilities by addressing gaps in services.

The Education of the Handicapped Act Amendments of 1986 (Public Law 99-457) was the most influential piece of legislation for children with disabilities and their families. Part H and Part B of this legislation established services for children from birth through 2 years of age and 3 to 21 years of age, respectively. Subsequent amendments to that law, the **Individuals with Disabilities Education Act of 1990 (IDEA)** (Public Law 101-476) further defined implementation of these services and reinforced the importance of prevention rather than remediation (Stephens & Tauber, 1996). IDEA legislation was updated in 2004 (Public Law 108-446) with key components of interest to occupational therapists. Among these are increased emphasis on transition services, involvement of parents, and support for emotional needs related to education of students. IDEA Part B conceptualizes occupational therapy as a "related service," an intervention that supports the educational goals of the child with a disability, not a medical service. IDEA Part C enables occupational therapy services from birth through 36 months as primary services that occur in the child's natural environment (Sandstrom, Lohman, & Bramble, 2009).

Medical Rehabilitation Referenced Legislation

Medical rehabilitation referenced legislation is intended to provide for the health of those constituencies covered by the legislation. The focus of this type of legislation is on medical care and the development of programs to meet the special health needs of persons with disabilities.

Public funds for rehabilitation services are typically available through either insurance or grant programs. "Between 1965 and 1975, legislation separated itself from protection and care legislation by redefining and broadening these concepts to include intervention, treatment, and therapy which focused on maintaining and restoring physical, social, vocational, and cognitive skills" (Fifield & Fifield, 1995, p. 58). Most significant were the Title XVIII (Medicare) and Title XIX (Medicaid) Amendments to the Social Security Act because they provided health insurance coverage to beneficiaries for services delivered in a wide range of settings, including hospitals, outpatient facilities, skilled nursing facilities, comprehensive rehabilitation facilities, home health agencies, hospices, and clinics (Reed, 1992).

Among other rehabilitation-related policy opportunities that can impact occupational therapy services are Medicaid Home and Community-Based Waivers. Designed as demonstration projects that eventually pay for themselves, such waivers involve a state application for portions of the Social Security Act to be "waived" to support innovative policy to enable community rather than institutional care (Centers for Medicare & Medicaid Services, 2009). States may have several of such waivers that address specific populations, such as the elderly who would be institutionalized without services enabled by the waiver, persons with autism, or other disabilities. There are waivers that propose alternatives to institutional care (typically section 1915(b) or 1915(c) of the

Social Security Act) and a statewide waiver that proposes a redesign of Medicaid services that is comprehensive in scope (section 1115) (CMS, 2005). Due to specific criteria about population access to institutional care, the populations that are most often targeted for 1915(c) waivers are children and adolescents, and the elderly.

The Deficit Reduction Act of 2005 has made it easier for states to provide services typically available only by applying for a waiver, without getting the formal waiver, if the services are for people with disabilities who meet the income criteria or for people over the age of 65 (Kaiser Family Foundation, 2006). For example, the *Money Follows the Person Demonstration* (MFP) is a Medicaid initiative that provides enhanced funding to states to provide more long-term care services in the community and fewer in institutional settings. An evaluation of the initiative identified successes with moving people from institutional to community settings and expanded services to facilitate transition. However, "identifying safe, affordable and accessible community housing for MFP participants is a major challenge for states" (Kaiser Family Foundation, 2009, p. 2). Therapists can research state Web sites or identify key policy makers on the state level to advocate a role for community-based occupational therapy services in these types of federal and state programs.

The Mental Retardation Facilities and Community Mental Health Center Construction Act of 1963 (Public Law 88-164) authorized construction of specially designed state facilities for the diagnosis, treatment, education, and training of people with disabilities, specifically individuals with mental retardation or mental illness. In addition, this act provided funding to establish community mental health centers, and to increase the accessibility and availability of mental health services to the public (Ellek, 1991; Reed, 1992).

The Workforce Investment Act (WIA) (P.L. 105-220, 404, 112 Stat. 936, 1148–49) supports many services that enable productive activity. These include vocational rehabilitation, training programs, and consultation to educational systems to support the transition of youth with disabilities to adulthood. States vary in which services they provide and program eligibility, so although there may be opportunities for occupational therapists, it is recommended that therapists communicate with the relevant state agency for specific information on which services are funded (Workforce Investment Act, 1998).

Civil Rights Referenced Legislation

Civil rights referenced legislation is intended to protect the lawful privileges of those constituencies covered by the legislation. The focus of this type of legislation is on equal protection under the law for all citizens. Social conflict during the 1960s resulted in an initial piece of legislation (Civil Rights Act of 1964) that asserted fundamental human rights and guaranteed numerous protections for all citizens. Subsequent legislative activities, such as the Architectural Barriers Act of 1968, Rehabilitation Act of 1973, and the Americans with Disabilities Act of 1990, included provisions to ensure the rights of people with disabilities. The Architectural Barriers Act of 1968 required all federal buildings to be accessible to persons with disabilities and included standards for accessibility that were later revised and incorporated into Section 504 of the Rehabilitation Act of 1973. Section 504, which provided the foundation for the Americans with Disabilities Act of 1990, prohibits discrimination on the basis of a disability by any program receiving or benefiting from federal financial aid. It also provided the first federal statutory definition of a disability, which has been used extensively in subsequent legislation.

Other legislation that incorporated civil rights provisions include the 1974 amendments to the Developmental Disabilities Act and the Education for All Handicapped Children Act (Public Law 94–142). The 1974 amendments to the Developmental Disabilities Act established protection and advocacy agencies in every state to ensure that state, public, or private service agencies did not violate the rights of persons with disabilities. The Education for All Handicapped Children Act of 1975 (Public Law 94-142) established the right of children with handicaps to a free and appropriate public education.

Perhaps the most significant disabilities legislation was the **Americans with Disabilities Act (ADA) of 1990** (Public Law 101-336). It expanded the nondiscrimination provisions primarily associated with the Rehabilitation Act of 1973 to include the private sector and public services. Previous legislation affected only government agencies and agencies receiving federal support (Fifield & Fifield, 1995; Reed, 1992; Stephens & Tauber, 1996). The *Olmstead v. L.C. Supreme Court* (*Olmstead v. L.C.* (98-536), 527 U.S. 581 [1999]) decision found that unnecessary segregation of people with disabilities in institutions could constitute discrimination based on disability (Center for an Accessible Society, 1999). This decision has spurred all levels of government to address access to community services. There are implications for persons with disabilities of all ages, including transition-aged youth moving from special education or government-sponsored mental health services to the broader community. Occupational therapists may be involved in direct or indirect community-based services relative to *Olmstead* issues of housing, employment, and rehabilitation needs.

Environment Referenced Legislation

Environment referenced legislation is intended to provide physical access to a variety of settings for those constituencies covered by the legislation. The focus of this type of legislation is on the accessibility and usability of programs for all persons but particularly for those with disabilities. Since the implementation of the Architectural Barriers Act of 1968 (Public Law 90-480), legislative provisions have extended the original focus of eliminating environmental barriers to buildings to include better access to information, services, and opportunities. Often, important community services were provided in locations and at times inconvenient to consumers but convenient to providers. The ideology for change has progressed from normalization and mainstreaming to full inclusion of persons with disabilities. The shift in the focus of control from the providers to the consumers was a direct result of the Independent Living Provisions of the 1973 Vocational Rehabilitation Act.

In the 1980s, the Education for All Handicapped Children Act (Public Law 94-142) focused on improving the fit between the person with a disability and the regular education environment. As a result, increased attention was placed on mainstreaming children with special needs and providing placement in the least restrictive environment.

The **Technology Related Assistance Act of 1988** (Public Law 100–407) expanded the definitions of assistive technology introduced and defined in the

Older Americans Act (1986) and in the Developmental Disabilities Act (1985) to include devices and services used to achieve independence, productivity, and integration (Fifield & Fifield, 1995, p. 63): "Since 1988, assistive technology has been an expanding provision included in the Individuals with Disabilities Education Act of 1990 and the 1992 amendments to the Rehabilitation Act. Advancements in assistive technology have made it feasible to implement many of the provisions of the Americans with Disabilities Act."

The Assistive Technology Act of 2004 (Public Law 108-364) was designed to increase access by persons with disabilities to technology devices and services. Among other things, it requires states to have an advocacy council to assure consumer directedness as well as to establish and monitor measurable goals.

The specific inclusion of environment relative to supporting health of populations is evidenced in the overarching goals of *Healthy People 2020*. In addition to goals related to prevention and removal of health disparities, *Healthy People 2020* supports goals that "create social and physical environments that promote good health for all" (U.S. Department of Health and Human Services, 2008, ¶11).

Consumer Referenced Legislation

Consumer referenced legislation is intended to provide for representation in decision making of those constituencies covered by the legislation. The focus of this type of legislation is on autonomy and the individual's right to self-determination.

Historically, society has viewed people with disabilities as different, often using negative descriptors. Throughout the 1970s and 1980s, the terms "handicapped" and "client" were used interchangeably when referring to people with disabilities. Both terms implied a dependent relationship in which the provider was the decision maker. The Developmental Disabilities Act of 1970 and the 1977 Rehabilitation Act amendments outlined provisions for increased consumer representation on policy and advisory councils, thus introducing the term "consumer" (Fifield & Fifield, 1995; Reed, 1992). The Education for All Handicapped Children Act strengthened the role of parents through the individual education plan process. According to Fifield and Fifield (1995), each successive reauthorization

of these pieces of legislation has aggressively strengthened the level and depth of consumer participation in planning, monitoring, setting priorities, and making decisions in the development of service delivery. Both the Technology Related Assistance Act of 1988 and the Americans with Disabilities Act of 1990 also strengthened consumer responsiveness by "using 'people first' language that addressed dignity, choice, and participation" (Fifield & Fifield, 1995, p. 64).

Federal and State-Level Policy and Community Practice

The roles of the federal and state governments vary in the policy making process. Traditionally, the role of the federal government has been to set broad parameters, such as overall policy goals and directions, with the role of the states to design and implement programs and services that meet federal guidelines according to population needs. The state's role in health policy historically involves financing some services, regulating health-care providers and organizations, and coordinating and implementing public health initiatives (Lipson, 1997). Additional health-related roles of the states include environmental protection, regulation of the sale of health insurance, state rate setting and licensing, and cost control (Weissert & Weissert, 2006). Occupational therapy practitioners need to be aware of both federal and state initiatives that may impact community practice. Federal policy may shape the direction of funding in terms of population, setting, and services. Examples of federal policy changes and their impacts have been identified in this chapter and include the Americans with Disabilities Act of 1990, and the *Olmstead* decision of 1999. Occupational therapists need to be aware of these changes so that they can assist populations to access needed services or rights/entitlements. In the case of the ADA, occupational therapists working with persons with disabilities in the community on employment or housing need to be aware of the appropriate federal department to access in case of a client complaint that may be a violation of the law. In the case of the *Olmstead* decision, occupational therapists working with persons with disabilities on aging in place need to be aware of how the state evaluates individuals relative to safety and resources that may be available, such as through state Medicaid waivers. In the case of state health policy, occupational therapists in community practice may provide services that are financed by the state through a waiver, such as services for people with autism, and so need to be aware of how to be included as a provider. Community occupational therapists may wish to be involved in public health initiatives such as disaster planning and again may benefit from volunteering on a local planning task force. Another area in which occupational therapists are affected daily by state policy is through the regulation of the profession. Occupational therapists can volunteer to serve on the state board of practice or relevant subcommittees.

State government is structured similarly to the federal government. Both have three branches of government: each state has a governor whose duties are similar to the president; both have a legislature that passes laws, allocates resources, and oversees the executive branch; and both have a similar process for a bill to become a law (Weissert & Weissert, 2006). Differences include revenue sources, the fact that states are required to have a balanced budget, and the fact that state elected officials have more direct responsibility to their constituents. The top two state funding areas are K–12 education and Medicaid. The fact that states must operate on a balanced budget may lead to cuts during times of economic challenge. Occupational therapists relying on state funding for community practice need to be informed about the process for influencing resource allocation to assure access to their services. For example, each state has a designated agency to provide vocational rehabilitation services through the department of education. Occupational therapists working with persons with disabilities on employment goals need to be aware of state priorities and funding challenges to advocate for access to critical services and supports for this population.

It is important for occupational therapists to be aware that although there are some consistencies, state policies can vary widely. This requires occupational therapy practitioners to develop key relationships at the local and state levels to monitor and advocate for issues of importance to community practice. For example, there are some mandated services, such as physician visits and hospital care, that must be provided by states offering Medicaid

services, and many optional services. Among optional services are occupational therapy, case management, personal care services, and home and community-based services. States differ in which optional services they provide, and many of the optional services include those provided in the community.

Advocacy Activities That Support Community Practice

Key leadership roles, such as board membership or volunteering to chair a community committee, enhance visibility of the professional and strengthen potential partnerships. Involvement with state and national professional associations can assist the community occupational therapist to stay abreast of key state and federal initiatives and assist the profession to participate in the policy making process. Collaboration or coalitions with other groups with a common interest can also assist with influence—the greater the numbers, the greater the potential impact. Examples of potential partners for community-based occupational therapists might be community health centers or their advocacy group, community behavioral health centers or their advocacy group, professional provider organizations, educational advocacy groups, disease-specific advocacy groups, consumer advocacy groups, and Centers for Independent Living.

Conclusion

Historically, federal legislation concerning persons with disabilities has developed from a focus on adults to a focus on children and policies that emphasize secondary prevention. Federal legislation has progressed from concerns primarily for physical disabilities to concerns for all types of disabilities, and expanded from assistance primarily for medical management to assistance that also includes non-medically based programs for citizens with disabilities that support them in the community context (Reed, 1992). Because community-based programs are unique to the community served and are often based financially and programmatically on a variety of local, state, and federal policies, practitioners shifting from the more traditional practice arena must research the environment of their intended practice to ensure optimum service provision to their clients. A readily accessible source for researching both current state and federal legislation that might impact occupational therapy practice is the American Occupational Therapy Association's Web site (www.aota.org).

In many community-based programs, the role of occupational therapy may not be clearly defined. It is then incumbent upon the practitioner to determine the role of occupational therapy. Both the roles and responsibilities should be based on the needs of the program recipients, the scope of occupational therapy practice, and applicable legislation/policy. In changing times and with changing societal needs, occupational therapists must be responsive to the needs of consumers and the community programs that serve them. According to Powell (1992, p. 562), "Occupational therapists must forge stronger bonds with consumers, increase consumer independence, and hasten consumer community integration to refocus and develop new programs."

Learning Activities

1. Discuss the differences in the terms "reimbursement" and "funding." For each, identify an example of federal legislation that provides this type of financial resource.
2. Describe key features of the Social Security Act, the Americans with Disabilities Act (ADA), the Individuals with Disabilities Education Act (IDEA), and the Technology Related Assistance Act that have implications for community-based occupational therapy practice.
3. Identify a community-based setting and discuss the policies that may affect practice in this setting.
4. Identify a community-based program and discuss the factors that an occupational therapy practitioner might consider in determining his or her role in that setting.
5. What resources are available to research legislative changes at the federal and state levels that may impact occupational therapy practice?

REFERENCES

Americans with Disabilities Act of 1990, Pub. L. 101-336, July 26, 1990, 104 Stat. 327 (42 U.S.C. 12101 et seq.).

Baum, C., & Law, M. (1998). Community health: A responsibility, an opportunity, and a fit for occupational therapy. *American Journal of Occupational Therapy, 52,* 7–10.

Brownson, C. (1998). Funding community practice: Stage 1. *American Journal of Occupational Therapy, 52,* 60–64.

Center for an Accessible Society. (1999). *Supreme Court upholds ADA 'Integration Mandate' in Olmstead decision.* Retrieved from http://accessiblesociety.org/topics/ada/olmsteadoverview.htm

Centers for Medicare & Medicaid Services (CMS). (2009). *Section 1915(b) Authority* [Online]. Retrieved from http://cms.hhs.gov/MedicaidStWaivProgDemoPGI/04_Section1915(b)Authority.asp

Civil Rights Act of 1964. Retrieved from http://ourdocuments.gov/doc.php?flash=old&doc=97

Ellek, D. (1991). The evolution of fairness in mental health policy. *American Journal of Occupational Therapy, 45,* 947–951.

Fifield, B., & Fifield, M. (1995). The influence of legislation on services to people with disabilities. In O. C. Karan & S. Greenspan (Eds.), *Community rehabilitation services for people with disabilities* (pp. 38–70). Boston: Butterworth-Heinemann.

Jacobs, K. (1996). The evolution of the occupational therapy delivery system. In *The occupational therapy manager* (pp. 3–48). Bethesda, MD: American Occupational Therapy Association.

Kaiser Family Foundation. (February 2006). *Deficit Reduction Act of 2005: Implications for Medicaid.* Retrieved from http://kff.org/medicaid/upload/7465.pdf

Kaiser Family Foundation. (2009). *Money follows the person: An early implementation snapshot.* Retrieved from http://kff.org/medicaid/7928.pdf

Kronenberg, F., Algado, S., & Pollard, N. (2005). *Occupational therapy without borders.* New York: Elsevier.

Lipson, D. J. (1997). State roles in health care policy: Past as prologue? In T. J. Lipman & L. S. Robins (Eds.), *Health politics and policy,* (3rd ed., pp.176-197). Albany, NY: Delmar Publishers.

National Collaborative on Workforce and Disability for Youth. (2008). *Disability Legislation.* Retrieved from http://ncwd-youth.info/resources_&_Publications/disability_Legislation/all_legislation.shtml

Powell, N. J. (1992). Supporting consumer-mandated programming for persons with developmental disabilities. *American Journal of Occupational Therapy, 46,* 559–562.

President's New Freedom Commission on Mental Health. (2003). *Achieving the promise: Transforming mental health care in America.* Retrieved from http://mentalhealthcommission.gov/reports/FinalReport/FullReport.htm

Reed, K. L. (1992). History of federal legislation for persons with disabilities. *American Journal of Occupational Therapy, 46,* 397–408.

Sandstrom, R. W., Lohman, H., & Bramble, J. D. (2009). Public policies addressing social disablement. In *Health services: Policy and systems for therapists,* 2nd ed. (pp. 63–70). Upper Saddle River, NJ: Pearson.

Stephens, L. C., and Tauber, S. K. (1996). Early intervention. In J. Case-Smith, A. Allen, & P. Pratt (Eds.), *Occupational therapy for children* (pp. 648–653). St. Louis: Mosby.

Stewart, D., and Law, M. (2003). The environment: Paradigms and practice in health, occupational therapy and inquiry. In L. Letts, P. Rigby, & D. Allen (Eds.),

Using environments to enable occupational performance (pp. 3–13). Thorofare, NJ: Slack.

U.S. Department of Health and Human Services. (1999). *Mental health: A report of the surgeon general*. Rockville, MD: U.S. Department of Health and Human Services, Substance Abuse and Mental Health Services Administration, Center for Mental Health Services, National Institutes of Health, National Institute of Mental Health. Retrieved from http://surgeongeneral.gov/library/mentalhealth/home.html

U.S. Department of Health and Human Services. (2008). *Phase I report: Recommendations for the framework and format of Healthy People 2020*. Retrieved from http://healthypeople.gov/hp2020/advisory/PhaseI/summary.htm

Weissert, C., & Weissert, W. G. (2006). States and health care reform. In *Governing health: The politics of health policy,* 3rd ed. Baltimore, MD: Johns Hopkins University Press.

Workforce Investment Act of 1998, Pub. L. No. 105-220, 404, 112 Stat. 936, 1148–49 (codified as amended at 29 O.S.C. 723 Supp. IV 1998).

World Health Organization. (2001). *International classification of functioning, disability and health.* Geneva, Switzerland: Author.

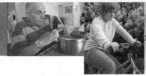
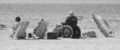
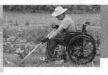

Community-Based Program Development

Chapter 5

Program Planning and Needs Assessment

Marjorie E. Scaffa, PhD, OTR/L, FAOTA, and Carol A. Brownson, MSPH

Planning is bringing the future into the present so that you can do something about it now. Failing to plan is planning to fail.

—Alan Lakein, author of *How to Get Control of Your Time and Your Life* (1989)

Learning Objectives

This chapter is designed to enable the reader to:

- Describe the processes of environmental scanning and trend analysis.
- Define the key steps in community health/health promotion program development.
- Describe three sources of data for needs assessments.
- Identify four factors that impact the selection of needs assessment strategies.
- Demonstrate understanding of the role of health behavior theories in community health/health promotion program planning.
- Define "goal" and "objective."
- Develop program objectives.
- Describe the five levels of the ecological approach to community health/health promotion programs.
- Develop implementation strategies at the different levels of intervention.
- Identify the purposes for each of the three levels of program evaluation.

Key Terms

Capacity assessment
Ecological perspective
Environmental scanning
Evidence
Evidence-based planning for health
Formative evaluation
Goal
Group processes
Impact
Interventions
Key informant
Needs assessment
Objectives

Outcome
Preplanning
Process evaluation
Program
Program development
Program planning
Secondary data
Societal levels
Stakeholders
Summative evaluation
Systematic reviews
Theory
Trend

Introduction

Program development, including planning and developing implementation and evaluation strategies, emerged in the 1980s as a key component of health education and health promotion (Timmreck, 1995, p. xv). With growing concerns about health care costs and access to care, health promotion and disease/injury prevention activities will likely play a major role in the future of health services. Planning, implementation, and evaluation skills are essential to the delivery of successful health promotion, health education, and prevention services.

Programs are distinguished from clinical services in that programs are primarily educational. A **program** is a "planned, coordinated group of activities, procedures, etc., often for a specific purpose or outcome; it addresses a specific need, problem or situation, shows what activities have taken place and reports what measurable changes have occurred" (Rutgers Cooperative Extension, 2007, p. 5). Sometimes referred to as **interventions,** programs are systematic efforts to achieve preplanned objectives such as changes in knowledge, attitudes, skills, and behaviors to maintain or improve function and/or health. These interventions can occur in a number of settings such as schools, work sites, community agencies, and health care environments.

Among the barriers to occupational therapists developing and/or providing health education and health promotion programs were lack of training in health promotion and in designing and implementing effective educational interventions (Johnson &

Jaffe, 1989, pp. 63–65). However, this lack of training should diminish as a result of occupational therapy educational institutions ensuring their curriculums are in compliance with current Accreditation Council for Occupational Therapy Education (ACOTE) standards, which became effective in 2008 (American Occupational Therapy Association [AOTA], 2006) and reflect the AOTA Centennial Vision (Baum, 2006).

The steps involved in developing community health and health promotion programs, beginning with trend analysis and environmental scanning, are described in this chapter. This is followed by a review of theoretical foundations and models on which programs can be based.

Environmental Scanning and Trend Analysis

Environmental scanning is "the acquisition and use of information about events, trends, and relationships in an organization's external environment, the knowledge of which would assist management in planning the organization's future course of action" (Choo, 2001, p. 1). The goal of scanning is to gain data, information, and knowledge to enable action. Environmental scans are often used as part of a strategic planning process. In its simplest form, environmental scanning is identifying one's information needs, searching for relevant information, and then using that information in decision making (Choo, 2001).

Environmental scanning is a tool for collecting data that can be used to design health programs tailored for specific communities (Rowel, Moore, Nowrojee, Memiah, & Bronner, 2005). Contextual factors can inhibit or facilitate individual and community health and are therefore an important aspect of a comprehensive needs assessment. This is particularly true for marginalized populations in which many health problems are related to environmental conditions.

Typically, an environmental scan examines a broad range of economic, social, political, and technological issues. Information is gathered from a variety of sources, and leading thinkers in the field are recruited to interpret the information and develop a variety of future scenarios. There is no single standardized methodology for conducting environmental scans. However, Choo (2001) identifies four modes of scanning, including undirected viewing, enacting, conditioned viewing, and searching. The "viewing" modes are more passive, whereas enacting and searching modes are purposefully active. Undirected viewing is noticing general characteristics or changes in the environment through informal information-seeking mechanisms. Conditioned viewing is value- and belief-driven and involves watching for specific characteristics or changes in the environment through routine information-seeking mechanisms. Enacting refers to exploring specific issues of concern through testing and experimentation and thereby gaining tacit knowledge. Searching refers to discovering detailed information through formal information-seeking mechanisms.

Analyzing trends allows one to anticipate change, recognize the implications, and take effective action. A **trend** is a general direction, tendency, or predictable sequence of events. Fazio (2008) outlines six steps in trend analysis:

1. Locate and gather sources of trend information, such as national and local newspapers, the Internet, television, magazines, etc.
2. Identify relevant articles and trend information, and take notes.
3. Categorize articles, trend information, and notes into broad categories, such as health, education, scientific research, economics, and local events.
4. Remove any items that you believe are not likely to impact occupational therapy practice.

5. Sort remaining articles, trend information, and notes into two groups, those that are likely to have a positive impact and those that are likely to have a negative impact on community-based occupational therapy practice.
6. Predict probable futures based on the trends discovered.

In order to plan and develop a viable and effective community program, environmental scanning and trend analysis is an important starting point. The information gathered through this process provides the basic foundation for the remainder of the program planning process.

Program Planning Principles

Program planning has been described as a process of establishing priorities, diagnosing causes of problems, and allocating resources to achieve objectives (Green, 1980). People have always planned, with or without a systematic method. As knowledge accumulates, planning continues to become more sophisticated. Although no one perfect model exists, Breckon, Harvey, and Lancaster (1994) point to seven principles common to all planning models.

Plan the Process

Preplanning is an important step that, if overlooked, can undermine the success of an otherwise effective intervention strategy. During the preplanning phase, consideration is given to who should be involved, when the planning should occur, what resources are needed, and what process will be followed. Internal and external resources are assessed, including attitudes, policies, available expertise, time, space, money, priorities, and fit with the organization's mission.

Plan With People

Experience has demonstrated the importance of involving clients in the planning process. Two community health promotion principles are encompassed here: (1) the principle of relevance and (2) the principle of participation. Similar to the concept of client-centeredness in occupational therapy, the principle of relevance, or "starting where the people are," exists when program planners begin by considering the perceived needs of community residents rather than those of the planners or their organizations.

Participation is considered essential for developing effective programs and is considered health enhancing. People meet and sustain their goals more effectively when they are actively involved in the process (Green & Kreuter 2005; Baker & Brownson, 1998; Minkler & Wallerstein, 1997). Participation can range from responding to requests for feedback on program plans to taking an active role in designing, implementing, and evaluating program activities.

Planning with people also encompasses the concept of collaboration. Program planning generally begins with a group of people who have a vested interest in the issues. Working with people and agencies who have shared interests and goals offers many advantages: resources and workload can be shared, duplication of effort can be minimized, and more creative problem solving can occur. The end result is a program that provides better service to the community.

Plan With Data

Sound planning decisions are based on a thorough knowledge of the health issue and associated factors, the service area or site, the target population, social and environmental support systems, and existing or former programs addressing the same issue. Much of the quantitative information can be gathered from existing sources, such as health departments, libraries, the National Center for Health Statistics, Chambers of Commerce, and health systems. Planners may also identify the need for additional data, perhaps more qualitative data that would help to identify attitudes, beliefs, or barriers. A review of available and gathered data provides a context in which planning and prioritizing can occur logically.

Plan for Performance

This principle speaks to long-range planning. Given that most serious health challenges will not completely disappear with one program, approaching the planning process with the idea of permanence, or sustainability, makes sense. This includes considering how the program might be staffed and financed after the initial intervention or how it might ultimately become incorporated as an integral part of an agency's services.

Plan for Priorities

The most effective programs are those that address the greatest need and are designed or known to have the greatest effect within given resources. Prioritization should flow naturally from planning with people and planning with data. Time for this activity needs to be built in to ensure continued community participation. A comprehensive needs assessment and input from all stakeholders helps to ensure that prioritization is directed by the stakeholders. **Stakeholders** are "persons who may or may not benefit directly by being involved in the potential program, but who may have a stake in the program's outcome and often the ability to influence that outcome" (Scaffa, Reitz, & Pizzi, 2010, p. 204).

Plan for Evaluation

Evaluation is a continuous process of asking questions, such as "Are we doing the right thing?" and "Are we doing things right?" and "What do we need to measure to know what and how we're doing?" These questions are usually answered through the systematic collection and analysis of program outcome data. Evaluation methods, depending on the goals and objectives of the program, should be built into the program design and spelled out in the program plan. Once the needed information is determined, record-keeping systems and evaluation instruments need to be selected and put in place to ensure that data are properly collected. The planning process should address who will be responsible for both data collection and analysis. It should also establish time frames for all steps.

Plan for Measurable Outcomes

The last of the seven planning principles is to match clearly articulated and measurable program objectives with data against which to judge program accomplishments. The format for the objective and the evaluation should match. For example, if the objective of a program is to reduce the risk of falling, then the outcome would be stated in terms of risk reduction, not reduced mortality or reduced hospitalization.

The Planning Process

A typical program planning process follows steps that are very similar to the occupational therapy process (Table 5-1). Program planning is a process

Table 5-1 Comparison of the Program Planning Process and Occupational Therapy Process	
Program Planning Process	**Occupational Therapy Process**
Preplanning (Exploration) • Identify/state the problem and the target population (also called "issue identification"). • Identify existing information regarding issue of concern. • Assess the internal and external resources and barriers. • Determine the goals of, and an approach for, the needs assessment.	Chart Review
Needs Assessment (Data Gathering and Analysis) • Collect relevant data. • Analyze and synthesize data. • Determine priorities. • Identify and evaluate alternative solutions. • Formulate an action plan.	Client Evaluation
Program Planning • Establish goals and objectives. • Develop the details of the intervention strategies, procedures, and time lines. • Develop a plan for evaluation. • Pretest materials and procedures.	Intervention Planning
Program Implementation • Implement/offer the program or service.	Intervention
Program Evaluation • Monitor and evaluate the program process, its impact, and ultimately the outcome. • Revise program as indicated and plan next steps (e.g., continue, terminate, and expand).	Re-evaluation and modification of intervention plan as appropriate
Sustainability Plan • Identify future sources of funding. • Build community capacity. • Cultivate supportive relationships.	Discharge Planning and Carryover to Home and Community
Dissemination Plan	Documentation
• Share the results with stakeholders, peers, and clients	

involving continuous cycles of needs assessment, planning the intervention, implementation, and evaluation (Dignan & Carr, 1992). Although these planning subtasks have discrete roles, in good programs they are interdependent and interwoven, using feedback at each step to revise or improve previous steps, as depicted in Figure 5.1 (Simons-Morton, Greene, & Gottlieb, 1995).

Preplanning

The pre-assessment or preplanning phase is an exploratory step during which existing data on the issue are identified and reviewed, resources are assessed, and the goals of the needs assessment are established. Identifying an issue to address can come from data, professional judgment, observation, existing literature, concerned individuals, or agencies.

Key questions of who, what, and why are answered. For example, *who* are the key players (e.g., service receivers, service providers, experts in the field, policy makers, agency representatives) with a vested interest in the issue; *what* do they hope will come from the needs assessment; and *why*—what prompted their concern, and how important is it (Soriano, 1995)? Answers to these questions will help define the key questions for the needs assessment. Planning often occurs through a group of

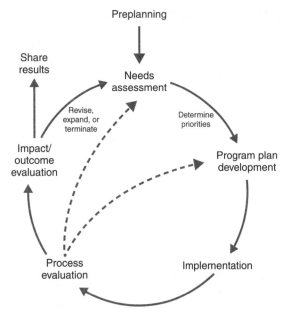

Fig. 5•1 The Cycle of Program Development.

stakeholders forming a planning committee. However broad or narrow the group, the perspectives of all stakeholders—particularly those of potential clients—must be considered and integrated into the planning process.

Every program planning initiative is influenced by factors that can support or inhibit the process. Considering these internal and external factors early in the process is important to avoid unnecessary pitfalls. First, a need must be analyzed for consistency or "fit" with the organization's mission. Assuming it fits, how important is the need relative to other issues? Is there a commitment of time and resources to see the project through? What is the potential for effecting a positive change? What do the other stakeholders want or expect? Are there other programs addressing this issue of concern?

Assessment of resources goes beyond the question of whether or not there is funding. Depending on the nature of the program being planned, other considerations may include location, space, materials, appropriately trained personnel, transportation for clients, and access to experts for certain phases of the process. Finally, preplanning should include an assessment of existing regulations and policies that might have an impact on the issue or the approach(es) being pursued.

Needs Assessment

The occupational therapist evaluates needs of clients daily in the delivery of direct care. In the context of program planning, however, a needs assessment is not intended to provide diagnostic information about individuals. Instead, the purpose is to make decisions about priorities for programs and services that affect groups of people.

A "need" is generally defined as the gap between the present state of affairs (what is) and some desired future state for a particular group with an identified issue (McKillip, 1987; Witkin & Altschuld, 1995). **Needs assessment** is "the regular systematic collection, assembly, analysis and dissemination of information on the health of a community" (Rowel et al., 2005, p. 527). Needs assessments are designed to prioritize issues and facilitate the development of interventions to address community concerns. In addition to identifying needs, this process also identifies available resources in a given population, discovers factors that contribute to the identified problem, establishes priorities, and devises criteria for interventions that will address the need (Witkin & Altschuld, 1995). If done properly, the needs assessment will lead to a clear set of program goals and objectives.

Profiling the Population and Community

One aspect of a needs assessment involves profiling the community in which the program is to be located. A community profile includes collecting both population demographics and social demographics. Population demographics refer to data about persons who reside within the selected community, such as age, race, ethnicity, education, religion, and income. Social demographics refer to data on the social and health problems of the population and existing resources in the community. Data collected may include housing, employment, crime, and health statistics (Fazio, 2008).

The next step in the community profiling process is to identify the service needs of the population. Understanding the problems in the community and the existing resources allows us to identify the gaps in services and develop a service profile. The service profile consists of a description of the population, data on the problem or unmet need, and information about the context in which the problem or unmet need occurs (Fazio, 2008). Positive community attributes and assets should also be identified. This is referred to as a community **capacity assessment** in which the capacities, skills, and strengths of individual community members, community organizations, and the community as a whole are identified (Scaffa, Reitz, & Pizzi, 2010). The community profile and the service profile provide the foundation for program development.

Data Collection

Key to the needs assessment process is the gathering of accurate and comprehensive information for making decisions about the best use of resources to resolve high-priority needs. Typically, in a needs assessment, information is gathered from key informants and stakeholders within the community. **Key informants** are persons, typically formal or informal leaders, who have expert knowledge about a phenomenon of interest. In the case of needs assessment, key informants provide information about the community, the population, local resources, and unmet needs. Key informants may be political figures, clergy, educators, social service providers, health care workers, school administrators, business leaders, and others who are influential in the community (Ritzer, 2007).

Methods for gathering data vary. Only a few of the potential methods will be briefly described here. Before collecting new data, a review of the scientific and intervention literature for background on the issue of concern and identification of strategies that have been used in similar situations are necessary.

Some common data sources and methods, such as secondary data, surveys, and group processes, are outlined in Table 5-2. The use of secondary data is one of the simplest and most cost-effective methods. **Secondary data,** also called archival data, are existing data collected by agencies for other purposes. Examples include birth and death records; census data; prevalence data on diseases, disability, illness, injury, and risk; demographic data; social indicators; and special surveys and reports. Secondary data are generally easy to obtain and particularly useful in the exploratory phase of the needs assessment process to determine what is already known about an issue. These data give a sense of the current status and give the planner an idea of what further information to gather. By themselves, secondary data do not constitute a needs assessment. To provide context and client

perspective, they are best used in conjunction with qualitative data.

Surveys, the most frequently used tool for gathering information for the needs assessment, are a cost-effective method for gathering information from large numbers of people who represent the target population. They may take the form of written questionnaires or interviews (in person, by telephone, or Web-based). Surveys should be administered to obtain information that does not exist elsewhere and should be designed so that inferences can be drawn about priorities and seriousness of needs. The most effective type of survey for a needs assessment asks people for their opinions based on their own experiences, background, expertise, or knowledge or for facts about themselves and others about whom they have direct knowledge (Witkin & Altschuld, 1995).

The specifics of survey methodology are beyond the scope of this chapter. While surveys look deceptively simple to construct, obtaining meaningful and reliable information requires considerable expertise in questionnaire development and administration. Questions need to be simple, straightforward, and carefully worded to elicit the desired information. The survey also must include people who are representative of the target audience and the stakeholders. Additionally, effort must be made to ensure that the method itself doesn't exclude segments of the population. Decisions need to be made about how the results will be analyzed. The survey also should be pretested on a sample of respondents. These tasks may require additional study (recommended is Witkin & Altschuld, 1995, Chapter 6) or the input of professionals with expertise in survey methodology.

Aside from surveys, **group processes** are the most frequently used method of collecting qualitative data for needs assessments (Witkin & Altschuld, 1995). Group processes provide face-to-face interactions with groups of stakeholders in a variety of discussion formats, most commonly open forums, focus groups, and nominal group processes. Group processes also provide direct interaction between the agency representatives and the target population, which can serve to build rapport. Like the other methods, group processes are most valuable when used in conjunction with other methods and sources. For further explanation of these techniques, the reader is referred to Witkin and Altschuld (1995), Krueger (2009), and Dignan and Carr (1992).

Table 5-2	**Overview and Comparison of Commonly Used Data Collection Methods for Needs Assessment**			
Data Source/ Method	**Description**	**Resulting Information**	**Advantages**	**Disadvantages**
Secondary (archival) data, i.e., records and logs, prior studies, demographic data, social indicators, risk-factor data, epidemiologic studies, census data, and rates under treatment	Existing data usually found in city, county, state, and national organizations and government bureaus	Quantitative data that help determine the status of a target population with regard to a need; may furnish information on causal or contributing factors	Relatively low in cost; generally available; minimal investment of time or staff; unbiased; complements other sources of data	No client input; possibly not representative for given target audience; technical assistance for statistical interpretation possibly needed
Survey methods, i.e., written questionnaire, face-to-face interview, telephone interview, and key informant interview	Techniques for gathering information directly from individuals using structured forms or protocols	Mainly qualitative— values, perceptions, opinions, judgments of importance, and observations	Client input achieved; quantitative data complemented	Generally more time- and labor-intensive than using secondary data sources
1. Written questionnaire			Easy to administer; relatively low in cost; time efficient; quantifiable; broad reach into community/ target population	Possible low return rates; may not be representative; not useful for people who are illiterate or not fluent in English; prone to design problems; technical assistance for questionnaire construction and data processing/analysis possibly necessary
2. Face-to-face interview			High response rate; greater flexibility for answers and interviewer probing; opportunity to observe non-verbal responses; ability to include people who are illiterate or who have vision problems; rapport building	Smaller sample size; costly in terms of time and travel; trained interviewers required; possible difficulty with scheduling; time consuming; opportunity for bias; possibility to raise client expectations; data more difficult to interpret and summarize;

Table 5-2	Overview and Comparison of Commonly Used Data Collection Methods for Needs Assessment—cont'd			
Data Source/ Method	**Description**	**Resulting Information**	**Advantages**	**Disadvantages**
				technical assistance for questionnaire construction and data processing/ analysis possibly necessary
3. Telephone interview			Easy to administer; no travel time and cost; perceived anonymity; fairly good response rate	Sampling challenges; may not be representative; not as suitable for long questionnaires; inability to observe non-verbal reactions; possible rise in client expectations; trained interviewers neces- sary to avoid bias; computer capability and technical assis- tance for question- naire construction and data processing/ analysis possibly needed
4. Key informant	Surveys (written and/or interview) of a select group of key commu- nity leaders, informal lay leaders, and pro- fessional persons who are aware of, and in touch with, the target population and the given issue		Limited number of participants necessary	Possible difficulty in identifying infor- mal leaders; biased results possible; participants may have vested interests
Group processes, i.e., community forums, focus groups, and nominal group processes	Techniques that involve small or large groups of stakeholders (e.g., service receivers, service providers, experts in the field, policy makers, and	Mainly qualitative— opinions and expert judgments; group perceptions and perspectives regarding values, importance of need; information on causes/ barriers; decisions	Opportunity for fluid, natural discus- sion around an issue; complemen- tary to other data	

Continued

Table 5-2   Overview and Comparison of Commonly Used Data Collection Methods for Needs Assessment—cont'd

Data Source/ Method	Description	Resulting Information	Advantages	Disadvantages
	agency represen- tatives) in vary- ing degrees of interaction	on priorities; feed- back or consensus on goals or courses of action		
1. Community forum	An open public meeting with all interested parties invited; a large group discussion	Ideas and input from a broad segment of the population	Broad range of views and concerns provided; natural discussion format; facilitation of dialogue among people with differ- ent viewpoints	Possibly not reflec- tive of opinions of general population; participation possibly low; domination by a few possible; difficult to analyze; logistics
2. Focus groups	Groups of 8 to 12 clients/ potential clients responding to a structured set of questions	Individual and group perspectives on a focused area or theme	Possible in-depth probing of themes	Skilled facilitators needed; technical assistance in data analysis possibly required; logistical challenges getting group together; groups variable, thus, more than one needed for reliable results
3. Nominal group process	The most structured of the group methods; a combination of written responses, voting, and dis- cussion used in small groups of 10 or less	Ranking by the group members of what they perceive to be the most important issues and/or solutions	Highly effective for getting at a large number of issues in a short amount of time; equitable participation	Expensive in terms of time and results; skilled leadership required; limited ability to generalize

Data from: Simons-Morton, B. G., Greene, W. H., and Gottlieb, N. H. (1995). *Introduction to health educa- tion and health promotion.* Prospect Heights, IL: Waveland. Soriano, F. L. (1995). *Conducting needs assessments: A multidisciplinary approach.* Thousand Oaks, CA: Sage. Witkin, B. R., and Altschuld, J. W. (1995). *Planning and conducting needs assessments: A practical guide.* Thousand Oaks, CA: Sage.

There is no inherently perfect or best method of data collection for needs assessment. The selection of methods depends on several factors (Soriano, 1995; Witkin & Altschuld, 1995), including:

- The characteristics of the target group and the survey respondents. For example, socioe- conomic factors, literacy, language, availability, and level of ability are among the factors that

may influence the manner in which informa- tion is gathered.

- The type of information desired. It makes sense to choose a combination of methods that yield different types of information, both qualitative and quantitative.

- Resources available (e.g., time, financial and human resources, and expertise). Trade-offs between the desired comprehensiveness of

the needs assessment and the resources available may be necessary.

- The amount of interaction desired with the audience. Some methods offer greater opportunity for dialogue with members of the target audience. Those same methods may be more costly or harder to analyze. Advantages and disadvantages of each approach should be considered.

Data Analysis and Interpretation

The data-gathering methods yield raw data. The next step is to analyze the data and use them in a practical way for planning. Even though the needs assessment is a form of survey research, the analysis is more of a planning tool than a statistical exercise. As such, the needs assessment relies less on inferential statistics and more on identification of need, risk, seriousness of a problem, and access to services (Timmreck, 1995). Once analyzed, the data should be presented to stakeholders in an easily understandable manner. Charts, graphs, and tables are useful techniques.

Interpretation of the data for planning purposes is the last step in the needs assessment process. The goal of this intermediate step is not to make final decisions about the intervention strategy but to interpret findings, set priorities regarding needs, suggest ways of addressing needs, weigh the alternatives based on a set of predetermined criteria, and propose a plan to implement the best solution (Witkin & Altschuld, 1995). This final step in the needs assessment process provides the direction and rationale for program planners to develop an effective intervention.

Program Plan Development

While needs assessments focus on the *ends* to be attained, the development of a program plan focuses on the *means* or solutions (Witkin & Altschuld, 1995). Ideally, the development of program components is based on a merging of the findings of the needs assessment, theories, and available resources (Simons-Morton et al., 1995).

The Role of Theories

Any time a program or service is planned, planners make assumptions about the causes of the problem and the best ways to effect change. If those assumptions are not made in terms of an explicit theory or theories, and there is no conceptual framework behind the choice of intervention, then there is no way to link the intervention to the intended outcome (Posavac & Carey, 1997). As a result, program design would be much less effective and evaluation would be less informative.

Simply stated, a **theory** is an explanation of why a phenomenon occurs the way it does (Freudenberg et al., 1995). Good theories complement practical skills and technologies by taking the program beyond simply conducting activities to actually solving problems. Theories can provide answers to a program developer's questions about *why* people engage or do not engage in specific health behaviors and *how* to engage people in changing and maintaining behaviors. Programs devised to address expected behaviors according to a theory help to determine *what* factors to focus on in the evaluation (Posavac & Carey, 1997; van Ryn & Heaney, 1992).

No single theory exists on which to base health education and health promotion programs. Populations, environments, cultures, and health issues vary broadly, so different theories or different combinations of theories may be useful in addressing a particular issue. Some theories focus on individual behavior; others focus on groups, organizations, or communities as the unit of change. The dominant theories currently used in health education have roots in social psychology and focus on health behavior at the individual level. These include the health belief model and the transtheoretical model. Bridging the individual, group, and community levels is social learning theory, also called social cognitive theory. (See Chapter 3 for a discussion of these and other theories that are useful for community program planning.)

Theories that address organizations and communities include organizational change theory (Butterfoss, Kegler, & Francisco, 2008), community organization and empowerment (Minkler, Wallerstein, & Wilson, 2008), diffusion of innovations (Oldenburg & Glanz, 2008), and media studies (Finnegan & Viswanath, 2008). These are not described here due to space constraints but are well described in the references noted.

Learning how to analyze a theory's fit with the issue or problem identified is challenging. According to Glanz and Rimer (2005, p. 6), "a working knowledge of specific theories, and familiarity with how they have been applied in the past improves

skill in this area." When selecting the best model, it is important to consider the characteristics outlined in Box 5-1 rather than prematurely selecting a theory that may be temporarily in vogue or a personal favorite. For more detail on the theories just described and others, and for a better understanding of their applications, the reader is referred to Glanz, Rimer, and Viswanath (2008) and Glanz and Rimer (2005).

Program Components

The general form of the written program plan includes:

- Goals
- Objectives
- Strategies
- Evaluation plan

Goals

Despite commonality of plan components, terminology is often confusing and used differently from one discipline to another. In health and social services planning, a **goal** is a quantified statement of a desired change in the status of a priority health need. Goals are long-term and broad in scope. As such, they are not directly measurable but should be considered attainable. Programs may have more than one goal.

Objectives

Objectives are used to reach goals. Unlike goals, objectives are specific, measurable, and performance

---

Box 5-1   A Good Fit: Characteristics of a Useful Theory

A useful theory makes assumptions about a behavior, health problem, target population, or environment that are:
- Logical;
- Consistent with everyday observations;
- Similar to those used in previous successful programs; and
- Supported by past research in the same area or related ideas.

From *Theory at a Glance: A Guide for Health Promotion Practice* (2nd ed., p. 7), K. Glanz & B. K. Rimer, (2005). Washington, DC: National Cancer Institute, U.S. Department of Health and Human Services, National Institutes of Health.

---

based. "They specify who, to what extent, under what conditions, by what standards, and within what time period certain activities are to be performed and completed" (Timmreck, 1995, p. 32). They outline the tasks and activities essential to accomplish the established goals. One goal may have several objectives, with each objective representing one aspect of accomplishing the goal. Well-written objectives typically answer the following questions:

- Who (clients/participants)?
- What (action/performance)?
- When (time frame)?
- How much (to what degree/standard of performance/level)?

For example, an objective might read: Within 6 months of completing the fall prevention course, 75% of participants will be continuing their balance exercises. Using the questions listed,

- "Who" refers to the participants of the fall prevention course.
- "What" refers to the action of continuing their balance exercises.
- "When" is identified as within 6 months of completing the course.
- "How much" is denoted as 75% of participants.

Programs that employ multiple approaches to reaching their goals may have different types of objectives. Some are directed at changes in the participants—their knowledge, behavior, or health status. Others may be directed at changes in resources or services. Examples of different types of objectives that pertain to the same goal are listed in Table 5-3.

Program plans may identify objectives by type and group them as such. Others may consider one type of objective as a "sub-objective" of another. The important element is that the program plan clearly identify its health objective(s); what the program will do to accomplish the objective(s); and what change in knowledge, skill, or behavior is expected in participants.

Strategies

The next task is to develop specific strategies for accomplishing the objectives that will be effective with the intended audience. Participation by members of the intended audience in the selection of methods is crucial to ensure that the methods are

Table 5-3 Different Types of Objectives for One Goal

Goal: By 2020, reduce injury from falls by half among older adults in Johnson County.

Objectives	Type
Within 2 years of the program's inception, admissions due to injury from falls in adults over age 60 will be reduced by 15% at Johnson County Hospital.	This is an example of a *health objective.* This objective specifies a change in health status (i.e., fewer injuries from falls). Health objectives define the specific health outcomes the program aims to accomplish and are sometimes referred to as "outcome objectives." There may be several for each goal.
By January 2015, the occupational therapist will reach 300 adults over age 60 through a fall prevention course taught in 15 senior housing complexes and nutrition centers in Johnson County.	This is an example of a *program objective.* It deals with the new service that is planned. These often address the "process" of the intervention.
By the end of the course, participants in the fall prevention program will be able to identify at least four risk factors for falls and develop an action plan for addressing their personal risks.	This is an example of a *learning objective.* It addresses knowledge, attitudes, or skills the program will attempt to effect to encourage specific behaviors in the intended population.
Within 6 months of completing the course, 75% of participants will be continuing their balance exercises at their goal level.	This is an example of a *behavioral objective.* Behavioral objectives, closely related to learning objectives, describe what the program will encourage people to do to reduce risk or improve health. Learning and behavioral objectives are sometimes called "impact objectives"; they do not directly address the health outcome but deal with factors that affect outcomes. They reflect the specific program strategies.
Home assessments will be provided to all interested clients who attend the fall prevention course.	This is an example of a *resource objective.* It addresses material support or essential services the program plans to provide.

acceptable and effective. Other factors to consider include literacy of the potential participants; degree of auditory or visual stimulation in their everyday lives; ways they customarily obtain information; cost; convenience; cultural relevance feasibility; and anticipated effectiveness (Dignan & Carr, 1992).

The most comprehensive programs go beyond the individual level, addressing systems that affect the ability of an individual to achieve work, leisure, and social participation goals. Socioecologic approaches to improving health recognize the interrelationships between people and their physical, social, cultural, economic, and political environments. Key to the **ecological perspective** in health promotion is that health behavior both influences and is influenced by the environment, known as reciprocal causation. This construct is well recognized in occupational therapy and evident in the theories and models of person-environment-occupation that guide occupational therapy practice (Law et al., 1997). In an ecological health promotion planning model, Simons-Morton et al. (1995) described five **societal levels** in which planners could intervene:

1. Intrapersonal: individual characteristics that influence behavior, such as knowledge, attitudes, beliefs, values, and personality
2. Interpersonal: family, friends, peers, and groups that provide social identity, support, and role definition
3. Organizational: agencies and their rules, regulations, policies, procedures, programs, and resources
4. Community: social networks, norms, trends, and standards that constrain or promote desired action

5. Public policy: local, state, and federal policies, laws, and programs that regulate or support desired action

An example of addressing the same health concern, physical activity for people with disabilities, from the five different levels is provided in Table 5-4.

Popular health promotion planning models that offer ecological frameworks for planning programs include PRECEDE-PROCEED (Green & Kreuter, 2005), social marketing (Storey, Saffitz, & Rimón, 2008), and MATCH (Simons-Morton et al., 1995). They address all societal levels and can be used to integrate diverse theories.

Some common intervention methods used at the different societal levels are described in Table 5-5.

Most occupational therapists and occupational therapy assistants are involved in smaller subpopulation interventions (levels 1 and 2), as opposed to working at changing systems, community norms, or policies (levels 3 to 5). Even at the interpersonal or group level, understanding and maintaining an ecological perspective of the issue is useful. It becomes a "mind-set" for viewing an issue of concern. At the very least, seeing clients as part of larger systems can provide guidance for improving transitions between and among programs and services and for identifying gaps. Having an ecological perspective also should encourage collaboration with agencies and systems that focus more clearly on other levels of intervention.

Trying to address all levels in one program initiative may not be feasible or even desirable. However, using their experience, knowledge, and expertise to influence others along the continuum can be very effective for occupational therapy practitioners. Encouraging advocacy; providing information to clients, employers, and policy makers; and joining community organizations and coalitions are examples of how one might extend his or her "reach" and leverage action at other levels. Doing so can also generate new partners and possibly new funding for programs that meet mutual goals (Brownson, 1998). Although not addressed in this chapter, another benefit of involvement at multiple levels is to expand occupational therapy's role in community, environmental, policy, and social arenas.

Evaluation Plan

Evaluation strategies are designed during the planning process before implementing interventions. The evaluation plan should be created with input from the key stakeholders, including potential participants or clients. Several steps for developing an evaluation plan are as follows:

1. Determine who will coordinate data collection and who will analyze it.
2. List the strategies, methods, or materials of interest for evaluation (i.e., the evaluation questions) and the anticipated results based on program standards and objectives.

Table 5-4 Ecological Health Promotion Model and Occupational Therapy

Level of Intervention	Potential Occupational Therapy Role
Intrapersonal/individual	Adapt physical activities/exercises for people with functional limitations to encourage fitness and promote health.
Interpersonal	Offer adapted exercise classes for specific populations; provide education to family members and friends.
Organizational	Work with existing gyms, YMCA/YWCAs, and exercise facilities to make their facilities accessible to people of all abilities; train staff.
Community	Work with appropriate health agencies and health professions to develop messages about the importance of physical activity for everyone; use appropriate channels to raise awareness; join others in advocating for accessible community facilities and transportation; offer professional consultation on adaptations and accommodations.
Government/policy level	Advocate for funding to support making public parks, trails, and facilities accessible to people with disabilities.

Table 5-5 Societal Levels and Methods Used

Societal Level	Method	Description
Individual/group level (educating, training, and counseling)	Lecture-discussion	Combination of prepared remarks by leader/facilitator and guided discussion or question-answer session
	Audiovisual aids	Compact discs, booklets, posters, flipcharts, models, display boards, YouTube slides, videotapes, computers, and interactive multimedia programs
	Peer group discussion	Use of small groups for discussion of topic common to group
	Simulation and games	Games, role-playing, dramatizations, case studies, storytelling, and songs
	Skill development	Explanation, demonstration, and practice of a psychomotor competency
	Mass media	Information provided through television, radio, texting, instant messaging, newspapers, magazines, billboards, direct mail (Dignan & Carr, 1992; AMC Cancer Research Center, 1994; Simons-Morton, Greene, & Gottlieb, 1995; Office of Cancer Communications, 1992)
Interpersonal level (educating, training, and facilitating)	Enhancing/developing social ties	Interpersonal relationships that provide emotional, instrumental, or informational assistance (Heaney & Israel, 2008)
	Use of natural helpers	Members of social networks that other members go to for advice, support, and other assistance (Eng & Young, 1992)
Organizational level (consulting, networking, training, and advocating)	Organizational development	Implementation of planned change within organizations (Goodman, Steckler, & Kegler, 1997)
Community level (marketing, organizing, developing, and advocating)	Media advocacy	The strategic use of mass media to increase public support for a social or policy initiative (Wallack, Dorfman, Jernigan, & Themba, 1993)
	Community coalitions	An alliance of organizations or individuals working together to achieve a common purpose (Butterfoss, Goodman, & Wandersman, 1993)
	Community organization	A set of processes and procedures "by which community groups are helped to identify problems or goals, mobilize resources, and develop and implement strategies to" solve a common problem or pursue a common goal (Minkler, Wallerstein, & Wilson, 2008, pp. 287–288)
	Community empowerment	A social action process through which "individuals, communities, and organizations gain mastery over their lives in the context of changing their social and political environment to improve equity and quality of life" (Minkler, Wallerstein, & Wilson, 2008, p. 295)
Governmental and policy level (advocacy, lobbying, and political action)	Policy development/advocacy	Changes in, or development of, local, state, or federal policies, programs, practices, regulations, and laws on behalf of a particular interest group or population

76   SECTION II | *Community-Based Program Development*

3. Construct "dummy" tables or charts to help visualize how the information collected might be organized and summarized to show results.
4. Make a list of all the information needed.
5. Develop a time line or work schedule for the remaining steps (6 to 11).
6. Identify the data collection techniques that are appropriate and feasible for the information needed (e.g., assessments, surveys, medical records, reports, questionnaires, observations, tests, interviews, etc.).
7. Identify sources of existing data that may be used, existing tools or instruments for data collection, and instruments that need to be developed.
8. Develop and test needed instruments.
9. Establish a data collection plan, including what will be collected, when, and by whom (this should be incorporated into the overall program time line).
10. Establish a data analysis plan, including time lines and responsible parties.
11. Develop a plan for disseminating the results, such as presentations, program reports, and papers. (Green & Kreuter, 1991; Dignan & Carr, 1992).

Programs can be evaluated at one or more of three levels:

1. Process,
2. Impact, and
3. Outcome.

Each level asks different questions, addresses different aspects of the program, and considers different indicators, as shown in Table 5-6. Note that, in this taxonomy, **impact** refers to the intermediate effects and **outcome** to the long-term effects of a program or process (Green & Kreuter, 2005). Others have delineated two levels of program evaluation: **formative** or **process evaluation,** which focuses on program development, and **summative evaluation,** which focuses on program results.

Evaluation designs range from simple to complex. The decision about the level and depth of evaluation to undertake is based on a number of factors, including the program's objectives, time, money, and expertise available, and management or funding agency priorities. Process evaluation, which should be done on every program, tends to be the least complex. As one moves along the continuum to measure the impact and outcome of a program, evaluation becomes more complex and costly in terms of time, money, and expertise

Table 5-6 Characteristics of and Distinctions Among the Levels of Program Evaluation

Level of Evaluation	What Is Being Evaluated	Time Frame for Evaluation	Outcome of Evaluation
Process	Program processes and procedures	Short-term—during and immediately following intervention	Feedback on program implementation (planned versus actual), audience participation and response, quality and appropriateness of materials, resources expended, staff response, etc.
Impact	Program objecttives	Intermediate—end of program and periodically thereafter	Feedback on changes in knowledge, attitude, behavior, and/or performance of participants; changes in environment; policies enacted, etc.
Outcome	Program goals	Long term—varies, depending on issue; may be years	Feedback on changes in health status—morbidity, mortality, disability, and quality of life

Data from: Dignan, M. B., and Carr, P. A. (1992). *Program planning for health education and health promotion* (2nd ed.). Philadelphia: Lea and Febiger. Green, L. W., and Kreuter, M. W. (1991). *Health promotion and planning: An educational and environmental approach* (2nd ed.). Mountain View, CA: Mayfield. Simons-Morton, B. G., Greene, W. H., and Gottlieb, N. H. (1995). *Introduction to health education and health promotion.* Prospect Heights, IL: Waveland.

required. Program evaluation strategies and designs are described in more detail in Chapter 7.

Planning With Evidence

Community-based programs should be developed, implemented, and evaluated using appropriate theoretical frameworks and program planning models applying principles of scientific reasoning (Brownson, Baker, Leet, & Gillespie, 2003; Glanz & Rimer, 2005). Program planning begins with the best evidence available. **Evidence** can be defined as data that informs decision making. Evidence is rarely constant; it is always emergent. The best available evidence of yesterday may be totally irrelevant today. Evidence may be quantitative, or numeric, and qualitative in the form of narrative. **Evidence-based planning for health** is the "application of the best available information derived from clinical, epidemiological, administrative, demographic and other relevant sources and consultations to clearly describe current and desired outcomes for an identified population or organization" (Ardal, Butler, Edwards, & Lawrie, 2006, p. 1). Epidemiological and demographic data is information about a population usually derived from a census or survey. Administrative data is information about services provided and the activities of the health care system. Consultation with experts can be a source of evidence. Expert opinion should be sought when formulating questions, identifying sources of information and evidence, and interpreting the findings (Ardal et al., 2006).

There is no single type of evidence that is most useful for planning health interventions. The type of information needed varies depending on the stage of the planning process. Decisions about program goals, objectives, and strategies should be based on established best practice, and interventions developed should have demonstrated effectiveness through research. Effectiveness means that the intervention chosen has better results than the alternatives, including no intervention.

The World Health Organization has developed five criteria for evaluating the quality of evidence. These are:

- proven validity of measurement instruments
- quantified reliability of measurement instruments

- comparability of measures over time and within populations
- an explicit data trail that clearly identifies how data was obtained and analyzed
- consultation with relevant experts and authorities to understand and accurately interpret the data (Murray & Evans, 2003).

According to Ardal et al. (2006), "an evidence base that has proven validity, quantified reliability, comparability, consultation with experts and an explicit data audit trail should lead to a plan that is valid, coherent and applicable" (p. 14). A plan is valid when the information and evidence gathered address relevant planning questions. A coherent plan is explains the differences in data and conclusions in a way that can be understood. A plan is applicable if it identifies how change can be measured, provides information that informs decision makers, and captures relevant situational realities.

Framing questions clearly is key to locating and using the right evidence. Finding and evaluating evidence can be time-intensive and requires some research expertise. **Systematic reviews** are often the most useful as they identify, assess, and synthesize research evidence from a number of individual research studies. A variety of sources of systematic reviews of research exist, some of which are listed in Box 5-2. Utilizing a range of information types and sources will create a comprehensive picture of the phenomenon of interest that results in a solid evidence base from which to make decisions and plan for the future.

Conclusion

To further establish the role of occupational therapy practitioners in community health, health promotion, and injury/disease prevention, more studies are needed to identify the occupational factors that affect health and well-being and to document the effectiveness of occupation-based community health and health promotion interventions. By being skilled in the steps of program development, from preplanning to publication, occupational therapy practitioners can strengthen their position in the provision of health education and health promotion programs and increase their marketability in the evolving health care arena.

Box 5-2 **Sources of Systematic Literature Reviews and Other Evidence**

- Best Practice Initiative (www.osophs.dhhs.gov/ophs/BestPractice)
- Campbell Collaboration Library (www.campbellcollaboration.org/library)
- Centers for Disease Control and Prevention (CDC) Recommends: The Prevention Guidelines System (www.phppo.cdc.gov/cdcRecommends/AdvSearchV.asp)
- Centers for Medicare and Medicaid Services (CMS) Healthy Aging Initiative- Evidence Reports (www.cms.hhs.gov/healthyaging/evidreports.asp)
- Clinical Evidence (www.clinicalevidence.bmj.com)
- Cochrane Collaboration (www.cochrane.org)
- ERIC Digests (www.eric.ed.gov)
- Evidence-Based Mental Health (www.ebmh.bmj.com)
- Joanna Briggs Institute Clinical Online Network of Evidence for Care and Therapeutics/JBI COnNECT (www.jbiconnect.org)
- National Guidelines Clearinghouse (www.guideline.gov)
- National Rehabilitation Information Center (www.naric.com)
- OT Seeker (www.otseeker.com)
- Substance Abuse and Mental Health Services Administration (www.samhsa.gov)
- The Community Guide (www.thecommunityguide.org/library)
- What Works Clearinghouse (www.whatworks.ed.gov)

Learning Activities

1. You have been contracted to provide occupational therapy services to children in a rural daycare setting. Many of the single, teenaged mothers have sought your advice on parenting. The day care manager has secured funding to develop a parenting class and has hired you to develop and implement the program. What steps would you take to assess need? Who would you involve? What questions would you want answered?

2. Write a goal, two learning objectives, and two behavioral objectives for this program.

3. How would you use occupational therapy constructs to shape an intervention strategy for the teen mothers?

4. For the same program, describe possible interventions at each of the five societal levels.

5. List several specific pieces of data you would collect to conduct a process evaluation of your program. Describe how you would record the data.

REFERENCES

AMC Cancer Research Center. (1994). *Beyond the brochure: Alternative approaches to effective health education.* CDC Cooperative Agreement U50/CCU806186–04.

American Occupational Therapy Association. (2006). *Accreditation Standards for a Master's-Degree-Level Educational Program for the Occupational Therapist.* Retrieved from http://aota.org/Educate/Accredit/StandardsReview/guide/Masters.aspx?FT=.msword

Ardal, S., Butler, J., Edwards, R., & Lawrie, L. (2006). Evidence-based planning: Module 3 in *The health planner's toolkit.* Ontario, Canada: Health System Intelligence Project.

Baker, E. A., & Brownson, C. A. (1998). Defining characteristics of community-based health promotion programs. *Journal of Public Health Management and Practice, 4*(2), 1–9.

Baum, C. (2006). Presidential address, 2006 Centennial challenges, millennium opportunities. *American Journal of Occupational Therapy, 60*(6), 609–616.

Breckon, D. J., Harvey, J. R., & Lancaster, R. B. (1994). *Community health education: Settings, roles, and skills for the 21st century.* Gaithersburg, MD: Aspen.

Brownson, C. A. (1998). Funding community practice: Stage 1. *American Journal of Occupational Therapy, 52*(1), 60–64.

Brownson, R. C., Baker, E. A., Leet, T. L., & Gillespie, K. N. (2003). *Evidence-based public health.* New York: Oxford University Press.

Butterfoss, F. D., Goodman, R. M., & Wandersman, A. (1993). Community coalitions for prevention and health promotion. *Health Education and Research Theory and Practice, 8*(3), 315–330.

Butterfoss, F. D., Kegler, M. C., & Francisco, V. T. (2008). Mobilizing organizations for health promotion: Theories of organizational change. In K. Glanz, B. Rimer, & K. Viswanth (Eds.), *Health behavior and health education: Theory, research, and practice* (4th ed., pp. 335–362). San Francisco: Jossey-Bass.

Choo, C. W. (2001). Environmental scanning as information seeking and organizational learning. *Information Research, 7*(1). Retrieved from http://InformationR.net/ir/7-1/paper112.html

Dignan, M. B., & Carr, P. A. (1992). *Program planning for health education and health promotion* (2nd ed.). Philadelphia: Lea and Febiger.

Eng, E., & Young, R. (1992). Lay health advisors as community change agents. *Family and Community Health, 151,* 24–40.

Fazio, L. S. (2008). *Developing occupation-centered programs for the community.* Upper Saddle River, NJ: Pearson, Prentice Hall.

Finnegan, Jr., J. R., & Viswanath, K. (2008). Communication theory and health behavior change: The media studies framework. In K. Glanz, B. Rimer, & K. Viswanth (Eds.), *Health behavior and health education: Theory, research, and practice* (4th ed., pp. 363–383). San Francisco: Jossey-Bass.

Freudenberg, N., Eng, E., Flay, B., Parcel, G., Rogers, T., & Wallerstein, N. (1995). Strengthening individual and community capacity to prevent disease and promote health: In search of relevant theories and principles. *Health Education Quarterly, 22*(3), 290–306.

Glanz, K., Rimer, B., & Viswanath, K. (Eds.). (2008). *Health behavior and health education: Theory, research, and practice* (4th ed.). San Francisco: Jossey-Bass.

Glanz, K., & Rimer, B. K. (2005). *Theory at a glance: A guide for health promotion practice* (2nd ed.). National Cancer Institute, U.S. Department of Health and Human Services, National Institutes of Health.

Goodman, R. M., Steckler, A., & Kegler, M. (1997). In K. Glanz, F. M. Lewis, and B. Rimer (Eds.), *Health behavior and health education: Theory, research, and practice* (2nd ed., pp. 287–312). San Francisco: Jossey-Bass.

Green, L. W. (1980). *Health education planning: A diagnostic approach.* Mountain View, CA: Mayfield.

Green, L. W., & Kreuter, M. W. (1991). *Health promotion and planning: An educational and environmental approach* (2nd ed.). Mountain View, CA: Mayfield.

Green, L. W., & Kreuter, M. W. (2005). *Health promotion and planning: An educational and ecological approach* (4th ed.). Mountain View, CA: Mayfield.

Heany, C. A., & Israel, B. A. (2008). Social networks and social support. In K. Glanz, F. M. Lewis, & B. Rimer (Eds.). *Health behavior and health education: Theory, research, and practice* (2nd ed.). San Francisco: Jossey-Bass.

Johnson, J. A., & Jaffe, E. J. (Eds.). (1989). *Occupational therapy: Program development for health promotion and prevention services.* New York: Haworth.

Krueger, R. A. (2009). *Focus groups: A practical guide for applied research* (4th ed.). Thousand Oaks, CA: Sage.

Lakein, A. (1989). How to get control of your time and your life. New York: Signet.

Law, M., Cooper, B. A., Strong, S., Stewart, D., Rigby, P., & Letts, L. (1997). Theoretical contexts for the practice of occupational therapy. In C. H. Christiansen & C. M. Baum (Eds.), *Occupational therapy: Enabling function and well-being* (2nd ed., pp. 73–102). Thorofare, NJ: SLACK.

McKillip, J. (1987). *Need analysis: Tools for the human services and education.* Newbury Park, CA: Sage.

Minkler, M., & Wallerstein, N. (1997). Improving health through community organization and community build-ing. In K. Glanz, F. M. Lewis, & B. Rimer (Eds.), *Health behavior and health education: Theory, research, and practice* (2nd ed., pp. 241–269). San Francisco: Jossey-Bass.

Minkler, M., Wallerstein, N., & Wilson, N. (2008). Improving health through community organization and community building. In K. Glanz, B. Rimer, & K. Viswanth (Eds.), *Health behavior and health education: Theory, research, and practice* (4th ed., pp. 287–312). San Francisco: Jossey-Bass.

Murray, C., & Evans, D. (2003). *Health system performance assessment, debates, methods & empiricism.* Geneva, Switzerland: World Health Organization.

Office of Cancer Communications. (1992). *Making health communications work: A planner's guide.* U.S. Department of Health and Human Services, National Cancer Institute, NIH Publication No. 92-1493.

Oldenburg, B., & Glanz, K. (2008). Diffusions of innovation. In K. Glanz, B. Rimer, & K. Viswanth (Eds.), *Health behavior and health education: Theory, research, and practice* (4th ed., pp. 313–333). San Francisco: Jossey-Bass.

Posavac, E., & Carey, R. (1997). *Program evaluation: Methods and case studies* (5th ed.). Upper Saddle River, NJ: Prentice Hall.

Ritzer, G. (2007). *Blackwell Encyclopedia of Sociology.* Retrieved from http://blackwellreference.com/public/book?id=g97814051 24331_yr2010_9781405124331

Rowel, R., Moore, N. D., Nowrojee, S., Memiah, P., & Bronner, Y. (2005). The utility of the environmental scan for public health practice: Lessons from an urban program to increase cancer screening. *Journal of the National Medical Association, 97*(4), 527–534.

Rutgers Cooperative Extension. (2007). Ten easy steps to program impact evaluation. Retrieved from http://nacaa.com/ampic/2007/presentations/ten_easy_ste ps_to_program_impact_evaluation.pdf

Scaffa, M. E., Reitz, S. M., & Pizzi, M. A. (2010). *Occupational therapy in the promotion of health and wellness.* Philadelphia: F.A. Davis.

Simons-Morton, B. G., Greene, W. H., & Gottlieb, N. H. (1995). *Introduction to health education and health promotion.* Prospect Heights, IL: Waveland.

Soriano, F. I. (1995). *Conducting needs assessments: A multidisciplinary approach.* Thousand Oaks, CA: Sage.

Storey, J. D., Saffitz, G. B., & Rimón, J. G. (2008). Social marketing. In K. Glanz, B. Rimer, & K. Viswanth (Eds.), *Health behavior and health education: Theory, research, and practice* (4th ed., pp. 435–464). San Francisco: Jossey-Bass.

Timmreck, T. C. (1995). *Planning, program development, and evaluation.* Boston: Jones and Bartlett.

van Ryn, M., & Heaney, C. A. (1992). What's the use of theory? *Health Education Quarterly, 19*(3), 315–330.

Wallack, L., Dorfman, L., Jernigan, D., & Themba, M. (1993). *Media advocacy and public health: Power for prevention.* Newbury Park, CA: Sage.

Witkin, B. R., & Altschuld, J. W. (1995). *Planning and conducting needs assessments: A practical guide.* Thousand Oaks, CA: Sage.

Chapter 6

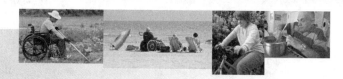

Program Design and Implementation

Joy D. Doll, OTD, OTR/L

Never doubt that a small group of thoughtful committed people can change the world. Indeed, it is the only thing that ever has.

—Margaret Meade

Learning Objectives

This chapter is designed to enable the reader to:
- Identify and discuss similarities and differences between intervention planning for individuals and the development of community-based programs.
- Describe the best practices to use in the development of a mission statement.
- Describe the characteristics of an effective team and the stages of team development.
- Identify and discuss issues related to program sustainability.

Key Terms

Advisory board
Board of directors
Direct costs
Goal
Grant
Indirect costs
Mission statement

Objective
Partnership
Sliding scale
SMART
Sustainability
Team
Vision statement

Introduction

Occupational therapists develop individualized intervention plans for their clients every day. Using clinical reasoning, the practitioner is able to determine which activities will enable clients to reach their goals. In community practice settings, the occupational therapy practitioner utilizes these same skills and applies them in the context of a community. Designing and implementing a program requires a similar thought process using reasoning skills to develop goals and objectives to implement a program. Many of the skills from practice with individuals can transfer to community practice. Yet,

program development requires an occupational therapy practitioner to use a systems approach instead of the traditional individual patient model (Fazio, 2008).

A general overview of program development and the needs assessment process was provided in Chapter 5. Details regarding developing a mission statement and an implementation plan with goals and objectives are shared in this chapter. Strategies for recruiting participants, developing teams, and establishing partnerships are reviewed. In addition, recommendations for budgeting, program management, and program sustainability are presented. The strategies described in this chapter utilize a systems approach based on the *Occupational Therapy Practice Framework* (American Occupational Therapy Association [AOTA], 2008) and clinical reasoning models.

Mission Statement

At this point in the process of developing and implementing a program, the occupational therapist should have a clear understanding of the community and the type of program that should be developed. The practitioner should review needs assessment data to ensure that the program has a clear focus. Often program planners will compose a vision statement prior to the development of a mission statement. A **vision statement** outlines the "ideal state or ultimate level of achievement to which an organization aspires" (Strickland, 2011, p. 103). A **mission statement** is "an organization's core, underlying purpose, or basis for its existence, focus and actions" (Strickland, 2011, p. 103). Companies and organizations utilize mission statements to guide employees in an overall plan and to make consumers aware of the purpose of the company. A mission statement goes beyond simply educating workers and consumers; it acts as the driving force or motivation behind decisions, actions, and program development. Mission statements also imply future direction, indicating what the program hopes to accomplish over time (Ohio Literacy Resource Center, 2007). When an organization is working in the community, the mission statement should be collective and inclusive of those the program will serve. Including community members in developing the mission statement is one strategy to insure buy-in to a program both at its inception and in the future.

The challenge to developing a mission statement is to describe a program and its values, purpose, and future direction in a few short sentences. In creating a mission statement, the occupational therapy practitioner can follow these best practices.

1. *Do some research.* The occupational therapy practitioner and any team members assisting in developing the mission statement should begin with finding current mission statements of organizations that the practitioner admires or believes are easy to understand. Mission statements can easily be found on Web sites or in company materials. For nonprofit organizations, the practitioner may want to explore existing mission statements of other non-profits as a starting point. The United Way can be a useful resource for identifying local nonprofit organizations.

2. *A mission statement is not a résumé repeated.* Its purpose is not to provide accolades to past successes or identify the reasons why the program was started. Instead, the mission statement should focus on the values and the premise of the program.

3. *Avoid emptiness.* A mission statement devoid of values lacks substance. The mission statement should be thoughtful and meaningful. It should elicit feelings of passion and offers an opportunity to articulate that passion for the program to others and those being served.

4. *Keep it short.* Mission statements should be a brief snapshot that captures the essence of the program or organization. Ideal mission statements are captured in a few easily recalled sentences.

5. *Be discipline-specific.* Professional identities guide values and are certainly relevant to the mission statement. The only caution here is to avoid jargon that might confuse people not familiar with occupational therapy terminology.

6. *Write clearly and concisely.* The occupational therapy practitioner should consider the literacy level of the audience when drafting the mission statement. Careful editing is important, as grammatical and syntax errors in the mission statement can detract from the program and its purpose.

7. *Ask others.* One of the best strategies to developing a good mission statement is to seek advice and feedback. This advice can come from peers or community members. Seeking feedback ensures that others understand the intent of the program, which is the ultimate goal of the mission statement. The occupational therapy practitioner can ask others the following questions to help them evaluate the mission statement:
   (a) Does the mission statement reveal the values of the program?
   (b) What future direction does this mission statement indicate for this program?

(c) Does the mission statement inspire? Why or why not?

Answers to these questions can provide feedback on the clarity and relevance of a mission statement.

8. *Do not settle.* Continue to revise the mission statement until all parties are satisfied and passionate about it (Voltz-Doll, 2008). When designing a program, it is important to be thoughtful about a mission statement as it is often one of the first aspects program participants may view. Furthermore, since the mission statement is included in reports and grant proposals, it needs to be representative of the program. Taking the time to ensure the mission statement clearly reflects the program can aid the program's sustainability.

Following the aforementioned best practices will aid the occupational therapy practitioner in developing a relevant and meaningful mission statement for the program. After the mission statement has been established, the next step in program design is to develop an implementation plan that includes the program goals, objectives, and activities.

Implementation Plan

Traditionally, when designing and implementing a program, the occupational therapy practitioner considers what will make the program work and also be sustainable. This thought process aids in the development of a structured and relevant implementation plan. An implementation plan includes the goals, objectives, activities, and desired outcomes of the program. The plan should also identify:

- who will be served by the program
- how the individuals being served will be recruited

Program qualifications should also be included that describe how and why an individual qualifies for the program and how an individual enters the program once qualification is determined.

Development of an implementation plan is important to identify specifically how program goals and objectives will be realized. The plan provides a holistic approach for identifying the program's purpose, program design, and implementation in one succinct document. According to Brownson, an implementation plan "spells out the details of the program and specifies who is responsible for each procedure and activity" (2001, p. 115). In the implementation plan, the details of who, what, when, where, and how need to be finalized for the program (Brownson, 2001; Chambless, 2003). The implementation plan usually contains a time line and persons responsible to address these goals to reach the program outcomes. An implementation plan allows the practitioner to map out the entire program in an effective and pragmatic manner. After completion, the implementation plan can be distributed to employees or even used for writing future grant proposals. Effective implementation plans help to ensure program success and sustainability. Table 6-1 outlines a sample program implementation plan.

Program implementation also requires thoughtful planning in order to maintain focus and ensure that activities are completed in a timely manner (Timmreck, 2003). Many organizations now use strategic planning for program implementation. Strategic planning is a common method, and facilitators with expertise in strategic planning can be hired to assist with the process. Ideally, implementation planning should be completed in a group environment to promote communication among team members, especially if a program is new and in development. Implementation planning provides an opportunity to clarify who will do what and when it will be done. Creating a document that outlines program activities ensures that all team members stay on track, communication flows smoothly, and the program goals and objectives are completed in an efficient manner. Implementation planning also allows the program team to plan and anticipate challenges in a proactive manner, which can impact program success and sustainability (Timmreck, 2003).

Program Goals and Objectives

In program development, a **goal** is defined as "a statement of a quantifiable desired future state or condition" (Timmreck, 2003, p. 32). Goals are written to be long-term and future-oriented, indicating a desired outcome (Brownson, 2001). Goals capture intended outcomes of the program, while objectives are more specific, identifying how goals will be met. **Objectives** are measurable, short-term, and usually contain a time

Table 6-1 Sample Implementation Plan

Objectives	Intervention Activities	Measurement Activities to Determine Outcomes	Short-Term Outcomes	Long-Term Outcomes
Describe scopes of practice by the end March	• Article on what constitutes scopes of practice • Internet research on licensing parameters for nurses / pharmacist/ physician • Simulated patient scenario where providers must refer to another professional • Interdisciplinary care plan	(a) Written exam (b) Care plan	(a) Knowledge of scope of practice/ pharmacist/ physician/ nurse with 95% accuracy (b) Utilization of team resource on care plan per "scopes rubric"	Increased confidence in referral to another professional
Develop a marketable educational module focusing on interprofessional ad hoc team function by the end of May	• Develop a marketing plan	(a) Count the number of courses using the material (b) Count the number of learners using the material	Modules incorporated into the curricula of medicine, nursing, pharmacy	Modules used in all schools at university
Develop and validate measurement tools related to individual professional performance	• Develop the instrument • Pilot the instrument with sufficient numbers to generate power to do measurement study	Conduct reliability study on instrument (e.g., item analysis, factor loading)	Obtain a reliability factor of X	Publish the instrument

Data from: Goulet, C. G., Begley, K., Gould, K., & Doll, J. D. (2008). *Interdisciplinary Team Skills Development for Health Professional Students.* Association for Prevention and Teaching. Awarded October 2008.

line for completion (Brownson, 2001; Timmreck, 2003). Goals and objectives are different but complementary. Goals and objectives should indicate the program's priorities, the program's intended outcomes, the communities' priorities, and the evaluation plan. A program can have multiple outcomes but should have a defined focus and prioritize the outcomes. Too many goals and objectives can make a program appear incoherent and disconnected, and poses challenges to successful completion. Drafting goals and objectives that are difficult to achieve makes a program appear disjointed and infeasible, which impacts program sustainability and the ability to garner support for the program, especially financially.

Occupational therapists are familiar with goal and objective writing related to intervention planning, but writing goals and objectives for a program requires a different perspective. Writing goals and objectives for a community program requires occupational therapy practitioners to think broadly and envision an overall outcome. In medical model patient care, the focus of goals is to enhance the well-being of an individual. In program planning for community practice, however, the focus is population-based, identifying how an intervention impacts a group of individuals (Edberg, 2007). In community settings, occupational therapists need an expanded thought process that incorporates a population-based approach. Although this aspect of goal writing can be challenging, the process of goal writing is similar to that in other practice areas, just applied more broadly.

The mnemonic SMART can aid in writing appropriate program objectives. **SMART** stands for:

S = Specific,
M = Measurement,
A = Attainable,
R = Relevant, and
T = Timely.

Program objectives should be specific to the program, identifying a measurable outcome. It is important that objectives are attainable and feasible considering time lines, resources, and staffing. Goals and objectives should also be developed with the targeted population to be served in mind and with a focus on the community needs gathered in the assessment. Written goals and objectives should align with community needs and wants to ensure success in meeting these goals and objectives. This concept follows the occupational therapy principle of client-centered practice applied to a program model (Brownson, 2001; Law, 1998). Goals and objectives that focus on community needs facilitate community buy-in and programmatic success. The SMART approach is useful not only when drafting objectives but also when evaluating the match between objectives and program activities (Weis & Gantt, 2004).

After drafting the goals and objectives, specific activities should be designed that address the goals and objectives. The program activities are specifically what will be done and the day-to-day activities of a program. Similar to therapeutic activities used to reach client goals, program activities are meant to achieve the desired program outcomes.

Another essential component of program planning beyond the goals and objectives is to identify programmatic roles. In the planning stage, the details of who will complete the program roles and responsibilities may not need to be identified, but thought should be given to potential roles and responsibilities required to make the program a success. Drafting job descriptions for both employees and volunteers provides program structure and ensures successful implementation. Time lines should also be discussed and developed.

Including all of these aspects in the implementation plan will ensure a stable and sustainable program design. Such a plan guides implementation and ensures that the program remains aligned with its mission and purpose. The implementation plan can be tied clearly to the evaluation plan and used to aid in garnering funds, such as grants. The plan should be dynamic and flexible enough to change but sufficiently stable to act as a road map for program implementation.

Participant Recruitment

A key aspect of successful implementation is the recruitment of program participants. Recruitment and retention of program participants must be considered in the planning process and is crucial in program design. Inattention to this step can negatively impact the use and success of the program, and ultimately not meet the community's needs. Establishing referrals requires the development of protocols and roles for each person involved in the program (Braveman, 2001). The development of policies and procedures for staff was already discussed; however, a policy and procedure should also be developed for recruitment of program participants. The recruitment and referral policy and procedure outline how community members will access and benefit from the services. If there are requirements or stipulations for admission to the program, these need to be identified. The target population should have been identified in the program development stage. Here, the practitioner is planning how to recruit participants, including qualifiers for program participation and marketing to potential clients.

In some cases, this step may require developing a marketing plan to identify methods for recruitment. The marketing plan may be referred to as a community awareness campaign depending on the program and target audience. Whatever the title, the marketing of services needs to be considered in the program design. When marketing, the occupational therapy practitioner should consider all necessary venues and utilize community resources such as partners, advisory boards, coalitions and community members, and participants. In the marketing plan development process, the occupational therapy practitioner should take into account the services being provided, who will benefit from these services, and who needs to know about the services (Braveman, 2001). For example, a nonprofit that offers a health equipment recycling program provides used health equipment to individuals in need. The main targets for marketing of this program are social workers, physical therapy practitioners, and occupational therapy practitioners. These individuals refer many clients who cannot receive health equipment through insurance and have been a successful target audience for the organization (Doll, 2009). Marketing or community awareness should be a thoughtful process because without customers, the program will not be a success.

Location and Space Issues

In addition to marketing and recruitment of program participants, location and space for program implementation are also issues to be addressed in program development (Braveman, 2001). For some, these will not be issues because the program is part of a larger organization that will donate or loan space for the program implementation. This is the case for a program implemented in a hospital practice setting where meeting rooms may be available for a community outreach program. Often these spaces will be free of charge if a case can be made to administrators that the program benefits the institution. Program managers may need to make a formal request for such space and should follow the policies of the institution with which they partner.

When designing a program, space and location are critical factors. If a paid space is necessary, it will be important for the occupational therapy practitioner to consider this when budgeting and determining program costs. The program manager will need to work with a realtor to find an appropriate space and location for the program. Collaborating with other institutions in the community may also be of benefit, allowing for shared costs of space.

For example, faith communities may be willing to donate space for health programming that benefits their constituents and the greater community (Swinney, Anson-Wonkka, Maki, & Corneau, 2001). Local nonprofit agencies may also be willing to share space or provide space at a reduced cost in exchange for lower fees for participants or just as goodwill to the community. Organizations that donate space can identify this as an in-kind donation, which may be of benefit to the organization. If lobbying an organization for space at a free or reduced cost, the occupational therapy practitioner should consider the benefits to the organization and be able to articulate them clearly. If necessary, a memorandum of understanding or a formal contract may need to be drafted to establish an agreement about space and its use.

When considering space for implementing a program, the program manager has to consider the needs of program participants. The program manager should consider liability issues, accessibility for participants, and the regulations and use of the space depending on program needs. Related to liability, insurance to cover the facility is important and should be included in the program budget. For program success, accessibility to the location and space are important. When considering accessibility, the occupational therapy practitioner needs to consider the program participants (Gitlow & Flecky, 2005). For example, if program participants are not able to drive, then considering a location close to public transportation is important. Beyond access to public transportation, the occupational therapy practitioner needs to consider accessibility to the space including ramps, elevators, accessible entrances, parking availability, and lighting. Locations such as faith communities may not be as accessible as other public facilities, so it is important to consider these factors when choosing a location for the program. Last, maintaining the space is important to consider in program planning. For example, if the space needs regular, professional cleaning, then this will need to be considered in the budget during program planning. Each location and space will come with regulations, and it is important to consider these in planning and in budgeting. Furthermore, the amount of time the space will be used is important to consider. In initial stages or with program growth, a change of space and location may be needed. It is important to consider the impact of such a change on both participants and program implementation.

Where to implement a program also will depend on the needs of the program and should be given thoughtful consideration during the planning process. Once a program has been implemented, challenges with space and location may arise that need to be considered. One method for strategizing is to build an assessment of the space and location into the program evaluation plan to continually assess the benefits and challenges of the place and location for the program.

Supplies and Equipment

Each program will have a need for unique supplies and equipment. During program planning, brainstorming a list of supplies and equipment is critical to ensure the program has what is required for successful implementation (Brownson, 2001; Fazio, 2008). Most programs require similar basic needs, such as computers and office supplies. However, programs will require specific supplies and equipment based on program demands. For example, in a grant-funded program using sensory rooms for suicide prevention for Native American youth, funds were used to purchase equipment to develop the sensory rooms along with basic office supplies.

Garnering supplies and equipment may be similar to garnering funds. Supplies may be donated, or equipment may already be purchased by an organization that will allow its use by a program. Otherwise, in the program development phase, the needed supplies and equipment will have to be identified and included in the budget.

Staffing and Personnel

The greatest resource of any program is the staff who make the program a success (Timmreck, 2003). When developing a program, it is important to consider what staffing and personnel are needed for successful program implementation. It is important to recognize that what is ideal for a program may not be feasible, and staff may be responsible for multiple roles. An occupational therapy practitioner may play many roles in a community setting. For a small program, the occupational therapy practitioner may be the program manager and the program evaluator. In a larger program, staff may be hired for specific roles in program management. It is important to analyze what staff members are needed for the program to be successful. If the program has a large budget, then a bookkeeper will be critical to help maintain records. Administrative and support staff may also be of benefit to help with appointments or with basic administrative tasks. If traditional occupational therapy services are offered and billing is necessary, then a staff member trained in billing and coding may be necessary. If the program experiences growth, then more staff may be needed.

Along with identifying and hiring staff, it will be important to set up an infrastructure for evaluating staff in order to ensure that personnel are successful in their ability to engage in their roles to make the program run smoothly. Staff members should be clear on expectations and their role in any paid or volunteer position. Performance review is important to ensure staff members are functioning in the way appropriate to the program (Family Planning Management Development, 1998).

One way to clearly define staff roles is to develop job descriptions. Job descriptions have multiple purposes; they can be used for hiring, employee orientation, employee supervision and performance review, and salary considerations. A job description traditionally includes the job title, supervisor, summary of the job duties, and the qualifications needed for the job. When developing job descriptions, the occupational therapy practitioner should start with the mission statement, which helps identify what values and goals are desired in employees. A potential job should be analyzed to identify the qualifications needed of a potential hire (Family Planning Management Development, 1998). Many samples of job descriptions exist on the Internet and can serve as a template for developing appropriate job descriptions for a program.

If paid staffing is not an option, volunteers may be another choice in helping to implement a program. The use of volunteers in program implementation is a popular model to leverage resources and build social capital for a program's success (Finlayson, Baker, Rodman, & Herzberg, 2002).

In academic-community partnerships, service-learning has been demonstrated as one approach that uses student volunteers to help with program implementation (Gitlow & Flecky, 2010). Programs can also tap into other volunteer programs like SeniorCorp or AmeriCorp to garner volunteers to aid in program implementation (Simon, 2002; Simon & Wang, 2002).

Compliance With Practice Regulations

As an occupational therapy practitioner, it is important to consider practice regulations. If using occupational therapy skills to design and implement the program, it is critical that the practitioner follow practice guidelines, including the differentiation of roles between the occupational therapist and occupational therapy assistant. Programs must fall within the occupational therapy scope of practice (AOTA, 2010b) and always follow the *Occupational Therapy Code of Ethics and Ethics Standards 2010* (AOTA, 2010a). If an occupational therapy practitioner has questions about whether the programs falls within occupational therapy regulations, the state licensure board should be contacted in order to ensure the program is in compliance. In the case that the program is engaged in billing and coding for services, reimbursement regulations should be followed at all times.

Financing Options

Start-Up Costs

When beginning a program, it is important to consider how initial funds will be acquired (Braveman, 2001; Timmreck, 2003). Depending on the program, start-up costs will vary. Prior to exploring start-up costs, a well-defined budget should be developed and finalized. When considering start-up costs, it is important to consider what is needed to initiate the program and whether these costs will be initial or ongoing. If the program plans on making a profit, then a business loan is an appropriate option to consider. On the other hand, if the program plans on simply making enough funds to cover program costs, then other funding sources, such as a grant or donations, may be more appropriate.

Funding Sources

When considering how to fund a community program, it is important to consider multiple factors, including the following:

- What is the funding needed for?
- Whom does the program plan to serve?
- What funding amount is needed to sustain the program?

Multiple funding sources exist, including donations, sponsorships, grants, and fees-for-service.

Funding can come from multiple sources depending on the program. In some cases, an institution may offer a program and cover the costs in accordance with its mission to serve the community. For a small program, such as a yoga program offered by an outpatient facility, the costs may be minimal and an institution may be willing to cover the expense of marketing if the occupational therapy practitioner is willing to donate his or her time.

Grants are another source of funding for program support. A **grant** is essentially a sum of funds donated to an organization to cover the costs of a program (Doll, 2010). The recipient of funds is accountable to the funding agency and has to follow the guidelines set forth by it, which often include specific accountability and reporting of program challenges and successes. Grants are typically available only to non-profit agencies that are categorized with a tax identification of 501(c)(3). Grant funds are available from a variety of sources, including local and federal government agencies and foundations. Grants are also available in various amounts, from very small amounts (e.g., $500) to millions of dollars, depending on the funding agency. Program development grants are often a source to start a program and are not regarded as a sustainable source of funding to support ongoing program implementation.

Programs may also benefit from donations. Donors receive tax benefits when donating to a tax-exempt organization, so this fact should be emphasized when seeking donations. When soliciting donations, it is important to be very clear about the purpose of the funds and to target individuals or organizations that have a specific interest in the program or participants of the program. Fund-raising may be another method for seeking donations for a program. It is important to remember that fund-raising and seeking donations can be time-consuming, so this must be considered when program planning.

Sponsorships are another possibility for garnering funds for a program. Typically, corporations are more willing to sponsor events than sponsor a program. When seeking sponsorships, it is important to clearly designate what sponsor monies will cover and how they will benefit the program. Benefits to sponsors should be considered. For example, if a sponsor provides a certain amount of funds, then the sponsor may receive free advertising on the program's Web site. Sponsorships are another consideration as source for funding a program or program event.

Establishing Fees for Service

Fees for service are another method to support a program during implementation and should be properly planned and included in the budget (Grossman & Bortone, 1986). In a fee-structured program, participants are required to pay a fee for services. Fees need to be realistic based on what the community can afford and what services are being offered. The program team will need to complete a careful analysis of costs and develop a fair and reliable fee structure (Shediac-Rizkallah & Bone, 1998). Another consideration is how to address the differing abilities of program participants to pay for services. In this case, a sliding scale fee may be an appropriate method for addressing the socioeconomic needs across program participants. A **sliding scale** fee identifies a program payment based on a participant's income. When implementing a sliding scale fee, records of participants' incomes must be maintained, which requires additional record keeping and bookkeeping for the program as well as processes to ensure confidentiality.

Another option is to define a flat fee for program participants that covers program costs. To explore appropriate fees for a program, research should be conducted on what similar programs charge for similar services rendered. This information can be ascertained by contacting similar programs or exploring program fees on program Web sites. If the program offers a service similar to that offered by a local occupational therapy practice, the occupational therapy practitioner may consider charging the same or similar fees. But if the service differs from the local practice, then fees should be competitive with similar programming. Another approach is to consult with an accountant who can provide guidance on appropriate fees to charge. It is important not to have fees beyond the ability of program participants to pay, or that are not competitive with similar programming.

Fees for service should be clearly outlined for program participants. In program planning, the timing and payment requirements should be established. If adjustments in fees for service are needed, this must be clearly communicated to program participants with adequate time for participants to determine whether they want to continue to receive program services. A rationale for fee increases is often important to ensure that program participants understand the need for the change.

Budgeting

The budget is another important component of program design and implementation. When creating a budget, the occupational therapy practitioner should consider what resources are needed for program implementation. Financial planning and budgeting should be an annual practice for the program, and budgets should be constantly monitored to ensure the program's viability. The operating budget outlines the program's financial plans for revenue, including monies and resources that come into the program as well as operating expenses to be paid out of the program's budget (Weis & Gantt, 2004).

When developing a budget, a thorough analysis of costs and income should be calculated. After determining the costs and income, the next step is to consider the balance between the two to ensure that the program at least attains a zero balance or has reserves in place to pay additional expenses (Weis & Gantt, 2004). Budgets are planned for the upcoming year as well as a proposed plan of the income and expenses of the program . If a program is new, the expenses and income should be recorded for completing the annual budgets in subsequent years. Program budgets should be in constant flux, adjusting to the expenses and income.

Budgets usually consist of two major components: direct costs and indirect costs (Gitlin & Lyons, 2004). **Direct costs** are those items in the budget that will be funded by the program's income. Common direct program costs include salary, benefits, equipment, consultants, travel, etc. **Indirect costs** are those costs required to implement the program, including overhead and administrative costs (Weis & Gantt, 2004). Indirect costs are typically held to a certain percentage of the budget to ensure the program can run. Examples of indirect costs include but are not limited to "rental fees, payment of utilities, equipment depreciation, providing security, and general maintenance of workspace" (Ingersoll & Eberhard, 1999, p. 133).

Budgets can be simple or complex, based on the program. A novice in program design and implementation might want to seek external assistance with budgeting. Programs often pay auditors to aid them in determining fiscal viability on an annual basis. Financial advisors are another resource for help in developing and managing a program budget.

Team Development

Due to its complicated nature, community practice cannot be done in isolation. Community programs require a team approach, making it necessary to create a strong team (Fazio, 2008). Developing a team to implement the program is an important aspect of program design and facilitates successful implementation. Being strategic with team development ensures that the program's implementation is not hindered by miscommunication or mistrust among team members. In this situation, the occupational therapy practitioner may lead the team or become a member of a developing or existing team.

A **team** consists of "two or more individuals with a high degree of interdependence geared toward the achievement of a goal or the completion of a task" (White & West, 2008, p. 3). Teams make decisions, solve problems, develop a focus, and accomplish outcomes. In community practice, the team will include not only the occupational therapy practitioner and other experts but also community partners and community members. Using a team approach provides different perspectives on program design and implementation, enhances program success and sustainability, and expands expertise and resources (Ruhs, 2000).

Teams require time to develop, going through a life cycle of forming, storming, norming, and performing in order to become effective (Blue et al., 2008). In the forming stage, team members begin by getting to know one another and establishing goals for the team. Team members begin to explore what tasks they will undertake as part of the team. In the storming stage, team members begin to voice their opinions about the team and its proposed tasks. Dysfunction can occur at this stage as team members negotiate goals and team member roles. However, this negotiation process is normal for a successful and effective team.

During the norming stage, team members come to an agreement about the expectations for the team and its members. Trust begins to develop, and team roles become clearly defined. In the performing stage, the team is able to complete goals successfully and effectively. The team is able to work together without conflict towards the team's goals (Blue et al., 2008; Cole, 2005). The stages of team development are described in Table 6-2.

Key activities of a team include communication, decision making, delegation, and problem solving (White & West, 2008). These activities should be collectively accomplished in the collaborative

Table 6-2	The Life Cycle of Team Development (Blue et al., 2008)
Stage	**Process**
Forming	• Team members get to know one another • Establish goals and tasks for team
Storming	• Team members begin to voice opinions • Dysfunction can occur with arguments about goals or team member roles
Norming	• Agreement of the team expectations • Trust develops • Team roles become clearly understood
Performing	• Shared leadership among team members • Tasks are completed effectively and efficiently

Doll, J. D. (2010). *Grant writing and program development: Making the connection*. Boston, MA: Jones and Bartlett.

model of a team in order to successfully design and implement a community program. Yet, working in a team is challenging. According to Patrick Lencioni, author of the *Five Dysfunctions of a Team,* teams become dysfunctional when there is an absence of trust, fear of conflict, lack of commitment, and inattention to results (2002). These factors can destroy a team, which ultimately destroys a program or the ability to address a community need. The team should be aware of these challenges and develop plans to remedy them as they arise.

A program team will look different for each program, but having a collaborative and cooperative team can lead to success and ensure that the program operates successfully. When building a team, the occupational therapy practitioner needs to identify who must be involved and when these individuals must be involved (Brooks, 2006). In some cases, bringing people in too late can be detrimental to the team and ultimately to program implementation.

Next, the team members should collectively define their purpose and goals for the program (Blue et al., 2008). In this process, the team members will communicate and begin to build trust with one another. Team members should take time to identify what each brings to the group. This activity will help in building trust early and in delegation of activities later. Group process is an important component of a team's development (Cole, 2005). Occupational therapy practitioners can use their expertise in group processes to aid in team development and sustainability.

In a team or group setting, power is shared. When working in a community program, this is an especially important aspect to emphasize. In the case where community members may be working with educated health care professionals, community members may feel inadequate, leading to a lack of active participation. The team leader can identify the strengths and contributions of each member in initial team-building activities and publicly recognize members for what each brings to the effort (Israel, Eng, Schulz, & Parker, 2005). Teams should celebrate together. The focus of a team should be not only to address needs but also to celebrate when a challenge has been successfully tackled collectively. Taking the time to celebrate is crucial to ensuring

ongoing commitment and making team members feel rewarded for their participation.

Teams need ongoing development and care, especially if members of the team change (Holtzclaw, Kenner, & Walden, 2009). Group dynamics always come with challenges, but overcoming these challenges is possible. The processes of the team need to be clearly defined, including communication, decision making processes, and problem solving. One suggestion is to develop a dynamic team commitment where team members identify each of the processes for the team to be successful. In this commitment, all members of the team agree how the team and its members should function, ensuring buy-in and dispelling common team challenges. As a team changes and develops, the team must revisit its purpose and mission frequently to ensure success and effective outcomes (Blue et al., 2008).

Establishing Partnerships

In community practice, it is rare that a program occurs without connections to other similar or complementary programs. Besides building a team of individuals to implement the program, program design and implementation should include building community partnerships. Community partnerships are an effective method for developing successful community programming. **Partnerships** are entities "formed between two or more sectors to achieve a common goal that could not otherwise be accomplished separately" (Meade & Calvo, 2001, p. 1578). Partnerships also help with marketing and recruiting participants that may be connected with other programs.

Collaboration is the foundation for partnerships, and successful collaboration is fundamental to a partnership's success (Ansari, Phillips, & Hammick, 2001; Fazio, 2008). Occupational therapy practitioners already understand the concept of partnership as discussed in literature related to client-centered practice (Law, 1998). In these discussions, the practitioner is in partnership with the client to ensure the client's therapeutic goals are addressed (Law, 1998; Sumsion, 1999). Community partnerships maximize resources by utilizing the strengths of a mobilized group of people.

In many cases, one program alone cannot address a need, but in collaboration, community needs can be addressed more efficiently. Furthermore, partnerships created to address health-related issues can "aim to create a seamless system of relevant healthcare services for the community" (Meade & Calvo, 2001, p. 1578).

Partnerships form between groups or organizations. Occupational therapy practitioners can be involved in multiple ways in community partnerships through academic-community partnerships, community coalition membership, advisory board membership, non-profit board membership, or simply as members of the community. Community partnerships, in themselves, can be complicated to develop and maintain (Becker, Israel, & Allen, 2005). As with the development of any team, a significant investment is required to develop trust and relationships and face the challenges necessary to collaborate effectively (Becker et al., 2005). Research has shown that developing and maintaining partnerships takes time, commitment, and open communication to develop the mutual trust required for true exchange in a partnership (Burhansstipanov, Dignan, Wound, Tenney, & Vigil, 2000; Kagawa-Singer, 1997; LaMarca, Wiese, Pete, & Carbone, 1996; Poole & Van Hook, 1997). The occupational therapy practitioner included in collaboration will need to commit the time and problem solving abilities needed to be an effective community partner.

Partnerships can be very formal or very informal, depending on the partners involved, the community need, and the program. If partnerships are formal, then the partners may develop a strategic plan identifying goals and objectives for the partners based on the program's mission (Becker et al., 2005). Formal agendas and meeting minutes should be maintained to track partners' efforts. In some cases, this documentation may be part of a program's evaluation plan and may provide valuable information for a grant report. Granting agencies that require partnerships will want documentation of the success of the partners in reaching their goals.

Developing community partnerships requires commitment. Occupational therapy practitioners can play a critical role in community practice using their expertise in occupation (Fazio, 2008). However, it is important to remember that there are many aspects of developing a community partnership. Partnerships should be thoughtfully developed and maintained, especially if a community is underserved. And, once a partnership is developed, it needs to be maintained.

Program Management

Programs are important to the communities they serve. In order to sustain programs and ensure they meet community needs, community members should be actively involved in the program. When designing and implementing a program, the practitioner should consider how community members will be involved in monitoring the program. Advisory boards are a model for including the community in program implementation and maintenance.

An **advisory board** is a collection of community members who provide feedback to a program (MacQueen et al., 2001). These individuals may be community stakeholders and/or community members. The advisory board is a resource to the program team and connects the team with community members. Prior to convening an advisory board, time should be taken to establish the role of the advisory board, the goals of the advisory board, and a description of the role of members on the advisory board. Advisory boards usually consist of experts who know the community and the organization, so these individuals can make recommendations and guide the organization or program. An advisory board demonstrates quality assurance and that the organization is listening to the voice of the community. When inviting individuals to participate in an advisory board, the leader of the advisory board needs to ensure that participants are individuals who will provide constructive and critical feedback, and also have the time to devote to advisory board activities. Advisory boards typically do not meet often and do not require a significant amount of time, which is a benefit when recruiting members. Advisory boards are not the same as a board of directors used in a non-profit model and do not necessarily require the same level of formality (Weis & Gantt, 2004). In some cases, a program may have a board of directors and an advisory board, depending on the program needs.

A **board of directors** is a group of individuals who guide the organization in its mission, finances, and programming. Non-profit agencies follow a model of including a board of directors to aid them in planning and ensuring financial viability for the organization. Each board of directors has traditional officer roles, including president, vice president, treasurer, and secretary. Members of a board of directors are volunteers who have expertise and can aid the organization. The members of a board are fiscally responsible for the agency they support both in monetary donations and in expert guidance. Depending on his or her role in relation to the board, the manager should know how to work with the board and communicate with board members as necessary. An executive director of a non-profit organization will work directly with the board, keeping them informed on the organization's functioning and development.

Program Sustainability

A program's sustainability is crucial and should be part of the program design and implementation. Community programs are not meant to be static and are ever evolving (Shediac-Rizkallah & Bone, 1998). **Sustainability** is more than simply having the funding to continue a program and includes other factors that influence the program's ongoing success. Program sustainability in communities means going beyond program implementation to connect with the community and build capacity to engrain the program into the community (Edberg, 2007). Sustainable community programs are "endurable, livable, adaptable, and supportable" (Akerlund, 2000, p. 354).

Programs terminate for many reasons, including poor or inadequate planning for program sustainability, sustainability has not been a program priority, the community lacks buy-in or support for the program, or fiscal barriers exist, such as lack of funding or poor economic times. Major problems exist when a program lacks sustainability. In some underserved and diverse communities, mistrust of outside individuals and sometimes mistrust of health care in general are part of the community's dynamics. Developing a program that suddenly ends when grant funding ends sends a message to the community that the program was not really created for their benefit (Jensen & Royeen, 2001). These actions can

lead to further mistrust and difficulty in forging future partnerships.

When addressing significant health issues in communities, sustainability can appear nearly impossible due to barriers and lack of resources. Yet, sustainability is possible if programs are well designed and complement the community's needs and capacities (Akerlund, 2000). Successful approaches to sustainability include ongoing evaluation, ongoing service development, program modification to meet community needs and desires, effective program marketing, and use of capacity building approaches (Gaines, Wold, Bean, Brannon, & Leary, 2004).

Community programs also need to be flexible to be successful. Community programs should respond not only to community needs but also to social, economic, and environmental conditions that impact both the community and the program (Brennan, Baker, & Metzler, 2008). Community programs are developed to address community needs, and sustainability is more likely when services are modified as community needs and desires change.

When addressing program sustainability, the following factors should be considered: effectiveness of the program, the relationship with the community, anticipated duration of the program, funding, and staff expertise. Program effectiveness is determined through an evaluation plan. Evaluation results will reveal if the program is really worth continuing, responds to community needs, or requires changes to be effective. In the case that the program is ineffective or the need is short-term, then sustainability might not be relevant (Glaser, 1981).

The length of the program is an important factor to consider. With most health-related community issues, a short-term solution will not be viable (Edberg, 2007; Timmreck, 2003). If the plan is to sustain the program for the long term, then goals and objectives need to be put into place that promote and suggest sustainability. If sustainability has not been considered in initial program development, the program team may need to go back to the drawing board of basic program development and redevelop components of the program for the long term.

The expertise of program staff is a very important factor in sustainability, especially because sustainability infers that programs change according to the community. Having staff that are flexible and able to offer expertise in multiple areas related to community issues is important in maintaining a successful program. Involving stakeholders from the community or hiring community members to implement the program enhances this aspect (Edberg, 2007). If funding the salaries of staff is difficult, then the program may choose to move towards a volunteer model instead of funding positions. This strategy will depend on the program, the access to volunteers, and the community needs (Akerlund, 2000).

Obviously, funding plays a role in the ability of a program to sustain itself. Multiple strategies can be considered when exploring financial sustainability of a program. If a program is grant funded, it must remain sustainable either by garnering outside funds or by implementing a fee for services. If seeking funds from external sources, the program team will need to have a plan in place to either search for future grant funds or engage in fund-raising efforts. A cost-benefit analysis should be done to be able to demonstrate to funders and donors the impact of the program and its relevance to be sustained (Akerlund, 2000). The strategies for fund-raising are many and will differ based on the program's structure and needs. The program team should also be aware of in-kind services, those that are provided free of cost to the program. Seeking in-kind services can aid in balancing a program budget (Akerlund, 2000). Fund-raising may seek not only funds but also services or supplies needed by the program. Fund-raising is often most successful when program staff have developed relationships with potential donors; sometimes this process is referred to as "friendraising" (Gottlieb, 2006).

Developing a Sustainability Plan

One of the best ways to ensure the long-term maintenance of the program is to develop a sustainability plan. The sustainability plan encompasses an overall strategy for program maintenance that includes specific goals for sustainability along with an action plan to address these goals (U.S. Department of Justice, 2005). A sustainability plan is meant to be an action plan outlining specifically what needs to be done and who needs to do it in order to maintain the program. The sustainability plan is similar to the implementation plan but is future oriented, focusing on what needs to be done to maintain the organization's viability. The plan should include goals, objectives, and action steps, including who will do what and a date for accomplishment. All the aspects of this plan should be focused and geared towards sustainability rather than program implementation.

Sustainability planning should include identifying the challenges to sustainability. One question to pose is: What could cause the program or organization to not be able to sustain itself? Addressing this question is difficult but essential to the core of any sustainability plan. Identifying the challenges to sustainability allows the program team to develop approaches to effectively address them (Akerlund, 2000; Conrad, 2008). Planning for sustainability is an essential process for a program's survival. One approach is to develop a committee or task group focused specifically on sustainability (Akerlund, 2000). In some cases, these individuals may be volunteers or members of the program team. Sustainability planning should involve a group of community stakeholders and those who have a vision for the future. This group should include individuals who have used the services and directly benefitted from them. Including input from community members ensures that the plan that is developed meets the needs and desires of the community, and aids in establishing sustainability. Also, the plan needs to be practical and feasible to ensure success. This means that it does not include raising community fees by an exorbitant amount nor propose strategies that will ultimately lead to challenges rather than success. The sustainability committee also needs to continually search for and garner resources that will support the program.

Conclusion

The occupational therapy practitioner needs to be thoughtful in the program design to ensure that once a program is implemented, it is viable and sustainable. Program design requires the development of the program's mission and implementation plan. Team building, sustainability planning, and budgeting are important components of program design to ensure successful implementation. Program design requires the occupational therapy practitioner to thoughtfully consider how the program will work, who will be involved, who will benefit from services, and how the program will be funded. In this process, the occupational therapy practitioner can take a programmatic idea and design a program that meets community needs to impact occupation and quality of life.

Learning Activities

1. Draft a mission statement for a potential program. Gather some mission statements from corporations or local organization via the Internet. Compare and contrast your drafted mission statement with those of other organizations.

2. Brainstorm the staff you need for your program idea. How many staff members do you need? What would you pay them? What qualifications do they need to implement the program?

3. Contact local programs similar to your program idea and set up an interview with an employee. Find out more about the program, including staffing, budgeting, and supplies and equipment. Compare the results of this interview to your initial program ideas.

REFERENCES

Akerlund, K. M. (2000). Prevention program sustainability: The state's perspective. *Journal of Community Psychology, 28*(3), 353–362.

American Occupational Therapy Association (2008). Occupational therapy practice framework: Domain and process, 2nd edition. *American Journal of Occupational Therapy, 62*(6), 626–683.

American Occupational Therapy Association. (2010a). *Occupational Therapy* Code of Ethics and Ethics Standards (2010). *American Journal of Occupational Therapy, 64*(Suppl.), S17–S26. doi: 10.5014/ajot2010.64S17-64S26

American Occupational Therapy Association (2010b). Scope of practice. *American Journal of Occupational Therapy, 64* (6), 389–396.

Ansari, W. E., Phillips, C. J., & Hammick, M. (2001). Collaborating and partnerships: Developing the evidence base. *Health and Social Care in the Community, 9*(4), 215–227.

Becker, A. B., Israel, B. A., & Allen, A. J. (2005). Strategies and techniques for effective group process in CBPR partnerships. In B. A. Israel, E. Eng, A. J. Schulz, & E. A. Parker (Eds.). *Methods in Community-Based Participatory Research for Health* (pp. 52–72). San Francisco: Jossey-Bass.

Blue, A. V., Hamm, T. L., Harrison, D. S., Howell, D. W., Lancaster, C. J., Smith, T. G., West, V. T., & White, A.

(2008). *Team Skills Handbook.* Charleston, SC: Medical University of South Carolina.

Braveman, B. (2001). Development of a community-based return to work program for people living with AIDS. *Occupational Therapy in Health Care, 13*(No. 3-4), 113–131.

Brennan, L. K., Baker E. A., & Metzler M. (2008). *Promoting Health Equity: A Resource to Help Communities Address Social Determinants of Health.* Atlanta: U.S. Department of Health and Human Services, Centers for Disease Control and Prevention.

Brooks, D. M. (2006). *Grant writing made easy.* Presentation made at the E-Tech Conference: Columbus, OH.

Brownson, C. A. (2001). Program development: planning, implementation, and evaluation strategies. In M. Scaffa, Ed. *Occupational Therapy in Community-Based Practice Settings* (pp. 95–118). Philadelphia: F.A. Davis.

Burhansstipanov, L., Dignan, M. B., Bad Wound, D., Tenney, M., & Vigil, G. (2000). Native American recruitment into breast cancer screening: The NAWWA project. *Cancer Education, 15,* 28–52.

Chambless, D. L. (2003). Hints for writing a NIMH grant. *The Behavior Therapist, 26,* 258–261.

Cole, M. B. (2005). *Group dynamics in occupational therapy: The theoretical basis and practice application of group intervention, Third Edition.* Thorofare, NJ: SLACK.

Conrad, P. (2008). To boldly go: A partnership enterprise to produce applied health and nursing services researchers in Canada. *Health Care Policy 3,* 13–30.

Doll, J. D. (2010). *Program development and grant writing in occupational therapy: Making the connection.* Boston: Jones and Bartlett.

Edberg, M. (2007). *Essentials of Health Behavior: Social and Behavior Health in Public Health.* Boston: Jones and Bartlett.

Family Planning Management Development. (1998). *The Health and Family Planning Manager's Toolkit.* Retrieved from http://erc.msh.org/toolkit/toolkitfiles/file/pmt33.pdf

Fazio, L. (2008). *Developing occupation-centered programs for the community* (2nd ed.). Upper Saddle River, NJ: Prentice Hall.

Finlayson, M., Baker, M., Rodman, L., & Herzberg, G. (2002). The process and outcomes of a multimethod needs assessment at a homeless shelter. *American Journal of Occupational Therapy, 56*(3), 313–321. doi: 10.5014/ajot.56.3.313

Gaines, S. K., Wold, J. L., Bean, M. R., Brannon, C. G., & Leary, J. M. (2004). Partnership to build sustainable public health nurse child care health support. *Family and Community Health, 27*(4), 346–354.

Gitlin, L. N. , & Lyons, K. J. (2004). *Successful Grantwriting: Strategies for Health and Human Service Professionals.* New York: Springer.

Gitlow, L., & Flecky, K. (2005). Integrating disability studies concepts into occupational therapy education using service learning. *American Journal of Occupational Therapy, 59*(5), 546–553. doi: 10.5014/ajot.59.5.546

Gitlow, L., & Flecky, K. (2010). *Service-learning in occupational therapy education.* Boston: Jones and Bartlett.

Glaser, E. M. (1981) Durability of innovations in human service organizations: a case study analysis. *Knowledge: Creation, Diffusion, Utilization, 3*, 167–185.

Gottlieb, H. (2006). *Friendraising: Community engagement strategies for boards who hate fundraising but love making friends.* Tucson, AZ: Renaissance Press.

Goulet, C. G., Begley, K., Gould, K., & Doll, J. D. (2008). *Interdisciplinary Team Skills Development for Health Professional Students.* Association for Prevention and Teaching. $2900. Awarded October 2008.

Grossman, J., & Bortone, J. (1986). Program development. In S.C. Robertson (Ed.), *Strategies, concepts, and opportunities for program development and evaluation* (pp. 91–99). Bethesda, MD: American Occupational Therapy Association.

Holtzclaw, B. J., Kenner, C., & Walden, M. (2009). *Grant writing handbook for nurses* (2nd ed.). Boston: Jones and Bartlett.

Ingersoll, G. L., & Eberhard, D. (1999). Grants management skills keep funded projects on target. *Nursing Economics, 17*, 131–141.

Israel, B. A ., Eng, E., Schulz, A. J., & Parker, E. A. (2005). Introduction to method in community-based participatory research for health. In Israel, B. A., Eng, E., Schulz, A. J., & Parker, E. A. (Eds.). *Methods in community-based participatory research for health.* San Francisco: Jossey-Bass.

Jensen, G. M., & Royeen, C.B. (2001). Analysis of academic-community partnerships using the integration matrix. *Journal of Allied Health, 30*, 168–175.

Kagawa-Singer, M. (1997). Addressing issues for early detection and screening in ethnic populations. *Oncology Nursing Forum, 24*(10), 1705–1711.

LaMarca, K., Wiese, K. R., Pete, J. E., & Carbone, P. P. (1996). A progress report of cancer centers and tribal communities: Building a partnership based on trust. *Cancer, 78*(Suppl. 7), 1633–1637.

Law, M. C. (1998). *Client-centered occupational therapy.* Thorofare, NJ: SLACK.

Lencioni, P. (2002). *The five dysfunctions of a team: A leadership fable.* San Francisco: Jossey-Bass.

MacQueen, K. M., McLellan, E., Metzger, D. S., Kegeles, S., Strauss, R. P., Scotti, R., Blanchard, L., & Trotter, R. T. (2001). What is community? An evidence-based definition for participatory public health. *American Journal of Public Health, 91*(12), 1929–1938.

Meade, C. D., & Calvo, A. (2001). Developing community-academic partnerships to enhance breast health among rural and Hispanic migrant and seasonal farmworker women. *Oncology Nursing Forum, 28*(10), 1577–1584.

Ohio Literacy Resource Center. (2007). *Leadership Development Institute: Personal Mission Statement.* Retrieved from http://literacy.kent.edu/Oasis/Leadership/mission.htm

Poole, D., & Van Hook, M. (1997). Retooling for community health partnerships in primary care and prevention. *Health and Social Work, 22*(1), 2–4.

Ruhs, B. (2000). *Successful grant writing tips and tactics.* Presented to the Massachusetts Department of Education Child Nutrition Programs.

Shediac-Rizkallah, M. C., & Bone, L. R. (1998). Planning for the sustainability of community-based health programs: conceptual frameworks and future directions for research, practice and policy. *Health Education Research, 13*, 87–108.

Simon, C. A. (2002). Testing for bias in the impact of AmeriCorps service on volunteer participants: Evidence of success in achieving a neutrality program objective. *Public Administration Review, 62*(6), 670–678.

Simon, C. A., & Wang, C. (2002). The impact of Ameri-Corps service on volunteer participants. *Administration and Society, 34*(5), 522–540.

Strickland, R. (2011). Strategic planning. In K. Jacobs & G. McCormack (Eds.), *The occupational therapy manager, 5th Edition.* Bethesda, MD: AOTA Press.

Sumsion, T. (1999). *Client-centered practice in occupational therapy.* Edinburgh: Churchill Livingstone.

Swinney, J., Anson-Wonkka, C., Maki, E., & Corneau, J. (2001). Community assessment: A church community and the parish nurse. *Public Health Nursing, 18*(1), 40–44. doi: 10.1111/j.1525-1446.2001.00040.x

Timmreck, T. C. (2003). *Planning, program development and evaluation* (2nd ed.). Boston: Jones & Bartlett.

United States Department of Justice. (2005). *Developing a sustainability plan for weed and seed sites.* Retrieved from http://ojp.usdoj.gov/ccdo/pub/pdf/ncj210462.pdf

Voltz-Doll, J. D. (2008). Professional development: Growing as an occupational therapist. *Advance for Occupational Therapy Practitioners, 24*(5), 41–42.

Weis, R. M., & Gantt, V. W. (2004). *Knowledge and skill development in non-profit organizations.* Peosta, IA: Eddie Bowers.

White, A., & West, V. (2008). An introduction to teamwork. Retrieved from http://academicdepartments.musc.edu/c3/presentations/teamskills_training.ppt

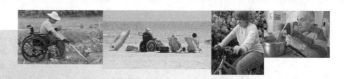

Chapter 7

Program Evaluation

David Ensminger, PhD, Marjorie E. Scaffa, PhD, OTR/L, FAOTA, and S. Maggie Reitz, PhD, OTR/L, FAOTA

What gets measured gets done. Measure the wrong things, and the wrong things get done.

—Michael Patton (2007, p. 110)

Learning Objectives

This chapter is designed to enable the reader to:

- Define program evaluation.
- Identify the purposes of program evaluation.
- Describe several approaches to program evaluation.
- Discuss the process of program evaluation.
- Describe the differences between experimental, quasi-experimental, and non-experimental evaluation designs.
- Discuss the appropriate use of qualitative methods in program evaluation.
- Identify the uses of evaluation results.
- Discuss the importance of disseminating the results of program development and evaluation.
- Identify the ethical considerations in designing and conducting evaluation research.

Key Terms

Appreciative inquiry approach	Objectives approach
Conceptual use	Outcome evaluation
Contingency perspective	Participatory approach
Efficiency evaluation	Process evaluation
Experimental designs	Process use
Formative evaluation	Program efficiency evaluation
4D Model	Program evaluation
Impact evaluation	Qualitative
Indicators	Quantitative
Instrumental use	Quasi-experimental designs
Logic models	Stakeholders
Managerial approach	Summative evaluation
Needs assessment	Symbolic use
Non-experimental designs	Utilization-focused approach

Introduction

Evaluation research, more commonly referred to as program evaluation, is used to make a judgment of merit, worth, or value of a program. Evaluation research optimizes the collection of relevant data for various stakeholder groups and then facilitates the use of this information for decision making and action (Johnson & Christensen, 2008). Fink (1993) defines **program evaluation** as "a diligent investigation of a program's characteristics and merits. Its purpose is to provide information on the effectiveness of projects to optimize the outcomes, efficiency, and quality of health care. Evaluations can analyze a program's structure, activities, and organization and examine its political and social environment. They can also appraise the achievement of a project's goals and objectives and the extent of its impact and costs" (p. 2).

Because evaluators seek to provide useful information to various stakeholder groups, the evaluator, unlike a "researcher," does not control all aspects of the evaluation. This is most evident in determining the questions for the evaluation. Evaluators rely on stakeholders to help develop the essential questions that will be answered in the evaluation. **Stakeholders** are "individuals, groups or organizations that can affect or are affected by an evaluation process and/or its findings" (Bryson, Patton, & Bowman, 2011, p. 1). The degree of stakeholder involvement is often dependent on the approach and can range from helping generate questions to full involvement in the collection, analysis, and reporting of results. Evaluators also differ from other researchers in that they consider the context to be a critical component of the research. As a result, there are limitations to generalizing results from an evaluation to other contexts. In addition, evaluators make value statements related to the merit or worth of the program based on the data.

The determination of a program's merit or worth is founded in the perspective that programs should have some level of accountability to stakeholders and the community at large. Although public perception of the need for evaluations generally focuses on accountability in terms of program effects and efficiency, evaluations also can be conducted to support the development and improvement of a program, or to further or deepen stakeholders' understanding of the program (Chelimsky, 1997). Although the notion of accountability suggests a decisive type of judgment, as will be explained in this chapter, the reporting of merit, worth, and value has different meanings depending on the purpose and focus of the evaluation as well as the approach used to conduct the evaluation.

Purpose of Program Evaluation

When designing or planning evaluations, evaluators work with key stakeholders to determine the main purpose of the evaluation, which often falls into one of two broad categories: summative or formative.

Although both lead to valuable information that can assist stakeholders in making decisions and taking actions regarding a program, it is often the nature of the decision or action being made that helps form the purpose of an evaluation. Formative evaluations are conducted when decisions or actions to be taken from evaluation results center on program improvement. Thus, **formative evaluations** provide credible and relevant information concerning a program's theoretical framework, design, activities, and operation. This information assists stakeholders in making changes that will lead to improvements in the program's activities, practices, processes, or operations.

Summative evaluations are conducted when decisions or actions to be taken from an evaluation center on continuing or discontinuing a program, increasing program size, or determining the effect of a program on a particular social problem or need. Thus, **summative evaluations** provide credible, valid information concerning the program's outcomes, impact, and effectiveness. The information from summative evaluations provides evidence that changes experienced by the clients of a program result from the program activities and not from other factors.

Focus of Program Evaluations

Evaluations tend to be conducted around five main foci (Rossi, Lipsey, & Freeman, 2004), which include:

- needs assessment
- program theory
- program implementation
- program impact
- program efficiency.

Even though these five focus areas are distinct, it is helpful to understand the relationships among them. Social programs are developed to address specific needs or problems within a community or society. In order for a program to be designed, there must be a clear, agreed-upon understanding and definition of the problem the program is to address. Needs assessments are conducted for this purpose. Once the problem is defined, programs must develop theories (often referred to as **logic**

models) that explain the cause-and-effect links between the problems, program activities, and outcomes.

Program theory evaluations help stakeholders develop a clear and agreed-upon model of how the program is intended to operate in order to address an identified social problem. To achieve their intended outcomes, programs need to be implemented as they are described within a program theory. Implementation evaluations focus on evaluating the fidelity of program implementation in terms of design and logic models. Programs that are implemented correctly should produce outcomes that address the social need or problem.

Outcome evaluations focus on the long-term effects of a program or process, establishing cause-and-effect relationships between the program and the outcomes or changes in the social problem or need. **Impact evaluations** assess the immediate effects of a program or process on the target population and typically measure the achievement of program objectives (Green & Kreuter, 2005). **Efficiency evaluations** are used to examine the costs and benefits of programs in terms of quality of their operations and the outcomes they produce. Efficiency evaluations are important because programs are often accountable to external stakeholder groups such as boards of directors, local communities, and governments that provide the program with resources and funding.

All five of these focus areas are important to address, and each lends itself to either summative or formative purposes. Needs assessments, program theory, and implementation generally have a more formative structure, whereas outcome, impact, and efficiency evaluations tend to have a more summative nature. Each focus will be examined in more detail in the following sections.

Needs Assessment

The main objective of **needs assessment** is to provide stakeholders with information that leads to a deeper understanding and working definition of the social problem or need. In addition, this type of evaluation should assess the extent of the problem in terms of incidence (how often it is observed or occurs in society) and prevalence (the distribution of the problem within society) as well as describe the target population and secondary populations that are affected

by the problem. The information from needs assessments provides the foundational information about the problem and population that helps determine the types of services needed in a program.

As stated previously, the nature of this information is formative, because this evaluation most often provides information that leads to the design and development of programs or improvement of existing programs to better address the defined need. Basic questions that drive this type of evaluation include:

- How often is this problem/need reported or observed in the community?
- How widespread is the problem within the community?
- What are the characteristics of the individuals who have this problem/need?
- How do different groups perceive the nature and the cause of the problem?
- What services would help reduce or eliminate the problem?

Through a needs assessment, the evaluator provides information that helps stakeholders better understand the nature of the social problem and use the data to design and implement programs or program activities to meet the identified need. The needs assessment process is discussed in more depth in Chapter 5 of this text.

Program Theory Evaluation

Program theory evaluation focuses on working with stakeholders to construct a clear description of how a program is intended to work. Program theory evaluations result in information that describes the causal links between the activities and events of the program and the outcomes these activities are intended to produce. Additionally, program theory evaluations describe the rationale behind how the program is intended to operate. Program theory evaluations often result in visual diagrams or logic models that represent the casual links between the problem, the program activities, and the program outcomes. See Figure 7.1 for an example of a logic model. Questions that drive program theory evaluations include:

- How well does the logic model describe the causal links between activities and outcomes?
- How well does the logic model fit with the current theories/practices used to address the problem?

Program Action-Logic Model

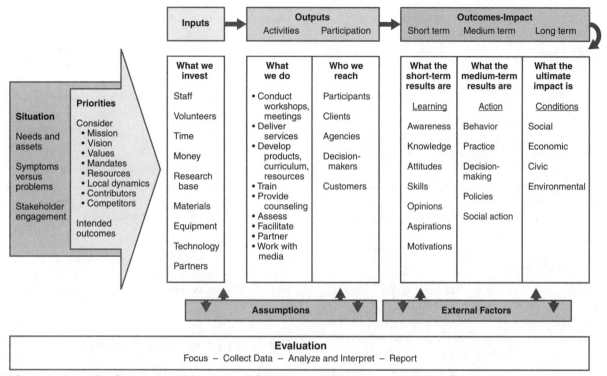

Fig. 7•1 Example of a Logic Model. (*Retrieved from University of Wisconsin-Extension-Cooperative Extension, Program Development and Evaluation Unit Web site: http://www.uwex.edu/ces/pdande/ evaluation/evallogicmodel.html Reprinted with permission.*)

- Does the service utilization display the correct order of activities to produce the desired outcomes?
- Does the organizational process plan provide adequate, accessible resources and qualified personnel to fulfill the utilization plan?

The aim of program theory evaluation is to provide information that allows stakeholders to better understand the theoretical foundations of a program and the causal links between program activities and program outcomes. In addition, the logic model should demonstrate the connections between needed resources and program operation.

Program Implementation Evaluation

Whereas program theory evaluations focus on what a program is intended to do, implementation (or process) evaluations provide information on the actual operation of the program (Stufflebeam, 2000). Implementation evaluations provide information on

the operation of a program, or how the program models are enacted on a daily basis. Implementation evaluations examine components of the program, such as the activities, events, functions, communication, and resources, with special focus on documenting and describing the actual practices of a program.

One purpose of implementation evaluation is to determine the level of program fidelity in relation to the program logic model. Program fidelity provides an opportunity for formative accountability by providing stakeholders with information about the degree to which the intended program (logic model) matches the actual program. These evaluations can provide useful formative recommendations to ensure the target population is being reached, program activities are being offered as designed, and program outcomes are being monitored.

Program monitoring involves the identification of key outcomes, and the systematic practice of collecting data to inform the stakeholders of the program's effectiveness in reaching these outcomes. Even though program monitoring can provide useful knowledge of the program's successes at achieving outcomes, it should not be mistaken for impact evaluation. Questions that drive implementation evaluations include:

- How well does the program reach its intended target populations?
- How well does the actual program match the impact theory and service utilization plan?
- What are the barriers that prevent the program from operating as intended?
- What factors facilitate the implementation of the program?
- How well do the organizational processes support the program?
- To what extent is the program reaching intended outcomes?

This focus relies on the evaluator providing information that allows stakeholders to identify areas where program operation does not fit with the program design, to identify areas where program activities can be improved, and to identify and establish means for ongoing data collection related to program activities and outcomes.

Program Impact Evaluation

Like program monitoring, program impact evaluations focus primarily on the goals, objectives, and immediate effects related to a program. However, in impact evaluations, evaluators try to employ the most rigorous methods for examining the cause-and-effect relationship between the program and the achievement of the program goals and objectives. Thus, impact evaluations attempt to measure program effects and have a summative purpose. Evaluators are seeking to provide valid evidence concerning the extent to which the program actually causes the measured or observed outcomes. In order to demonstrate this, a comparison group that did not receive the program is needed to determine what would have happened if the intervention had not been implemented.

Outcomes can be affected by a number of other variables aside from the program intervention. For example, changes in economic or social conditions can influence health outcomes. Other programs with similar objectives may be targeted to the same population at the same time, which could influence the outcome. In addition, the normal development and maturation of participants, particularly children, could contribute to the outcome. Likewise, some program participants may have already been predisposed to the outcomes being measured and would have realized those positive outcomes without being exposed to the program interventions. The questions that drive impact evaluations include:

- What effect does the program have on the social problem?
- To what extent can program outcomes be directly linked to program activities?

In summary, a well-conducted impact evaluation provides the foundation for sound policy making. It describes whether or not the program had an impact as well as how much of an impact and on whom.

Program Efficiency Evaluation

Where impact evaluations focus on determining the cause-and-effect relationship between the program and its outcomes, **program efficiency evaluation** focuses on the merit or worth of a program from the standpoint of its financial benefits and costs. In this type of evaluation, evaluators must develop a method for explaining the benefits and costs of a program in monetary terms. Program efficiency evaluations often take two main forms: benefits analysis and cost-benefits analysis. In benefits analysis, evaluators look for ways of representing program outcomes in terms of monetary benefits (e.g., reduction in cost of future services needed by clients, increase in income of clients, reduction in program costs compared to other programs, increase in human and social capital). When conducting benefits analysis, the evaluator must be able to show links between the outcomes of the program and the identified benefits. The merit or worth of the program is determined by the benefits the program provides.

In cost-benefits analysis, the evaluator compares the benefits of the program determined in a benefits analysis to the actual costs of the program. When conducting cost analysis, evaluators must examine all the costs associated with running the program, not simply the costs associated with direct services to the client (e.g., material resources, operation expenses, salary and benefits of employees, loss of work days for clients in program). Questions that drive efficiency evaluations include:

- What are the monetary values of the program outcomes?
- How do the benefits of the program compare to the cost of running the program?
- Which program is more cost-effective to run?

This focus requires the evaluator to provide information that informs the stakeholders about the observed benefits of a program in relation to measured costs.

Approaches to Program Evaluation

The field of program evaluation has been influenced by diverse epistemologies, beliefs, methodological views, values, and perspectives (Fitzpatrick, Sanders, & Worthen, 2004). These influences have shaped the approaches used by evaluators today. These varying approaches provide foundational perspectives of how evaluations can be conducted for different purposes. The authors of this chapter do not favor one approach but instead encourage evaluators to employ a contingency perspective (Shadish, Cook, & Levinton, 1991) when determining the methods and activities to be carried out in an evaluation.

The **contingency perspective** advocates the use of different approaches to evaluation based on important information such as the nature of the program being evaluated, the context of the evaluation, the informational needs and intended use of the evaluating results by stakeholders, programmatic resources, and the specific evaluation questions. In order to apply a contingency perspective, evaluators must have an understanding of the broader evaluation approaches used in the field.

Although many specific models of evaluation exist (e.g., Discrepancy Evaluation, CIPP [Context, Input, Process, and Product], Utilization Focused), these models fit into one of the broader approaches to evaluation. Several of these approaches will be discussed in the second half of this chapter, including

the objectives approach, managerial approach, participatory approach, utilization-focused approach, and appreciative inquiry (AI) approach.

All evaluation approaches are concerned with the values and merit, or worth, of programs. However, they can differ in what elements of evaluation are emphasized (e.g., which stakeholders have more input, what information or data provides greater evidence, or what methods for collecting information are more important) and how program value is determined. These approaches emphasize different aspects of the evaluation process or the program; it is important to note that each approach has its unique set of strengths and weaknesses. Evaluators should have an understanding of each approach so they can effectively modify or combine approaches in order to meet the needs of stakeholders.

Objectives Approach

Mistakenly viewed as the main goal of all evaluations, the **objectives approach** emphasizes the determination of the achievement of stated goals and objectives in the program design. Specific evaluation models that emphasize this approach include the Tylerian approach, Discrepancy Evaluation, and Metfessel and Michael's Evaluation Paradigm (Fitzpatrick et al., 2004).

The main activities in this approach are determining the goals and objectives of the program, including the development of specific operational definitions (i.e., specific behavioral or observational definitions) of the objectives. Whereas stakeholders may be involved in determining the objectives and providing operational definitions, typically in this approach the objectives are determined based on the mission and goals of the program, and in some cases specific objectives may already exist as part of the program documentation.

Once the objectives are determined, a method for measuring the objectives is agreed upon. The evaluator then collects the data from these measurements and compares the data collected to the specific goals and objectives. If a specific criterion of success has been established for an objective (e.g., 75% of program participants will report using bicycle helmets upon program completion), then data collected is compared to the predetermined criterion.

Discrepancies between the observed data and the stated objectives are interpreted to provide either formative or summative information to stakeholders. For the objectivist approach, program value is directly related to the achievement of stated objectives, and quantitative methods are frequently used to measure program outcomes.

Strengths associated with this approach include:

- it is easy to understand and carry out,
- objectives are a clear and easy way to define a program's success, and
- information concerning achievement of program objectives is relevant to most stakeholder groups.

Although this approach has many advantages, it also has limitations. Weaknesses associated with this approach include:

- program merit or worth is limited to the program objectives,
- no value is set for the objectives themselves,
- outcomes or program values not related to objectives are often overlooked,
- information concerning program planning and implementation is ignored, and
- in many cases stakeholder involvement may be minimal (Fitzpatrick et al., 2004).

Although this approach is simple and provides valuable information about a program, it often provides limited information that stakeholders can use to improve programs. Even though objectives might be a part of an evaluation plan, few evaluators rely solely on this approach when conducting an evaluation.

Managerial Approach

Similar to the objectives approach, the **managerial approach** does include examining program objectives; however, it looks beyond programmatic outcomes and views the informational needs of managers as a critical aspect of evaluation. This approach emphasizes providing useful information to managers or program directors in order to improve their decision making. Evaluations must provide information about how the program operates, not simply if objectives are being reached. In order to assist managers, the managerial approach evaluates the context, planning, structure, resources, implementation, and organizational factors that impact a program. Specific evaluation models associated with this approach include the CIPP, UCLA Model (Fitzpatrick et al., 2004), and Evaluability Assessment (Wholey, 2004).

Stufflebeam's (2000) CIPP model provides a comprehensive example of this approach and employs four different types of evaluation to provide managers with information related to specific decisions. The CIPP acronym represents the major constructs in this model: context, input, process, and product evaluation. Context evaluations assist with decisions regarding program planning, while input evaluations are used for decisions concerning program structure. **Process evaluation,** also referred to as formative evaluation, assesses, analyzes, and documents the development and implementation of a program or strategy to determine if the program activities were conducted as planned. Process evaluations are used for decisions surrounding program implementation, and product evaluations inform managers' decisions about program outcomes and objectives. The purpose of these evaluations is to provide quick, ongoing, and useful information to managers for the purpose of ongoing program improvement.

In the managerial approach, program value is determined by the managers or program directors and is reflected in the decisions they make based on evaluation results. The decisions made by managers can take either a formative tone and focus on program improvement, or a summative nature and result in program expansion or program elimination. Both qualitative and quantitative research methods may be utilized, depending on the nature of the evaluation questions. **Qualitative** approaches use language or narrative as raw data in order to study people's thoughts, experiences, and perspectives. **Quantitative** approaches use numbers as raw data in order to test hypotheses and establish cause-effect relationships (Barker, Pistrang, & Elliott, 2002). The managerial approach to evaluation is closely related to the field of human performance technology and performance improvement in business and industry. Many of the specialized models of performance improvement and quality assurance used in business and industry (e.g., Six Sigma, Lean, and Total Quality

Management [TQM]) share core aspects with the managerial approach to evaluation.

The strengths of the managerial approach include:

- collecting useful information to make informed decisions for the purpose of program changes,
- focusing of evaluation activities on specific program aspects (e.g., planning, structure, implementation), and
- emphasizing timely ongoing feedback through the life cycle of the program.

The emphasis on a single stakeholder group's needs (i.e., managers) makes this approach undemocratic. Other potential limitations include the possibility that important information may not be gathered if the manager does not see its importance, or the manager may fail to make decisions even when presented with relevant information (Fitzpatrick et al., 2004). Additional weaknesses include the fact that it can be costly to carry out an evaluation on all aspects of a program, and that important decisions may be made in advance, which may ignore the organic nature of programs.

Participatory Approach

The **participatory approach** emphasizes the formative purpose of evaluation. Similar to the managerial approaches in that both types emphasize the need to provide information for program improvement, the participatory approaches consider the information needs of all stakeholder groups rather than emphasize the information needs of managers. The involvement of all stakeholders is viewed as essential to the evaluation process in order to gain multiple perspectives of the program. Of all the approaches, the participatory approach places the most value on democratic principles, viewing the knowledge of those who carry out program activities (i.e., front end users), clients, and program supervisors as critical when gathering information about a program and determining the merit or worth of the program.

Specific examples of this approach include Utilization Focused, Responsive, and Empowerment evaluations (Fitzpatrick et al., 2004). Along with multiple perspectives, the inclusion of multiple stakeholders in the evaluation process increases the likelihood that evaluation information will be used. Participatory evaluators seek to determine the critical information needs of the various stakeholder groups and then plan evaluations that will provide the needed information to these stakeholders in order to promote program improvement. Whereas the managerial approach applies a top-down perspective, the participatory approach uses a bottom-up perspective of program change. One important outcome of participatory evaluations is increased dialogue among the various stakeholder groups that results in broader perspectives of the program, deeper understanding of the program, and promotion of social justice through the inclusion of marginalized populations in the evaluation process. Program merit and worth is often a result of the evaluator's interpretation and presentation of multiple perspectives, and perceived value of the program from the various stakeholder groups. This approach favors qualitative methods and reports that provide detailed descriptions of the program and the various stakeholders' accounts of the program.

The strengths of this approach include:

- involving a variety of stakeholder groups,
- recognizing that programs serve people and are run by people,
- bringing to light multiple accounts of the program,
- placing importance on the democratic processes and the need for stakeholder dialogue,
- considering the complexity of programs, and
- recognizing that one of the contextual elements of evaluations is that different stakeholder groups will have different evaluation questions and need different information.

Weaknesses associated with this approach include the:

- subjective nature of these evaluations,
- emphasis on qualitative methods causing concerns of evaluator bias, and
- extensive cost and time associated with qualitative data collection and analysis (Fitzpatrick et al., 2004).

Participatory evaluations require evaluators who are skilled at qualitative research practices. Skilled qualitative researchers are trained in carrying out evaluation studies that will stand up to methodological criticism, questions concerning validity of the evaluation results, and evaluator bias.

Utilization-Focused Approach

The **utilization-focused approach** is not a specific evaluation methodology but rather a process for including the users in the design of the evaluation process and focusing on their intended purposes and uses of the evaluation results. The basic premise of utilization-focused evaluation (U-FE) is that the results of evaluative processes should be judged by their utility, usability, and use or actual application of the findings (Patton, 2008). An important step in designing utilization-focused evaluations is to identify the intended users of the assessment results and how best to meet the needs of these users. The goal of U-FE is to generate valid, useful, consistent, and credible information that provides data to guide action. U-FE shifts attention from the program to be evaluated to the users and stakeholders who will utilize the program evaluation data. U-FE is highly situation- and context-specific, and choices made in developing evaluation strategies are based on utility. A U-FE is grounded in the perspectives, values, and interests of program participants and stakeholders and can serve a variety of purposes (e.g., formative, summative, cost-effectiveness) and focus on processes, impacts, and/or outcomes. U-FE research often uses mixed methods, employing both quantitative and qualitative data collection strategies. According to Patton (2002), "intended users of evaluation are more likely to use evaluations if they understand and feel ownership of the evaluation process and findings" (para. 4); in this way U-FE is a very participatory process. The primary tasks of U-FE are outlined in Box 7-1.

In addition to improving the usability of evaluation results, U-FE also appears to impact programs and organizations that have participated in its process. Participation in the evaluation process can result in individual and collective changes in attitudes, thinking, acting, and organizational culture as a result of learning. These changes, referred to as process use, may in fact be more long lasting than the mere utilization of the evaluation results

Box 7-1   Steps in the Utilization-Focused Evaluation Process
• *Program/Organizational Readiness Assessment*: Determine if the key players in the organization understand and are interested in U-FE.
• *Evaluator Readiness and Capability Assessment*: Determine if the evaluator has the skills to conduct U-FE and is committed to the underlying philosophy.
• *Identification of Primary Intended Users*: Find and recruit persons who are credible, knowledgeable, teachable, and interested in using the results of the evaluation and assess the characteristics of these primary intended users.
• *Situational Analysis*: Identify, understand, and adapt to situational factors (barriers and supports) that may affect the use of evaluation results.
• *Identification of Primary Intended Uses:* Make decisions about the purposes of the evaluation, what types of data are needed, and how the evaluation results will be used.
• *Focusing the Evaluation*: Actively involve users in identifying evaluation priorities and questions.
• *Evaluation Design*: Involve users in decisions about evaluation methods, assessment instruments, and responsibilities for data collection.
• *Simulation of Use:* Create and implement a simulation using fabricated findings to determine the usability of the evaluation results.
• *Data Collection:* Involve intended users and other stakeholders in the data collection process and provide interim results as appropriate.
• *Data Analysis:* Organize the data to make them understandable and relevant for the users, and facilitate data interpretation among users to increase their understanding of the implications of the results.
• *Facilitation of Use:* Work with the primary users to identify what they have learned in the evaluation process and to implement the findings in meaningful ways.
• *Meta-evaluation*: Determine if the evaluation met the needs of the users and the extent to which the results were utilized.

Data from: Patton, M. (2008) Utilization-focused evaluation (4th ed). Thousand Oaks, CA: Sage.

(Patton, 2004). Patton (2007) identifies six types of process use:

- Infusing evaluative thinking into organizational culture

- Enhancing shared understandings within the program
- Supporting and reinforcing the program intervention
- Instrumentation effects
- Increasing participant engagement, self-determination, and sense of ownership
- Program and organizational development (p. 110).

Appreciative Inquiry Approach

An **appreciative inquiry** (AI) **approach** to evaluation focuses on organizational and program assets as opposed to the identification of problems and deficits. The evaluation process attempts to discover what is working particularly well and then envision what the future might be like if these positive attributes were to manifest themselves more frequently. AI is grounded in social constructivism, which reflects a belief that there is no single, objective reality, but that many realities exist based on individuals' perceptions and shared understandings.

Cooperrider and Whitney (2000) described five principles for the practice of AI. These include:

- The *constructivist principle:* acceptance that multiple realities exist
- The *simultaneity principle:* inquiry and change are simultaneous and therefore inquiry is intervention
- The *poetic principle:* an organization or program is continuously authoring its own story and can take the plot line in any direction at any time
- The *anticipatory principle:* the image an organization or program has about its future guides its current actions
- The *positive principle:* by focusing on positive experiences, participants become more motivated, inspired, and engaged.

The most common method for conducting AI is referred to as the **4D Model** (Discovery, Dream, Design, and Destiny). The discovery phase of the process involves participants sharing stories about their peak experiences and *appreciating what is* currently good about the program or organization. Out of these stories, key themes are identified. In the dream phase, participants imagine themselves and their organization functioning at its best and envision *what might be,* developing a broad and holistic vision of a desirable future. In the design phase, the dream or vision is operationalized into *what should be* and co-constructed through the development of goals, strategies, processes, collaborations, and systems. The destiny phase involves implementing the strategies, monitoring progress, sustaining the change, and engaging in new AI dialogues. The 4D process is on-going, iterative, cyclical, and highly participatory in nature (Coghlan, Preskill, & Catsambas, 2003).

AI has the potential to contribute to evaluation practice in many ways. Coghlan et al. (2003) provide a list of situations in which AI might be most useful. These include:

- "Where there is a fear of or skepticism about evaluation"
- "When change needs to be accelerated"
- "When dialogue is critical to moving the organization forward"
- "When relationships among individuals and groups have deteriorated and there is a sense of hopelessness" and
- "Where there is a desire to build a community of practice" (p. 19).

The Process of Planning and Conducting Evaluations

Planning an evaluation is best done prior to program implementation. The creation of an evaluation plan involves:

- identifying stakeholders
- developing evaluation questions
- determining data needs, and
- choosing evaluation methods and instruments.

Identifying Stakeholders

Stakeholders may include:

(a) persons having authority over the program, such as funders and advisory boards,
(b) persons having responsibility or oversight for the operations of the program, such as program managers and administrators,

(c) persons who benefit from the program, including program participants and their families,

(d) persons who may be disadvantaged by the program in some way, and

(e) members of the general public who may have a direct or indirect interest in the outcomes of evaluation.

Involving stakeholders in the evaluation process "is presumed to enhance the design and implementation of evaluations and the use of evaluation results in decision-making" (Bryson et al., 2011, p. 1). Failure to incorporate the interests and needs of stakeholders in the evaluation process frequently leads to useless findings and other poor outcomes. However, in order to make stakeholder participation practical, decisions must be made about which stakeholders will be the primary users of the evaluation findings. Identifying the stakeholders who should be involved in the evaluation requires knowledge about:

- who cares about the program,
- who has potential influence over the program,
- who has resources to support the program,
- who will use the evaluation findings, and
- how they will use the findings.

Stakeholders should have a high level of interest in the outcome of the evaluation and substantial power to affect change. Not all stakeholders will participate equally, some may only desire information, some may want to be consulted, others will be involved, and a few will collaborate as decision makers (Bryson et al., 2011).

Developing Evaluation Questions

The most difficult task in evaluation is often the development of clear, useful, and researchable evaluation questions. The information needs of program developers and managers change with varying organizational and environmental conditions. Resources may limit the scope of the evaluation, and therefore evaluation questions must be chosen carefully and prioritized. Resource constraints may also impact evaluation design, data collection strategies, and scope of the inquiry. Logic models can be used to identify program components and outcomes, to generate evaluation questions, and to

organize evaluation activities. A basic logic model was previously illustrated in Figure 7.1.

Rossi et al. (2004) identify three types of logic models: impact theory, service utilization, and organizational processes. Impact theory logic models visually display the change processes produced by the program. Construction of impact models includes the identification of program goals, objectives, inputs, and outputs, as well as the primary, secondary, and tertiary outcomes of the program. Once identified, the evaluator works with the stakeholders to construct a model that represents the process of how program activities work to produce the intended change. Emphasis is placed on illustrating the causal links between activities and outcomes. Activities typically do not provide direct links to outcomes; instead, activities often address some condition associated with the problem or need (Rossi et al., 2004). Also, models can form virtuous cycles (Rogers, 2000) with some outcomes serving not only as effects but also as causes to future outcomes.

Service utilization logic models show the movement of clients through a program. These models often take on the appearance of a flowchart that represents the pathway of clients as they progress through the program. The models also show the activities, events, outcomes, and decision points from the clients' perspective.

Organizational processes logic models are constructed to display the links between organizational resources (e.g., financial, personnel, material) and the associated program activities, events, and outcomes. These models represent the resources needed to operate a program as it is described in the impact theory and the service utilization logic models. In addition, organizational processes logic models also provide an illustration of how auxiliary program activities, such as fund-raising, political liaison, marketing, and personnel management, work to support the function of the program.

Determining Data Needs

Evaluation questions influence the research design, types of impact, outcome data to be collected, and data collection methods. Short-term impact measures often assess knowledge, attitudes, skills, and opinions. Intermediate-term impact measures target behavior change, and longer-term outcome measures address changes in social, economic, and health conditions. In some cases evaluation data will include program attendance and changes in knowledge, attitudes, values, behaviors, and health outcomes. It is critical to choose impact and outcome indicators that will answer the evaluation questions. **Indicators** are observable and measurable milestones toward an outcome target. According to the American Occupational Therapy Association (2008, pp. 662–663), occupational therapy outcome indicators include:

- Occupational performance
- Adaptation
- Health and wellness
- Participation
- Prevention
- Quality of life
- Role competence
- Self-advocacy
- Occupational justice

In addition to determining what types of data are needed for the evaluation, the timing of data collection is a consideration. Typically, baseline or pre-test data is collected prior to program implementation, post-test data is collected immediately after the intervention has been completed, and follow-up data is collected at intervals following the post-test in order to determine if the program effects are lasting. Figure 7.2 provides an outline for developing the data collection aspect of the evaluation plan.

Choosing Evaluation Methods

Evaluation methods should be appropriate for the evaluation questions being asked. The proposed methods should be practical, cost-effective, and ethical. Typically, evaluation designs fall into two categories: quantitative designs and qualitative designs. These approaches may be combined in a mixed-methods approach either sequentially or concurrently. Combining the methods can mitigate the weaknesses of each.

Quantitative Designs

Quantitative approaches to program evaluation generally fall into the three broad categories listed here, beginning with the least complex.

- **Non-experimental designs** (e.g., *cross-sectional designs, cohort studies*) involve participants serving as their own controls. Evaluation measures are gathered on participants before and after the intervention program.
- **Quasi-experimental designs** (e.g., *nonequivalent control group design, interrupted time-series design*) compare two groups. The group that is receiving the intervention is matched to a population that is similar demographically but is not receiving the program. Data are collected from both groups at the same time points and compared.
- **Experimental designs** (e.g., *randomized controlled trial*) randomly assign people to two groups. One group receives an intervention and the other does not. Data are collected from both groups at the same time points and compared (Crosby, DiClemente, & Salazar, 2006; Shadish, Cook, & Campbell, 2002).

Impact evaluations typically consist of studies that involve either experimental or quasi-experimental designs. These types of evaluations resemble traditional

Outcome	Indicator(s)	Source of Data (program participants, records, census, etc.)	Method of Data Collection (survey, interviews, observation, etc.)	When Data will be Collected (baseline, post-intervention, follow-up with dates)	Person Responsible for Collecting Data
1.					
2.					
3.					

Fig. 7•2 Evaluation Data Collection Plan.

quantitative research studies that test hypotheses and attempt to control for confounding variables that might arise as alternative explanations for the cause-and-effect relationships. Because evaluations occur in the context of the program, evaluators want to minimize any disruption to the normal operation of the program when conducting impact evaluations. These types of evaluations can be difficult to design depending on the contextual constraints of the program.

Whereas impact evaluations seek to have the most rigorous design (i.e., randomized, pretest-posttest control group design), in many instances the ability to randomly assign clients to control or experimental groups is not possible. Often evaluators are faced with selecting the quasi-experimental design that will fit best with the program. Most often this involves the use of a nonequivalent group pretest-posttest design. When employing these designs, evaluators must minimize the threats to internal validity that arise from selection bias inherent in this design (Johnson & Christensen, 2008). Most often evaluators will employ matching techniques or proximity scores as a means of equating the two groups (Shadish et al., 2002). The main goal of these types of research designs is to measure treatment effects (Shadish et al., 2002). While evaluators seek the most stringent designs when conducting the impact evaluations, contextual limitations often result in the use of weaker quantitative designs such as single group pretest-posttest designs, single group posttest-only designs, and time-series designs. These designs do not control for many of the threats to internal validity (Johnson & Christensen, 2008), and, as a result, evaluators must address the limitations of these designs when reporting program impact. These weaker designs are better suited for program monitoring because they tend to measure either outcome levels (the measurement of an outcome at a particular time) or outcome change (the difference between outcomes measured at two different times).

Qualitative Designs

The purpose of qualitative evaluation is "to capture the perspectives of program participants, staff and others associated with the program" (Patton, 2002, p. 151). A qualitative evaluation approach provides an in-depth perspective on phenomena that are not easily quantifiable. It is especially useful when the evaluator wants to understand not only what worked but also why it worked. Qualitative methods are particularly suited to analysis and interpretation of the contexts within which programs are operating. Qualitative assessment can produce a deeper, fuller understanding of the program and its effects. This is done by collecting firsthand, direct observation of naturally occurring situations in naturally occurring settings. Qualitative methods in evaluation use an inductive approach to data gathering and interpretation. It is a holistic, naturalistic orientation, searching for themes in the evaluation data and attempting to understand the lived experience of program participants. A qualitative approach to evaluation can illuminate what happened, to whom, and with what outcomes. There are many benefits to qualitative evaluation, such as providing information about context and meaning.

There are many ways to collect qualitative data, including interviews, focus groups, observation, and review of documents. If the evaluation seeks to understand what the program participants experienced, what they believe, or how they feel, then interviews are a good data collection strategy. Interviews can be conducted individually face-to-face, over the telephone, online, or with multiple people in a focus group. Semi-structured interviews using open-ended questions tend to produce the most useful information. If the evaluation seeks to identify what people do during given time frames, observation is a good data collection strategy to use.

Observations should be carried out in a variety of contexts, across multiple time periods. Recording observation data in field notes is recommended. If the evaluation seeks to understand the mission, history, and activities of an organization or agency, then document reviews can be a useful data collection approach. Documents to review may include mission statements, policies and procedures, brochures, Web site content, and meeting minutes (FRIENDS National Resource Center for Community-Based Child Abuse Prevention, 2009).

Utilizing Evaluation Results

Use refers to how "real people in the real world apply evaluation findings and experience the evaluation process" (Patton, 2002, para. 1). There are several types of use, including instrumental, conceptual, process, and symbolic. **Instrumental use** refers to using evaluation results to inform action. This is the most common type of use referred to in the evaluation literature. **Conceptual use** refers to the impact of evaluation processes on decision makers' thought processes about a current or future program. **Process use** occurs when cognitive and behavioral changes result as a function of participating in the evaluation process, and **symbolic use** is the use of evaluation data for political gain (Johnson, 1998).

Rossi et al. (2004) outline several guidelines for maximizing the utilization of evaluation results, including:

- Evaluation results should be timely and readily available.
- Evaluation results should be understandable to stakeholders and decision makers.
- Dissemination plans should be explicit and part of the evaluation design.
- Utilization of results should be assessed.

Communicating Evaluation Results

Evaluation results can and should be disseminated in a variety of ways, depending on the information needs of the audience. Reporting evaluation results serves several purposes, including:

- Providing a basis for further program development and quality improvement
- Generating support for continuing or expanding programs
- Enhancing public relations, and
- Demonstrating good stewardship of funds.

There are typically a number of different audiences for evaluation findings. These may include: stakeholders, program staff, program participants, funders, collaborating agencies, professional organizations, elected officials, and business groups, among others. The presentation of evaluation results should include the focus of the evaluation, the processes used, and the strengths and limitations of the evaluation. Dissemination involves communicating the procedures and lessons learned from an evaluation in a timely and unbiased way. Communication may take the form of verbal presentations, written reports, or visuals in the form of graphics or photographs.

One particularly effective method for presenting evaluation results for community-based programs is the "success story." A good success story captures the attention of the audience, provides a compelling story, describes specific outcomes, and is based on reliable and valid data. A success story consists of four parts: the situation, the response, the results, and the evidence. The situation refers to the problem, concern, or issue that needed to be addressed. Describe the situation and its impact locally. The response refers to the program characteristics, who participated and benefited, and the services provided. The results section of the success story describes the outcomes, what changed and for whom, and what was learned. Finally, the evidence component refers to how the program and its outcomes were evaluated and how the results are known to be accurate and credible (University of Wisconsin-Extension, Cooperative Extension, 2009).

Ethical Issues in Community-Based Program Evaluation

Appropriately used evaluation approaches in community-based practice can enhance efficacious community-centered needs assessments, program development, program implementation, and program evaluation. However, inadequate, misused, or incorrectly targeted evaluations can result in community alienation, wasted expenditure of limited resources, and missed opportunities for enhancing quality of life (Reitz, Pizzi, & Scaffa, 2010). Poorly developed or implemented program evaluations would be in conflict with one or more of the profession's core values and attitudes, which include "altruism, equality, freedom, justice, dignity, truth, and prudence" (AOTA, 2010, p. S17). In addition, the principles from the AOTA *Occupational Therapy Code of Ethics and Ethics Standards (2010)* apply to all aspects of the program evaluation process, including:

- Selecting the appropriate evaluation approach and outcome measures (Principle 1 Beneficence)

- Obtaining IRB approval from all applicable institutions (Principle 1 Beneficence, Principle 3 Autonomy/Confidentiality, and Principle 5 Procedural Justice)
- Avoiding conflicts of interest (Principle 1 Beneficence, Principle 7 Fidelity)
- Acquiring and using current assessments/outcome measures and upholding copyright laws (Principle 1 Beneficence)
- Ensuring compliance with established program evaluation protocol and anonymity/confidentiality as appropriate (Principle 1 Beneficence, Principle 3 Autonomy/Confidentiality)
- Training program staff and evaluators to ensure competency (Principle 2 Nonmaleficence)

- Reporting accurate results to participants and stakeholders in a timely manner (Principle 1 Beneficence, Principle 6 Veracity), and
- Securing evaluation materials and resulting data (Principle 3 Autonomy/Confidentiality).

In addition to official documents of the American Occupational Therapy Association (AOTA), groups such as the Joint Committee on Standards for Educational Evaluation can offer guidance regarding the appropriate use of evaluation (Yarbrough, Shulha, Hopson, & Caruthers, 2011). In Table 7-1, portions of the program evaluation standards developed by this group are compared to the AOTA *Occupational Therapy Code of Ethics and Ethics Standards (2010)* and the *NBCOT Candidate/Certificant Code*

Table 7-1 Program Evaluation Standards

Program Evaluation Standards	Occupational Therapy Code of Ethics and Ethics Standards (2010)	NBCOT Code of Conduct (2010)
Utility Standards		
U1-Evaluator Credibility	Beneficence (1D, 1E,1G) Procedural Justice (5E, 5F, 5G) Veracity (6A)	Accuracy & Veracity (3) Procedural Justice (4) Nonmaleficence (6)
U2-Attention to Stakeholders	Beneficence (1B) Social Justice	Nonmaleficence (6)
U3-Negotiated Purposes	Beneficence (1B, 1C)	Accuracy & Veracity (3)
U4-Explicit Values	Beneficence (1B) Autonomy/Confidentiality (3A)	Nonmaleficence (6)
U5-Relevant Information	Beneficence (1B, 1C)	Nonmaleficence (6)
U6-Meaningful Processes & Products	Beneficence (1B) Autonomy/Confidentiality (3A)	Nonmaleficence (6)
U7-Timely & Appropriate Communicating & Reporting	Beneficence (1A, 1B, 1C) Veracity	Accuracy & Veracity (3) Nonmaleficence (6)
U8-Concern for Consequences & Influence	Beneficence (1D) Nonmaleficence (2A) Autonomy/Confidentiality (3A)	Nonmaleficence (6)
Feasibility Standards		
F1-Project Management	Beneficence (1F, 1N)	Accuracy & Veracity (3)
F2-Practical Procedures	Beneficence (1B, 1C) Procedural Justice (5N) Fidelity (7A)	Accuracy & Veracity (3)
F3-Contextual Viability	Social Justice (4D, 4F)	Accuracy & Veracity (3) Nonmaleficence (6)
F4-Resource Use	Procedural Justice (5K) Fidelity (7H)	Procedural Justice (4)

Table 7-1 Program Evaluation Standards—cont'd		
Program Evaluation Standards	**Occupational Therapy Code of Ethics and Ethics Standards (2010)**	**NBCOT Code of Conduct (2010)**
Propriety Standards		
P1-Responsive & Inclusive Orientation	Autonomy/Confidentiality (3A) Social Justice (4C, 4F)	Nonmaleficence (6)
P2-Formal Agreements	Autonomy/Confidentiality (3J) Social Justice (4F) Procedural Justice (5I)	Accuracy & Veracity (3) Procedural Justice (4)
P3-Human Rights & Respect	Nonmaleficence (2A, 2C, 2I, 2J) Autonomy/Confidentiality (3B, 3G, 3H) Social Justice (4D) Fidelity (7A)	Procedural Justice (4) Nonmaleficence (6)
P4-Clarity & Fairness	Autonomy/Confidentiality (3B) Social Justice (4D) Veracity (6A)	Accuracy & Veracity (3)
P5-Transparency & Disclosure	Autonomy/Confidentiality (3G, 3H) Veracity (6A)	Accuracy & Veracity (3) Procedural Justice
P6-Conflicts of Interest	Beneficence Fidelity (7E, 7F)	Accuracy & Veracity (3)
P7-Fiscal Responsibility	Procedural Justice (5K)	Accuracy & Veracity (3)
Accuracy Standards		
A1-Justified Conclusions & Decisions	Procedural Justice (5P) Veracity	Accuracy & Veracity (3)
A2-Valid Information	Veracity	Accuracy & Veracity (3)
A3-Reliable Information	Procedural Justice (5P) Veracity	Accuracy & Veracity (3)
A4-Explicit Program & Context Descriptions	Procedural Justice (5P) Veracity	Accuracy & Veracity (3)
A5-Information Management	Veracity (6A)	Accuracy & Veracity (3)
A6-Sound Designs & Analyses	Beneficence (1D, 1F, 1G)	Accuracy & Veracity (3)
A7-Explicit Evaluation Reasoning	Beneficence (1G) Veracity	Nonmaleficence (6)
A8-Communication & Reporting	Social Justice (4D) Veracity (6)	Accuracy & Veracity (3)
Evaluation Accountability Standards		
E1-Evaluation Documentation	Beneficence (1F) Veracity (6A, 6C, 6D)	Accuracy & Veracity (3)
E2-Internal Metaevaluation	Beneficence (1F, 1N)	Accuracy & Veracity (3)
E3-External Metaevaluation	Beneficence (1N) Procedural Justice (5B)	

Data from: The standards in column 1 are from "The Program Evaluation Standards: A Guide for Evaluators and Evaluation Users, 3rd ed.," by D. B. Yarbrough, L. M. Shulha, R. K. Hopson, & F. A. Caruthers, 2011, Washington, DC: Sage. Copyright 2011 by Joint Committee on Standards for Educational Evaluation. The principles in column 2 are from "Occupational Therapy Code of Ethics and Ethics Standards," by the Ethics Commission of the American Occupational Therapy Association, 2010, *American Journal of Occupational Therapy, 64*(6), 151–160. Copyright 2010 by the American Occupational Therapy Association. The principles in column 3 are from the *Certification Renewal Handbook 2010* (p. 22), by the National Board for Certification in Occupational Therapy, 2010, Gaithersburg, MD: Author. Copyright 2010 by National Board for Certification in Occupational Therapy.

of Conduct (2010). As can be seen from this table, evaluation is complex and open to a variety of possible ethical concerns. The terminology used in the AOTA *Occupational Therapy Code of Ethics and Ethics Standards* is used to describe the content of the NBCOT principles so that parallels can be seen between these two documents.

In community-based practice, the client can be an individual, a portion of a community, or an entire community. The same standards that apply when evaluating individuals carry over to working with communities. When the client is an entire community or portion of a community, such as in program development, implementation, and evaluation, an additional layer of complexity becomes evident due to the involvement of people from a variety of professional backgrounds and other numerous stakeholders. All stakeholders may not have the same motives or ethical framework. The AOTA *Occupational Therapy Code of Ethics and Ethics Standards (2010)* can be used to help support ethical participation in important projects aimed at addressing societal needs. Performing due diligence to ensure all actions taken support community rights and autonomy is an ethical necessity. Whereas it may be relatively simple to match an assessment to an individual, locating an assessment or developing an outcome measure that is well suited for a broad array of individuals within a program or community can be complicated. For example, individuals in the community may have significantly differing reading levels, languages and language skills, visual acuity, and activity tolerance. Any of these differences can make it challenging to select an appropriate measure to be part of an evaluation approach for use with all program participants or community members. It is essential to avoid selecting approaches that exclude portions of the community based on a desire to reduce time, effort, or expense. Program evaluation teams must be open to using multiple methods in order to provide all program participants or community members with the opportunity for inclusion in program development and program evaluation.

Conclusion

Program evaluation uses systematic processes for collecting, analyzing, and interpreting data in order to provide information to program stakeholders and make statements concerning the merit, worth, and value of a program. Evaluations tend to be completed for one of two main purposes: formative (i.e., evaluations to inform decisions or activities related to program improvement) or summative (i.e., evaluations to inform decisions or activities related to the expansion, termination, or funding of programs).

Evaluations often have one of five main areas of focus: needs assessment, program theory, program implementation, program impact, or program efficiency. Each focus area provides unique and valuable information regarding the program, although all five are related to program improvement or accountability. Although these approaches provide good foundational knowledge for planning, all evaluations should be program-specific and based on important information, such as: the nature of the program being evaluated, the context of the evaluation, the informational needs and intended use of the evaluation results by stakeholders, programmatic resources, and the specific evaluation questions.

Learning Activities

1. Identify and list at least five school or community health programs in which you or a family member has participated over the years. Which of these programs had a program evaluation component? Was this program evaluation formative or summative in nature?
2. How would you improve upon the program evaluation process for one of the programs you have identified? Or, if you do not remember any of the programs having an evaluation component, describe at least one potential summative evaluation strategy.
3. Design a formative program evaluation plan for a course that you are currently taking.
4. You have conducted a backpack awareness campaign at a middle school for the past two semesters. This year you wish to conduct an evaluation in order to gather data to support a request to the county school board for funding, including a salary for yourself, to implement a countywide program. You are concerned about your conflict of interest in gathering the data. How can you ensure that the data is collected and that you are in compliance with the AOTA *Occupational Therapy Code of Ethics and Ethics Standards (2010)*?

REFERENCES

American Occupational Therapy Association. (2008). Occupational Therapy Practice Framework: Domain & Process, 2nd Edition. *American Journal of Occupational Therapy, 62*(6), 625–683.

American Occupational Therapy Association. (2010). Occupational Therapy Code of Ethics and Ethics Standards (2010). *American Journal of Occupational Therapy, 64*(Suppl.), S17–S26. doi: 10.5014/ajot2010.64S17-64S26

Barker, C., Pistrang, N., & Elliott, R. (2002). *Research methods in clinical psychology: An introduction for students and practitioners.* Hoboken, NJ: Wiley & Sons.

Bryson, J. M., Patton, M. Q., & Bowman, R. A. (2011). Working with evaluation stakeholders: A rationale, step-wise approach and toolkit. *Evaluation and Program Planning, 34*(1), 1–12.

Chelimsky, E. (1997). The coming transformation in evaluation. In E. Chelimsky & W. Shadish (Eds.), *Evaluation for the 21st century: A handbook.* Thousand Oaks, CA: Sage.

Coghlan, A. T., Preskill, H., & Catsambas, T. T. (2003). An overview of appreciative inquiry in evaluation. *New Directions for Evaluation, 100*, 5–22.

Cooperrider, D. L., & Whitney, D. (2000). A positive revolution in change: Appreciative inquiry. In D. Cooperrider, P. F. Sorensen, D. Whitney, & T. F. Yaeger, (Eds), *Appreciative Inquiry: Rethinking Human Organization Toward a Positive Theory of Change.* Champaign, IL: Stipes.

Crosby, R. A., DiClemente, R. J., & Salazar, L. E. (2006). *Research methods in health promotion.* San Francisco: Jossey-Bass.

Fink, A. (1993). *Evaluation fundamentals: Guiding health programs, research, and policy.* Newbury Park, CA: Sage.

Fitzpatrick, J. L., Sanders, J. R., & Worthen, B. R. (2004). *Program evaluation: Alternative approaches and practical guidelines* (3rd ed.). Boston: Pearson.

FRIENDS National Resource Center for Community-Based Child Abuse Prevention. (2009). *Using qualitative data in program evaluation: Telling the story of a prevention program.* Chapel Hill, NC: Author.

Green, L. W., & Kreuter, M. W. (2005). *Health promotion and planning: An educational and ecological approach* (4th ed.). Mountain View, CA: Mayfield.

Johnson, R. B. (1998). Toward a theoretical model of evaluation utilization. *Evaluation and Program Planning, 21*, 93–110.

Johnson, R. B., & Christensen, L. (2008). *Educational research: Quantitative, qualitative, and mixed approaches* (3rd ed.). Thousand Oaks, CA: Sage.

National Board for Certification in Occupational Therapy. (2010). NBCOT® Candidate/certificant code of conduct. In *Certification renewal handbook 2010.* Gaithersburg, MD: Author. Retrieved from http://nbcot.org/index.

php?option=com_content&view=article&id=271& Itemid=110

Patton, M. (2002). Utilization-focused evaluation (U-FE) checklist. Retrieved from http://www.eepsea.org/uploads/user-S/10905198311Utilization_Focused_Evaluation.pdf

Patton, M. (2004). The roots of utilization-focused evaluation. In M. Alkin (Ed.), *Evaluation roots: Tracing theorists' views and influences.* Thousand Oaks, CA: Sage.

Patton, M. (2007). Process use as a usefulism. *New Directions for Evaluation, 116*, 99–112.

Patton, M. (2008). *Utilization-focused evaluation* (4th ed.). Thousand Oaks, CA: Sage.

Reitz, S. M., Pizzi, M. A., & Scaffa, M. E. (2010). Evaluation principles in health promotion practice. In M. E. Scaffa, S. M. Reitz, & M. A. Pizzi (Eds), *Occupational therapy in the promotion of health and wellness* (pp. 157–172). Philadelphia: F.A. Davis.

Rogers, P. (2000). Program theory: Not whether programs work but how they work. In D. L. Stuffelbeam, G. F. Madaus, & T. Kelleghan (Eds.), *Evaluation models: Viewpoints on educational and human services evaluations* (2nd ed., pp. 209–232). Boston: Klewer.

Rossi, P., Lipsey, M. W., & Freeman, H. E. (2004). *Evaluation: A Systematic Approach* (7th ed.). Thousand Oaks, CA: Sage.

Shadish, W. R., Cook, T. D., & Campbell, D. (2002). *Experimental and quasi-experimental research designs for generalized causal inference* (2nd ed.). Boston: Houghton-Mifflin Harcourt.

Shadish, W. R., Cook, T., & Levinton, L. C. (1991). *Foundations of program evaluation: Theories of practice.* Thousand Oaks, CA: Sage.

Stuffelbeam, D. L. (2000). The CIPP model for evaluation. In D. L. Stuffelbeam, G. F. Madaus, & T. Kelleghan (Eds.), *Evaluation models: Viewpoints on educational and human services evaluations* (2nd ed., pp. 274–317). Boston: Klewer.

University of Wisconsin-Extension, Cooperative Extension. (2009). Using your evaluation: Communicating, reporting, improving. Retrieved from http://4h.uwex.edu/evaluation/results.cfm

Wholey, J. (2004). Evaluability assessment. In J. Wholey, H. P. Hatry, & K. E. Newcomer (Eds.), *Handbook of practical program evaluation* (2nd ed.). San Francisco: Jossey-Bass.

Yarbrough, D. B., Shulha, L. M., Hopson, R. K., & Caruthers, F. A. (2011). Program evaluation standards. In *Program evaluation standards: A guide for evaluators and evaluation users* (3rd ed.). Washington, DC: Sage. Retrieved from http://www.jcsee.org/program-evaluation-standards

Chapter 8

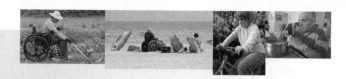

Entrepreneurship and Innovation in Occupational Therapy

Marjorie E. Scaffa, PhD, OTR/L, FAOTA, Michael A. Pizzi, PhD, OTR/L, FAOTA, and Wendy M. Holmes, PhD, OTR/L

It is time to build a system around your heart. Build a system around your passion . . . go and build what you know you must build.

—Kiyosaki (1999, p. 129)

Learning Objectives

This chapter is designed to enable the reader to:
- Identify the characteristics of entrepreneurs.
- Describe the various aspects of the entrepreneurial process.
- Identify the similarities and differences between intrapreneurship, social entrepreneurship, and business entrepreneurship.
- Compare and contrast for-profit and non-profit businesses.
- List the steps in developing a small health care business.
- Describe the components of a typical grant proposal.

Key Terms

Business plan
Contract
Diffusion
Entrepreneur
Environmental scan
Grant

Intrapreneur
Marketing
Social entrepreneur
Strategic planning
SWOT analysis

Introduction

As occupational therapy services expand to diverse populations and settings, therapists are required to develop new and innovative models of service delivery. These models may take the form of a new occupational therapy business, private practice, or program developed to meet the needs of a particular client group or community. A business opportunity must be recognized and nurtured; establishing a business requires a steadfast vision and perseverance. The skills, characteristics, and roles of occupational therapy practitioners mirror those of entrepreneurs.

The word "entrepreneur" derives from the French *entreprendre*, to "undertake" (Kuratko & Hodgetts, 1995, p. 4). Commonly, an entrepreneur is described as a person who starts or owns his own businesses (Allen, 1999; Bhide, 2000), or as "someone who undertakes to make things happen" (Kirby, 2004, p. 511) whether within a business or non-profit organization.

Being an entrepreneur has been a recognized role within the profession for many years. Historically, the American Occupational Therapy Association (AOTA) defined an **entrepreneur** as an occupational therapy practitioner who is self-employed on a part- or full-time basis (AOTA, 1993). More currently, the *2010 Occupational Therapy Compensation and Workforce Study* (AOTA, 2010) provides information about occupational therapy practitioners who identify themselves as self-employed or contractors. Approximately 27.4% of the respondents were self-employed on a part- or full-time basis (AOTA, 2010). Over time, the percentage of individuals who were self-employed part-time increased at a greater rate than the percentage of those who were self-employed full-time. The study results indicate that self-employment levels for occupational therapists (28.1%) and occupational therapy assistants (23.1%) are at the highest rates since 1993. Most of the respondents who classified themselves as self-employed were independent contractors, agency contractors, or owners/co-owners of a private practice (AOTA, 2010).

Foto (1998) described an occupational therapy entrepreneur as one who is "actively involved in organizing, launching, and operating not only new models of practice, but also profit-making businesses" (p. 765). Others in the profession described entrepreneurs as practitioners who possess the ability to identify and respond to new opportunities that are innovative (Loukas, 2000). No matter the definition, Pazell and Jaffe (2003) stated, "Industry leaders admit that occupational therapy practitioners who are functioning as entrepreneurs are a poorly researched and ill-represented group" (p. 223).

Research on entrepreneurship, intrapreneurship, and social entrepreneurship, and application to occupational therapy, will be described in this chapter. In addition, basic steps in starting for-profit and non-profit businesses, marketing, strategic planning, and grant writing will be discussed.

Research on Entrepreneurs

As an evolving field of study, one that Low describes as "in its adolescence" (2001, p. 17), the literature presents and discusses entrepreneurship from a variety of perspectives, several of which will be discussed here.

The Entrepreneurial Mind-Set

Bygrave (1997) discussed the contribution of personal attributes to the development of an entrepreneur. He suggested certain personality characteristics, such as decisiveness, determination, and a desire for control, are commonly associated with entrepreneurs. However, while certain traits such as vision, perseverance, and energy are deemed as important for success, Cunningham and Lischeron (1991) report, "there is little evidence to suggest that certain traits are associated with successful entrepreneurs" (p. 48).

Despite the differing opinions, the suggestion that certain personality traits or characteristics are typical of entrepreneurs and markedly different from non-entrepreneurs is a premise basic to the psychological (Cunningham & Lischeron, 1991; Kirby, 2004) or the trait schools of thought about entrepreneurs (Kuratko & Hodgetts, 1995). Particularly, the personal values of honesty and responsibility, a risk-taking propensity, creativity, locus of control, the desire for autonomy, and the need for achievement, among others, are all variously considered to be fundamental to successful entrepreneurship (Cunningham & Lischeron, 1991; McClelland, 1961). More specifically, Schmit, Kihm, and Robie (2000) developed a personality assessment that measures five major personality characteristics thought to be integral to entrepreneurs: openness, extroversion, agreeableness, conscientiousness, and neuroticism.

In brief, observations of entrepreneurs point to the identification of multiple characteristics common to their mind-set and motivation. However controversial this approach is, it is now thought that these characteristics can be inherent to the individual or acquired through study and practice.

The Entrepreneurial Process

A second perspective broadly addresses the activities and events of entrepreneurship. The entrepreneurial process has been well documented and is typically rational, controlled, and systematic. From the economic perspective, an entrepreneur notices or identifies a new opportunity, gathers all relevant information pertinent to developing the opportunity, systematically evaluates the alternatives, and finally chooses the option that maximizes economic viability and success (Corner-Doyle & Ho, 2010).

In the 1980s, Gartner (1985, 1989) and others proposed a change in orientation in research away from the entrepreneur and his or her intentions (Carland, Hoy, Boulton, & Carland, 1984; Carland, Hoy, & Carland, 1988) to a focus on the complexity of the organization or venture creation. In support of this shift, Gartner stated, "if we are to understand the phenomenon of entrepreneurship in order to encourage its growth, then we need to understand the process by which new organizations are created" (1989, p. 62). A case in point is Bygrave's (1989) entrepreneurial events model. This model considers personal, environmental, social, and organizational elements influencing the entrepreneurial process, beginning with the generation of the innovative idea to the implementation and growth of the entrepreneurial venture. Further, the model's author acknowledges a triggering event, such as a change in employment or personal circumstances, as a significant ingredient to the innovative idea or opportunity becoming a reality.

Understanding the relationship between the required skills and successful behaviors of entrepreneurs to new development and successful innovation is integral to the entrepreneurial process. The entrepreneur requires skills to identify the need for a new product or unmet service and to recognize the situation as an available opportunity for development. Once the entrepreneur chooses to respond to the opportunity, a plan to address the identified gap is created. Often, entrepreneurs approach this phase with enthusiasm or a strong sense of purpose (Farrell, 2001; Smilor & Sexton, 1996). Along the way, the entrepreneur needs to communicate his or her vision to gain the necessary resources and support for launching and growing the new enterprise from a start-up endeavor to a stable business (Bhide, 2000). Consequently, the ability to tolerate uncertainty, to recognize the unexpected as potential opportunities, to communicate effectively, and to navigate change are thought to be critical to the entrepreneurial process (Bhide, 2000; Drucker, 1985; Smilor & Sexton, 1996).

Opportunity recognition is an important element of the entrepreneurial process. Successful entrepreneurs or entrepreneurial organizations not only recognize opportunities but also capably take advantage of them to reach their goals. To better understand how entrepreneurs make decisions, Keh, Foo, and Lim (2002) studied how specific cognitive factors affect the assessment of a possible entrepreneurial opportunity. The authors surveyed the founders of medium-sized companies to gather information about how the individuals perceived the risk of an opportunity in relationship to the cognitive constructs of overconfidence, belief in the law of small numbers, planning fallacy, and illusion of control. The study results indicated that the entrepreneurs' evaluation of an opportunity and its associated risks was influenced primarily by the individual's cognitive beliefs in small numbers and the illusion of control. Consequently, the study participants acted after considering just a few similar cases or examples or relied on minimal valid information to draw conclusions for action. As well, the participants demonstrated a propensity to believe their skills and abilities could control most situations and outcomes, thereby underestimating the risk associated with the opportunity.

More recently, a second model for the entrepreneurial process has been recognized, that of effectuation. A key premise to this viewpoint is that entrepreneurs begin with "a set of means" (Corner-Doyle & Ho, 2010, p. 4), their skills, knowledge, and resources, and consider how those means might address a particular issue or need. As such, this view of the process is conducive to addressing both social and economic opportunities. Opportunities and outcomes can then be shaped, adapted, and influenced by the passion and vision of the entrepreneur rather than waiting to be identified or recognized.

Beyond opportunity recognition and the entrepreneur's orientation to the promising prospect, external resources available to facilitate the development of new organizations or ventures are also crucial. Specht (1993) categorized these resources into social, economic, political, infrastructure development, and market emergence factors, all of which influence the potential success of the entrepreneurial event.

Intrapreneurship

A third perspective of entrepreneurship further explores the entrepreneurial process within organizations, commonly termed intrapreneurship (Cunningham & Lischeron, 1991; Pinchot, 1985). Intrapreneurship focuses on the innovation, creativity, and resulting behaviors within organizations rather than on the individual entrepreneur. Pazell and Jaffe (2003) defined an **intrapreneur** as an individual "who harnesses the resources within an organization to develop, improve, promote, extend, or enhance a new or existing program" (p. 223). Intrapreneurship is not found in all organizations or corporations. Cunningham and Lischeron (1991) reported that some organizations are more successful in creating an environment that allows its members to act in an entrepreneurial fashion, while others lose employees to their own ventures. "The success of the intrapraneurial model seems to depend on the abilities of the organizational level participants to exploit entrepreneurial opportunities" and whether managers "see the need to exploit these opportunities" (p. 54). More specifically, Kuratko and Hodgetts (1995) advised that innovation within organizations requires the development of explicit goals, systems for feedback and reinforcement, an organizational emphasis on personal responsibility, and a process for linking rewards to results (p. 121).

Social Entrepreneurship

The vast majority of entrepreneurship research focuses on the entrepreneur and the profit-making venture or business. This wealth of information applies to those individuals providing innovative services under the auspices of for-profit companies or businesses. However, many professionals provide services for community-based, not-for-profit, voluntary, or service organizations. The entrepreneurial process in these settings generated a new direction of research focusing on the social entrepreneur and the social entrepreneurial process.

The mission of social entrepreneurs differs from that of business entrepreneurs and influences the entrepreneurial process as a result (Mort, Weerawardena, & Carnegia, 2002). "**Social entrepreneurship** leads to the establishment of new social organizations or not-for-profits and the continued innovation in existing ones" (p. 79). Much as the mission of an entrepreneur with a for-profit focus is to provide a superior product, service, or value to its customers, the mission of a social entrepreneur may be to provide superior value or services to his or her clients or to find "effective ways to harness commercial forces for social good" (Dees, 2000, p. 67). Similarly, a social entrepreneur

may advocate for social changes that will make a positive difference to the community or the organization's clients (Prabhu, 1999). Commonly, social entrepreneurship may also involve for-profit ventures within social service or not-for-profit organizations to assist in achieving the organization's mission and sustaining its service base.

Researchers purport that social entrepreneurs share common characteristics and behaviors with business entrepreneurs. Nga and Shamuganathan (2010) studied the characteristics that influence the intentions of social entrepreneurs in relationship to the five major traits of entrepreneurs proposed by Schmit, Kihm, and Robie (2000). They found that agreeableness, openness, and conscientiousness had a positive influence on all aspects of the social entrepreneurship endeavor, further suggesting the spirit of social entrepreneurship may be promoted among "future would-be" entrepreneurs.

Barendsen and Gardner (2004) studied a group of social entrepreneurs in an effort to identify if and how they are different from business entrepreneurs and service professionals. The authors found the social entrepreneurs' personal histories and belief systems about their obligation, and ability to create positive change in society, were atypical. However, the greatest ongoing challenge faced by the entrepreneurs was carrying out their vision of the needed changes while meeting the financial obligations and realities of keeping their organizations solvent. This challenge appeared to be more demanding than for either the business entrepreneurs or service professionals participating in the study.

Spear (2006) conducted an exploratory study of six small to medium-sized enterprises to further the research on social entrepreneurship. Among the six firms, entrepreneurship was collectively practiced and distributed among employee teams along with external stakeholders such as customers rather than by one champion individual. The motivation for business decisions was varied but included ideological aspects, and decisions were negotiated and "mediated through professionals, advisers, or support organizations" (p. 408). The author's findings offer a broader, collective view about social entrepreneurship, suggesting multiple models of social entrepreneurship are common. In summary, social entrepreneurship appears to be a viable role within small and large organizations or businesses.

Corner-Doyle and Ho (2010) studied the entrepreneurial process of social entrepreneurs, in particular the stage of opportunity recognition. Four patterns emerged among the social entrepreneurs studied. First, the pattern of opportunity development was multifaceted, complex, and did not follow the typical linear steps of commercial entrepreneur endeavors. Second, the opportunity benefited from the collective efforts of multiple individuals with skills, talent, and a passion for a social issue. Third, the experience each of the individuals brought to the endeavor affected the success and outcome. Finally, the fourth pattern described a moment of "spark" (p. 655) or inspiration that related to but was separate from the recognition of an opportunity. These findings suggest the social entrepreneurship process may be more collective, fluid, and spontaneous in nature.

Research leading to a better understanding of the relationship between the entrepreneur and the entrepreneurial process will ultimately influence entrepreneur training and educational programs. Drucker (1985) described innovation as "the specific tool of entrepreneurs, the means by which they exploit change as an opportunity for a different business or a different service. It is capable of being presented as a discipline, capable of being learned, capable of being practiced" (p. 19). Hundreds of how-to books, courses, and academic programs are available to develop the knowledge and skills for entrepreneurism. However, Kirby (2004) argued that all too often, programs "educate 'about' entrepreneurship and enterprise rather than 'for' entrepreneurship" (p. 514). He emphasized that course content and learning activities need to capitalize on the learner's entrepreneurial attributes and creative ways of thinking and behaving, in addition to teaching the principles and practices of entrepreneurship. Applying the entrepreneurial process, one or more individuals sharing a common ideology can be a powerful force for positive change within an organization or community.

Entrepreneurship and Innovation

Among the multiple skills required of an entrepreneur, the ability to effectively create, transform, and promote a new venture or service is critical to success.

Consequently, the entrepreneurial process is inextricably linked to the process of innovation. Van de Ven, Polley, Garud, and Venkataraman (1999) describe this progression as a journey that "from initiation to implementation or termination can vary greatly in number, duration, and complexity. Whatever its scope, the journey is an exploration into the unknown process by which novelty emerges" (p. 3). The study of how individuals learn about, accept, and implement new, innovative ideas or practices inherently includes the examination of the process by which changes are diffused.

Rogers (2003) defined **diffusion** as "the process by which an innovation is communicated through certain channels over time among the members of a social system" (p. 35). Diffusion research examines the multiple facets of this process, such as the rate and consequences of adoption by others and the factors that affect the adoption in a variety of social and cultural settings. The four main elements of the diffusion process Rogers identified include:

1. the innovation
2. the communication channels
3. time
4. social system.

The characteristics of the innovative idea, product, or service itself influence how individuals perceive it when considering its adoption. Customarily, individuals weigh the perceived complexity, usability, and advantages of an innovation before trial. However, a common development during the trial and adoption period is the re-invention or modification of the innovation to better suit the individual's purposes, frequently contributing to the sustainability of the innovation (Rogers, 2003, p. 183). The communication process and channels by which persons learn about an innovation vary widely and frequently include the mass media and the Internet. However, research demonstrates the power of interpersonal communication between individuals with similar interests and values as equally important to successful diffusion.

Next, the element of time considers the speed by which the decision to adopt occurs, along with the characteristics of the persons who adopt the innovation. Rogers (2003) classified these individuals as innovators, early adopters, early majority, late majority, and laggards (p. 22), depending on when each group embraces the innovation. Rogers (2003) suggested that innovativeness is the cornerstone of the diffusion process and associated certain characteristics with each of the adopter categories. "The salient value of the innovator is venturesomeness, due to a desire for the rash, the daring, and the risky" (p. 283). In contrast, the early adopters are more conservative than innovators and yet serve as leaders and role models by embracing the innovation. "In one sense, early adopters put their stamp of approval on a new idea by adopting it" (p. 283).

Occupational therapy entrepreneurs meet the definitions of innovators and early adopters as proposed by Rogers (2003) or of change agents. As change agents, occupational therapists frequently promote innovative social changes for the benefit of their clients or service systems. Zaltman and Duncan (1977) suggested, "One of the basic functions performed by a change agent is to establish a link between a perceived need of a client system and a possible means of satisfying that need" (p. 187). Early adopters also function as change agents and, in so doing, demonstrate effective communication of the vision and the ability to motivate and influence others; both entrepreneurs and leaders share similar attributes.

Occupational Therapy Entrepreneurship

The delivery of entrepreneurial occupational therapy services often requires the ability to identify an opportunity and address an unmet need through new practice methods (Fazio, 2001; Jacobs, 2002). Alternatively, occupational therapy practitioners may already possess knowledge and skills that upon self-reflection are suitable to addressing a particular cause or social need within their communities. They may turn their talents and resources to developing an innovative service that best addresses an identified social need (Corner-Doyle & Ho, 2010).

Four occupational therapy entrepreneurs were asked seven basic questions about their businesses. The practices of each of the entrepreneurs were very different from one another and included wellness coaching, ergonomics, a mental health practice, and a community health non-profit organization. All of the practices were innovative and used principles of occupational therapy as preparatory skill and knowledge. A qualitative analysis was conducted of the interview content, and four general themes emerged:

1. identification of trends,
2. characteristics of effective entrepreneurs,
3. the importance of research, skill building, and planning, and
4. the benefits and barriers involved in starting a new business.

Identification of Trends

While the entrepreneurs approached their businesses from different angles, networking within and outside of occupational therapy was important to identify trends. Reading literature related to each of their business ideas also was a means of identifying trends. Each recognized that by following trends and developing new knowledge in their area of interest, they could best meet community needs and expand their businesses to include a wide array of customers. One entrepreneur stated, "I have always been a person who followed the trends to obtain ideas for how the world works, what people were following and how that translated for the profession of occupational therapy. That, combined with my personal history (living in a family with chronic disability), provided creative ideas for developing new and innovative projects" (M. Pizzi, personal communication).

Characteristics of Effective Entrepreneurs

The characteristics of entrepreneurs derived from the interviews varied widely; however, there were five qualities of an entrepreneur that all interviewees stated in different forms. These include:

1. Be visionary and future oriented.

   One of the entrepreneurs stated: "I stayed attuned to shifting markets and trends by reading and networking with a diverse array of individuals from different professions. I realized that there was an opportunity to use my skills and expertise in ergonomics to develop a consulting practice in this area" (K. Jacobs, personal communication).

2. Maintain optimism.

   The entrepreneurs agreed that to make a business succeed, one must have a "can-do" attitude and spirit. Pushing through barriers and obstacles is part of entrepreneurship, and having the right person-business-attitude fit is vital to establishing a business that works for you. One entrepreneur stated that it is "the ability and confidence to say yes I can do that then figure out how to do it well [furthers your business]" (L. Learnard, personal communication). Another entrepreneur takes her can-do attitude from Goethe, "Whatever you can do, or dream, you can begin it," and the Nike slogan, "Just do it" (K. Jacobs, personal communication).

3. Be a risk-taker.

   All of the entrepreneurs are risk-takers, but calculated risk-takers. They weren't afraid to begin something for which they had great passion because of some obstacles or perceived barriers. One of the entrepreneurs stated it concisely by saying, "If it feels right to YOU, and is part of the vision for who YOU are in the world, both personally and professionally, then go for it!" (M. Pizzi, personal communication).

4. Take advantage of opportunities.

   Being open to seeing opportunities is the cornerstone to a successful business. Communicating effectively, networking, and approaching people and situations with your ideas can expand your business. The entrepreneurs view the possibilities in every situation and with every person they meet as potential business. One entrepreneur stated that in order to take advantage of opportunities, an entrepreneur needs to "step outside of the traditional occupational therapy practice arenas and take advantage of opportunities that span across professional boundaries" (M. Scaffa, personal communication).

5. Be persistent.

   Barriers and obstacles can occur daily with a new business. Persistence in strategically placing your ideas in the marketplace, networking, and communicating, while at the same time understanding that everything takes time, can help your business grow. Not allowing negativity to alter your vision and being persistent about having others recognize the value of your product are important factors in business expansion.

One entrepreneur stated, "Problems will occur if you are not being willing to adapt to changing situations; it is important to continue to work on your practice and to always launch new products and ideas" (L. Learnard, personal communication).

Importance of Research, Skill Building, and Planning

This theme centered on developing a business plan and doing the research necessary for a successful business. Unlike traditional occupational therapy practice, starting a business requires other skills that often are not in the skill set of practitioners. Taking the time to develop this skill set will enable one to enhance the likelihood of developing exactly what it is one envisions. Business plans were created by two of the entrepreneurs, while a third developed a strategic plan and another developed community relationships to disseminate information about the business to have consumers purchase the products being offered. Three of the four entrepreneurs engage in fee-for-service payment, meaning that an agreement is reached for a fee for the service/product, sometimes a written contract is developed, and payment is in the form of cash after the service/product is delivered. Several community resources were identified that could assist with research, skill-building, and planning. These include the Small Business Administration (SBA), the Chamber of Commerce, business and management courses offered by local colleges, and support groups for new entrepreneurs.

Benefits and Barriers to Starting a New Business

In addition, the entrepreneurs described the benefits and obstacles involved in starting one's own business. These are described in Table 8-1.

Starting a New Business: The Basics

There are many advantages to starting one's own business, but not all occupational therapists have entrepreneurial characteristics and most have little, if

Table 8-1	Benefits and Obstacles in Starting a Business	
Benefits	**Obstacles**
Autonomy; taking control of your business future	Limited resources (primarily financial)
The challenge (to create something meaningful that contributes to individuals and society)	Limited time (to dedicate to the business; feeling pulled in many directions)
Focus on creating value that contributes to improving quality of life	Lack of vision for the business and its growth (sometimes feeling overwhelmed and subsequently unwilling to move forward)
Feeling good about what you do and the process of doing it	Trying to be all things to all people and being unable to delegate
Financial rewards (with yourself in control of making that happen)	Unwilling to adapt to changes in trends, business needs, and personnel needs

any, training in business. Therefore, it is critical to identify and utilize experts knowledgeable in business, accounting, and law. If the business will be marketed as occupational therapy, the services provided should conform to the legal scope of practice in the licensure law of the state in which the business will operate (Glennon, 2007).

Types of businesses and legal structures are highly variable. It is important to determine the best organizational structure for the unique needs of one's business. Starting a business can be a daunting process. It is critical to understand all aspects of the business in as much detail as possible. The aim of this chapter is not to provide the reader with a definitive strategy for starting a business, as there are other excellent resources for this purpose. However, some general principles to consider when embarking on a business venture will be presented.

For-Profit or Non-Profit?

The first decision to be made in starting a business is to determine whether it will be a for-profit or non-profit organization. There are many differences between these two types, and each has unique benefits and liabilities. First, the purposes are usually different. The purpose of a for-profit company is to generate profits for the owner(s) and shareholders. The purpose of a non-profit is typically charitable, religious, or educational. An individual or shareholders do not own a non-profit; it is owned by the public. The board of directors directs and operates the non-profit but does not own it. Another difference is the

source of revenue. For-profit businesses generate income through the sales of products or services. Non-profit businesses also can sell products and services, but they also are allowed to solicit donations and apply for grants from the government and private foundations (Fritschner, 2006).

The legal structures also may be different. A for-profit business can be a sole proprietorship, partnership, limited liability company (LLC), or corporation. A non-profit can never be a sole proprietorship but can be set up as an LLC, corporation, or trust, depending on state laws. For-profit companies pay federal taxes, state and local income taxes, sales taxes, property taxes, and employment taxes on employees. Non-profits are often referred to as tax-exempt because they do not pay federal taxes and may also be exempt from some state taxes depending on the laws in each state. However, non-profit companies must pay employment taxes on employees.

In for-profit businesses, profits are usually distributed to the owners or shareholders in the form of dividends. Non-profit businesses can "make a profit," meaning they can accumulate earnings in excess of their expenses. However, these "profits" must be put back into the non-profit organization and cannot be distributed as dividends. The excess funds can be used to purchase equipment and supplies, provide staff training, or increase salaries and benefits, or be retained for future charitable use. If a for-profit company is dissolved, then the assets are distributed to the owners. If a non-profit is dissolved, its assets must be distributed to other non-profit organizations or to the government (Fritschner, 2006). In either case, both non-profit organizations and for-profit businesses are incorporated entities.

Incorporation Process

Articles of incorporation provide the legal description of the business or non-profit organization. Establishing a legal entity protects the board of directors, staff, and volunteers from liabilities such as lawsuits or debts. When the business or non-profit organization is formalized in this way, it is assigned an EIN, or employer identification number, which allows the establishment of a bank account and the ability of the entity to own property. In addition, it allows a non-profit organization to solicit funds in the form of donations and apply for grants that are often restricted to entities with a 501(c)(3) designation of tax-exempt status. A format for articles of incorporation is presented in Box 8-1.

It is important to obtain a copy of requirements for incorporation from the state in which the business or non-profit organization will be located. Each state has its own policies and procedures regarding incorporation, and these can usually be obtained from the Office of the Secretary of State.

Starting a For-Profit Business

Richmond and Powers (2004) outline 15 steps for starting a health care business (Box 8-2). These steps apply to all types of businesses to some degree and provide a useful framework for planning. There are four basic types of legal structures used in for-profit businesses. These are a sole proprietorship, a partnership, an LLC, and a corporation. The simplest for-profit business to develop is a sole proprietorship. This is a business with one owner and no employees. A sole proprietorship is a useful structure for a small private practice, a consulting business, or an independent contractor. The benefits of this type of structure are that it is easy to form, the owner is in total control, he or she receives all income, certain business expenses can be deducted from income taxes, and there are few record-keeping requirements. However, the owner assumes all liability risks and has all legal and operational responsibilities (Richmond & Powers, 2004).

Box 8-1 **Format for Articles of Incorporation**

- Article I: Name of the business or non-profit organization
- Article II: Street address of the business or non-profit organization and mailing address of registered agent (usually the president)
- Article III: Name and address of each incorporator or founding board member
- Article IV: Purpose of the business or non-profit organization and mission statement
- Article V: Membership of the non-profit organization and mission statement
- Article VI: Meetings of the non-profit organization membership (if applicable)
- Article VII: Committees
- Article VIII: Board of Directors
- Article IX: Officers and Duties
- Article X: Amendments to the Articles
- Article XI: Dissolution of Assets
- Article XII: Limitation on Activities (if applicable)

Data from: Fritschner, A. (2006). *An easy, smart guide to starting a nonprofit.* New York: Barnes & Noble Books.

Box 8-2 **15 Steps for Starting a Business**

- Perform a self-assessment and identify business opportunities
- Create a vision statement
- Develop a mission statement
- Describe your business concept
- Adopt a legal structure
- Develop an organizational structure
- Research and register your business name
- Write a business plan
- Develop a marketing plan
- Solicit advice from experts
- Complete start-up tasks
- Hire staff
- Implement and manage business operations
- Manage financial operations
- File quarterly and annual reports

Data from Richmond, T. & Powers, D. (2004). *Business fundamentals for the rehabilitation professional.* Thorofare, NJ: SLACK.

Partnerships have two or more owners and may or may not have employees. Written partnership agreements stating the roles, responsibilities, and liabilities of each partner are essential. This structure is useful for group practices, for joint ventures with separate businesses sharing space and overhead expenses, and when one prefers to take on a financial partner rather than a loan. The benefits of a partnership are that it is relatively easy to set up, liability risks and operational tasks are shared, and there are more opportunities for growth. The disadvantages are that decision making is shared and disagreements between partners can harm the business. In addition, each partner is individually and jointly responsible for the actions of the other (Richmond & Powers, 2004).

LLCs allow the owners the liability protection of a corporation while retaining the operational flexibility of a sole proprietorship or partnership. Each state has specific LLC restrictions, and some states do not permit occupational therapists and other health care providers to establish an LLC business structure. Some of the advantages of an LLC are that it is easier to establish than a corporation, there is no personal liability for business debt, there is less recordkeeping and paperwork required, and business losses can be used as a tax deduction on personal income taxes. Two major factors in the success of a for-profit company are a comprehensive business plan and effective marketing.

Corporations are the most complicated business structures, but they also afford the most protection against liability for the owners. Corporations have multiple owners or stockholders. The persons with the largest shares of stock have the most control over business decisions. A corporation has a board of directors and officers, has bylaws and articles of incorporation, and is subject to extensive governmental regulation. There are several types of corporations, for example, the C corporation, the S corporation, and the professional service corporation (PC). Each of these has different tax implications, so an accountant and an attorney should be consulted to determine the most advantageous structure for your business.

Developing a Business Plan

According to entrepreneurs, a business plan can take various forms, depending on the type of business in which one chooses to engage. According to Jaffe and Epstein (1992), "how successful the business's products will be depends on how thoroughly the prospective entrepreneur has researched and analyzed the business plan" (p. 638). A **business plan** is a road map or blueprint for a business and includes the goals of the business and a description of how the business is going to organize its resources in order to achieve the desired outcomes (Richmond & Powers, 2004). A business plan should be a work in progress that is reviewed and modified on a frequent and routine basis to guide business decisions both large and small. To establish this plan, Richmond and Powers devised five areas in which the entrepreneur needs to focus. The entrepreneur must:

- Perform a market assessment.
- Develop a mission statement.
- Develop a business concept.
- Develop business goals.
- Develop the plan.

Market assessment helps entrepreneurs examine the geographic region of their products, the clientele, and their needs. The Internet has provided occupational therapy entrepreneurs with the world as their market; however, it is wise to develop product lines slowly and create your niche before expanding globally.

Mission statements are broad ideas of the purpose of the business. "Once a mission statement has been developed, it should serve as a guiding principle for practice. It should meet today's needs and tomorrow's prospects" (Jaffe & Epstein, 1992, p. 639). The development of mission statements is discussed in greater detail in Chapter 6.

A business concept defines specifics of the business. For example, if you wish to offer wellness consultation services to underprivileged families, you would describe your specific location of services, the types of services offered, how often services can be offered, and costs of services. These details are important for you to focus your practice and will later help with marketing those services.

Business goals are those you develop initially and can change as your business grows. As an entrepreneur, a typical business goal is to be financially stable. Meeting your costs can be a goal versus having to turn a profit in a specific amount of time. Another goal can be one of philanthropy, whereby the business works towards giving to the community. Philanthropic goals and financial goals do not have to be mutually exclusive.

The plan is the organizational plan, or structure, of the business. This includes the types of people one might employ (if any), bookkeeping practices, and strategies to financially manage the business. There are many books and other resources for entrepreneurs in developing plans that fit their needs. Local chambers of commerce and the SBA are also available to assist one with resources.

Even though occupational therapy is a service-oriented profession, developing a clear, focused plan and marketing one's services and products are critical to the success of the business. **Marketing** refers to the "communications activities the organization will undertake in order to attract service users" (Fritschner, 2006, p. 200). The goals of marketing include creating consumer awareness of the product or service, building name recognition, and meeting financial goals. MacStravic (1977) outlined five components of social marketing:

- Identification of constituencies
- Assessment of the marketing environment and its problems
- Selection and evaluation of marketing objectives
- Design of a marketing strategy
- Planning, implementation, control, and evaluation of marketing efforts (as discussed in Gilkerson, 1997).

Developing a plan and possessing knowledge of how to implement that plan and market your services can turn a great idea into a successful practice. Karen Jacobs (1998), past president of the American Occupational Therapy Association, stated that the "use of a marketing approach will allow practitioners to approach the health care environment proactively and be ready to meet the changing needs and wants of the marketplace. In all times of change, there is great opportunity" (p. 620).

Starting a Non-Profit Organization

Non-profits are often referred to as agencies, foundations, associations, and organizations. There are four types of non-profits: public non-profits, private foundations, membership-supported non-profits, and service non-profits. Funding for public non-profits comes from the constituencies the non-profit serves. For example, the American Red Cross and the United Way receive monies from the public in order to provide services. Public non-profits can provide educational, advocacy, community, cultural, and health services. Private foundations exist to distribute money to charities. Typically, private foundations derive their funding from a single, private source, frequently wealthy philanthropists, such as the Carnegie Foundation. Membership-supported non-profits can receive funds from the general public, but what makes them unique is that their members help to financially support them. Environmental groups, labor unions, fraternities, and sororities fit into this category. Service non-profits provide services to the general public, such as schools and hospitals, and receive their funding from a variety of sources (Fritschner, 2006).

Starting a non-profit organization is much the same as starting a for-profit business. The tasks for starting a non-profit organization are listed in Box 8-3. The first stage is the idea phase. It is important to research the services or products one hopes to deliver. Is there a need that is not being met by other community agencies? The second stage is to gather people who share one's vision and commitment. These are people who will become the board of directors, officers, and volunteers. The third stage is determining the form or legal structure for the non-profit. Considerations at this stage include size of the organization, perceived liabilities, and tax-exempt status. Next is the development of a strategic plan, followed by publicity and a fund-raising campaign. Finally, there must be a plan for growth and continued development of the organization.

Three major factors in the success of a non-profit organization are strategic planning, fund-raising, and grant writing.

Strategic Planning

Strategic planning is a systematic process of setting long-term organizational goals and priorities, identifying organizational activities, and predicting potential outcomes. Strategic planning "is an ongoing, continuous process, which must adapt to environmental changes, both external and internal" (Smith, Bucklin & Associates, 2000, p. 5). A strategic plan is a realistic agenda for action that operationalizes the organization's mission statement and focuses the

---

Box 8-3 Tasks Involved in Setting Up a Non-Profit Organization

- Meet with volunteers and discuss what type of services and products the organization will provide and who will be in charge of various operational functions. A board of directors must be established and officers elected. Create a mission statement and choose a name for the organization.
- Develop the organization's articles of incorporation. These describe the non-profit's legal structure and how it will be operated.
- File the articles of incorporation with the state in order to establish the organization as a legal entity. Be prepared to pay a filing fee.
- Apply to the Internal Revenue Service (IRS) for an Employer Identification Number (EIN). This can be done online. This number identifies the non-profit and affords the organization the legitimacy to establish a bank account in its name.
- File an application for non-profit tax-exempt status with the IRS (referred to as 501(c)(3) status). This allows the organization to receive tax-deductible contributions and avoid paying federal income tax.
- Create a logo and acquire stationery that displays your logo, mailing address, and other contact information.
- Set up a corporate bank account and acquire a mailing permit from the post office for bulk mailings.
- Create a Web page to enhance the credibility and visibility of the non-profit organization. Register your domain name as.org, which is the identifier for a non-profit, rather than .com.

---

organization's energies toward high-yield objectives and activities. A well-designed strategic plan will:

- establish priorities,
- guide program activities,
- allocate resources, and
- establish mechanisms to assess the organization's accomplishments.

The steps in the strategic planning process include:

- conducting an environmental scan and analysis,
- setting broad organizational goals,
- establishing strategic objectives, and
- developing an operational plan.

An environmental scan and analysis is the first step in strategic planning. It is important for the planners to understand the trends and issues that impact the organization and how the environment may facilitate or hinder the accomplishment of the organization's mission. An **environmental scan** identifies trends in a variety of spheres, including demographic, economic, technological, political, professional, and educational. An internal scan of the organization's financial and human resources, technological capabilities, and culture is also an important source of information. Sometimes this approach is referred to as a **SWOT analysis**, where "S" refers to strengths and assets, "W" to weaknesses and limitations, "O" to opportunities, and "T" to threats. Once the organization's strengths, weaknesses, opportunities, and threats are identified, a strategic plan can be developed to address these factors. An example of a SWOT analysis is provided in Box 8-4. Trends that have a high probability of occurrence and potentially may have a significant impact on the organization should be considered critical issues to be addressed in the strategic plan (Smith, Bucklin & Associates, 2000). The second step in strategic planning is setting broad organizational goals. These goals are generally derived from the mission statement and represent the purpose of the organization.

The third step in strategic planning is setting strategic objectives, those "major accomplishments the organization hopes to achieve in a defined time frame," usually three to five years (Smith, Bucklin & Associates, 2000, p. 19). Strategic objectives support the mission and goals of the organization, provide direction, and afford a means for measuring outcomes. These objectives should be realistic, meaningful, and measurable. Strategic objectives identify what is to be accomplished. The next step is to operationalize the strategic objectives; this involves specifying how the objectives will be achieved. An operational plan describes the tasks to be accomplished, who is responsible, what resources are required, when the objectives will be achieved, the anticipated results, and how these results will be measured. Finally, the strategic plan is implemented, monitored, and adjusted as necessary.

Fund-Raising

There is a science and an art to fund-raising. The science is applying fund-raising models and using available data and research to target fund-raising

Box 8-4	**SWOT Analysis Example: A Senior Center Wishing to Expand and Provide Health Promotion Services**

Strengths/Assets
- Stable, experienced staff
- Good reputation in the community
- Adequate financial resources for current services
- Well networked with other non-profit agencies
- Member of the Chamber of Commerce

Weaknesses/Limitations
- Inadequate space to expand
- Lack of finances to build a new facility
- Limited parking
- Location not on public transit routes

Opportunities
- Recent hospital downsizing producing unused space
- Increasing older adult population
- University collaboration for potential student training
- Lack of local services for older adults with dementia or mental disorders

Threats
- Current economic recession
- Inadequate political support
- Competition from medically based health services

efforts. The art consists of developing and nurturing interpersonal relationships with potential donors and funders. Funding for non-profit organizations can come from a variety of sources, including individual donors, corporate donors, bank loans, grants, contracts, online fund-raising, and other fund-raising events. The most viable non-profit organizations bring in dollars, goods, and services from multiple sources. The vast majority of donations, approximately 75%, comes from individuals; therefore, it is imperative to cultivate a donor base (Fritschner, 2006).

Developing a donor base occurs in phases. The first phase, prospecting, is where a list of potential donors is developed. These potential donors are then prioritized based on how much they might donate and the probability of successfully soliciting a donation. Each potential donor is invited to observe and participate in the activities of the organization, and then a request for a donation can be made. When a donation is solicited, it is important that it is solicited from the right person, for the right amount of money, at the right time, and for the right purpose. This is called the Rule of Rights in fund-raising. In-person solicitation is always more effective than fund-raising through the mail. Thanking the donor, acknowledging the contribution publicly, and informing the donor about how the money was spent will improve the likelihood the donor will choose to donate again (Fritschner, 2006).

Corporations are often interested in donating funds to non-profits that serve the local communities in which their employees live and work. In addition,

corporate donations are tax deductible, often produce publicity, and generate goodwill for the corporation. Typically, corporations are not interested in funding annual operating costs but will provide start-up funds for new projects or programs. In lieu of money, some corporations will provide in-kind donations, often in the form of goods and services. Corporations represent approximately 5% of the dollars, goods, and services donated nationwide (Fritschner, 2006). For example, a homeless shelter needing a vehicle in order to provide transportation to and from medical appointments and job interviews may receive an in-kind donation of a van from a car dealership.

Another source of funding for start-up ventures is small business loans. Small business loans are available to 501(c)(3) non-profit organizations that have at least a 3-year operating history. Just like any other business loan, repayment with interest on a schedule is expected, and the interest rate is typically similar to that of a for-profit business.

Online fund-raising usually takes the form of selling some product to the general public; however, online donation solicitation is also an option. To take advantage of the Web as a source of funds, it is necessary for the organization to be able to process credit card payments. Another option is to collaborate with brand name companies that donate a portion of their online sales proceeds to charitable organizations.

Many non-profits sponsor special fund-raising events. These may include dinners, concerts, theatrical productions, auctions, and sports outings, with the type of event limited only by one's imagination. In addition to garnering revenue from ticket sales, non-profits may also solicit sponsorships from corporations. Fund-raising events are time- and labor-intensive, with costs often approximating 50% of the revenue generated. However, they are useful in publicizing the work of the non-profit, increasing its visibility, and cultivating new donors (Smith, Bucklin & Associates, 2000).

Grant Writing

Foundations provide nearly 12% of the funds provided to non-profits. Most foundations require a grant proposal from the organization that is compatible with the mission and purpose of the foundation. There are a number of different types of grants, and these are listed in **Box 8-5**. It is important to identify the type of grant and the appropriate foundation from which to solicit funds before writing a grant proposal (Fritschner, 2006).

There are five basic types of foundations:

1. Independent family foundations, established by persons of wealth

---

Box 8-5 Types of Grants

- *Start-up grants:* also called "seed money"; grants that are used to partially fund new programs or projects in order to attract other donations
- *Program grants:* grants that are used for a specific program within an organization
- *Continuing support grants:* grants that can be renewed for a number of years
- *Consulting grants:* grants that are used to hire consultants for a project
- *Conference grants:* grants that are used to send organization board members or staff to continuing education workshops, or to plan and implement conferences or seminars for others
- *Research grants:* grants that provide funding for basic or applied research, usually provided to or through hospitals and universities
- *Challenge or matching grants:* grants that provide partial funding but require other donors to match the funding in order to receive the grant
- *Endowment:* monetary gift, or grant, to be invested, the income from which can be used to fund projects and support the non-profit organization

Data from: Fritschner, A. (2006). *An easy, smart guide to starting a nonprofit.* New York: Barnes & Noble Books.

---

2. Corporate foundations, sponsored by large companies
3. Community foundations, designed to serve a particular geographic region
4. Special-purpose foundations, focused on a specific area of interest
5. General-purpose foundations, typically national in scope and supporting a variety of activities with no geographic limitations (Smith, Bucklin & Associates, 2000).

Information about foundation funding can be obtained from the Foundation Center (www.fdncenter.org) and the Council on Foundations (www.cof.org).

In addition to foundation sources, funding can be obtained from state and federal government agencies. The Catalog of Federal Domestic Assistance is the primary source of information about federal funding opportunities. Government agencies may offer funds in the form of grants or contracts. **Grants** are funds awarded for a specific purpose based on the submission of an original creative proposal. **Contracts** are also awarded for a specific purpose, but in this case the government agency has already outlined the scope of services to be provided and non-profit organizations are invited to bid competitively on the project (Scaffa, 2001). Funding for occupation-based health promotion projects may be available from the following federal agencies:

- Centers for Disease Control and Prevention
- Department of Education
- Department of Health and Human Services
- Department of Housing and Urban Development
- Department of Labor
- Department of Transportation
- National Institutes of Health
- Public Health Service
- Veterans Administration.

Grant funding is often a non-profit organization's primary source of support. Grants are considered "soft money," meaning the funding is available for only a specified period of time, usually a year, occasionally for 3 years, and rarely for up to 5 years. No single grant or contract provides a permanent revenue stream, and therefore it is imperative that non-profit staff and volunteers develop, or contract for, grant writing capabilities.

Grant Proposals

Grant proposals typically consist of the following:

- Introduction
- Statement of need
- Goals and objectives
- Program activities
- Program evaluation strategies
- Budget and personnel
- History of organization and prior funding
- Summary or conclusion
- Appendices of supporting materials (Fritschner, 2006).

Although the introduction is the first thing the funder will read, it is typically one of the last components of the grant proposal you write. To ensure that the introduction is a complete synopsis of the full grant proposal, it is typically written at the same time as the conclusion.

The most efficient strategy is to write a basic grant proposal with all of the above components. Then this information can be "cut and pasted" into any grant proposal format for any funding source. The first step is to identify and describe the need for the particular project or service that is being proposed. The statement of needs provides data that is specific to the problem and population being addressed and the geographic area the project is designed to serve. Basically, it answers the question, "Why is this project important and necessary?"

The second step is to identify the goals and objectives of the program or project. These define what is to be achieved. A goal is a general statement regarding expected outcomes, while an objective is a specific statement that defines the goal in measurable terms. Goals represent the final destination; objectives specify how the goals will be achieved. Examples of goals and related objectives can be found in **Box 8-6**. The objectives should support the achievement of the goals, and the goals should address the needs identified in the statement of needs. Basically, this section answers the question, "What is to be accomplished by this project?" Describing program activities is the third step in the grant writing process. These activities are designed to accomplish the specified program objectives. Typically, there are several program activities for each objective. This section of the proposal often includes a time line for completion of the program activities and a list of staff,

---

Box 8-6 Sample Grant Goals and Objectives

Goal:

Increase the ability of teachers, school counselors, clergy, health-care professionals, emergency response personnel, and human resource and personnel directors of local businesses to effectively respond to the mental health needs of persons affected by disaster.

Objectives:

Workshop participants will demonstrate:

- Increased knowledge of the symptoms of post-traumatic stress disorder (PTSD) and the critical incident stress model
- Improved identification and referral of persons in need of mental health services
- Effective use of appropriate interventions for persons experiencing critical incident stress or PTSD.

Goal:

Enhance the mental health of individuals affected by disaster.

Objectives:

Support group participants will demonstrate:

- Reduced symptoms of critical incident stress and PTSD
- Increased use of adaptive coping strategies in response to critical incident stress
- Decreased use of maladaptive coping strategies in response to critical incident stress.

---

equipment, and supplies that are necessary to implement the activities. It answers the question, "What activities will be done to achieve the objectives?"

Program evaluation, the fourth step, is an extremely important component of a grant proposal. Funders want to know that their money is well spent, how program effects will be measured, and which program goals and objectives were achieved. The program evaluation describes how and when progress will be measured and what assessment tools will be used. Program evaluation assesses what was done, the activities, and the effects of those activities or outcomes. It answers the question, "Did the program accomplish what it set out to achieve?"

The fifth step, describing the budget and personnel, provides support for the amount of funding that is being requested. It answers the question, "How will the money be spent?" Funders want to see that you have accurately estimated the costs of implementing the program. This requires the grant writer to collect cost information for salaries, rent, utilities, equipment, and supplies. Some people speculate that if the costs are underestimated and the total costs are lower, then the grant is more likely to be funded. However, this is typically not true. Funders frequently know the costs of doing business, and proposals that claim to be able to implement programs at significantly below market costs are deemed unrealistic and likely to fail. It is useful to have the assistance of an accountant in the preparation of a budget for a grant proposal. When describing personnel by name, mention only those who will play a major role in the project, and list their relevant credentials and qualifications. The rest of the project staff can be identified by categories, such as childcare workers, bus drivers, tutors, and others (Fritschner, 2006).

Finally, the last step is to write the introduction and summary or conclusion for the grant application. These two sections are extremely important, as they are the first and last impressions the proposal reader will have of the project or program. If the introduction is not well written, clear, and interesting, the reader may choose not to continue or to peruse only superficially. A poorly written introduction is often a death sentence for a grant proposal. The introduction and the conclusion contain basically the same information, and they provide a concise overview of the project as a whole. Fritschner (2006) recommends that the introduction use action words and the conclusion use more of an emotional appeal. The introduction and conclusion should include a brief statement of the problem, how the program will address the problem, the non-profit organization's qualifications, and the amount of money needed. Including the name of the foundation or funding source in both the introduction and conclusion is highly recommended. This personalizes the grant proposal and engages the funding sources as co-participants.

In addition, certain documents may be requested for the appendices of supporting material. Supporting material may include: letters of support and endorsement from key community stakeholders, newspaper clippings regarding the problem to be addressed by the program, resumes of key program staff members, copies of assessments and program evaluation tools, and the IRS tax-exempt letter designating the organization as a 501(c)(3) corporation (Fritschner, 2006).

Conclusion

Entrepreneurship, like occupational therapy, is both a science and an art (Kiyosaki, 1999). Occupational therapy practitioners who aspire to become business owners should take courses and immerse themselves in the science of business management and leadership. The art of entrepreneurship is best learned through mentoring. Surrounding oneself with innovative thinkers, leaders, and business owners is one of the keys to success. Finding an entrepreneurial role model is extremely useful.

Entrepreneurship is developing rapidly in the profession of occupational therapy, yet the process of entrepreneurialism is not well defined nor understood. This process and the need for continued research were presented in this chapter along with the characteristics, steps, and strategies for developing entrepreneurship. Occupational therapy practitioners are typically creative, adaptive, and relationship builders. These characteristics provide a solid foundation for becoming entrepreneurs.

Learning Activities

1. Identify an entrepreneur in your business or health-care community. Arrange to interview him or her to discover how and why this individual chose to become an entrepreneur, what personal qualities this person brings to the entrepreneurial role, and the challenges and rewards to being an entrepreneur.
2. Visit the Small Business Administration (SBA) Web site and review the business plan template (http://web.sba.gov/busplantemplate/BizPlanStart.cfminformation). Using an idea for a community-based, occupational therapy service, write a mission and vision statement for your business idea that would meet those elements of a business plan.
3. Go to the following site to take the Entrepreneur Risk Assessment Quiz from the Georgia State University Small Business Center (www2.gsu.edu/~wwwsbp/entrepre.htm).

Continued

Complete the quiz, note your score, and visit the Answer Sheet to interpret your score and see if you possess the personal characteristics necessary to succeed in business.

4. With a group of your classmates, identify an unmet need for occupational therapy services in your community. Visit either the Grants.gov or The Foundation Center Web site to see if you can identify a government agency or foundation with funding criteria that match the proposed new services. Note whether a request for a proposal (RFP) or funding announcement is available for your idea.

REFERENCES

Allen, K. R. (1999). *Growing and Managing an Entrepreneurial Business.* New York: Houghton Mifflin Company.

American Occupational Therapy Association. (1993). Occupational therapy roles. *American Journal of Occupational Therapy, 48,* 1087–1099.

American Occupational Therapy Association. (2010). *2010 Occupational Therapy Compensation and Workforce Study.* Bethesda, MD: Author.

Barendsen, L., & Gardner, H. (2004, Fall). Is the social entrepreneur a new type of leader? *Leader to Leader, 43–50.*

Bhide, A. V. (2000). *The origin and evolution of new businesses.* New York: Oxford University Press.

Bygrave, W. D. (1989, Fall). The entrepreneurship paradigm: A philosophical look at its research methodologies. *Entrepreneurship: Theory and Practice, 14*(1), 7–26.

Bygrave, W. D. (1997). *The portable MBA in entrepreneurship.* New York: John Wiley & Sons.

Carland, J. W., Hoy, F., Boulton, W., & Carland, J. A. C. (1984). Differentiating entrepreneurs from small business owners: A conceptualization. *Academy of Management Review, 9,* 354–359.

Carland, J. W., Hoy, F., & Carland, J. A. C. (1988, Spring). "Who is an entrepreneur?" Is a question worth asking. *American Journal of Small Business, 33–38.*

Corner-Doyle, P., & Ho, M. (2010). How opportunities develop in social entrepreneurship. *Entrepreneurship: Theory & Practice, 635–659.*

Cunningham, B., & Lischeron, J. (1991). Defining entrepreneurship [Electronic version]. *Journal of Small Business Management, 29,* 45–61.

Dees, J. G. (2000, January-February). Enterprising nonprofits [Electronic version]. *Harvard Business Review, 55–67.*

Drucker, P. F. (1985). *Innovation and entrepreneurship: Practice and principles.* New York: Harper & Row.

Farrell, L. C. (2001). *The entrepreneurial age: Awakening the spirit of enterprise in people, companies, and countries.* New York: Allworth Press.

Fazio, L. S. (2001). *Developing occupation-centered programs for the community: A workbook for students and professionals.* Upper Saddle River, NJ: Prentice-Hall.

Foto, M. (1998). Competence and the occupational therapy entrepreneur. *The American Journal of Occupational Therapy, 52*(9), 765–769.

Fritschner, A. (2006). *An easy, smart guide to starting a nonprofit.* New York: Barnes & Noble Books.

Gartner, W. B. (1985). A conceptual framework for describing the phenomenon of new venture creation [Electronic version]. *Academy of Management Review, 10*(4), 698–708.

Gartner, W. B. (1989). "Who is an entrepreneur?" Is the wrong question [Electronic version]. *Entrepreneurship: Theory and Practice, 13*(4), 47–68.

Gilkerson, G. (1997). *Occupational therapy leadership: Marketing yourself, your profession and your organization.* Philadelphia: F.A. Davis.

Glennon, T. J. (2007). Putting on your business hat. *OT Practice, 12*(3), 23–25.

Jacobs, K. (2002, June 24). Navigating the road ahead. *OT Practice, 7,* 24–30.

Jacobs, K. (1998). Innovation to action: Marketing occupational therapy. *American Journal of Occupational Therapy, 52*(8), 618–620.

Jaffe, E. G., & Epstein, C. F. (1992). *Occupational therapy consultation: Theory, principles and practice.* St. Louis: Mosby.

Keh, H. T., Foo, M. D., & Lim, B. C. (2002, Winter). Opportunity evaluation under risky conditions: The cognitive processes of entrepreneurs. *Entrepreneurship Theory and Practice, 125–148.*

Kirby, D. A. (2004). Entrepreneurship education: Can business schools meet the challenge? *Education & Training, 46*(8/9), 510–519.

Kiyosaki, R. T. (1999). *Rich dad's cashflow quadrant.* New York: Time Warner.

Kuratko, D. F., & Hodgetts, R. M. (1995). *Entrepreneurship: A contemporary approach* (3rd ed.). Fort Worth, TX: Dryden Press.

Loukas, K. M. (2000, June). Emerging models of innovative community-based occupational practice. *OT Practice.* Retrieved from http://aota.org/featured/area2/links

Low, M. B. (2001). The adolescence of entrepreneurship research: Specification of purpose. *Entrepreneurship Theory and Practice, 25*(4), 17–25.

MacStravic, R. E. (1977). *Marketing health care.* Germantown, MD: Aspen.

McClelland, D. C. (1961). *The Achieving Society.* Princeton, NJ: Van Nostrand.

Mort, G. S., Weerawardena, J., & Carnegie, K. (2002, July). Social entrepreneurship: towards conceptualization [Electronic version]. *International Journal of Nonprofit and Voluntary Sector Marketing, 8*(1), 76–88.

Nga, J. K. H., & Shamuganathan, G. (2010). The influence of personality traits and demographic factors on social entrepreneurship start up intentions. *Journal of Business Ethics, 95,* 259–282.

Pazell, S., & Jaffe, E. G. (2003). Entrepreneurial ventures. In G. L. McCormack, E. G. Jaffe, & M. Goodman-Levy (Eds.). *The occupational therapy manager* (pp. 219–255). Bethesda, MD: American Occupational Therapy Association.

Pinchot, G. (1985). *Intrapreneuring: Why you don't have to leave the corporation to become an entrepreneur.* New York: Harper and Row.

Prabhu, G. N. (1999). Social entrepreneurial leadership [Electronic version]. *Career Development International, 4*(3), 140–145.

Richmond, T., & Powers, D. (2004). *Business fundamentals for the rehabilitation professional.* Thorofare, NJ: SLACK.

Rogers, E. M. (2003). *Diffusion of innovations* (5th ed.). New York: Free Press.

Scaffa, M. (2001). *Occupational therapy in community-based practice settings.* Philadelphia: F.A. Davis.

Schmit, M. J., Kihm, J. A., & Robie, C. (2000). Development of a global measure of personality. *Personal Psychology, 53,* 153–193.

Smilor, R. W., & Sexton, D. L. (Eds.). (1996). Leadership and entrepreneurship: Personal and organizational development in entrepreneurial ventures. Westport, CT: Quorum Books.

Smith, Bucklin & Associates (2000). *The complete guide to nonprofit management* (2nd ed.). New York: John Wiley & Sons.

Spear, R. (2006). Social entrepreneurship: A different model? *International Journal of Social Economics, 33*(5/6), 399–410.

Specht, P. H. (1993). Munificence and carrying capacity of the environment and organization formation. *Entrepreneurship: Theory and Practice, 17*(2), 77–86.

Van de Ven, A. H., Pelloy, D. E., Garud, R., & Venkataraman, S. (1999). *The Innovation Journey.* New York: Oxford University Press.

Zaltman, G., & Duncan, R. (1977). *Strategies for planned change.* New York: John Wiley & Sons.

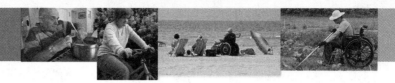

Children and Youth

Chapter 9

Early Intervention Programs

Donna A. Wooster, PhD, OTR/L, and Abigail Baxter, PhD

Article 27: Every child has the right to a standard of living adequate for [her/his] physical, mental, spiritual, moral and social development.

—United Nations Children's Fund, n.d.

Learning Objectives

This chapter is designed to enable the reader to:

- Identify the components of Early Intervention (EI) programs.
- Discuss the role of the occupational therapist in EI programs.
- Identify and describe appropriate areas for evaluation and assessment instruments for early intervention occupational therapy services.
- Discuss the importance of family involvement in early intervention.
- Identify best practice in occupational therapy early intervention services.

Key Terms

Amplification
Early Intervention (EI)
Ecological evaluation
Eligibility
Family-centered

Food neophobia
Individualized family service plan (IFSP)
Natural environments
Service coordinator
Solution-focused questions

Introduction

Early Intervention (EI) is a federally supported program implemented by states for children age birth to 3 years who have a disability. Federal funding is available to states that have developed EI service systems. States that have taken federal dollars for EI are mandated to implement a "statewide, comprehensive, coordinated, multidisciplinary, interagency system of early intervention services for infants and toddlers with disabilities and their families" (Individuals with Disabilities Education Improvement Act [IDEIA], 2004, p. 5). Even though EI is not a federally mandated program, each state has developed an EI system based on federal guidelines designed to address its specific needs and resources. Occupational therapists should seek information specific to the state(s) in which they practice.

The primary purpose of EI services is to identify children with disabilities or delayed development who may be eligible for services and to provide necessary services to promote the family's ability to care for the child. The components of the programs are detailed in the IDEIA. Part A describes the general purpose and provisions of the act, including definitions. Part B covers centers and services to meet special needs of individuals with disabilities aged 3–21 years, and Part C defines infants and toddlers with disabilities (birth through age 2). The components requiring a Free Appropriate Public Education (FAPE) are in parts A and B, which mandate the provision of education for all children with disabilities between the ages of 3 and 21 years.

Improvements in the legislation have occurred over time. A more inclusive environment for the infants and toddlers with disabilities was mandated. Services were required to be provided in **natural environments** (i.e., places children would normally find themselves, depending on age and activity). These include home, day care provider's home, day care center, nursery school, and playgrounds. Parents have input guiding the team in the choice of location(s) of service delivery. Service provision also should be provided in these inclusive environments. More recently, the IDEIA 2004 required that EI services be evidence-based. In addition, the IDEIA emphasized measureable results and pre-literacy and language skill development.

In this chapter the authors discuss the need for, and purpose of, EI and the legislatively mandated components of EI programs. The role of the occupational therapist in EI services is described, including evaluation, intervention, and family involvement. In addition, a case study illustrates the major points of the chapter.

EI Programs

The number and percentage of children birth to age 3 being served in EI has increased over the past 20 years. Estimates suggest that these trends will continue. In the past, parents were urged to place children with disabilities in institutions. Changes in society have contributed to the expectation that families will care for their child at home regardless of the child's disability. Some families need intense interventions and supports to competently handle this level of care. Research suggests that professionals can help families by providing information, emotional support, and continuous services (Anderson & Telleen, 1992; Hebbeler, Spiker, Bailey, Scarborough, Mallik, & Simconsson et al., 2007).

Medically fragile children now have longer life expectancies than they did in the past (Fitzsimmons, 1993; Gortmaker & Sappenfield, 1984). Although the total size of the population of children with disabilities and chronic illness probably will remain stable, the longer life span will result in families with needs that will change over time as the child grows (Wallace, Biehl, MacQueen, & Blackman, 1997).

Societal trends, such as recessions and international crises and conflicts, also can impact the number of families in need. For example, job relocation and deployment of servicemen and servicewomen are both factors that may result in having fewer family members living close by who could be resources. Additionally, many children with disabilities may live in poverty, dysfunctional families, and disadvantaged communities (Thompson, 1992). Poverty is associated with increased risk for disability and increased hospitalizations for problems related to chronic health conditions (Newacheck, 1989; Wissow, 1988), thus placing children with disabilities at greater accumulated risk.

Components of Early Intervention

There are three components of EI programs. These components include identification, eligibility determination, and evaluation.

Identification

Each state must establish a system to identify children who may be eligible for services and refer them to the EI system. Children with suspected developmental delays or a disability may be identified through a variety of sources, including occupational therapists, parents, physicians, other health providers, and community agencies. Professionals must seek verbal approval from the parents to make a referral. A central phone number (usually an 800 number) is typically available for referrals.

Eligibility Determination

One component of each statewide system is establishment of the local lead agency. This appointed agency varies from state to state and may be part of the state health department, education department, or another department. The local lead agency schedules the evaluation with the parents to determine eligibility. **Eligibility** refers to whether or not the child qualifies, under the state's criteria, to receive EI services. States must serve children "who are experiencing developmental delays" in accordance with the state's definition of developmental delay and children with "a diagnosed physical or mental condition that has a high probability of resulting in developmental delay" (IDEIA, 2004, p. 100). Once written parental consent is obtained, the evaluation process is initiated. The evaluation can be done by a variety of trained professionals. The evaluation scores will be used to determine eligibility for services. A specific level of developmental delay (such as 25%) in one or more areas, or two standard deviations below the norm in any two areas, may constitute eligibility. In some states, professional opinions of high risk may qualify the child.

Evaluation

The IDEIA 2004 includes specific information about the evaluation process. Multidisciplinary evaluations must be done within 45 days of referral and given in the native language or type of communication that suits the family. Best practice research indicates that the evaluation of a child in multiple environments or contexts increases the reliability of the evaluation (Miller, 1994). If possible, occupational therapists should conduct observations of the child at home and in the community, including day care or nursery school and other natural environments. Factors that may be evaluated include response to different environments, effects of peer role models on performance, solitary versus group function, and social-emotional and communication skills with children as well as adults other than the parents. Gathering information across environments will help the occupational therapist to match the child's abilities with the requirements of the occupation and the features of the environment to enhance performance.

A variety of factors, such as the child's age, gender, ethnic background, native language, culture, and information needs of the family and team, influences the selection of assessment tools. Assessments must be standardized test instruments that assess performance in five areas:

1. motor,
2. cognitive,
3. social-emotional,
4. communication, and
5. adaptive development.

Assessment instruments must not be culturally biased. Many states indicate a specific instrument as the assessment tool of choice and allow other informed clinical opinions to be expressed in writing to support the findings. Parents should be included in the evaluation process to provide information about the abilities of their child. Assessments of family needs also are conducted.

The EI program is primarily an educational model with teachers as the primary evaluators and providers. EI teams must have many other professionals, including occupational therapists, physical therapists, speech language pathologists, audiologists, nurses, and others, available. One team member, usually a teacher, may perform the primary assessment. This person administers assessment tools and then, based on test findings across the five areas, calls in other services such as speech or occupational therapy.

Another format is the arena-style evaluation. Multiple service providers gather to simultaneously observe the evaluation being conducted by one or two primary evaluators. Each team member records information and discusses the child's abilities. The team members discuss the observations and write a joint evaluation report. A child may be determined eligible for EI services based on the test scores. A report is written following the evaluation, and if the child is eligible for services an individualized plan is developed based on the assessment information. The results and observations of the evaluation are used to make referrals to appropriate service providers. For example, if the child scored low on adaptive and fine-motor skills, then a referral is usually made for occupational therapy services.

Individualized Family Service Plan (IFSP)

Once eligibility has been established, a written plan, called an **individualized family service plan (IFSP),** must be developed by the team. This process is summarized in Box 9-1 and includes the development of child and family goals. Only one IFSP is developed despite the involvement of a number of agencies. Family members are key participants in the development of the IFSP. All services required by the child must be documented in the plan, including which community agency will provide the service. The service providers, the frequency of intervention, the family goals, and the resources that will be involved are specified in the plan. Expected measurable outcomes are clearly stated. This process will identify the child's needs, family resources, priorities, concerns, and supports. At the conclusion of the process, which

also includes the appointment of a service coordinator and a family meeting, the nature and extent of services will be delineated. The IFSP is reviewed every 6 months (or more frequently if required) and must be evaluated once a year. Outcomes can be modified or changed at any time if the parent desires.

Occupational therapy may be a primary service provider for the infant/toddler under the IFSP plan (Decker, 1992). Occupational therapy may be the only service provider or may be part of a team of providers. Each plan is customized to the needs of the child and the family. Any child with an identified need for occupational therapy must receive the service. Occupational therapy is one of the "big five" EI services, and more than a third of infants and toddlers receiving EI services receive occupational therapy services (Hebbeler et al., 2007).

The **service coordinator** functions as a consultant to the parents and service providers. The service coordinator may be involved in training parents and other family members and professionals, coordinating appointments with medical personnel, participating in the team IFSP process, and establishing links with service providers. In addition, the service coordinator assists the family in planning for the transition to public school when the child is 3 years of age. The service coordinator is responsible for implementing the IFSP. An occupational therapist also could serve in the role of the service coordinator, which would decrease the number of professionals involved.

Parents have many rights associated with the IFSP process. The parents may review records at any time and can consent to share medical information with the IFSP team. A parent who is dissatisfied with the service provision or finds the documented IFSP services are not being provided has the right to due process. This is a legal proceeding that involves a hearing conducted by an impartial mediator to resolve disputes. This clearly illustrates the rights of the family in planning for the needs of their child who is receiving EI services.

Box 9-1	**The Individualized Family Service Plan (IFSP) Process**

The IFSP process gathers information on the following.
• Child's current status.
• Family resources, priorities, and concerns.
• Major measureable outcomes expected.
• Specific services—frequency, duration, provider, and dates to initiate.
• Description of natural environment in which services will be provided
• Need for other services, for example, medical.
• Name of service coordinator.
• Steps to support transition at age 3.

Team Members

Members of the EI team usually consist of the parents, teachers, therapists, and other individuals, including a variety of contracted service providers, working with the child. There are 14 early intervention services, as shown in Box 9-2. The occupational therapist can be one member of this team. The team's primary goal is to provide the needed services to the family as documented in the IFSP. Each team is formed based on the needs of the family. Teams that have a clear, focused statement of purpose, goals, and philosophies function more effectively (Briggs, 1993).

Transition Planning

Transition planning must be part of any IFSP. In transition planning, families and service providers should discuss the possible options for the child after he or she can no longer be served by an EI team. Possible options include the local school system, a private preschool, a child care center, Head Start, or other community services for young children. The discussion of options should occur early and referrals to other programs should be made at least 6 months before the child's third birthday. Approximately 60% of children served in EI transition into preschool special education services. If the family wants the child to be considered for such a placement, the local education agency (LEA) will determine preschool programs that are available to the child. The IFSP team works closely with the family to notify the future placement staff of any special equipment that will be required in the preschool environment. If possible, when given parental permission, the EI occupational therapist should contact the school

occupational therapist personally to facilitate the transition. This may be helpful to provide pertinent information about techniques and procedures that have worked well, such as positive reinforcers, the amount and course of progress, and the intervention approach. If a meal-time protocol has been developed, providing it to the preschool program staff will improve continuity.

Transitioning into the preschool-based setting is stressful to families. The model changes from a family-friendly model to a special education school-based model. EI teams should assist parents in developing assertiveness and advocacy skills to request necessary services for their child. If the family is relocating, the occupational therapist might offer to make a videotape of the current feeding/toileting/dressing programs and routines. This facilitates carryover of desired techniques. If possible, adaptive equipment should be sent with the child and family. If that is not possible, team members can make a list of specific equipment and purchasing information for the parents and the new team.

Occupational Therapy Services in EI

Occupational therapists may assume many roles in the EI process. They can be part of the evaluation team, provide direct services, provide consultation to other team members in a transdisciplinary model, or fulfill any combination of these roles (Hanft, 1989). The occupational therapist working in early intervention needs to have good background knowledge of assessment tools for children and common therapeutic interventions. Some best practice guidelines for occupational therapy in EI are listed in Box 9-3.

Occupational Therapy Evaluation

Evaluations must be nondiscriminatory; be performed by qualified and trained personnel; and include informed opinion, review of the child's pertinent medical records, and the child's overall developmental level. Depending on if any other evaluations have been conducted by the EI team members, occupational therapists must determine the scope of the occupational therapy evaluation process depending on

---

Box 9-3 Best Practice Guidelines for Occupational Therapy in Early Intervention

- Regard parents as partners in decision making.
- Use a clear, open, and collaborative communication style with all team members.
- Share responsibilities for service implementation with team members.
- Use knowledge to improve performance and functional outcomes.
- Deliver cost-effective quality intervention.
- View child's abilities in context of natural environments.
- Incorporate carryover into natural daily routines.
- Use amplification and solution-focused questions.

---

the child's needs, diagnosis, medical concerns, and family priorities. Selected assessment instruments should demonstrate high validity and reliability; include comprehensive health, social, behavioral, and environmental components; and involve the family as equal partners with the professionals (Hanson & Lynch, 1989).

Children, especially those about 6–10 months of age, may experience stranger anxiety and therefore need more warm-up or adjustment time with the occupational therapist before actual testing begins. Allowing the parents to initially remain with the child is important. Also, during this time, the child should be approached slowly with time allowed for gradual interaction and play. Performance will be negatively affected when a child is crying or afraid.

Parent Interview

A parent interview is an essential element of the evaluation process of a young child. The purpose of the interview is to obtain needed information, including:

- parents' perspective of their needs for caring for this child,
- the child's condition and interventions to date,
- an understanding of family daily routines and structure,
- identification of resources available to the family, and
- the family's story of hopes and wants for their child.

Open-ended questions or requests are often better to facilitate retrieval of this information than close-ended questions. Requests such as "Tell me what a typical day is like for you and your child" or "Describe for me the feeding process for your child" will elicit a much more detailed response. The use of narratives and life stories provides a view that encompasses the child within the family and community context.

During the interview with the parent, the message that families are competent and in control of their child's life must be conveyed. One way to do this is to ask solution-focused questions (Andrews & Andrews, 1993). **Solution-focused questions** are worded such that they assume the family is already working toward improving the situation, giving the family credit for their efforts. For example, "I have noticed how carefully you position your child's head and arms when you place him in the infant seat. This is great. Do you do this in any other tasks or positions as well?" Another example is "Turning off the TV during feeding really seemed to help your daughter concentrate on feeding. Have you noticed other things you do that help her pay attention?" Important information, as well as trust building, can be gained from this approach. This interview provides a framework for understanding the child as an occupational being in the context of his or her family and his or her physical, social, economic, and cultural world.

Observation

Observation is a key element of the evaluation process that guides interpretation and planning and begins the minute the destination is reached. The occupational therapist examines the community and home environments, the parent-child and child-child interactions, and the family caregiving routines and play experiences. Observations usually are made in a variety of areas, including the:

- quality of the movement of the infant,
- interactions and communication between the infant/child and others,
- safety, accessibility, and opportunities provided in the home environment,
- daily routines and the amount and types of structure provided,
- caregivers' responsiveness and stress, and
- opportunities provided and resources available.

The concept of amplification may be a useful strategy for occupational therapists. **Amplification** is a process of "noticing, describing, and discussing an interactive event between family member and child that is likely to promote child change" (Andrews & Andrews, 1993, p. 42). This means that the occupational therapist discusses his or her observations with the family regarding any communication attempts the child makes and the responses of the parents that reinforce the child's behavior. This encourages the parents to notice and respond to nonverbal communication attempts. For example, during lunch, the occupational therapist might comment, "I just saw your child visually attend to you and move his head toward the spoon. Try placing the spoon just in front of his mouth again this time, and see if he moves that way again." This encourages the parent to attend to nonverbal communication and reinforces the child's efforts. This may be the first recognition of interaction, which can facilitate bonding between the child and parent.

Looking at the family's normal daily routine also is important. Families will be better able to carry over positioning and exercises if they are taught how to fit them into their established daily routine (Pretti-Frontczak & Bricker, 2001). Examples include suggesting to the parent(s) to

- perform range of motion exercises during diaper changes,
- incorporate an undressing routine just before bath time,
- implement sensory calming techniques after dinner time to promote calming down for sleep, and
- plan rough-and-tumble play with one parent or family member while another is cooking dinner.

Ecological Evaluation

Ecological evaluation determines the skills needed to be successful in various environments. The home environment will have its own opportunities and obstacles for the child to navigate. A child may have freedom to move about and play in childproofed safe areas requiring little supervision while provided with developmentally appropriate toys. In another home environment, the child may be restricted to a very small play area such as a playpen for her or his own safety. The opportunities for outdoor play may vary significantly as may the types of equipment, toys, and presence of other children. The routines at home are often different than those allowed in a child care center. For example, a child care setting may require the child be able to move from his chair to sit in a circle on carpet squares, remove outer clothing and place it on a hanger, request to go to the bathroom, play safely on the playground with other children moving about, and obtain lunch or snacks from a lunch box. These are very different routines than in the home environment. Each environment will require different skills, thus task analysis is helpful for determining a child's abilities and needed modifications or adaptations.

Play

Play is assessed by occupational therapists because it is the primary occupation of children. A variety of assessments are available to assist the occupational therapist in gaining specific information about baseline play performance and skills. Most children are motivated to play and have play preferences. Often a play history is conducted to find out the child's typical play and preferences (Takata, 1974). This is an interview designed to determine both the quality and quantity of the child's play experiences, interactions, environments, and opportunities across time. There is great diversity in the play environments, play opportunities, toys, peers, and promotion of play skills. Not all children have equal play opportunities. Culture influences the adults' view about what is appropriate play for children, what should be provided, and what is acceptable. Intervention techniques are easily embedded into play routines to improve the skills, participation level, and satisfaction of the child's play experiences.

Play Assessments

The Transdisciplinary Play Based Assessment, Second Edition (TPBA2) is an observation-based, transdisciplinary assessment tool (Linder, 2008). The team evaluates the child in normal play in a natural environment. Data is collected on normal developmental sequences of skill acquisition in the areas of cognition, social-emotional, communication, and sensorimotor skills. Procedures for conducting a transdisciplinary arena-type assessment are included.

The Revised Knox Preschool Play Scale is for children from birth to 6 years of age (Knox, 1997). Four areas of play are examined:

1. space management,
2. material management,
3. pretense/symbolic, and
4. participation.

This requires play observation both indoors and outdoors in natural environments with peers over a minimum of two 30-minute observations. More detailed descriptions of the evaluation process and interpretation of play assessments can be found in the work of Parham and Fazio (2008).

The Test of Playfulness (ToP) has been designed specifically to evaluate components of play related to suspension of reality, source of motivation, and perception of control. This tool can be used with children from 18 months–18 years old (Skard & Bundy, 2008). Free play is observed and then the test is scored. The test is recommended to evaluate the play skills of children with autism spectrum disorders and those whose delay interferes with their spontaneity and playfulness (Skard & Bundy, 2008). In conjunction with the ToP, the Test of Environmental Supports is often administered.

The Test of Environmental Supports (TOES) assesses the environmental support for a child's motivation for play (Bronson & Bundy, 2001). This assessment is helpful for reviewing the relationships between the child's motivation, caregiver supports, playmates, toys and objects, spaces, and the environment (Skard & Bundy, 2008). Scores are only interpreted on a per item basis, and discussion with caregivers can lead to ideas for needed environmental modifications and other adaptations to promote play in that particular environment.

Sensory Processing and Neuromotor Status

Sensory processing and neuromotor status are important components for the occupational therapist to evaluate. Understanding the body language of premature babies is especially important for therapists and parents to interpret the behaviors appropriately and avoid under- and overstimulation. Hussey (1988) has developed a helpful manual to consult when working with premature infants.

An examination of infant states, infant behaviors, and infant responses to the environmental demands is important for the occupational therapist to consider. The Infant-Toddler Symptom Checklist (Degangi, 1995) and the Infant-Toddler Sensory Profile (Dunn, 2002) are useful tools to examine the infant's responses to sensory stimulation, including need for and avoidance of stimulation.

A newly developed tool called the Newborn Behavioral Observations (NBO) will be helpful to therapists who work with newborn infants up to the age of 4 months (Nugent, Keefer, Minear, Johnson, & Blanchard, 2007). This assessment is an individualized, infant-focused, family-centered assessment for use in examining communication and interactions between infant and parent. This assessment consists of 18 neurobehavioral observations that describe the infant's capacities and behavioral adaptations. It is designed to help parents identify the infant's unique capabilities and vulnerabilities. Occupational therapists can help parents learn to understand and interpret the infant's behaviors so parents can in turn respond in ways to meet their child's developmental needs.

Additionally, the Infant Neurological International Battery (INFANIB) is useful for infants from birth to 18 months and includes examination items in the categories of spasticity, head and trunk, vestibular functions, legs, and French angles (passive movement at a single joint) (Ellison, 1994). It is based on observation and includes a rating scale. The scores reflect an infant's neuromotor status and may be useful to the occupational therapist by identifying specifics about distribution of abnormal tone and poor quality of motor responses (Ellison, 1994).

Occupational Therapy Interventions

Kellegrew (2000) determined that the self-care routines of children with disabilities were often related to the value mothers placed on the routines, the time afforded to conduct them, and the goals established. She also determined that on a daily basis, mothers make small adjustments in the home routines that shape the opportunities for skill development offered to their children. Practices regarding adaptive skills and social-emotional skills are very much dependent on the culture of the family. Views regarding child rearing vary greatly, including the involvement of other children in family decisions, the types of foods and the social climate of meals, hygiene, clothing habits and choices, behavioral expectations, and disciplinary actions and methods. A child's ability to participate in religious ceremonies, cultural activities, and school activities may be especially important for families. In the following section, intervention strategies for feeding, dental care, dressing, and toilet training are shared.

Feeding

Feeding is an especially important performance area to evaluate in infants and toddlers because good nutrition is essential for adequate growth and development. This is one of the key areas in which occupational therapists must be well versed for EI practice. It is indicated that approximately one third of all children with a developmental disability will develop a feeding problem significant enough to interfere with their nutrition, medical well-being, or social inclusion (Sullivan, Lambert, Rose, Ford-Adams, Johnson, & Griffiths, 2000). Infants who have motor delays, immature central nervous systems, or gastrointestinal abnormalities may experience significant difficulties with feeding.

Feeding is an experience rich in sensory stimulation that also demands internal processing to coordinate breathing, digestion, postural control, and alignment. Feeding problems are often a result of multiple issues such as anatomical abnormalities, motor dysfunction, sensory dysfunction, medical complications, psychological conditions, growth abnormalities, difficulty with social interactions, or behavioral issues. Some infants who take more than 30 minutes to suck a bottle may actually be burning more calories than they ingest. Morris and Klein (2000) suggest that sensory or medical problems that interfere with feeding develop into more complex emotional and behavioral issues. The occupational therapist working in EI must have a detailed understanding of normal feeding development, experience with pediatric feeding issues, and knowledge of common interventions.

Most children's hospitals have feeding teams available to conduct feeding evaluations. These teams are multidisciplinary and take a holistic view, involve the parents, and typically have the medical resources available for a comprehensive evaluation (Wooster, Brady, Mitchell, Grizzel, & Barnes, 1998). These teams provide the safest environment to evaluate the medically complex and fragile child. Occupational therapists should develop a link with the nearest feeding team for referrals and consultations. A thorough evaluation must be conducted when an infant is at risk for aspiration. Infants at risk for aspiration often demonstrate apnea, bradycardia, and an arching or stiffening of the body during meals. Toddlers may present with coughing, wheezing, congestion, wet burps or wet hiccups, frequent swallowing with negative facial expressions, vomiting, difficulty with sleeping, or hoarse voice. Coughing and gagging during meals that persists for several weeks, repeated bouts of pneumonia, and chronic chest congestion require immediate comprehensive feeding team evaluation (Rudolph & Link, 2002).

Feeding intervention involves establishing safe and appropriate feeding programs that meet the child's nutritional and hydration needs and can be competently carried out by family members in a reasonable amount of time. Most young infants are fed very frequently, and even preschoolers eat six times a day when meals and snacks are considered. Interventions with infants often begin with non-nutritive sucking and oral-motor programs to normalize tone, build tolerance for touch in the facial and mouth areas, and promote oral motor skills. Knowledge about positioning options is especially important as positioning continues to change as the infant grows and gains head control. Respiratory issues may promote the infant to push into abnormal patterns to protect or increase the size of the airway. The ideal position for the older infant involves a firm base of support with hips symmetrical and neutral, adequate trunk support, feet support, and neutral head and neck with slight chin tuck. This is often difficult to achieve without additional supports.

Most toddlers become somewhat pickier in their eating patterns; however, some children with disabilities will exhibit significant food refusal or selectivity. **Food neophobia** is a fear of new foods. Many children between the ages of 2 and 3 exhibit this behavior, but it diminishes by age 5 (Ernsperger & Stegen-Hanson, 2004). They will need repeated presentations of new foods before the foods will be accepted.

Children with food selectivity accept a very limited number of foods; may avoid entire food groups; may avoid specific textures, temperatures, or flavors; or may refuse to eat foods that are not presented in the same manner such as the size, shape, or plate. Complete evaluation of the sensory system and sensory preferences is warranted to determine if hyper- or hyposensitivities are part of this problem.

Some children are unable to focus on feeding because of distractions in the environment. An observation guide can help identify potential distractions. Wooster (1999) developed a feeding observation guide to assist the occupational therapist when observing meal times with parents and infants. A parent meal time questionnaire was developed by Morris and Klein (2000). In addition, Wooster (2000) described more specific feeding interventions for children with nonorganic failure to thrive.

Adaptive equipment may include a variety of types of bottles, nipples, and cups to promote safe nutritional intake and improve sucking skills. As the infant grows older, finger feeding and then feeding with utensils will be introduced. Additionally, more children are able to drink from straws at much earlier ages than previously recorded in the literature (Hunt, Lewis, Reisel, Woldrup, & Wooster, 2000). There are many more pieces of adaptive equipment to consider, which include spoons, cups, bowls, plates, and forks. Morris and Klein (2000) offer guidelines for choosing a variety of pieces of feeding adaptive equipment. Positioning is usually more upright, and a variety of commercial products such as high chairs and booster seats are commonly used and may offer opportunities for adaptations. Some styles of high chairs offer a slight tilt as well as more than one tray size and height adjustment. A more physically involved child may still need to be held or positioned well in a customized seat.

A pre-feeding program may be designed to normalize any abnormal tone and promote cheek, lip, and tongue movement and sensory stimulation prior to eating. If adaptive equipment is required, it is set up and ready for the feeding process. Parents should be key members and engage in the decision making to keep meal times manageable. The feeding program and specific techniques should be demonstrated and practiced; the parent should carry this out with the therapist present and garner feedback for revisions of the process. The feeding program should be documented for the child's record, with copies for the parent and therapist. Feeding programs should be closely monitored and updated regularly.

Effective feeding strategies include:

- minimizing the negative effects of medical influences,
- improving oral motor function,
- establishing appropriate positioning,
- modifying the environment as needed,
- promoting appetite and desire to eat,
- promoting eating as a pleasurable and desirable experience,
- providing adaptive equipment as indicated, and
- ensuring adequate nutritional and hydration needs are consistently met.

Not all children will consume enough calories by mouth; therefore, supplemental feedings may need to continue. The acquisition of skills for oral eating and saliva control are often valued by parents and may allow children to participate in culturally significant events, such as tasting their own birthday cake or participating in a religious event.

Dental Care

Children with developmental disabilities are at high risk to develop dental disease. Many children have dental alterations or malocclusions that make chewing more difficult and increase risk for decay. Dental decay is related to the presence of bacteria. Children who fall asleep after nursing or drinking a bottle are at great risk. A high, narrow palate may become a place where food particles lodge. The three most important factors for protecting already formed teeth from decay are maintaining good oral hygiene, limiting ingestion of carbohydrates, and eliminating or reducing cavity-causing bacteria (Acs, Ng, Helpin, Rosenberg, & Canion, 2007).

Young infants can be introduced to a soft baby toothbrush that fits over the adult's finger. This is used for sensory stimulation of the gums and cleaning of the gums and emerging teeth. Next, a NUK brush set is introduced to get the infant used to longer, brush-like instruments being placed in the mouth. This includes a set of three instruments that start out larger and round and end with one resembling a toothbrush. Once this is tolerated well, the child can be transitioned to a regular, soft child-sized toothbrush. Most children under the age of 6 do not have the dexterity to adequately brush their teeth. Children should be encouraged to participate by holding and moving the toothbrush; however, an adult needs to go over the entire mouth area to provide adequate cleaning. A child who is willing to use a battery operated toothbrush may do a more thorough job. Children need to establish the dental hygiene routines as part of their daily self-care skills.

Dressing

Parents will be dressing and undressing children several times daily for diaper changes and cleanliness. Children with specific medical conditions or those that require extensive procedures daily may do best with limited clothing or clothing that is adapted to allow easy access for parents to get to a gastrostomy tube (G-Tube), that is large or flexible enough to go around or over braces or casts, or that has enlarged neck holes to make it easier to get overhead. Some infants, especially in colder winter months, may respond negatively to being undressed. Discuss with the parents their comfort level with these procedures and the need for any clothing adaptation to speed up the process and minimize the discomfort to the child.

There are multiple opportunities each day for practicing undressing and dressing in the natural context. Going outside in winter often requires putting on a sweater, jacket, or coat and removing these when we return inside. Going to the bathroom promotes the partial removal of pants and underpants to the knees and then back up. Sometimes parents find it easiest to adapt the clothing by eliminating all fasteners and choosing elastic-waist, loose-fitting clothes that are quickly pulled down. Bath time promotes the removal of clothing and afterwards putting on sleepwear. A child who wants to go swimming may be motivated to help participate in changing into a swim suit. Children are encouraged by parents to partially participate in the dressing process as much as time allows. Infants may lift and arm or leg and push it into a sleeve by their first birthday. This process needs to be facilitated and practiced in children with disabilities.

A thorough evaluation and an understanding of the dressing routines will help the occupational therapist provide the appropriate interventions and expectations for parents. Many evaluations for children under age 3 include adaptive skills as components, such as the Hawaii Early Learning Profile-Revised (Furuno, O'Reiley, Hosaka, Zeisloft, & Allman, 1997), the Early Learning Accomplishment Profile (Glover, Preminger, & Sanford, 1988), and the Carolina Curriculum for Infants and Toddlers (Johnson-Martin, Attermeier, & Hacker, 2004). The Pediatric Evaluation of Disability Inventory is useful for children 6 months up to age 7 and evaluates self-care, social, and mobility skills (Haley, Coster, Ludlow, Haltiwanger, & Andrellos, 1992). The Wee-Fim has recently been revised to include two versions that evaluate self-care, mobility, and cognition (Hamilton & Granger, 2000)

Toilet Training

Toilet or "potty" training is a skill often introduced during the second year of life. It is a complex task and involves identification of sensory signals, communication, positioning (usually sitting up), and active control of muscles. Bowel control is usually achieved first. As the infant's bowel or bladder fills, the muscles relax and release automatically and the infant urinates or defecates. However, as the toddler gains control over these functions, the cerebral cortex sends signals to inhibit the reflexes and the child takes over the control. This skill is often identified as a hallmark of development.

There are multiple books written about a variety of potty training programs for parents to consider; however, none are targeted specifically for the child with a disability. This process takes fine-tuning and sometimes months to master in a normally developing child with the motor control and cognition to achieve it. A child with a disability may require a medical evaluation to determine if a bladder problem exists and if the bladder is trainable before potty training can begin. A child with a disability to the corticospinal tract or spinal cord may be unable to inhibit the autonomic nervous system, resulting in difficulty in gaining this control.

Positioning is a key component of potty training. The youngest children are often placed on small, stable floor-sitting potty chairs as the standard in-home toilets are too high. Children with motor delays and abnormal tone will need the occupational therapist to evaluate positioning needs for the potty chair. Adaptations may need to be made to a commercially available chair, or a customized potty chair will be required to promote correct sitting alignment. Often a tray is helpful to provide some arm stability, which can assist with sitting up and is useful to place communication cards or devices to indicate when "all done." At times, trays are helpful to restrict the child's access to touching the feces.

Tracking success is helpful for both the parent and the child. Often a daily chart with stickers is used to promote success and provide visual reinforcement for the child. The parents may need to track more carefully the accidents and determine if the timing of placement on the potty chair needs adjusting. Often when clock changes are made to accommodate daylight savings time, the adults need to remember the child's body is still on the old schedule and will need time to make the adjustments. Parents must want to work on this skill and be committed for success to be achieved.

After toileting, children need to learn the routine of hand washing. Some children can easily move to the sink, use a step stool, and begin to learn the steps of hand washing. Often a hand washing song is used to promote an adequate scrubbing time. Some children may need to clean their hands with antibacterial germ products while seated on the toilet. These routines need to be established early on in the process to minimize the risk of infection and help children establish the connection between the two tasks. Shepherd (2005) offers a variety of strategies for improving participation in self-care tasks, including simple picture sequences, task adaptations, environmental modification, clothing adaptation, and task analysis with interventions for toileting skill development.

Family Involvement in Intervention

A **family-centered** philosophy is based on the assumption that the parents know best. This philosophy is consistent with occupational therapy practice (American Occupational Therapy Association, 2008). The parents, viewed as partners with the service providers, are expected to be advocates for their child. The role of service providers is to meet the needs of the family by providing the information and instruction designated as important by the parents. Accepting parental reports as reliable information, allowing parents to help define goals, letting parents lead the discussions, and allowing parents to have questions ready for the team to problem solve together are all aspects of family-centered care.

Simeonsson and Bailey (1990) identified a hierarchy of parental involvement, representing a continuum from passive to active participation, for EI. Families will fluctuate in the levels, depending on the environmental demands and their coping abilities at the time. At the lowest level is *elective noninvolvement,* in which the family chooses not to be involved in the child's care. *Information seeking* is another level of involvement in which the family focuses on gathering information and developing skills. *Partnership* is when the family views themselves in a reciprocal interaction and decision making process with the health care providers. At the highest level, the family assumes the role of *advocacy* for their child. Some families may need the help of the therapist to teach them how to be advocates for their own needs and empower them to make decisions for themselves and their child. Identifying the level at which the family is functioning, at a given time, will assist the occupational therapist in determining appropriate caregiving roles within the family.

The nature of the activity can also affect which family members are available to help. Every parent needs time for personal hygiene, meal preparation, and care of siblings. The therapist can demonstrate ways the child can be placed in a safe and independent play position when a parent is most likely to be busy. Siblings can be involved by showing them ways to play with and monitor the child. This, of course, depends on the ages and abilities of the siblings.

Parent and Caregiver Instruction

Occupational therapy home programs need to be designed specifically for each child and fit within the family routines and context. Research indicates home programs are important for children with disabilities (Schreiber, Effgen, & Palisano, 1995). A well-designed home program includes therapeutic interventions that are embedded within everyday routine tasks to ease the caregiver strain and to promote the child's functional skills (Anderson & Schoelkopf, 1996; Hinojosa, 1990; Rainforth & Salisbury, 1988). Programs that have assisted parents in their interactions with the child have had better outcomes than services focused exclusively on the child (Bonnier, 2008; Hebbeler et al., 2007).

Caregiver instruction and written directions increase the likelihood of carryover by the caregivers (Simon, 1988). Parent instruction is an ongoing process that includes modeling the practice of skills and specific behaviors, and includes feedback on performance. Case-Smith and Nastro (1993) found that mothers preferred the use of written handouts with pictures of specific activities. Often, simple, clear diagrams, placed in strategic locations, can be great aids to reinforce these activities. For example, placing pictures near the changing table (and just inside the diaper bag) demonstrating how to relax the child with high tone, the best position for the child during diaper changing, and some simple range of motion exercises may be most effective. Feeding documentation is placed in the appropriate area of the home, such as in the kitchen on the refrigerator. It may include a photograph of best positioning, needed equipment, and a bulleted reminder of techniques to promote feeding skills. Practicing techniques with parents and interested family members can provide reassurance.

Conclusion

Community-based EI practice can be isolating at times, and unique and challenging at other times.

In this chapter, the authors reviewed the need for and role of occupational therapists in EI, the evaluation process, and strategies for intervention. The skills required of an EI occupational therapist include skilled observation and evaluation, flexibility in scheduling, good time management, knowledge of community agencies and resources, awareness of cultural and religious diversity, and excellent communication skills.

Therapists who desire to work in EI should consider their abilities and seek additional continuing education. Experience with children and youth, an understanding of medical testing, and knowledge of pediatric assessment tools are helpful. Knowledge of standardized and nonstandardized assessment tools and their use is essential. Familiarity with basal and ceiling age criteria, administering and scoring, and the interpretation of test scores is also important. Awareness of the expertise that occupational therapy and other service providers bring to the EI team is important as well. Each state has created competencies that must be met by all early intervention team members. Specific continuing education and experiences are usually required but can vary by state.

CASE STUDIES

CASE STUDY 9•1 Juan

Juan is a 22-month-old toddler with developmental delay. He has just been referred to early intervention by his pediatrician. Juan lives in a small apartment with his parents. His mother stays at home to care for him and she is currently 4 months pregnant. The language spoken at home is Spanish; however, both parents know some English. Parental concerns include Juan's lack of eye contact, not eating more foods, getting upset with noises, and difficulty taking him to unfamiliar environments. His mother reports he can finger feed, eats fewer than 10 different foods on a regular basis, and only drinks room temperature water. Some days he will just play with his food, and his mother then attempts to feed him. He has lots of toys but plays with the same toys each day, mostly dropping them, throwing them, or lining them up in a pattern. He wakes up two to three times per night. His mother has been leaving him in his crib, and sometimes he will go back to sleep. Lately he is starting to try to climb out, and the parents are concerned he will get hurt. They want to transition him to a bed before their new baby is born but do not want him roaming around the apartment at night. They sometimes bring him into their bed, but he is restless and does not go back to sleep. When outside, he runs around and sometimes spins around. He likes the sandbox and will sit and watch the sand fall through his fingers. He loves television, especially *Diego,* but the TV volume must be low and he wants to stand right at the screen. Your observation of play identifies repetitive play patterns, lining up of toys, lack of eye contact, inconsistent response to his name, and some self-stimulation with hand flapping.

Continued

CASE STUDY 9•1 Juan
cont'd

CASE STUDY 9•1 Discussion Questions

1. Which of Juan's behaviors are indicative of possible sensory dysfunction?
2. Which assessment tools could an occupational therapist utilize to further evaluate Juan's occupational performance and developmental level for sensory, motor, self- care, and play skills? Why did you select these tools?
3. Research the "red flag" warning signs of autism in toddlers. Does Juan demonstrate any of these, and if so, which ones?
4. What occupations would you observe as part of your skilled observation?
5. What suggestions might you make to help with Juan's sleeping difficulties and safety?

Learning Activities

1. Design a "therapy kit" to keep in your car. Name what equipment, supplies, and forms you would include in the kit.
2. Research how to refer a child for early intervention services in your area.
3. Identify local resources that would be available to help the early intervention occupational therapist.

REFERENCES

Acs, G., Ng, M.W., Helpin, M. L, Rosenberg, H. M., & Canion, S. (2007). Dental care: Promoting health and preventing disease. In Batshaw, M., Pellegrino, L., & Roizen, N. (Eds.), *Children with disabilities* (6th ed.). Baltimore: Paul H. Brookes.

American Occupational Therapy Association. (2008). Occupational therapy practice framework: Domain and process (2nd ed.). *American Journal of Occupational Therapy, 62,* 625–683.

Anderson, J., & Schoelkopf, J. (1996). Home-based intervention. In Case-Smith, J., Allen, A. S., & Pratt, P. N. (Eds.), *Occupational therapy for children* (3rd ed., pp. 758–765). St. Louis: Mosby-Year Book.

Anderson, P., & Telleen, S. (1992). The relationship between social support and maternal behavior and attitudes: A meta-analytic review. *American Journal of Community Psychology, 20*(6), 753–774.

Andrews, M., & Andrews, J. (1993). Family centered techniques: Integrating enablement into the IFSP process. *Journal of Childhood Communication Disorders, 15,* 41–46.

Bonnier, C. (2008). Evaluation of early stimulation programs for enhancing brain development. *Acta Pediatrica, 97,* 853–858.

Briggs, M. (1993). Team talk: Communication skills for early intervention teams. *Journal of Childhood Communication Disorders, 15,* 33–40.

Bronson, M., & Bundy, A. (2001). A correlational study of the Test of Playfulness and the Test of Environmental Supports. *Occupational Therapy Journal of Research, 21,* 223–240.

Case-Smith, J., & Nastro, M. (1993). The effect of occupational therapy intervention on mothers of children with cerebral palsy. *American Journal of Occupational Therapy, 46,* 11–817.

Decker, B. (1992). A comparison of the individualized education plan and the individualized family service plan. *American Journal of Occupational Therapy, 46*(3), 247–252.

Degangi, C. (1995). *Infant toddler symptom checklist.* San Antonio, TX: Therapy Skill Builders/Psychological Corporation.

Dunn, W. (2002). *Infant toddler sensory profile.* San Antonio, TX: Therapy Skill Builders. Psychological Corporation.

Ellison, P. H. (1994). *The INFANIB: A reliable method for the neuromotor assessment of infants.* Tucson, AZ: Therapy Skill Builders.

Ernsperger, L., & Stegen-Hanson, T. (2004). *Just take a bite.* Arlington, TX: Future Horizons.

Featherstone, H. (1980). *A difference in the family: Life with a disabled child.* New York: Basic Books.

Fitzsimmons, S. (1993). The changing epidemiology of cystic fibrosis. *Journal of Pediatrics, 122,* 1–9.

Furuno, S., O'Reilly, K., Hosaka, C. M., Zeisloft, B., & Allman, T. (1997). *Hawaii Early Learning Profile-Revised.* Palto-Alto, CA: Vort.

Glover, M. E., Preminger, J., & Sanford, A. (1988). *The early learning accomplishment profile.* Chapel Hll, NC: Kaplan Press.

Gortmaker, S. L., & Sappenfield, W. (1984). Chronic childhood disorders: Prevalence and impact. *Pediatric Clinics of North America, 31,* 3–18.

Haley, S. M., Coster, W. J., Ludlow, L. H., Haltiwanger, J., & Andrellos, P. (1992). *Administration manual for the Pediatric Evaluation of Disabilities Inventory.* San Antonio, TX: Psychological Corporation.

Hamilton, B. B., & Granger, C. U. (2000). *Functional Independence Measure for Children. (Wee-Fim-II).* Buffalo, NY: Research Foundations for the State University of New York.

Hanft, B. E. (1989). Nationally speaking—early intervention issues in specialization. *American Journal of Occupational Therapy, 43,* 431–434.

Hanson, M., & Lynch, E. (1989). *Early Intervention: Implementing child and family services for infants and toddlers who are at risk or disabled.* Austin, TX: Pro Ed.

Hebbeler, K., Spiker, D., Bailey, D., Scarbourough, A., Mallik, S., & Simeonsson, R., et al. (2007, January). *Early intervention for infants and toddlers with disabilities and their families: Participants, services, and outcomes. Final report of the National Early Intervention Longitudinal Study (NEILS).* Retrieved from http://sri.com/neils/pdfs/NEILS_Final_Report_02_07.pdf

Hinojosa, J. (1990). How mothers of preschool children with cerebral palsy perceive occupational and physical therapists and their influence on family life. *Occupational Therapy Journal of Research, 10*(3), 144–162.

Hunt, L., Lewis, D., Reisel, S., Woldrup, L., & Wooster, D. (2000). Age norms for straw drinking abilities. *Infant-Toddler Intervention: A Transdisciplinary Journal, 10*(1), 1–8.

Hussey, B. (1988). *Understanding my signals.* Palo Alto, CA: VORT Corporation.

Individuals with Disabilities Education Improvement Act of 2004, Pub. L. No. 108-446, §1431 et seq. (2004, December). Retrieved from http://copyright.gov/legislation/pl108-446.pdf

Johnson-Martin, N., Attermeier, S. M., & Hackler, B. (2004). *The Carolina curriculum for infants and toddlers with special needs* (3rd ed.). Baltimore: Brooks.

Kellegrew, D. (2000). Constructing daily routines: A qualitative examination of mothers with young children with disabilities. *American Journal of Occupational Therapy, 54,* 252–259.

Klein, M. D. (1983). *Pre-dressing skills.* Tucson, AZ: Communication Skill Builders.

Knox, S. (1997). Development and current use of the Knox Preschool Play Scale. In L. D. Parham & L. S. Fazio (Eds.), *Play in occupational therapy for children* (pp. 35–51). St. Louis: Mosby/Year Book.

Linder, T. (2008). *Transdisciplinary play based assessment* (2nd ed.). Baltimore: Paul H. Brookes.

Miller, L. J. (1994). Journey to a desirable future: A value-based model of infant and toddler assessment. *Zero to three, 14*(6), 23–26.

Morris, S. E., & Klein, M. D. (2000). *Pre feeding skills* (2nd ed.). San Antonio, TX: Therapy Skill Builders/Harcourt Health Sciences.

Newacheck, D. W. (1989). Adolescents with special health needs: Prevalence, severity, and access to health services. *Pediatrics, 84,* 872–881.

Nugent, J. K., Keefer, C. H., Minear, S., Johnson, L. C., & Blanchard, Y. (2007). *Understanding newborn behavior and early relationships: The Newborn Behavioral Observations (NBO) system handbook.* Baltimore: Paul H. Brookes.

Parham, L., & Fazio, I. (2008). *Play in occupational therapy for children* (2nd ed.) St. Louis: Mosby.

Pretti-Frontczak, K., & Bricker, D. (2001). Use of the embedding strategy during daily activities by early childhood education and early childhood special education teachers. *Infant-Toddler Intervention: The Transdisciplinary Journal, 11*(2), 111–128.

Rainforth, B., & Salisbury, C. (1988). Functional home programs: A model for therapists. *Topics in Early Childhood Special Education, 7*(4), 33–45.

Rosenbaum, P, King, S., Law, M., King, G., & Evans, J. (1998). Family-centered service: A conceptual framework and research review. *Physical and Occupational Therapy in Pediatrics, 18,* 1–20.

Rudolph, C., & Link, D. T. (2002). Feeding disorders in infants and children. *Pediatric Clinics of North America: Pediatric Gastroenterology and Nutrition, 49,* 97–112.

Schreiber, J. M., Effgen, S. K., & Palisano, R. J. (1995). Effectiveness of parental collaboration on compliance with a home program. *Pediatric Physical Therapy, 7,* 59–64.

Shepherd, J. (2005). Activities of daily living and adaptations for independent living. In J. Case Smith (Ed.), *Occupational therapy for children* (5th ed.). St Louis: Elsevier Mosby.

Simeonsson, R. J., & Bailey, D. B. (1990). Family dimensions in early intervention. In S. J. Meisels and J. P. Shonkoff (Eds.), *Handbook of early childhood intervention.* Cambridge, MA: Cambridge University Press.

Simon, G. (1988). Parent errors following physician instruction. *American Journal of Diseases of Children, 142,* 415–416.

Skard, G., & Bundy, A. (2008). Test of playfulness. In L. Parham & L. Fazio (Eds.), *Play in occupational therapy for children* (2nd ed.). St. Louis: Mosby Elsevier.

Sullivan, P. B., Lambert, B., Rose, M., Ford-Adams, M., & Griffiths, P. (2000). Prevalence and severity of feeding and nutritional problems in children with neurological impairment: Oxford Feeding Study. *Developmental Medicine and Child Neurology, 42,* 674–680.

Takata, N. (1974). Play as prescription. In M. Riley (Ed.), *Play as exploratory learning.* Beverly Hill, CA: Sage.

Thompson, T. (1992). For the sake of our children. In T. Thompson & S. Hupp (Eds.), *Saving our children at risk: Poverty and disabilities.* Newburg Park, CA: Sage.

United Nations Children's Fund (n.d.). The rights of the child—II of II. [Photo essay]. Retrieved from http://unicef.org/photoessays/30556.html

Wallace, H., Biehl, R., MacQueen, J., & Blackman, J. (1997). *Mosby's resource guide to children with disabilities and chronic illness.* St. Louis: Mosby.

Wissow, L. (1988). Poverty, race, and hospitalization for childhood asthma. *American Journal of Public Health, 78,* 777–782.

Wooster, D. (1999). Assessment of nonorganic failure to thrive. *Infant-Toddler Intervention, 9*(4), 353–371.

Wooster, D. (2000). Intervention for nonorganic failure to thrive. *Infant-Toddler Intervention, 10*(1), 37–45.

Wooster, D. M., Brady, N. R., Mitchell, A., Grizzle, M. H., & Barnes, M. (1998). Pediatric feeding: A transdisciplinary team's perspective. *Topics in Language Disorders, 18*(3), 34–51.

Chapter 10

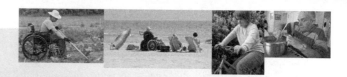

Community-Based Services for Children and Youth With Psychosocial Issues

Laurette Olson, PhD, OTR/L, FAOTA, and Courtney S. Sasse, MA EdL, MS, OTR/L

Policymakers and service providers in health, education, social services, and juvenile justice have become invested in intervening early in children's lives: they have come to appreciate that mental health is inexorably linked with general health, child care, and success in the classroom and inversely related to involvement in the juvenile justice system.

—U.S. Department of Health and Human Services [USDHHS], 1999, p. 133)

Learning Objectives
This chapter is designed to enable the reader to:
- Describe common mental health disorders of youth and the behavioral characteristics associated with those disorders.
- Identify useful assessment tools for children and youth with mental health problems.
- Describe interventions that are appropriate to address the mental health problems of children and youth.
- Understand the role of after school programs and summer camps for the development of children and youth.
- Discuss potential roles for occupational therapy practitioners in community-based services for children and youth with psychosocial issues.

Key Terms
After school programs (ASPs)
Culturally inclusive climate
Effortful control
Emotion-related self-regulation
Parent-child activity group

Self-regulation
Sensory modulation programming
Supportive parenting
Temperament

Introduction

Prior to addressing the occupation-based mental health needs of children and youth in community practice, a practitioner must first recognize the breadth and depth of these needs and then understand the most common mental health disorders seen in children and youth. Information about the prevalence of mental health issues, the most common mental health disorders that an occupational therapist may encounter in community-based practice, and occupation-based evaluation and intervention for psychosocial issues will be provided in this chapter. Occupational therapy practitioners may encounter children and youth diagnosed with mental health disorders or youth at risk for developing mental health disorders in a variety of community settings, including schools, after school programs (ASPs), or settings such as day treatment programs, group homes, or residential treatment facilities (Estes, Fette, & Scaffa, 2005).

Unstructured and unsupervised time spent outside of school places at-risk children in danger of academic, behavioral, and social-emotional isolation. This increases the likelihood of behavior problems, drug use, and risky behavior, as well as the likelihood of occupational deprivation. Two community-based services that support the healthy development of children, families, and youth—ASPs and summer camps—are highlighted in this chapter.

Mental Health Disorders in Children and Youth

Mental health disorders are more prevalent among children and youth than previously acknowledged (O'Connell, Boat, & Warner, 2009). A recent U.S. epidemiological study found that in a nationally representative sample of children ages 8–15 years, 8.6% of the children were diagnosed with attention-deficit/hyperactivity disorder (ADHD), 3.7% with mood disorders, 2.1% with conduct disorders, 0.7% with panic or generalized anxiety disorder, and 0.1% with eating disorders (Merikangas, Brady,

Fisher, Bourdon, & Koretz, 2010). Blanchard, Gurka, and Blackman (2006) similarly reported that approximately 36% of parents in a national survey of children's health had concerns about depression and anxiety in their children. About one-fourth of parents surveyed identified fears about substance abuse or eating disorders in their offspring. These parental concerns are critical to consider as health and educational professionals develop community-based services. To address these parental concerns, occupational therapy practitioners collaborate with other health or education professionals in designing preventative or health promotion programming for youth. Occupational therapists also might organize psycho-educational group programs for parents to address ways parents might use co-occupations to reduce their children's risk of developing mental health disorders (Olson, 2010).

The most common mental disorders in children and youth are outlined in Table 10-1, including Attention Deficit Disorder, disruptive behavior disorders (Oppositional Defiant Disorder and Conduct Disorder), and Major Depressive Disorder. Suicidality is a significant concern in this population. The U.S. Surgeon General (USDHHS, 1999) reported that 90% of children and youth who committed suicide had a diagnosable mental

Table 10-1 Common Mental Health Disorders among Children and Youth			
Disorder	**Symptoms**	**Comorbid with**	**Negatively impacts**
ADHD	• Hyperactivity • Short attention span • Impulsivity • Insufficient behavioral inhibition • Poor organizational skills	• Learning disabilities • Depression • Anxiety • Oppositional defiant disorder • Sensory processing disorders	• Academic performance • Interpersonal/peer relationships • Sleep cycles • Ability to adapt to change
Conduct Disorder (CD)	Poor emotional and behavioral regulation resulting in: • Aggressive behaviors that violate social norms • Bullying behavior • Destruction of property • Harming people or animals • Stealing • Truancy • Running away from home	• Negative mood states (depression) • ADHD • Limited frustration tolerance	• Academic performance • Interpersonal/peer relationships • Ability to adapt to change • Social problem solving

(continued)

Table 10-1   Common Mental Health Disorders among Children and Youth—cont'd

Disorder	Symptoms	Comorbid with	Negatively impacts
Oppositional Defiant Disorder (ODD)	Poor emotional and behavioral regulation resulting in: • Negative, hostile, and defiant behavior lasting more than 6 months • Noncompliance and argumentativeness with caregivers	• Negative mood states (depression) • ADHD • Limited frustration tolerance • Substance abuse	• Academic performance • Interpersonal/peer relationships • Ability to adapt to change • Social problem solving
Major Depressive Disorder (MDD)	• Depressed and/or irritable mood • Loss of interest/pleasure in everyday activities • Changes in appetite and sleep patterns • Low energy levels • Poor concentration • Low self-esteem • Feelings of hopelessness	• ADHD • Anxiety • ODD • CD	• Academic performance • Interpersonal/peer relationships • Participation in play/leisure • ADL performance

Data from: American Psychiatric Association (2000), David-Ferdon & Kaslow (2008), Hathaway & Barkley (2003), Reynolds & Lane (2009), Speltz et al. (1999), USDHHS (1999).

health disorder at the time of their death, with Major Depressive Disorder being the most common. Many of these youth, at the time of suicide, also had a concurrent anxiety disorder. Interpersonal conflicts and poor communication patterns with parents are considered important risk factors that lead to suicide attempts in vulnerable youth.

In addition to children formally diagnosed with mental disorders, there are numerous children at risk for mental health issues due to adversities related to poverty, family stress, and exposure to traumatic events. These children are not typically identified with a mental health disorder but may exhibit some of the behaviors consistent with one or more disorders. Childhood adversities that are risk factors for mental health dysfunction include: interpersonal loss (e.g., parental death or divorce), parental maladjustment (e.g., mental illness, substance abuse, criminality, and violence), harsh parenting (e.g., physical abuse, sexual abuse, or neglect), and serious physical illness or family economic adversity. Costello, Erkanli, Fairbank, and Angold (2002) reported that more than 25% of youth in the U.S. have been exposed to a traumatic event by the age of 16, and many youth

have had multiple exposures to traumatic events, including sexual or physical abuse, witnessing community violence, or experiencing natural disasters such as Hurricane Katrina. Children respond in varied ways to these experiences, and some may show symptoms of post-traumatic stress disorder, anxiety, depression, or disruptive behavior disorders. Reports on the long-term impact of trauma suggest that many of these children still experience functional deficits into adulthood (Silverman, Ortiz, Viswesvaran, Burns, Kolko, Putman, & Amaya-Jackson, 2008).

Children with difficult temperaments may encounter social and behavior difficulties and be at risk for mental health issues (Dodge & Pettit, 2003; Greene & Doyle, 1999). **Temperament** refers to a person's inborn natural style and habitual way of responding to people, places, and things. Temperament includes such dimensions as activity level, intensity, adaptability, persistence, mood, distractibility, and sensory threshold. According to Chess and Thomas (1996), typical temperamental patterns include easygoing or flexible, active or feisty, slow to warm up or cautious, and difficult. Children with a difficult temperament are children who may have irregular sleep and eating patterns, high activity levels, and intense negative moods. They are more irritable, are less flexible and adaptable, and more easily give up on tasks than children with positive affectivity. Building on the earlier work of Chess and Thomas (1996), recent research suggests that temperament consists of "constitutionally based individual differences in emotional, motor, and attentional reactivity, as measured by the latency, intensity, and recovery of response, and self-regulation—processes such as effortful control and executive attention that modulate reactivity" (Rueda & Rothbart, 2009, p. 20). **Effortful control** refers to "the ability to inhibit a dominant response in order to perform a subdominant response, detect errors, and engage in planning" (Rueda & Rothbart, 2009, p. 20). In a number of studies, temperament has been associated with patterns of coping (Rothbart & Bates, 2006).

Dyson, Olino, Durban, Goldsmith, and Klein (2012) conducted a study of temperament in preschoolers that was observational in nature as compared to many of the prior studies that were based on parental report. Through factor analysis, a five-factor model of temperament was generated that consisted of:

- sociability
- positive affect/interest
- dysphoria
- fear/inhibition
- constraint versus impulsivity (Box 10-1).

Children with high negative emotionality tend to experience high levels of arousal in response to novel or stressful situations and use avoidant coping strategies. Avoidant coping involves attempting to escape the stressful situation and/or avoiding thinking about the problem. Children with higher levels of positive emotionality and effortful control tend to be support seeking and use active cognitive coping. Active cognitive coping involves problem solving strategies and cognitive reappraisal. Support seeking refers to the use of social supports to solve the problem and/or to reduce negative affect (Rueda & Rothbart, 2009). It is important for parents to understand temperament as an innate characteristic and to learn strategies for helping their children express their temperament in ways that promote occupational adaptation.

Box 10-1 Components of Temperament in Preschoolers

Children will have more or less of each of the following factors, the configuration of which describes temperament:

Sociability

Reflects the degree to which the child initiates and/or dominates interpersonal relationships, and his or her level of need for affiliation

Positive Affect/Interest

Refers to the child's degree of engagement in tasks and level of positive affect

Dysphoria

Reflects the child's degree and dominance of negative affect, particularly anger and sadness

Fear/Inhibition

Refers to the child's level of anticipation or expectation of potential loss or punishment

Constraint versus Impulsivity

Constraint reflects the child's ability to inhibit a dominant response and the tendency to be compliant, adhere to rules, and respect authority.

Impulsivity refers to reactive undercontrol and the inability to delay or wait for a desired goal or object.

Data from: Dyson, M. W., Olino, T. M., Durbin, C. E., Goldsmith, H. H., & Klein, D. N. (August 22, 2012). The structure of temperament in preschoolers: A two-stage factor analytic approach. *Emotion.* doi: 10.1037/a0025023.

Evaluation of Children and Youth in Community-Based Settings

Occupation-based assessments are an important part of an interdisciplinary assessment of children at risk or those identified with mental health issues. Occupational therapists have developed a number of tools that provide insight into the occupational participation, interests, and goals of parents and children. The Short Child Occupational Performance Evaluation (SCOPE) (Bowyer, Ross, Schwartz, Kielhofner, & Kramer, 2005) is an assessment tool that provides an occupational therapist with a broad overview of a child's occupational participation. It is structured to systematically evaluate factors that facilitate or restrict occupational participation. The SCOPE is grounded in the

Model of Human Occupation (MOHO) (Bowyer, Ross, Schwartz, Kielhofner, & Kramer, 2005) and focuses assessment on the key constructs of skills, volition, habituation, and the environment. It is simple to use and supports the development of occupation-focused interventions. The Pediatric Interest Profile (Henry, 2000), also based on MOHO constructs, is a simple and time-efficient assessment that provides an understanding of children's play interests and participation. It is a self-report tool that facilitates discussion of the youth's leisure activities.

The Coping Skills Inventory (Zeitlin, 1985) is an observation instrument that is useful in assessing children's behavior patterns and skills that support a child's coping strategies to meet personal needs and adapt to environmental demands. It frames the styles of coping strategies that children use into active versus passive, productive versus nonproductive, and flexible versus rigid styles. Williamson and Szczepanski (1999) developed a frame of reference for utilizing coping assessments and interventions within an occupational therapy framework.

The Behavior Rating Inventory of Executive Functioning (BRIEF) (Gioia, Esquith, Guy, & Kenworthy, 2000) includes caregiver and self-rating assessments that provide therapists with important information about children's executive functions that are important for behavioral and emotional regulation, including attention, flexibility, and emotional control.

Sensory processing assessments such as the Sensory Profile (Dunn, 1999), Sensory Profile School Companion (Dunn, 2006), and Adolescent/Adult Sensory Profile (Brown & Dunn, 2002) also are helpful in better understanding children and youth responses to everyday sensory input. When working with youth at risk or diagnosed with a mental health disorder, it is important to interpret the results of any sensory processing assessment in light of the particular youth's trauma and attachment histories. Deficits that may appear to be sensory-based may be rooted in past exposure to trauma and/or inadequate caregiving.

In addition to standardized assessments, it is important that occupational therapists interview caregivers about the strengths and challenges the caregivers experience in co-occupation with their children with mental health disorders. Occupation-based family assessments can be an effective and critical complement to other family-based assessments. Occupational therapists also should include observing youth in some of their everyday occupations as part of the assessment process, especially those activities that have been identified by youth or their caregivers as ones that are challenging for the youth. Occupational therapists offer excellent skills in analyzing tasks and matching the clients' skills and those occupational tasks. In this way, the need for skill development and/or task or environmental adaptations or supports can be identified.

Considerations in Designing Interventions for Children and Youth

Cognition (David-Ferdon & Kaslow, 2008; Dishion & Stormshak, 2007; Eyberg, Nelson, & Boggs, 2008), and coping and emotional regulation skills (Silverman et al., 2008) are supported by evidenced-based literature and are considered mediators of positive change for children with mental health disorders. **Emotion-related self-regulation** refers to "the process of initiating, avoiding, inhibiting, maintaining, or modulating the occurrence, form, intensity, or duration of internal feeling states, emotion-related physiological attentional processes, motivational states, and/or the behavioral concomitants of emotion in the service of accomplishing affect-related biological or social adaptation or achieving individual goals" (Eisenberg & Spinrad, 2004, p. 338).

Self-regulation, the ability to modulate emotion, self-soothe, delay gratification, and tolerate change in the environment, is the subject of a great deal of developmental research (Clark, Woodward, Horwood, & Moor, 2008). Children with a difficult temperament are more likely to exhibit deficits in self-regulation that are related to temperament, including attention, approach, avoidance, inhibition, and typical mood state. Eisenberg, Valiente, Fabes, Smith, Reiser, and Shepart (2003) found that teaching self-regulation strategies to youth prone to negative emotional states is likely to increase the youths' social competence. Degnan, Calkins, Keane, and Hill-Soderlund

(2008) examined how maternal behavior influences a child's level of frustration, reactivity, emotion regulation, and socially appropriate behavior. They found mothers might escalate their children's reactivity by maternal control, though children demonstrating less innate regulatory capacities appeared to need increased structure and direction from mothers. When children have difficulty regulating emotions, behavior problems interfere with learning new skills as their behaviors alienate them from peers and adults. As a result, these children may have fewer opportunities to learn and practice socially appropriate behaviors in their everyday environments (Hauser-Cram, Warfield, Shonkoff, & Krauss, 2001).

The developmental research literature also provides key insights for occupational therapy practitioners preparing to provide services for children with mental illness and their families. Vondra and Barnett (1999) suggest that parenting impacts an infant's developing neurological system. They found that infants who are insecurely attached to their caregivers have higher cortisol levels than infants who are securely attached to their caregivers. High cortisol levels are present when a person experiences stress. A principal hypothesis within attachment theory is that parental sensitivity impacts the quality of a parent-child attachment relationship. Pettit, Bates, and Dodge (1997) identified supportive parenting as key to children's health and positive development. They correlated supportive parenting with positive school adjustment and potentially buffering children from the negative effects of family adversity. **Supportive parenting** is demonstrated in a number of ways, including parent to child warmth, proactive teaching, inductive discipline, and positive involvement with children. The emphasis placed on different features of supportive parenting may vary depending on family context and culture.

LeBel, Champagne, Stromberg, and Coyle (2010) reviewed the literature on the effects of trauma on an individual's capacity to process and integrate sensory information and regulate emotional states. Early trauma negatively impacts children's abilities to sustain or develop secure attachment relationships. Children experiencing trauma are vulnerable to living in a dysregulated state of arousal. This dysregulation may be accompanied by symptoms of sensory sensitivity to sounds, touch, and/or movement, and as a result children may experience frequent sensations of flight, fight, or freeze. Koomar (2009) identified connections between assessment and intervention methods used within a sensory integration framework with those used within an attachment-informed trauma framework.

Davis-Kean, Huesmann, Jager, Collins, Bates, and Lansford (2008) found links between beliefs about one's ability to perform a task (i.e., self-efficacy) and actual ability to perform a task. Children who have positive beliefs about their own skills relative to a particular task or activity are more likely to succeed at the task than children who have negative beliefs about their own capacities. Davis-Kean et al. (2008) suggest that a primary way to change children's behaviors related to task performance and peer relationships is to change their belief system. They recommend that intervention focus on children's beliefs about their capacities and the effectiveness of their behavioral strategies, as these beliefs are in formation and are more amenable to change in childhood. In this way, children's beliefs about their capacities might be supportive of more positive and successful behaviors.

Hauser-Cram et al. (2001) found that mastery motivation (i.e., persistence on problem-posing tasks) was a positive predictor of change in children with disabilities, including growth in mental age and mastery of daily living skills. Bandura (1995) stated that mastery promotes positive emotions. If children understand their errors, they are more likely to persist at a task, which supports developmental progress. In the study by Hauser-Cram et al. (2001), children who showed greater growth in mental age and in social and communication skills had mothers who were more responsive and growth promoting in parent-child interactions.

Intervention Approaches for Community-Based Programming

Two of many possible approaches in community-based interventions are described below. These examples provide a sampling of the wide array of programs that can be developed and customized to meet the mental health needs of children and youth, families, and communities.

Interventions to Develop Self-Regulation

Augustyniak, Brooks, Rinaldo, Bogner, and Hodges (2009) identified self-regulation capacities as a central underpinning of social competence. In promoting children's self-regulatory capacities, an occupational therapy practitioner may apply Williams and Shellenburger's (1994) structured psychoeducational group approach to helping children become aware of how sensory input impacts one's level of arousal and physiological state. It is then important to teach children how to use that knowledge to regulate their own physiological state for successful participation in their daily activities.

Conte, Snyder, and McGuffin (2008) favor developing youth's internal coping methods, as opposed to using passive or strictly behavioral approaches for controlling the aggressive behavior of youth with mental illness. Children with mental illness often experience intervention as being forced on them. In response to a staff member's demand or limit, the child's behavior may escalate as the child feels threatened and fears restraint. In support of youth developing self-regulatory capacities and learning strategies for coping with stress, occupational therapists have applied sensory processing strategies (Champagne, 2010; Champagne, Koomar, & Olson, 2010). They recommend use of sensory processing strategies as a trauma sensitive intervention to help an individual restore a sense of personal control and safety. Key components of **sensory modulation programming** are assessing, exploring sensory tendencies and preferences, creating sensory diets, modifying physical environments, and educating caregivers (LeBel et al., 2010).

Koomar (2009) stated that it is important that occupational therapists be trained to recognize the symptoms of trauma and dissociation in order to avoid incorrect assumptions about behaviors being due to underlying sensory modulation or integration deficits. Children with trauma backgrounds are triggered by specific sensory experiences associated with past abuse. Children with sensory modulation disorders may be moved into a state of overarousal by specific categories of sensation, regardless of the object or person producing the sight, sound, smell, etc. The origin of children's behavior affects intervention choices. Occupational therapists can be important team members intervening with children with trauma by using their knowledge of sensory organizing and modulating methods with these children. Developing protective spaces and introducing sensory comforts supports children with trauma by lowering their state of arousal, which can enable their participation in classroom activities and social activities. Though sensory strategies may help ameliorate the behavioral symptoms of trauma and related sensory modulation dysfunction, it is important to make decisions about interventions with these children based upon observations of the child, along with information about history of trauma and attachment disorders (Koomar, 2009).

An occupational therapy practitioner may intervene by teaching children with behavior disorders self-management strategies such as self-monitoring and self-evaluation. Jenson, Olympia, Farley, and Clark (2004) found that teaching children how to actively recruit feedback and praise from adults was very effective in creating more positive social environments for these children in academic settings. These researchers also stated that it is critical for students to match their own self-evaluations to their teachers' evaluations of their behavior. When these students were positively reinforced for close matches in their evaluation of their own behavior with their teachers' evaluations, students were more successful in modifying their behavior in ways that led to positive feedback from adults (Jenson et al., 2004).

Interventions to Increase Social and Task Competence

Jackson and Arbesman (2005) reviewed the evidence related to activity-based interventions for children and youth and reported that these interventions aid in improving peer and social interaction. Activity group participants developed increased ability to respond to adult direction, and comply with social norms and expectations. In addition, they exhibited increased task-focused behavior. They identified effective interventions, such as direct instruction for targeted skill development, the use of activities to teach and encourage the practice of new skills, the use of peers to model and promote practice of new skills, supportive adults to coach and reinforce appropriate behavior, and sufficient length of time to provide opportunity to experience interventions and practice-emerging skills.

Occupation-based groups can be structured to support children's development of self-efficacy and their positive beliefs about their own abilities to succeed in their everyday tasks. Bandura (1995) describes four pathways to self-efficacy: mastery experiences, vicarious experiences, social persuasion, and physiological and emotional state regulation. Occupation-based groups can be structured to provide all of these experiences.

Occupational therapy practitioners may also apply psychoeducational group methods to their interventions. Delucia-Waack (2006) provides clear guidance on the application of these group methods for children and youth. When leaders use a psychoeducational group approach, they focus on applying learning theory to first teach group members specific skills or strategies for everyday occupational participation, such as social skills or coping with bullies. Leaders provide a brief lesson and then give members the opportunity to discuss and then practice skills within the safety of the group. After exploring skills in activities with peers, group members then discuss how the skills learned and practiced might be useful in their everyday lives beyond the group. Williamson and Dorman (2002) demonstrate the use of psychoeducational methods in an occupation-based group designed to teach children skills for social participation. Psychoeducational group methods also are helpful as preparatory strategies to support children's participation in a task-oriented group.

Larson, Hansen, and Moneta (2006) explored how a variety of organized youth activities promote different developmental skills. For example, they identified the potential of team sports for supporting youth's development of capacities for goal setting, sustaining effort, and managing emotion. Their analysis of service learning youth activities suggested that well-run programs support interpersonal development and facilitate youth's connections to adult networks.

Family-Based Interventions

Leaders in the treatment of children with serious mental health disorders (American Association of Children's Residential Centers, 2009) advocate moving beyond intervening with children to also actively partnering with families in meaningful ways to support children's mental health functioning (Estes, Fette, & Scaffa, 2005). Research on depression, disruptive behavior disorders, and ADHD has identified interventions that support the development of parenting skills and family competence as key elements in effective mental health interventions. The American Association of Children's Residential Centers (2009) reports that family members of youth with mental illness exhibit a preference for hands-on assistance to support their skill development for engaging with their children with mental illness as opposed to traditional psychotherapeutic methods. Affronti and Levinson-Johnson (2009) advocate that programs designed to provide services for youth with serious mental health issues support family competence by actively engaging parents in positive activities and program events.

The literature related to children with ADHD and disruptive behavior disorders addresses the importance of breaking negative cycles of interaction and building positive interaction between these children and their parents. Olson (2006a) describes **parent-child activity group** interventions that support parents in learning how activity and their approach to co-occupation with their children can support or hinder interaction with their children. In the process of interacting together in a therapeutic environment, parents and children realize and begin to apply new ways of interacting with each other beyond the therapeutic group sessions.

Parent-child occupation-based groups, in the early stages of the change process, ease tensions that often exist between children with mental health disorders and their caregivers, increase children's interest and motivation for participation in play in the presence of their caregivers, and increase parents' expectations for positive and playful interactions with their children. Parents and children ready to change their everyday patterns of interacting are facilitated by a parent-child group that provides them with strategies and activities that can be practiced and transferred to home and community environments. A leader of an occupation-based parent-child group structures the therapeutic group environment so that parents and children experience successful and positive play that is under their own control.

The leader assists parents and children in adapting activities to support the full participation of both. A leader tactfully cues both parents and children in actively listening to one another's verbal and non-verbal cues as is developmentally and therapeutically appropriate. Olson (2006b) emphasizes that it is important for a group leader to carefully choose activities that promote positive interaction, as well as ways of facilitating conversation between parents and children.

In a qualitative study of one parent-child group that included children hospitalized with psychiatric disorders and their parents, Olson (2006c) reported that parents and children stated the group provided them with an opportunity to interact in a positive way. This was important to both parents and children, to lessen the impact of recent negative experiences with each other that had been argumentative, aggressive, or hostile.

After School Programs

After school programs (ASPs) can be key community services for supporting positive social development and preventing negative developmental trajectories, especially for children from low-income families (Marshall et al., 1997; Morrison, Storino, Robertson, Weissglass, & Dondero, 2000; Posner & Vandell, 1994). Children from low-income families who participated in a high-quality ASP demonstrated better grades, peer relations, and emotional adaptation (Posner & Vandell, 1994). Academic performance and conduct were negatively correlated with amount of time spent in outdoor unorganized activities. Posner and Vandell (1999) also conducted a longitudinal study looking at children in grades 3 through 5. It was concluded that African American children who received higher grades in third grade were more likely to participate in structured outdoor activities after school, as well as more likely to participate in after school extracurricular activities. These successful children were less likely to have participated in unstructured and unsupervised after school activities. In addition, teachers reported that children who participated in after school activities in the third grade adjusted better in the fifth grade.

Miller (2003) described the Harvard Family Research Project that included a meta-analysis of ASPs. Youth who participated in ASPs demonstrated significant positive changes in their feelings and attitudes towards school, their self-confidence, and their demonstration of positive social behaviors. These youth also exhibited a decrease in negative behaviors, including aggression, noncompliance, and disruptive conduct. The researchers emphasized that ASPs that used evidence-based skill training approaches were consistently successful in producing positive outcomes for youth, while programs that did not use evidenced-based skill training approaches failed to demonstrate success.

Similarly, researchers also suggest that structured, well-organized after school activities have a powerful impact on youths' transition to adulthood. Larson (2007) reported connections between youth participation in productive out-of-school activities and school completion, adult employment, and civic participation. Youths participating in extracurricular activities along with their peer network were less likely to drop out of school and to get involved in antisocial activities. This is especially true among youth at highest risk for persistent antisocial behavior due to multiple disadvantages (Mahoney, 2000).

ASPs can provide youth with an alternative environment that is more aligned with their interests, motivations, and needs than their academic environment during school hours. Effective youth activity programs are highly organized and structured to include regular meeting times, competent adult leadership, and an emphasis on increasingly complex skill building within group activities.

Mehsy (2002) advocates that leaders of ASPs create **culturally inclusive climates** so that all youth, regardless of gender, race, ethnicity, religion, or sexual orientation, feel welcome in the program. A number of concrete suggestions are offered to guide ASP developers in ways to increase youth's cultural literacy and competency, and civic and moral development. Organized activities can encourage youth to explore and share different aspects of their cultural and ethnic background or engage youth in activities and dialogues that examine and challenge media portrayals of different cultural groups or foster examination of their own and their peers' family and cultural values and beliefs.

ASPs can promote social development by providing critical opportunities for youth to socialize outside of their primary peer group in school or in their neighborhood. Youth can learn and practice positive conflict resolution and learn cooperative behaviors by working in teams. An after school group activity designed to enhance social skills is outlined in Box 10-2. Civic and moral development can be supported through the examination of family, cultural, and peer group values and beliefs; the sharing of moral dilemmas; and presentations about the way in which different cultures might apply their values to solving the dilemmas. Youth also might be engaged in activities such as surveying their local communities about current social and political issues or volunteering their time and skills to support the functioning of their communities.

Family-Based Programming in ASPs

ASPs have the potential for strengthening the link between schools and families. Out-of-school programs that engage families have shown that parents are more involved in children's education and school. Parents and children in such programs also demonstrate improved relationships and report fewer arguments and increased trust in one another. ASPs with family engagement also have improved program outcomes for children socially and academically. Barriers to engaging parents included limited professional resources for designing programs to engage families, and inadequate monetary resources for staffing and implementing programs. In one study of ASPs, only 27% had family engagement programming (Kakli, Krieder, Little, Buck, & Coffey, 2008).

Kakli et al. (2008) surveyed urban African American and Latino parents whose children participated in ASPs in low-income neighborhoods. These parents reported that spending more time with their children would make them better parents, but they also stated that they were faced with multiple challenges in their communities and had little support beyond their immediate families. In response to these research findings, Kakli et al. (2008) advocate for rethinking ways to support low-income, urban parents of children participating in ASPs. They have suggested that ASPs include complementary learning experiences for families, including engaging parents in advocacy, leadership, event organization, parenting workshops, and activities with their children.

Box 10-2 Example of an After-School Group

Healthy Snacks and Edible Art Group
Goals:
Participants will:
• Demonstrate the social skills necessary to work as a group, including following group rules, taking turns in shared activities, and simple, social problem solving skills.
• Learn to follow simple recipes for healthy snacks.
Overall Group Plan:
In the first group session, the leaders introduce the theme of the group and share potential recipes with group members. The leaders then address the importance of rules for getting along and having fun. Group members are guided in articulating key rules and making a group rules poster. The group leaders give group members choices for recipes for creating a healthy snack that requires minimal to no cooking. Child-friendly recipes, such as making a banana-pear caterpillar and an edible scooter snack made from pretzels, string cheese, and vegetables, are used.

In subsequent group sessions:
1. Group members read a chosen recipe. The leaders demonstrate key components of the recipe and provide simple pictured and printed instructions.
2. The children and leaders identify which key food preparation skills are needed, which skills group members already have, and which they need to learn or need an adult to do.
3. They identify key social skills that are needed for group members to work together and have fun while successfully creating healthy snacks/edible art.
4. Children follow the recipes working parallel or in teams of two.
5. Children and leaders work out social and task problems as a group.
6. Children with the help of group leaders take a picture of the healthy snack creation.
7. Children and leaders share the snack with each other and/or wrap up snacks to bring home.
8. Each child puts a copy of the recipe in his or her individual healthy snack recipe book.
9. Children work with leaders to clean up the group room.
10. Group members discuss what happened in the group, what they learned, and what was important to remember for future group sessions. They also discuss what they learned that they could use at home or at school.

Interactions with families in ASPs typically focus on problems rather than child and family assets. Though it is important to engage parents in individual and group program activities to address problems, it also is important to engage them in ways that facilitate use and further development of their strengths and assets. Parents are most often invited to general information sessions, parent-support or parenting training groups, or GED classes, but they are less often provided with formal opportunities to participate in group activities with their own children. Providing opportunities to enjoy activities with their children while also expanding their repertoire of inexpensive family activities is one way to accomplish this goal. Parents of low-income children who attend ASPs have limited or no access to programs that support and provide opportunities for them to engage in productive activities with their children in the company of other parents and children. Program staff may wrongly assume that if parents are not proactive in engaging with the ASP, they are uninvolved and do not care about their children's learning. When parents are invited to participate in engaging, supportive, and proactive family-based activities, they are more likely to respond and interact with program staff.

In addition, engaging parents with their children in family-based activities is consistent with the research on the importance of parent-child relationships. According to the Institute of Medicine, positive development in children is associated with emotionally responsive parent-child relationships (O'Connell et al., 2009). A hypothesis of attachment theory is that parental sensitivity influences the quality of parent-child attachment. Parent-child occupation-based groups engage parents in enjoyable, productive, and meaningful interactions with their children, while also providing opportunities for communicating and understanding their own children. Parents participating in one urban, occupation-based Family Night Program provided as part of an ASP for low-income families reported that what they enjoyed most was the opportunity to sit down as a family to do projects and talk together. They reported that they had the chance to observe their children's creativity and hear the ideas of their children. Though parents were acquainted with other families participating in the ASP Family Night Programs, they stated that they had not sat down and interacted with these families before the Family Night Program. They reported that they enjoyed the sense of community that was typically lacking in their neighborhood.

Some parents also reported that their parent-child activity experiences within these groups were in contrast to their experiences with their children at home, where television and children's individual use of computers were dominant activities (Olson, Agunwa, Anderson, & Evangelista, 2011). In addition to promoting increased parent-child interaction, occupation-based family night programs might also serve as a vehicle to engage and support families as children make, develop, and experience physical and school-based transitions. Dishion, Shaw, Connell, Gardner, Weaver, and Wilson (2008) highlighted the unique opportunities that natural transitions in child development provide for helping families promote health and reduce developmental risks for children. Entry into kindergarten or middle school and physical maturation of preadolescents are events in a child's life that make demands on youth and require families to reorganize in response to the changes in youth and societal or community demands. Dishion et al. (2008) note that parents may be more open to interventions and support during these transitions, and stress the importance of identifying and promoting positive parenting practices to prevent children's problem behavior. Occupation-based activities can be structured so that parents have the opportunity to not only learn and practice positive parenting practices but also experience the power and benefit of these practices as they interact with their children in mutual activity.

Summer Camps

Over the past few decades, there has been an increase in focus on developing summer camp experiences for children with disabilities (Briery & Rabian, 1999; Gieri, 2001; Michalski, Mishna, Worthington, & Cummings, 2003; O'Mahar,

Holmbeck, Jandasek, & Zukerman, 2010) as well as including children with disabilities in camps with typically developing children (Brannan, Fullerton, Arick, Robb, & Bender, 2003). In a summer camp, children with disabilities, like other children, have a chance to be viewed in a different light than they are in their home community. The children and adults they meet at camp are meeting them for the first time or see them only in the summer. Therefore, the developmental struggles or behavioral challenges that the children may have experienced over a number of years at their schools or in their communities are irrelevant to their new companions.

For parents of children with disabilities, summer camps can provide respite from caregiving responsibilities, an opportunity to learn about children's potential for functioning away from home, and new strategies for supporting children's independence and skill development at home. In addition to a 3-week camp experience for youth with learning and emotional disabilities, Michalski et al. (2003) described a program that provided parents with opportunities to learn strategies to support their children in applying new skills learned at camp to their home and community environments. Participating parents reported significant gains in children's skills related to social participation, including cooperation, responsibility, and self-control in follow-up telephone interviews.

Conclusion

A significant number of children in the United States suffer from mental health adversities and disorders. These issues develop or are exacerbated by child and environmental factors such as unstructured time spent outside of school. Occupational therapy practitioners are well suited for collaborating with other professionals in identifying and analyzing the barriers to children's and youth's mental health functioning, as well as for providing occupation-based interventions that support their physical and mental health and those of their caregivers. Occupational therapy practitioners have a great deal to offer as consultants and in-service

trainers within community-based programs such as ASPs, summer camps, and group homes. There also is a great need for the staff of these programs to understand children's behavior and learn ways to support children's underlying capacities for self-regulation. Self-regulation has been related to adaptive functioning in children from low-income families (Buckner, Mezzacappa, & Beardsle, 2009). An occupational therapist might lead a short-term self-regulation group and then provide consultation and intermittent in-services for staff, so that self-regulation strategies become a routine practice within programming.

Though many community-based programs typically do not have the funding to have occupational therapy practitioners as group leaders or as staff members, ASPs and other similar programs can offer excellent fieldwork or service learning opportunities for occupational therapy students working under the supervision of occupational therapists. Bazyk and Bazyk (2009) described the outcomes of preventative occupation-based groups, developed by graduate students. Through the group the children develop social-emotional competencies while also being exposed to new leisure occupations. Qualitative data collected suggested that children found the groups to be fun and that they learned how to work together and share. Children also stated that they learned how to express their feelings and respond in healthy ways when they became angry. Olson (2010) provides guidance in developing and implementing groups for children.

Blanchard et al. (2006) emphasize the importance of participation in everyday activities as critical for children's development, as well as for their quality of life and life outcomes. They call on health professionals and communities to put more focus on finding creative ways to more fully and productively engage children with developmental issues, including emotional and behavior disorders, in everyday life within their communities. This is at the core of an occupational therapy practitioner's skill set. It is crucial that occupational therapy practitioners step forward to meet the challenge along with other health professional groups and community leaders.

CASE STUDIES

CASE STUDY 10•1 Sean and Serena

Sean is a 9-year-old boy in the third grade who was recently discharged from a residential facility for children with serious emotional disturbances. He previously has been diagnosed with Attention Deficit Disorder and Oppositional Defiant Disorder. He has experienced a number of childhood adversities. His parents divorced when he was a toddler. His mother suffered from postpartum depression after his birth and attempted suicide. She was briefly hospitalized after his birth. After Sean's parents divorced, he and his mother moved into a shelter and received public assistance until she moved in with a new boyfriend when he was 3 years old. Sean was placed in the care of his maternal grandparents when he was 4 years old due to physical abuse by his mother's boyfriend. He returned to his mother's care 1 year later after she completed court mandated parenting classes and psychiatric counseling. Sean was placed in a special education class at the start of kindergarten and was diagnosed with ADHD.

In second grade, Oppositional Defiant Disorder was added to his diagnoses. When Sean was 8 years old, he was again removed from his mother's care due to physical abuse on the part of his mother. After being placed in foster care for 1 month, he threatened to commit suicide by jumping off the roof of his foster home. He was then hospitalized for 3 months and subsequently was placed with his foster family again. He attends school and after-school care and receives intensive individual and family counseling four times per week with his social worker and foster care counselor. Sean's therapy team coordinates their schedules so that two of the days of the week they are able to provide his interventions at the ASP site and coordinate interventions with the ASP staff. The occupational therapist is the member of Sean's team, whose role is to coordinate services.

Sean presents as distractible and disorganized with loose, illogical thinking. He is argumentative, disrespectful, defiant, and non-compliant with adult caregivers. He is easily provoked to verbally and physically attacking peers. His psychological testing indicates that his intelligence falls in the low end of average, but his performance suggests that his mental health issues may have limited his IQ score, and he may have high average intelligence.

Serena is a 7-year-old African American girl who attends the second grade at the same school that Sean attends and participates in the ASP that is offered at their elementary school. Serena lives with her mother in a one-bedroom apartment close to her elementary school. Ms. Smith, Serena's mother, had a long-term relationship with Serena's father Mr. Murphy, but never married him. She terminated the relationship 2 years ago after experiencing verbal and physical abuse for many years. Mr. Murphy lives in the neighborhood but rarely sees Serena. He works intermittently and is known to have a drug and alcohol problem. Ms. Smith works as a waitress in a local coffee shop.

Serena's teacher describes her as often impulsive and inattentive in class. Serena enjoys group activities and seeks out friendship, but she tends to get into difficulty with her peers. She has difficulty waiting her turn and grabs materials from peers when she wants them. When she gets frustrated during group activities on the playground, she frequently becomes verbally aggressive with peers and storms away from her peer group.

As part of fieldwork education experiences embedded with their academic education, graduate occupational therapy students from one occupational therapy program provide a series of occupation-based groups for the ASP that Serena and Sean attend. The ASP director assigned Serena to two occupation-based groups: Healthy Snacks and Edible Art, and Girls' Friendship and Crafts group. See Box 10-2 for the Healthy Snacks and Edible Art Group Protocol; see Box 10-3 for the Girls' Friendship and Crafts Group Protocol.

Serena enthusiastically participated in both groups with six female peers over the course of the school year. Serena initially became embroiled in verbal altercations with a few of her fellow group members over small differences, such as position in line prior to group or taking turns in activities. Group rules were developed, displayed, and reviewed at each group session. For the first four sessions of each group, Serena and a few of her peers received at least one time-out because of a verbal altercation between two girls. To help group members to learn to consciously manage their impulsivity in social interactions, a behavior self-rating form was created and used in both occupation-based groups (Table 10-2). Each group member filled out an individual form at the end of each group session. The group leaders then facilitated a discussion about the girls' overall cooperation with each other. As the girls became accustomed to the rating form, the leaders also encouraged the girls to positively reinforce one another as the girls demonstrated the positive behaviors addressed in the form. Over the course of 2 months of group participation, Serena was successful in participating in most group activities and was able to resolve disagreements with fellow group members within the structure of the group. Serena's teacher also reported that Serena was developing more positive peer interactions within class, especially with her fellow group members.

Sean participated in the occupation-based cooking group where he could learn to bake a variety of desserts while also learning to collaborate and negotiate with a small group of peers. Although Sean is often distracted during other activities, following recipes that are task specific has improved his ability to focus his attention. He seems proud of his culinary efforts.

CASE STUDY 10•1 Discussion Questions

1. Compare and contrast Sean and Serena's problems and how they affect each child with regard to their occupational performance.
2. What strengths are noted in these children? How might potential strengths be highlighted?
3. What interpersonal skills should a child of Sean's age demonstrate?
4. How might home life have contributed to problems with coping, communication, and peer interaction?
5. In what ways might the occupational therapist collaborate with the special education teacher, other teachers, family members, and parents to address Sean and Serena's academic problems? What behavioral suggestions can you make to the occupational therapy students who will work with Sean and Serena in the ASP?

Box 10-3 Girls' Friendship and Crafts Group

Goals:

Participants will:
1. Demonstrate key social skills for supporting the development of friendship including turn taking.
2. Demonstrate key task skills for participating in simple craft activities.
3. Seek help from adults and peers when challenged by a group activity.
4. Help peers when peers are challenged by a group activity or part of a group activity that is not as challenging to them.

In the first group session, the leaders introduce the theme of the group and lead a discussion with the girls on what kind of craft activities would best represent friendship. The leaders make a few suggestions, such as making friendship bracelets, group picture frames, group banners, and keepsake boxes, and then facilitate the girls brainstorming their own ideas and preferences. The leaders then facilitate a discussion about the importance of group rules for getting along and having fun. Group members are then guided in articulating key rules and in making a poster of group rules.

In subsequent group sessions:
1. An activity from the list developed by the group is introduced and demonstrated.
2. Group members discuss how the activity relates to friendship and their friendships or developing friendships with each other.
3. The children identify what is going to be easy to do in the activity and what is likely to be difficult or challenging. The leaders facilitate a discussion about how the girls will ask for help if they need help. Group members also discuss how they might help one another.
4. As social or task challenges arise, children and group leaders discuss and choose potential solutions to address the challenges.
5. Group members complete projects and then clean up.

After completing the activity of the day, group members discuss what occurred in the group, what they learned, and what is important to remember for future group sessions. They also discuss how they might use what they learned at home or at school.

Table 10-2 Girls' Self-Rating Behavior Scale for Occupation-Based Groups

Behavior	3	2	1
I respected the personal space of the other girls and took my place in line.			
I waited my turn to speak and listened to the other girls when they were speaking.			
I took turns in our group activity.			
When I had a problem, I worked with the leaders and other group members to solve it.			
I followed our group rules.			

3) means that I was a star and regularly demonstrated the behavior throughout the group without a leader or other group member reminding me.

2) means that I demonstrated the behavior most of the time and needed a reminder or two.

1) means that I had trouble with this behavior today and need to work on it for our next group session.

Learning Activities

1. Conduct an online search to locate a local chapter of a family self-help group for children with mental health disorders. Call the chapter and ask whether you can attend a meeting or get in touch with a local member so that you might learn about the daily life experiences of families that include children with mental illness. How could an occupational therapist assist the parent(s) that you meet?

2. Learn about the services available in your local community for children with mental health disorders. Develop a proposal for enhancing the services in your community by offering occupational therapy services.

3. Choose a low-income school or community in the geographic area in which you live and explore what ASPs are available for children. Identify what one program offers to the participating children. What are the strengths of the program? What are the gaps? What might an occupational therapy practitioner add?

4. Complete an online search for summer camps for a child with a particular disability for whom an occupational therapist would likely provide services (e.g., ADHD, Autism, Oppositional Defiant Disorder). Review the daily routines and occupational opportunities offered to children at the camp. What supports are offered to the children at the camp to support their occupational functioning? If there is an occupational therapist working at the camp, what is his or her role? If not, what potential roles might an occupational therapist fill?

REFERENCES

Affronti, M. L., & Levinson-Johnson, J. (2009). The future of family engagement in residential care settings. *Residential Treatment for Children and Youth, 26,* 257–304.

American Association of Children's Residential Centers. (2009). Redefining residential: Family-driven care in residential treatment—Family members speak. *Residential Treatment for Children and Youth, 26,* 252–256.

American Psychiatric Association. (2000). *Diagnostic and statistical manual of mental disorders, IV-TR.* Arlington, VA: Author.

Augustyniak, K. M., Brooks, M., Rinaldo, V. J., Bogner, R., & Hodges, S. (2009). Emotional regulation: Considerations for school-based group interventions. *Journal for Specialists in Group Work, 34*(4), 326–350.

Bandura, A. (1995). Exercise of personal and collective efficacy in changing societies. In A. Bandura (Ed.), *Self-efficacy in changing societies* (pp. 1–45). New York: Cambridge University Press.

Bayzk, S., & Bayzk, J. (2009). Meaning of occupation-based groups for low-income urban youth attending afterschool care. *American Journal of Occupational Therapy, 63,* 69–83.

Blanchard, L. T., Gurka, M. J., & Blackman, J. A. (2006). Emotional, Developmental, and Behavioral Health of American Children and Their Families: A Report From the 2003 National Survey of Children's Health. *PEDIATRICS, 117*(6), e1202–e1212.

Bowyer, P., Ross, M., Schwartz, O., Kielhofner, G., & Kramer, J. (2005). *The Short Child Occupational Profile (SCOPE) (version 2.1).* Model of Human Occupation Clearinghouse, Department of Occupational Therapy, College of Applied Health Sciences, University of Illinois at Chicago, Chicago.

Brannan, S. A., Fullerton, A., Arick, J. R., Robb, G. M., & Bender, M (2003). *Including youth with disabilities in outdoor programs: Best practices, outcomes, and resources.* Champaign, IL: Sagamore.

Briery, B. G., & Rabian, B. (1999). Psychosocial changes associated with participation in pediatric summer camp. *Journal of Pediatric Psychology, 24*(2), 183–190.

Brown, C. E., & Dunn, W. (2002). *Adolescent/Adult Sensory Profile.* San Antonio, TX: PsychCorp.

Buckner, J. C., Mezzacappa, E., & Beardsle, W. R. (2009). Self-regulation and its relations to adaptive functioning in low-income youths. *American Journal of Orthopsychiatry, 79* (1), 19–30.

Champagne, T. (2010). Occupational therapy in high-risk and special situations. In M. K. Scheinholtz (Ed.), *Occupational therapy in mental health: Considerations for advanced practice* (pp. 179–197). Bethesda, MD: AOTA Press.

Champagne, T., Koomar, J., & Olson, L. (March 2010). Sensory processing evaluation and intervention in mental health. *OT Practice, 15*(5), CE1–7.

Chess, S., & Thomas, A. (1996). *Temperament: Theory and practice.* New York: Brunner/Mazel.

Clark, C. A., Woodward, L. J., Horwood, L. J., & Moor, S. (2008). Development of emotional and behavioral regulation in children born extremely preterm and very preterm: Biological and social influences. *Child Development, 79*(5), 1444–1462.

Conte, C., Snyder, C., & McGuffin, R. (2008). Using self-determination in residential settings. *Residential Treatment for Children and Youth, 25*(2), 307–318.

Costello, E. J., Erkanli, A., Fairbank, J., & Angold, A. (2002). The prevalence of potentially traumatic events in childhood and adolescence. *Journal of Traumatic Stress, 15*, 99–112.

David-Ferdon, C., & Kaslow, N. J. (2008). Evidence-based psychosocial treatments for child and adolescent depression. *Journal of Clinical Child and Adolescent Psychology, 37*(1), 62–104.

Davis-Kean, P. E., Huesmann, L. R., Jager, J., Collins, W. A., Bates, J. E., & Lansford, J. E. (2008). Changes in the relation of self-efficacy beliefs and behavior across development, *Child Development, 79*(5), 1257–1269.

Degnan, K. A., Calkins, S. D., Keane, S. P., & Hill-Soderlund, A. L. (2008). Profiles of disruptive behavior across early childhood: Contributions of frustration reactivity, physiological regulation, and maternal behavior. *Child Development, 79*(5), 1357–1376.

DeLucia-Waack, J. L. (2006). *Leading psychoeducational groups for children and adolescents.* Thousand Oaks, CA: Sage.

Dishion, T. J., Shaw, D., Connell, A., Gardner, F., Weaver, C., & Wilson, M. (2008). The family check-up with high-risk indigent families: Preventing problem behavior by increasing parents' positive behavior support in early childhood. *Child Development, 79*(5), 1395–1414.

Dishion, T. J., & Stormshak, E. A. (2007). *Intervening in children's lives: An ecological, family-centered approach to mental health care.* Washington DC: American Psychological Association.

Dodge, K. A., & Pettit, G. S. (2003). A biopsychosocial model of the development of chronic conduct problems in adolescence. *Developmental Psychology, 39*(2), 349–371.

Dunn, W. (1999). *Sensory profile.* San Antonio, TX: PsychCorp.

Dunn, W. (2006). *Sensory PROFILE SCHOOL COMPANION USER'S MANUAL.* San Antonio, TX: PsychCorp.

Dyson, M. W., Olino, T. M., Durbin, C. E., Goldsmith, H. H., & Klein, D. N. (2012). The structure of temperament in preschoolers: A two-stage factor analytic approach. *Emotion, 12*(1), 44–57.

Eisenberg, M., & Spinrad, T. L. (2004). Emotion-related regulation: Sharpening the definition. *Child Development, 75*(2), 334–339.

Eisenberg, N., Valiente, C., Fabes, R. A., Smith, C. L., Reiser, M., Shepard, S. A.,...Cumberland, A. J. (2003). The relations of effortful control and ego control to children's resiliency and social functioning. *Developmental Psychology, 39*, 761–776.

Estes, R., Fette, C., & Scaffa, M. E. (2005). Effecting successful community re-entry: Systems of care community based mental health services. *Residential Treatment for Children and Youth, 23*(1), 133–150.

Eyberg, S. M., Nelson, M. M., & Boggs, S. R. (2008). Evidence-based psychosocial treatments for children and adolescents with disruptive behavior. *Journal of Clinical Child and Adolescent Psychology, 37*(1), 215–237.

Gieri, J. (2001). Happy Camping. *Exceptional Parent, 31*(3), 46–48.

Gioia, G. A., Esquith, P. K., Guy, S. C., & Kenworthy, L. (2000). *Behavior Rating Inventory of Executive Functioning (BRIEF).* Lutz, FL: Psychological Assessment Resources.

Greene, R. W., & Doyle, A. E. (1999). Toward a transactional conceptualization of oppositional defiant disorder: Implications for assessment and treatment. *Clinical Child and Family Psychology Review, 2*(3), 129–148.

Hathaway, W. L., & Barkley, R. A. (2003). Self regulation, ADHD & child religiousness. *Journal of Psychology & Christianity, 22*(2), 101–115.

Hauser-Cram, P., Warfield, M. E., Shonkoff, J. P., & Krauss, M. W. (2001). Children with Disabilities. *Monographs of the Society for Research in Child Development, 66*(3, Serial No. 266).

Henry, A. D. (2000). *Pediatric Interest Profiles: Surveys of play for children and adolescents.* San Antonio, TX: Therapy Skill Builders.

Jackson, L. L., & Arbesman, M. (2005). *Occupational therapy practice guidelines for children with behavioral and psychosocial needs.* Bethesda, MD: AOTA Press.

Jenson, W. R., Olympia, D., Farley, M., & Clark, E. (2004). Positive psychology and externalizing students in a sea of negativity. *Psychology in the Schools, 41*(1), 67–79.

Kakli, Z., Kreider, H., Little, P., Buck, T., & Coffey, M. (2008). *Focus on families! How to build and support family-centered practices in after school.* Joint Publication of: United Way of Massachusetts Bay, Harvard Family Research Project, and Build the Out-of-School Time Network.

Koomar, J. (2009). Trauma and attachment—informed sensory integration assessment and intervention. *Special Interest Section Quarterly Sensory Integration, 32*(4), 1–4, American Occupational Therapy Association.

Larson, R. W. (2007). From "I" to "we": Development of the capacity of teamwork in youth programs. In R. K. Silbereisen & R. M. Lerner (Eds.), *Approaches to positive youth development* (pp. 277–292). Los Angeles: Sage.

Larson, R., Hansen, D., & Moneta, G. (2006). Differing profiles of developmental experiences across types of organized youth activities. *Developmental Psychology, 42*(5), 849–863.

LeBel, J., Champagne, T., Stromberg, N., & Coyle, R. (March 2010). Integrating sensory and trauma-informed interventions: A Massachusetts state initiative, Part 1. *Special Interest Section Quarterly Mental Health, 33*(1), pp. 1–4, American Occupational therapy Association.

Mahoney, J. L. (2000). School extracurricular activity participation as a moderator in the development of antisocial patterns. *Child Development, 71*(2), 502–516.

Marshall, N. L., Coll, C. G., Marx, F., McCartney, K., Keefe, N., & Ruh, J. (1997). After-school time and children's behavioral adjustment. *Journal of Developmental Psychology, 43*(3), 497–514.

Mehsy, C. (2002). *Cultural competency: The role of after school program in supporting diverse youth.* Colorado Trust After-school Initiative Colorado Foundation for Families and Children.

Merikangas, K. R., He, J. P., Brody, D., Fisher, P. W., Bourdon, K., & Koretz, D. S. (2010). Prevalence and treatment of mental disorders among US children in 2001–2004 NHANES. *Pediatrics, 125*(1), 75–81.

Michalski, J. H., Mishna, F., Worthington, C., & Cummings, R. (2003). A multi-method evaluation of a therapeutic summer camp program. *Child and Adolescent Social Work Journal, 20*(1), 53–76.

Miller, B. M. (2003, May). *Critical hours: Afterschool programs and educational success.* Commissioned by the Nellie Mae Education Foundation. Brookline, MA: Miller Midzik Research Associates.

Morrison, G. M., Storino, M. H., Robertson, L. M., Weissglass, T., & Dondero, A. (2000). The protective function of after-school programming and parent education and support for students at risk for substance abuse. *Evaluation and Program Planning, 23*(3), 365–371.

O'Connell, M. E., Boat, T., & Warner, K. E. (2009). *Preventing mental, emotional and behavioral disorders among young people: progress and possibilities.* Washington, DC: National Academies Press. Retrieved from http://nap.edu/catalog.php?record_id=12480

O'Mahar, K., Holmbeck, G. N., Jandasek, B., & Zukerman, J. (2010). A camp-based intervention targeting independence among individuals with spina bifida. *Journal of Pediatric Psychology, 35*(8), 848–856.

Olson, L. J. (2006a). *Activity group in family-centered treatment: Psychiatric occupational therapy approaches for parents and children.* Binghamton, NY: Haworth.

Olson, L. J. (2006b). Parent-child activity groups reconsidered. *Occupational Therapy in Mental Health, 22*(3/4), 103–119.

Olson, L. J. (2006c). A qualitative research study of one parent-child activity group. *Occupational Therapy in Mental Health, 22*(3/4), 49–82.

Olson, L. J. (2010). Developing and implementation of groups to foster social participation and mental health. In S. Bayzk (Ed.). *Occupational therapy's role in promoting mental health and social participation in children and youth.* Bethesda, MD: AOTA Press.

Olson, L. J., Agunwa, M., Andersen, C., & Evangelista, M. (2011). *Developing an occupation-based family night program for an afterschool program.* Unpublished manuscript.

Pettit, G. S., Bates, J. E., & Dodge, K. A. (1997). Supportive parenting, ecological context, and children's adjustment: A seven-year longitudinal study. *Child Development, 68*, 908–923.

Posner, J. K., & Vandell, D. L. (1994). Low-income children's after-school care: Are there beneficial effects of after-school programs? *Child Development, 65*, 440–456.

Posner, J. K., & Vandell, D. L. (1999). After-school activities and the development of low-income urban children: A longitudinal study. *Development Psychology, 35*(3), 868–879.

Reynolds, S., & Lane, S. L. (2009). Sensory overresponsivity and anxiety in children with ADHD. *American Journal of Occupational Therapy, 63*, 433–440.

Rothbart, M. K., & Bates, J. E. (2006). Temperament. In W. Damon, R. Lerner, & N. Eisenberg (Eds.), *Handbook of child psychology.* Hoboken, NJ: Wiley.

Rueda, M. R., & Rothbart, M. K. (2009). The influence of temperament on the development of coping: The role of maturation and experience. *New Directions for Child and Adolescent Development, 124,* 19–31.

Silverman, W. K., Ortiz, C. D., Viswesvaran, C., Burns, B. J., Kolko, D. J., Putnam, F. W., & Amaya-Jackson, L. (2008). Evidence-Based psychosocial treatments for children and adolescents exposed to traumatic events. *Journal of Clinical Child and Adolescent Psychology, 37*(1), 156–183.

Speltz, M. L., DeKlyen, M., Calderon, R., Greenberg, M. T., & Fisher, P. A. (1999). Neuropsychological characteristics and test behaviors of boys with early onset conduct problems. *Journal of Abnormal Psychology, 108*(2), 315–325.

U.S. Department of Health and Human Services. (1999). *Mental Health: A Report of the Surgeon General.* Rockville, MD: U.S. Department of Health and Human Services, Substance Abuse and Mental Health Services Administration, Center for Mental Health Services, National Institutes of Health, National Institute of Mental Health. Retrieved from http://surgeongeneral.gov/library/mentalhealth/toc.html

Vondra, J. I., & Barnett, D. (1999). Atypical attachment in infancy and early childhood among children at developmental risk. *Monographs of the Society for Research in Child Development, 64*(3, Serial No. 258).

Williams, M. S., & Shellenberger, S. (1994). *How does your engine run?* Albuquerque, NM: TherapyWorks.

Williamson, G. G., & Dorman, W. J. (2002). *Promoting social competence.* San Antonio, TX: Therapy Skill Builders.

Williamson, G. G., & Szczepanski, M. (1999). Coping frame of reference. In P. Kramer & J. Hinojosa (Eds.), *Frames of reference for pediatric occupational therapy,* 2nd ed. Baltimore: Lippincott, Williams and Wilkins.

Zeitlin, S. (1985). *Coping inventory.* Bensonville, IL: Scholastic Testing Service.

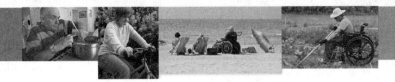

Productive Aging

Chapter 11

Driving and Community Mobility for Older Adults

Wendy B. Stav, PhD, OTR/L, SCDCM, FAOTA

Leave sooner, drive slower, live longer.
—A highway safety billboard message

Learning Objectives

This chapter is designed to enable the reader to:

- Identify the contribution of driving and community mobility to occupational engagement, quality of life, and health.
- Describe the occupational and health consequences of not being mobile in the community.
- Discuss the importance of developing referral pathways in the development of a driving rehabilitation program.
- Identify funding sources for driving rehabilitation services.
- Discuss credentialing for driving rehabilitation programs and personnel.
- Identify the range of occupational therapy community mobility interventions.

Key Terms

Community mobility
Driving
Driving rehabilitation
Occupational enabler

Paratransit
Transportation alternatives

Introduction

Community mobility is a critical necessity to occupational engagement and fulfillment of life as an occupational being. The American Occupational Therapy Association (AOTA) defines **community mobility** as "moving around in the community and using public or private transportation, such as driving, walking, bicycling, or accessing and riding in buses, taxi cabs, or other transportation systems" (2008a, p. 631). Attention to community mobility in the United States is largely focused on driving due to a constellation of factors, including the geographic dispersion of most communities, the automobile dependent culture, the lack of transit infrastructure in most areas, and the need to access the community in order to engage in several areas of occupation. **Driving** falls within the domain of community mobility (AOTA, 2008a) and refers specifically to the operation of an automobile, incorporating motor performance skills to manipulate the vehicle controls, sensory perceptual performance skills for awareness of the driving environment, and cognitive performance skills to maneuver safely throughout a variety of contexts (Pierce, 2002). The driving rehabilitation practice area is currently a high-profile area of specialization due to steady research funding since the 1990s, politically motivated agendas and advocacy related to senior driver licensing guidelines, and emotionally charged driving outcome decisions for both families and older adults. The purpose of this chapter is to discuss issues related to driving and community mobility for older adults.

According to the 2000 census data there were over 49 million people with some type of long-term condition or disability, with almost 14 million of them over the age of 65 (Waldrop & Stern, 2003). Diagnosis with a disabling condition may not hinder occupational engagement, but for many (18 million), their condition was so disabling it was difficult to travel outside of the home. The inability to travel outside of the home is particularly problematic for almost 14 million adults age 65 or older (Waldrop & Stern, 2003). There is clearly a need for occupational therapy practitioners to be involved in driving rehabilitation; however, the limited number of programs and specialized workforce in driving rehabilitation and community mobility

do not address the needs of many aging individuals who do not possess the cognitive, physical, and/or sensory performance skills to operate an automobile. The community is the ideal setting in which to address driving and community mobility in its entirety to enable seniors to remain mobile and actively engaged in their communities.

Contributions of Driving and Community Mobility

Driving and community mobility play a vital role in the performance of several other areas of occupation, including Instrumental Activities of Daily Living (IADL), education, work, leisure, and social participation (AOTA, 2008a, p. 628). Although community mobility is classified as an IADL, it is often necessary to be mobile in the community in order to engage in other IADL such as care of others, care of pets, child rearing, financial management, health management, home establishment and management, religious observance, and shopping (AOTA, 2008a, p. 631). Individuals must travel to medical appointments, places of worship, and retail establishments to obtain goods and services for successful engagement in IADLs. Older adults often continue to engage in educational occupations in the form of lifelong learning programs, museum trips, and seminars and lectures offered by community centers. Travel to the venue of learning in order to actively participate in these educational pursuits is a necessary first step. Work also is an area of occupational engagement for older adults as many individuals maintain their employment for personal or financial reasons or enlist in volunteer activities. These occupations may require an individual to travel through the community. Engagement in leisure and social participation occupations often requires access to the community whenever the venue is outside of the individual's home. For instance, individuals who engage in book club meetings, the theater, and bridge clubs must travel to congregate with others for engagement. The ability to access services located in the community and engage in occupations contributes to a person's life, well-being, and quality of life (Glass, de Leon, Marottoli, & Berkman, 1999). The ability to travel within one's community allows for access to and participation in several areas of occupation and elevates driving and community mobility beyond a single category of IADL. Driving and community mobility are **occupational enablers** because they enable engagement in other areas of occupation (Stav & Lieberman, 2008).

Engagement in driving or community mobility is not required for engagement in sleep and rest. However, one must engage in sufficient sleep and rest in order to safely engage in driving and community mobility. There are precautionary measures related to sleep and driving in that individuals who are sleep deprived, have a sleep disorder, or are excessively drowsy due to medication or illness should refrain from engaging in driving or community mobility until the sleep issues have been resolved (Vanlaar, Simpson, & Robertson, 2008).

Consequences of Not Engaging in Community Mobility

Although it is important to recognize the contribution of community mobility to engagement in occupation, occupational therapy practitioners should also be aware of the implications of not engaging in community mobility. Due to the depth and breadth of potential negative outcomes following driving cessation, practitioners and family members should carefully consider the individual's community access needs, available support network, and transportation options to allow for continued engagement in the community when making decisions about driving retirement or taking away the car keys from an older adult.

The inability to be mobile within the community severely limits access to necessary community-based resources such as the grocery store, pharmacy, and medical offices. Decreased access to these necessary destinations can have far-reaching implications, including limited nutritional intake, poor or nonexistent medication management, and insufficient contact with health care providers to manage health needs. Individuals without community mobility are further limited in their community access to nonessential but desired and meaningful destinations for religious observance, shopping, socialization, leisure pursuits, work and volunteer responsibilities, and

educational pursuits. Although travel into the community for engagement in these occupations is not life-sustaining, the lack of engagement in meaningful occupations can lead to occupational deprivation and can ultimately affect quality of life, life satisfaction, and health (Glass et al., 1999). Marottoli and colleagues (1997) examined the health of older adults and found an increase in depressive symptoms as individuals ceased driving. It is possible that the emotional and psychological connection to driving is so strong that the loss of driving resulted in depressive symptoms. However, it is more likely that the loss of driving caused a decrease in occupational engagement, which reduced quality of life and resulted in depressive symptoms. There is evidence suggesting that engagement in physical, cognitive, social, leisure, and religious activities; ADL and IADL; and work/volunteering is associated with or even results in improved health compared to a lack of engagement (Stav, Halleran, Lane, & Arbesman, 2012). This body of evidence informs occupational therapy practitioners that it is important to promote community mobility so older adults can continue to be actively engaged in occupations and subsequently experience improved health outcomes.

Alternatives to Driving

It seems that the obvious solution to support older adults who can no longer drive would be to transition them to one of the many transportation alternatives. **Transportation alternatives** are modes of transportation other than a person's private automobile that promote travel within the community. These may be publicly or privately funded and operated and can include bus or train transit, paratransit, shared ride programs, volunteer driver programs, shuttles, jitneys, fee-for-service rides such as taxis, or senior transportation services. **Paratransit** refers to flexible transportation that does not follow regular schedules or fixed routes and often provides curb-to-curb service. The option of transitioning a senior to a transportation alternative is often not a viable option for several reasons. The most common problem with transportation alternatives is existence of services in the location of origin, the destination, or both. Although large metropolitan areas typically have a full transit infrastructure and possibly even a subway or rapid transit system, they exist in only a limited number of cities in the United States. Most of the geographic area of the United States is rural or suburban with limited or no existing transit system. The presence of a fixed-route transit system, such as a bus or subway, is not sufficient to meet the needs of an aging traveler if the origin or destination is not along that fixed route; therefore, other modes of transportation would be necessary.

The existence of transportation services alone will not support community mobility if the individual is unable to use the service. The very same performance skills that hinder the ability to safely operate a motor vehicle can also impede use of transportation alternatives. For example, a visually impaired person may be unable to read a bus schedule, complete a paratransit or accessible transportation application, or travel from the point of drop-off to the destination independently. Similarly, an older adult with physical limitations that prevent operation of vehicle controls may not be able to ascend or descend the steps on a bus, manipulate money or a bus pass allowing ridership, or have the endurance to wait at a bus stop. A person lacking the cognitive performance skills to safely drive on public roadways may not be able negotiate bus or train transfers, remember to call 24 hours in advance to schedule a ride, or plan the timing of a bus route to arrive at a destination on time. All of the performance impairments that caused an older adult to cease driving must be taken into consideration when choosing the transportation alternative that best fits the individual's community travel needs.

Characteristics of the context such as climate, distance, and zoning may be detrimental to a person's community mobility. Extremes in weather, either very hot or very cold, can encumber a traveler's ability to walk to and from pick-up and drop-off locations and wait for buses or transfers. Travelers also may have to endure long rides if they live in more rural areas and have to travel farther or if fixed routing extends trip durations. A person living in the back of a senior community and one mile from the front gate may have to walk to a community shuttle stop to use the community shuttle service for transport to the community entrance, only to wait for an extended period of time at the transit bus stop for the next transit bus for travel to the destination.

It is also difficult logistically for older adults to manage community needs using transportation alternatives. A fixed route or even a scheduled transportation service will not wait for travelers to complete their business to provide a ride home. Instead, the vehicle continues providing transportation services to other users while riders are grocery shopping, receiving medical care, or watching a show at the theater. From a resource use perspective this is an efficient manner to provide the most services for the maximum number of consumers. However, from the traveler's perspective it results in long wait times and unexpected delays for return trips home. An older adult using transit to travel to the grocery store may be using a bus operating on a 45-minute loop, which allows a person 45 minutes to complete his or her business and return to the front of the store for the return trip home. If complications arise and the person's business lasts slightly longer than the duration of the loop, the person needs to wait for up to the full duration of another loop for his or her return trip. If this were the only implication, it is surmountable; however, it typically sets off a chain reaction of missed transfers, extended periods of time subjected to the climatic conditions, fatigue from waiting and holding purchases, and possibly even spoiled or melted food.

In addition to the complications of travel using transportation alternatives, there are secondary issues for consideration when an older adult is not able to travel using a private automobile. Access to restrooms can become a problem for older adults, particularly males with prostate involvement, as buses used for public transportation typically do not have restrooms. There is also no opportunity to stop or reroute in response to restroom needs because travel is occurring with others or on a fixed route. The previously described scenario with difficulty grocery shopping can ultimately result in poor nutrition due to difficulty carrying large quantities of food or fresh foods that have potential for spoiling. Dairy products, fresh meat, and heavy fruits and vegetables are often sacrificed for lightweight prepared foods with lower nutritional value for ease of transport home. Choosing lighter weight, preserved foods in a single shopping trip may be preferred to multiple smaller shopping trips per week due to the duration of each trip on transit, which can last as long as 3 hours depending on distance and required waiting and transfers.

Rather than brave the elements, endure long wait times, negotiate transfers, and pre-plan multi-step outings, many older adults choose to remain home and do without the services, resources, socialization, and occupational engagement awaiting them in the community. The result can be social isolation, neglected health care, poor nutrition, depression, and reduced quality of life. Occupational therapy practitioners should interrupt the path to these negative health outcomes by addressing driving and community mobility at a community level.

Driving and Community Mobility Practice

In 2006, the 30 million licensed drivers over the age of 65 represented 15% of all licensed drivers in the United States (National Highway Traffic Safety Administration [NHTSA], 2009). Crash data from 2007 revealed that older adults accounted for 196,000 of the injuries in traffic crashes and comprised 14% of all traffic-related fatalities for the year (NHTSA, 2009). Although older adult crash, injury, and fatality rates are disproportionately higher compared with those of their younger counterparts when controlled for annual miles driven, stereotypical age-related driving changes are not the cause. Rather, the rates represent the high incidence of age-related illnesses that impair driving performance and the increased frailty and fragility of an aging body, which make it more difficult to sustain the energy forces of a crash (Eberhard, 2008). Occupational therapy can play a role in reducing the crash, injury, and fatality statistics by determining driving capability for drivers with age-related performance issues, providing intervention strategies to improve performance or compensate for impairments, or using individual or population-based injury prevention approaches to reduce injuries and fatalities in the event of a crash. This role is fulfilled through the specialty practice area of **driving rehabilitation,** which is the therapeutic approach focusing on the occupation of driving with consideration for the person's (driver and passengers') performance skills, the context in which driving takes place, and the activity demands of performing the occupation.

Driving Rehabilitation Program Development

Driving rehabilitation programs are inherently community-based because the occupations of driving and community mobility occur in the community. There are several models for program development to support a community-based perspective representing different settings or host agencies. The most common venues for driving rehabilitation programs are hospital-based programs, private practice settings, and university-based programs (Finn, Gross, Hunt, McCarthy, Pierce, & Redepenning, 2004). These settings, including the typical outpatient department of hospital-based programs, offer access and connections to the community for a seamless transition back to driving.

The core principles of health program development apply to driving rehabilitation programs with the addition of considerations for the high cost of equipment, specialty trained personnel, automobile insurance and liability issues, and state-based credentialing or designation (Stav, 2004). Despite the similarities in program development principles, individuals and facilities working to develop or sustain a driving rehabilitation or community mobility program encounter several barriers. The top six barriers, client willingness/ability to privately pay for services, funds to develop a program, access to trained specialists to provide services, third-party reimbursement to pay for services, concerns about risk and liability, and time to address driving, were identified by more than 50% of the 2,800 study respondents (Stav, Snider-Weidley, & Love, 2011). These issues function as barriers to increasing the capacity of programs to meet the community mobility needs of older adults. An expert consensus panel was convened to generate strategies to overcome the barriers. The outcome of the panel was an online resource toolkit (AOTA, n.d.).

Referral Pathways

Developing a driving or community mobility program is only the first step in meeting the community mobility needs of older adults. The next critical step is developing a comprehensive referral network. Because the establishment of these referral relationships is important and often time-consuming, it is recommended that new programs invest time and effort developing a referral network before becoming operational (AOTA, 2008c). Continued efforts to sustain and further build referral pathways are necessary even for established programs due to the location of most community mobility programs outside of an existing health care network.

The strategies used to establish and maintain referral pathways are largely marketing techniques incorporating education about older driver safety and "red flag" issues that should trigger a concern about safety and a subsequent referral. The first strategy involves gathering and disseminating information about the program and services offered; other types of programs and services available, such as AARP's Safe Driving Program; the laws related to licensure in the state; medical reporting guidelines; ethical guidelines for physicians and occupational therapy practitioners; and pertinent evidence related to driving with specific medical conditions (AOTA, 2008c). Providing information to potential referral sources about whom to refer and on what basis establishes a sound foundation and eliminates questions about responsibility. Informing other departments within your facility or health care network is equally important as it facilitates access to and

timeliness of services for clients while supporting the business of the facility. Marketing materials should be developed to create an easy, seamless referral. Beyond the obvious brochures, materials containing the program's name and contact information, such as pens, key chains, sticky notes, and magnets, are easily available, so referring practitioners do not have to search for information to make the referral.

Many referrals originate from sources other than physicians when social service workers, first responders, friends, family, and neighbors recognize the potential for risk with an older driver. Presenting educational and marketing materials to a large range of individuals and agencies is an excellent mechanism to raise awareness, dispel myths, and inform the public and providers about appropriate referrals. The range of health care disciplines, community practitioners, and community organizations that can be targeted for educational marketing efforts are identified in Box 11-1.

Traffic incidents involving older adults are presented in the local media through print or television. It is in the best interest of older adult consumers of driving and community mobility services as well as the program to establish a relationship with local

---

Box 11-1   Targets for Education and Marketing Efforts

Health-Care Providers
- Neurologists
- Physiatrists
- Geriatricians
- Ophthalmologists
- Optometrists
- Neuro Optometrists
- Behavioral Optometrists
- Orthopedists
- Endocrinologists
- Cardiologists
- Internists
- Occupational Therapists
- Physical Therapists
- Speech Language Pathologists
- Nurses
- Social Workers
- Case Managers

Community Practitioners
- Department of Transportation
- Department of Insurance
- Medical Advisory Board at Driver Licensing Agencies
- Department of Children and Families
- State/County/Municipal Crisis Lines
- Municipal Planning Organizations
- Law Enforcement
- Fire Rescue
- AAA
- AARP
- Jewish/Catholic Family Services
- Risk Management Professionals
- Traffic Lawyers
- Traffic Court Judges
- Case Managers
- Managed Care Groups
- Food/Grocery Delivery
- Pharmacies
- Automobile Dealerships

Community Organizations
- Senior Centers
- Offices on Aging
- Community Centers
- Civic Organizations
  - Lions Club
  - Rotary Club
  - Kiwanis
  - Masons
- Support Groups
  - Stroke
  - Diabetes
  - Multiple Sclerosis
  - Alzheimer's/Dementia
  - Parkinson's
- Neighborhood Alliances
- Political Organizations
- Religious Social Groups

news outlets to serve as a credible, trustworthy source of information (AOTA, 2008c) rather than fueling the stereotypes that are so frequently sensationalized. Once these relationships are established, reporters will seek the professional advice of personnel in the program as it makes for a more credible story. After these relationships have been nurtured, the interaction becomes mutually beneficial for the program and the reporter, resulting in special interest stories, information pieces, and coverage of community-based events.

Funding

Reimbursement for driving rehabilitation services is limited due to Medicare's recognition of driving as "not medically necessary" (AOTA, 2008b). Other reimbursement sources include the Veterans Administration system, Medicaid in select states, and, to a lesser extent for older adults, workers' compensation and state vocation rehabilitation agencies (AOTA, 2005b). The scarcity of third-party reimbursement for driving rehabilitation services has led to the majority of payment for services being out-of-pocket. This creates obvious inequities and potential for occupational injustice for those who cannot afford the costly services, but clients and their family members with sufficient resources typically find the means to pay for services because driving is a critical occupation in most people's lives.

Community mobility services outside of the private automobile are often fiscally supported by a transportation agency through mandated paratransit services or grant-funded programs to enhance accessibility. Grant-funding opportunities are available to support additional programs and services through agencies such as United We Ride, which is an interagency federal national initiative geared toward coordinating transportation services (2006), or foundations that support senior health and mobility, including the Beverly Foundation (2009) and the Robert Wood Johnson Foundation (2009). Practitioners can also take creative measures to establish a fund for driving and community mobility services through legislation that taps into steady transportation-related revenue streams, such as a gas tax or additional fees on moving violations. Monies generated from a fraction of a cent on every gallon of gas sold in a state or from one additional dollar on every speeding ticket quickly add up to

support continued community mobility for all members of the community.

Credentialing of Programs and Personnel

To add credibility to a driving or community mobility program and assure legal operation, it is essential to secure the credentialing required by the state and valued by referring entities. There are two levels of credentialing; one is related to legitimizing the program or facility, and the other is credentialing the practitioners working in the program. Credentialing the facility or the program is mandated by some states to provide a mechanism of regulation and protect the public. Not all states have such mandates, but states that do require such regulation mandate the program be designated as a driving school or other officially recognized entity capable of providing driving instruction to new drivers. Operation of a program without the necessary credentialing is neither legal nor ethical. Parties interested in establishing a new program should inquire with the state agency authorized to grant the credential, which is typically the state Department of Motor Vehicles, Driver Licensing, Highway Safety, or Education.

Some states additionally mandate the personnel who work in the driving rehabilitation program to be credentialed as certified driving instructors. The regulations vary considerably from state to state, ranging from no required credential to a weekend course to graduate-level coursework. Similar to operating a program without the required credential, it is neither ethical nor legal to practice without the required certification in a state that mandates such a designation. It is therefore imperative that practitioners seek the correct information about required credentialing, which can typically be found within the same agency that oversees credentialing of a program.

There are certification programs for personnel that are voluntary but can add to the credibility of a program and serve as a selling point for referrals. Efforts to designate those practitioners who specialize in driving rehabilitation from generalists have resulted in certification programs. The Association of Driver Rehabilitation Specialists (ADED), an interdisciplinary organization, enacted the first certification program in 1995 (ADED, 2007). The certification designates individuals as certified driver rehabilitation specialists and awards a credential of CDRS. The

CDRS credential indicates health care providers, driver educators/instructors, and equipment dealers who have met the certification requirements to "plan, develop, coordinate and implement driver rehabilitation services for individuals with disabilities" (ADED, 2009, p. 1). Individuals who meet the educational and experiential criteria and pass the certification exam are awarded the CDRS credential.

A certification program was developed by the AOTA and initiated in 2006. The certification, available only to occupational therapists and occupational therapy assistants, designates individuals as specialty certified in driving and community mobility and awards a credential of SCDCM, or SCADCM for occupational therapy assistants (AOTA, 2009). The SCDCM or SCADCM identifies occupational therapy practitioners who focus their practice on driving and community mobility as opposed to generalist practice. Earning the credential requires individuals to meet the experiential criteria and complete the reflective portfolio application according to the established competencies in the practice area (AOTA, 2009). The SCDCM or SCADCM certification program is based on a professional development program that is grounded in the AOTA Standards of Continuing Competence (AOTA, 2005a). Neither the CDRS nor the SCDCM/SCADCM is required to practice in the area of driving rehabilitation. Although not required, a specialization credential is preferred as it demonstrates focused knowledge and experience and adds credibility when working with other team members and state agencies.

Role of Occupational Therapy Practitioners in Interventions

Consistent with the *Occupational Therapy Practice Framework,* occupational therapy practitioners provide driving and community mobility intervention services to three different levels of client: the person, organizations, and populations (AOTA, 2008a). Interventions to the person as a client focus on individual people or families with limitations in engagement in community mobility or driving or who have a need to access other community-based occupations. Practitioners working with organizations seek to support transportation services provided by the organization, improve safety of those traveling with that organization, and improve access and use of transportation services. Interventions aimed at serving a population are largely focused on injury prevention through educational initiatives and policy development or refinement. The following are examples of interventions in the area of driving and community mobility for older adults across the three levels.

Interventions With the Person

One of the most widely used functions of driving rehabilitation services for older adults is determination of medical fitness for driving through a comprehensive evaluation. Driving evaluations typically consist of a clinical assessment portion during which vision, cognition, and motor performance are measured to identify risk factors and potential problems while driving. The second portion of the evaluation is a behind-the-wheel assessment that measures driving performance in a naturalistic environment. Following both portions of the assessment, the occupational therapist synthesizes the results combined with the individual's history, progressive nature of the diagnosis, and potential for rehabilitation, and makes a determination about medical fitness to drive (Stav, Hunt, & Arbesman, 2006). As a result of the evaluation, recommendations are made to the individual, the family, the referring physician, and often to the state Medical Advisory Board. The permission or requirement to report to the state, confidentiality of that report, and practitioner immunity from legal action depend on state laws and vary considerably across the United States. A listing of each state's medical reporting guidelines can be found in the *American Medical Association's Physician's Guide to Assessing and Counseling Older Drivers* (Wang, Kosinski, Schwartzberg, & Shanklin, 2003) and should be referred to prior to filing reports with the state Medical Advisory Board.

Following the evaluation, many older drivers are referred for interventions to facilitate a return to driving. For individuals who have rehabilitation potential to improve performance skills for a safe return to driving, interventions are provided to remediate the deficit areas. This type of intervention may be focused on one or more of the performance skill areas to improve sensory perceptual skills, motor and praxis skills, emotional regulation skills, cognitive skills, or communication and social skills. In circumstances in which the client's performance skills cannot improve due to a permanent or progressive condition, the interventions may address training in the use of adaptive strategies or adaptive equipment to support a return to driving. The decision to implement these adaptive interventions should be made carefully and incorporate consideration of the client's abilities for new learning (Stav et al., 2006) and ability to pay for the recommended assistive technology and training sessions. Because Medicare does not reimburse for driving rehabilitation services in most states (AOTA, 2005b), clients must pay out of pocket for all vehicle modifications and training sessions, which can cost over $2,000 depending on the equipment needed and the extent of training required.

There are instances when it is no longer safe for an individual to drive and transportation alternatives must be utilized to remain mobile in the community. In such cases, occupational therapy practitioners may facilitate community mobility planning for driving retirement, offer travel training to build new skills in the use of transportation alternatives, or provide support and assistance in the completion of paratransit applications. All of these interventions take into the consideration the individual's community mobility needs, the context of the community, and the capacity of performance skills to negotiate different transportation alternative systems. Specific interventions may include route planning, money management, or transfers on and off a vehicle to ensure independence in community mobility, so clients may focus their energies on the occupations to which they are traveling. Professional training in the practice of travel training is available nationwide through Easter Seal's Project ACTION (2009).

Regardless of the person's ultimate mode of transportation, the occupational therapy practitioner may use advocacy strategies to help the client achieve optimal transportation. Advocacy efforts can include promotion of access on a transit system, requests for funding for adaptive equipment, or support for continued licensure but will always focus on the ultimate goal of endorsing community mobility in support of occupational engagement in the community.

Interventions With Organizations

Occupational therapy practitioners may provide interventions on a larger scale to an entire organization to assist the organization in providing safe, effective, and efficient community mobility to its clients. Organizations that may utilize an occupational therapy practitioner either as an employee or a consultant might include transportation agencies, senior centers, community centers, or places where older adults travel for leisure, such as the movie theater. The range of services provided includes ensuring access to the transit, determining ridership eligibility, and training of personnel.

All public transportation agencies must meet accessibility guidelines set by federal law with regard to accessible transportation services for those who cannot benefit from fixed-route transit services (Americans with Disabilities Act of 1990, 1991). Based on the legal requirements, occupational therapists may work for the transit company to ensure continuous accessibility of bus stops and buses to maximize ridership among travelers with disabilities. Particular attention is paid to roadway shoulders, integrity of sidewalks, curb cuts, curb heights, and shelters at bus stops.

Some individuals are unable to use existing fixed-route services because they cannot travel to bus stops, negotiate the ingress and egress of the vehicle, nor plan transfers between multiple vehicles and routes. These individuals may be eligible for accessible transportation services for all their travel needs, only some trips, or only under certain conditions such as inclement weather with ice and snow. Because the door-to-door service provided through paratransit is substantially more expensive than fixed-route transit, agencies are often concerned about eligibility of riders and limiting use of paratransit to only those who cannot use the fixed-route system. This concern has led to the involvement of occupational therapy practitioners, who evaluate potential or existing users to determine eligibility for the costly service. The role of the occupational therapist may lead to simplification of the eligibility application process as the evaluations can be customized to assess only the performance skill areas affected by the diagnosis rather than maintaining a broad reaching evaluation protocol for every potential rider.

Organization-based interventions with transit companies may also include the training of personnel with regard to wheelchair management, safety with wheelchair tie-downs, wheelchair lifts, and behavioral management with riders. The training may extend to include sensitivity training for employees who work in scheduling, paratransit application processors, and transport personnel specific to cognitive issues, sensory loss, and privacy. These same approaches might be used with other organizations that provide transportation to older adults, such as senior centers, to ensure fluid operation of their transportation so travelers can arrive at their destinations and engage in the intended occupation.

Interventions With Populations

Interventions with populations are far-reaching as they aim to address an issue of all members of a group who might be defined by a geographic region, diagnostic category, or experience. The approaches tend to be preventative in nature and in the area of traffic safety are usually aimed at reducing crashes, injuries, and fatalities. Carfit is one very focused example of a population-based intervention and functions as a community-based educational program developed to address driver-vehicle fit and vehicle safety feature use among older drivers in the United States. CarFit is a community-based program offering assessments of driver-vehicle fit to older drivers along with education to promote safe use of vehicles (American Automobile Association [AAA], AARP, AOTA, 2008). The primary purpose of CarFit is to relay safety information, and it does not address any evaluative functions to determine driver performance (AAA et al., 2008). The three objectives of CarFit agreed upon by all three collaborating agencies and addressed by hundreds of volunteers all over the United States are:

1. promote continued safe driving and mobility among older drivers by focusing attention on senior driver placement in their vehicle,
2. create an open environment that promotes conversations about driving, and
3. provide information, education, and community-based resources to older drivers

in a non-threatening, quick, and easily accessible manner. (AAA et al., 2008, p. 4)

CarFit uses a 12-point checklist to guide measurements and observations of older adults sitting in their vehicles and a mechanism for open communication with recommendations specific to the areas of need. Although the program does examine one individual at a time, it is not intervention based but provides structured education to older drivers throughout the United States. Other similar opportunities for population-based educational intervention exist within several traffic safety initiatives, such as Buckle-Up America, Drive Well Toolkit: Promoting Older Driver Safety and Mobility in Your Community, and Child Passenger Safety for grandparents who transport grandchildren.

On a macro level, occupational therapy practitioners can provide services in the area of policy development related to both driving and community mobility. Several states have state-wide special interest groups that meet regularly to discuss and modify policies related to driver licensing, license renewal, medical reporting, roadway design, transportation infrastructure, transportation disadvantage, and the role of occupational therapy in determining medical fitness to drive. Involvement in these groups offers an opportunity to influence policy, change laws, and elevate the perception of occupational therapy in addressing senior mobility issues. Even without the operation of these groups, occupational therapy practitioners can educate and lobby for their legislators to write and modify laws for the inclusion of occupational therapy as a valuable resource in community design, medical fitness to drive, and review of driving licensing standards for medically involved drivers.

On a smaller scale, although still population based, occupational therapists can influence population-based occupational engagement by working with community planners and collaborating with municipal planning organizations. These entities decide on zoning and placement of a community's infrastructure. An occupational therapy perspective is valuable in understanding the occupational patterns and needs of the senior members of a community to making suggestions related to sidewalk width, curb cuts, crosswalk timing, angle of intersections, inclusion of protected left turn signals and left turn lanes, and the location of residential versus recreational and commercial areas to minimize driving burdens and optimize walking and biking opportunities. Many of these recommendations have already been suggested on a federal level through the Federal Highway Administration's *Highway Design Handbook for Older Drivers and Pedestrians* (2001); an occupational therapist can ensure the need to follow the recommendations due to the effects of aging on performance and when capacity for engagement in activity is known.

Conclusion

Community mobility is a vital area of occupational engagement that contributes to productive, healthy aging for community-dwelling older adults. Not only does community mobility serve as a means to travel from point A to point B but it also allows for engagement in other areas of occupation. Because of the significant impact of this one occupation on the health of older adults, occupational therapists should pay particular attention to facilitating or sustaining the community mobility of older adults.

The range of therapeutic services related to driving and community mobility is substantial and includes evaluations and interventions specific to driving a private automobile, identifying appropriate transportation alternatives and training in the use of those services, supporting the services provided by transit agencies through accessibility and personnel training, and injury prevention initiatives to improve the health and safety within an entire population. The role of the occupational therapy practitioner does not end with the provision of clinical or consultative services in the area of driving and community mobility. Other skills such as marketing, education, and establishment of referral pathways and collaborative relationships are essential. Practitioners working in the area of driving and community mobility describe their programmatic successes as being heavily dependent on these skills (Stav, 2012). Occupational therapy practitioners should hone their skills that support programs for successful endeavors in the community-based practice of driving and community mobility.

CASE STUDIES

CASE STUDY 11•1 Mr. Martin

Mr. Martin is a 78-year-old gentleman who sustained a left cerebral vascular accident and subsequent right ankle fracture 3 months ago. He was referred to a driving rehabilitation program after he expressed a desire to return to driving. An occupational profile reveals that Mr. Martin is married with three adult children and five grandchildren. He was active in his grandchildren's lives through attendance at their sporting events and after-school activities, and through the responsibility of picking them up after school three days per week. The family car was driven primarily by Mr. Martin to travel to medical appointments for him and his wife, grocery shopping, and other outings. Mrs. Martin had limited her driving in recent years because she felt her skills were slipping and had come to rely heavily on her husband for community mobility. Mr. Martin also enjoyed an active golf hobby with friends every Sunday afternoon, weather permitting. The primary stated client goal is to "return to driving so I can be myself again." Assessments revealed intact cognition; adequate vision within the state guidelines but a mild left visual field cut; right upper extremity use within functional limits; and mildly impaired right lower extremity function due to sensory impairment, mildly increased extensor tone, and decreased range of motion due to the fracture. A behind-the-wheel assessment revealed that Mr. Martin has a strong foundation in driver safety, is aware of his limitations, but is not able to safely operate an automobile with the manufacturer's equipment. Driving rehabilitation services are recommended for intervention to return Mr. Martin to driving.

CASE STUDY 11•1 Discussion Questions

1. What areas of occupational loss may Mr. Martin and his significant others experience as a result of his driving limitations?
2. What types of interventions would be the most appropriate for Mr. Martin?
3. What strategies could be used to facilitate Mrs. Martin's community mobility?

CASE STUDY 11•2 Mrs. Brown

Mrs. Brown is a 69-year-old woman recently diagnosed with early stages of dementia whose physician is concerned about her driving safety and propensity for getting lost. Her neurologist referred her to an occupational therapist to evaluate potential and develop a community mobility plan. Through the occupational profile, Mrs. Brown's social history was revealed and it became apparent that she has limited family support as she is a widow, has no children, and lives alone in an apartment with her two cats. However, she does have a niece who lives in town. Since her husband passed away 6 years ago, Mrs. Brown has been active in the community in a part-time volunteer position at the library two afternoons per week when she reads to preschool children and assists with scheduling of outside groups that use library meeting space. In addition, she has been an active member of her church, fulfilling the role of ministering to the sick in their homes or at the hospital. Clinical assessments of Mrs. Brown's performance indicates she has strengths in motor and praxis skills, visual perceptual skills, and communication skills as well as a strong desire to be independent in community mobility. She does present with limitations to independence due to impaired memory, organizational skills, and judgment, with slightly decreased attention span. Mrs. Brown's community mobility performance was assessed both in driving her car and negotiating the local transit system for the first time. She was able to operate her motor vehicle with adequate safety, which is not surprising as she is just in the first stages of dementia; however, she expresses concern about her own abilities. Mrs. Brown was able to navigate to the grocery store and library using the local transit system in her small suburban town. She expressed comfort riding the bus and locating her destinations because she knows the streets so well after living in town all her life.

CASE STUDY 11•2 Discussion Questions

1. Who will be impacted by Mrs. Brown's limited community mobility and in what ways?
2. What are your concerns for Mrs. Brown regarding use of a fixed-route transit system?
3. What intervention strategies would you recommend to support Mrs. Brown's continued community mobility?
4. How could you support a transit agency in providing transportation services for riders with a range of disabling conditions?

Learning Activities

1. Create a list of community transportation resources available to older adults in your community with names, contact information, eligibility, cost, scheduling guidelines, and travel limitations such as distance, days, and hours of operation.
2. Consider a typical week in your life and the community mobility used to engage in a full week of occupations. List all the occupations in which you engage that require community mobility and identify the mode of transportation used (private automobile, fixed-route transit, taxi, train, etc.). Generate a plan to continue your engagement in all the listed occupations if you could NOT use your private automobile.
3. Identify the stakeholders and potential referral sources in your area if you were to develop a driving or community mobility program, along with strategies to establish a collaborative relationship.

REFERENCES

American Automobile Association, AARP, & American Occupational Therapy Association. (2008). *CarFit technician manual.* Washington, DC: American Automobile Association.

American Occupational Therapy Association. (2005a). Standards for continuing competence. *American Journal of Occupational Therapy, 59,* 661–662.

American Occupational Therapy Association. (2005b). Statement: Driving and community mobility. *American Journal of Occupational Therapy, 59,* 666–670.

American Occupational Therapy Association. (2008a). Occupational therapy practice framework: Domain and process,

2nd edition. *American Journal of Occupational Therapy, 62*(6), 625–683.

American Occupational Therapy Association. (2008b). *Pros and Cons of Medicare Payment for Specialty Driving Programs.* Retrieved from http://aota.org/olderdriver/docs/pros_cons.pdf

American Occupational Therapy Association. (2008c). *Tips on setting up referral pathways.* Retrieved from http://aota.org/olderdriver/tips.html

American Occupational Therapy Association (2009). *AOTA specialty certification in driving and community mobility: Occupational therapist candidate handbook.* Available from http://www.aota.org/Practitioners/ProfDev/Certification.aspx

American Occupational Therapy Association (n.d.). *Driving rehabilitation program development toolkits.* Available from http://aota.org/Older-Driver/Professionals/Toolkit/Programs.aspx

Americans with Disabilities Act of 1990, Pub. L. No. 101-336, § 2, 104 Stat. 328 (1991).

Association of Driver Rehabilitation Specialists. (2007). *History: Association for Driver Rehabilitation Specialists.* Retrieved from http://driver-ed.org/i4a/pages/index.cfm?pageid=119

Association of Driver Rehabilitation Specialists (2009). *Candidate handbook.* Available from http://www.driver-ed.org/files/public/ADED_Certification_Exam_handbook_2009.pdf

Beverly Foundation. (2009). *Beverly Foundation.* Retrieved from http://beverlyfoundation.org/

Easter Seals. (2009). *Project ACTION.* Retrieved from http://projectaction.org

Eberhard, J. (2008). Older drivers' "high per-mile crash involvement": the implications for licensing authorities. *Traffic Injury Prevention, 9*(4), 284–290.

Federal Highway Administration. (2001). *Highway design handbook for older drivers and pedestrians (FHWA-RD-01-103).* McLean, VA: United States Department of Transportation.

Finn, J., Gross, M., Hunt, L., McCarthy, D., Pierce, S. L., Redepenning, S., et al. (2004). *Driving evaluation & retraining programs: A report of good practice, 2004.* Bethesda, MD: American Occupational Therapy Association.

Glass, T. A., de Leon, C. M., Marottoli, R. A., & Berkman, L. F. (1999). Population based study of social and productive activities as predictors of survival among elderly Americans. *British Medical Journal, 319*, 478–483.

Marottoli, R. A., Mendes de Leon, C. F., Glass, T. A., Williams, C. S., Jr., Berkman, L. F., et al. (1997). Driving cessation and increased depressive symptoms: Prospective evidence from the New Haven EPESE. *Journal of the American Geriatrics Society, 45*, 202–206.

National Highway Traffic Safety Administration. (2009). *Traffic safety facts 2007 data: Older population* (No. DOT HS 810 992). Washington, DC.

Pierce, S. L. (2002). Restoring Competence in Mobility. In C. T. M. Radomski (Ed.), *Occupational therapy for physical dysfunction* (5th ed., pp. 665–693). Baltimore: Lippincott, Williams & Wilkins.

Robert Wood Johnson Foundation. (2009). *Robert Wood Johnson Foundation.* Retrieved from http://rwjf.org/

Stav, W. B. (2004). *Driver rehabilitation: A guide for assessment and intervention.* San Antonio, TX: Psychological Corporation.

Stav, W. B. (2012). Developing and implementing driving rehabilitation programs: A phenomenological approach. *American Journal of Occupational Therapy, 66*(1). doi: 10.5014/ajot.110.000950

Stav, W. B., Hallenen, T., Lane, J., & Arbesman, M. (2012). Systematic review of occupational engagement and health outcomes among community-dwelling older adults. *American Journal of Occupational Therapy. 66*(3), 301–310.

Stav, W. B., Hunt, L., & Arbesman, M. (2006). *Driving and community mobility for older adults: Occupational therapy practice guidelines.* Bethesda, MD: AOTA Press.

Stav, W. B., & Lieberman, D. (2008). From the desk of the editor. *American Journal of Occupational Therapy, 62*(2), 127–129.

Stav, W. B., Snider-Weidley, L., & Love, A. (2011). Barriers to developing and sustaining driving and community mobility programs. *American Journal of Occupational Therapy, 65*(4), e38–e45. doi: 10.5014/ajot.2011.002097

United We Ride. (2006). *United we ride.* Retrieved from http://unitedweride.gov/

Vanlaar, W., Simpson, H., & Robertson, R. (2008). A perceptual map for understanding concern about unsafe driving behaviours. *Accident; Analysis and Prevention, 40*(5), 1667–1673.

Waldrop, J., & Stern, S. M. (2003). *Disability status: 2000* (No. C2KBR-17). Washington, DC: United States Census Bureau.

Wang, C. C., Kosinski, C. J., Schwartzberg, J. G., & Shanklin, A. V. (2003). *Physician's guide to assessing and counseling older drivers.* Washington, DC: National Highway Traffic Safety Administration.

Chapter 12

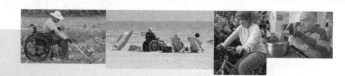

Adult Day Services Programs and Assisted Living Facilities

Courtney S. Sasse, MA EdL, MS, OTR/L

How does one keep from "growing old inside"? Surely only in community. The only way to make friends with time is to stay friends with people.... Taking community seriously not only gives us the companionship we need, it also relieves us of the notion that we are indispensable.

—Robert McAfee Brown

Learning Objectives

This chapter is designed to enable the reader to:

• Appreciate the impact of the geographic and demographic shifts in families in the United States
• Identify legislation and regulatory bodies that affect nursing homes, assisted living facilities, and adult services centers.
• Describe the various models of providing services for older adults in day care programs and assisted living facilities.
• Describe emerging roles for occupational therapy practitioners in adult day services programs and assisted living facilities.
• Discuss ways that adult day services programs and assisted living facilities can enhance and support successful aging for older adults, families, and communities.

Key Terms

Adult Day Services Centers/Programs (ADCs)
Assisted Living Facilities (ALFs)
CARF International
Continuing Care Retirement Community (CCRC)
Independent Living Community (ILC)

Individualized Services Care Plan
Productive aging
Successful aging
The Joint Commission

Introduction

There is increasing emphasis in the literature on productive and successful aging as the "baby-boomers" advance toward old age. **Productive aging** typically refers to "a broad perspective of aging that focuses on all valuable contributions that the elderly make to our society through paid and unpaid work and other occupational roles" (Gerson & Patterson,

1997, p. 11). This concept emphasizes productivity across the aging continuum as a means of increasing quality of life. **Successful aging** is a more inclusive term that includes "reaching one's potential and arriving at a level of physical, social and psychological well-being in an old age that is pleasing to both self and others" (Gibson, 1995, p. 279). Successful aging focuses on optimization of well-being by building strengths rather than a deficits-based, medical model of aging. The goal of adult day services centers (ADCs) and assisted living facilities (ALFs) is to enable successful aging by providing services needed by older adults. These programs are relatively new developments and have not always been available to seniors.

Assisted Living Facilities (ALFs) are residential facilities that provide assistance with activities of daily living (ADLs) for people who do not require the skilled nursing or medical care available in nursing homes (United States Department of Health and Human Services, (2011). The level of service in ALFs is generally limited to routine general protective oversight and supportive services. Although nursing homes were once considered as one of few options for care of the elderly and disabled, more diverse and client-centered choices have evolved (Board of Scientific Counselors of the National Center for Health Statistics [BSCNCHS], 2009; Love, 2010). In the 1990s, with changing demographics and an increasing number of older adults living away from their extended families, came the emergence of assisted living facilities (ALFs). Other factors contributing to the recent proliferation of ALFs include the aging of the baby-boom generation, a higher divorce rate, a lower birth rate, and the increasing number of households with dual earners. The increase in women entering the workforce has led to less care availability within the home for family members who are elderly or have complex medical needs (Bruce, 2006).

Regulatory and Accrediting Agencies

Because the typical ALF does not provide the extent of medical care that is required in nursing homes, ALFs are less stringently regulated than nursing homes. They are typically regulated by local and state governments (Golant, 2004). Regulation serves to protect the public and assure a minimum quality of services. However, nursing homes, ALFs, adult day services centers, and independent living communities may also be accredited. Accreditation is a process by which an agency, program, or institution demonstrates compliance with standards that exemplify best practices. Accreditation agencies include The Joint

Commission, formerly the Joint Commission on Accreditation of Healthcare Organizations (JCAHO), and CARF International, formerly the Commission on Accreditation of Rehabilitation Facilities (McCormack, 2011; MetLife Mature Market Institute [MMMI], 2009).

The Joint Commission is a private, independent nonprofit organization that provides voluntary accreditation for almost 18,000 hospitals and other health care agencies in the United States. Facilities are encouraged, if not required, by state governments to attain accreditation from The Joint Commission as a condition of licensure and receipt of Medicare reimbursement. **CARF International** is a private, nonprofit organization that focuses primarily on human services organizations. CARF International is widely recognized for accrediting programs and services in community agencies, such as adult day services centers and ALFs. The purpose of CARF is to "promote the quality, value, and optimal outcomes of services through a consultative accreditation process that centers on enhancing the lives of the persons served" (McCormack, 2011, p. 570). The American Occupational Therapy Association (AOTA) has a long and well-established relationship with CARF International, and the two agencies have collaborated on the development and revision of CARF standards, best practices, and the definition of quality performance indicators in a variety of rehabilitation contexts (McCormack, 2011).

Continuum of Care and Program Models

A multidimensional approach to assessing, evaluating, treating, and supporting the elderly, those with chronic disabilities, or those who wish to maintain health and well-being but who are unable to age-in-place is needed. To meet the needs of older adults in the community, the continuum of care consists of many options with differing levels of support. Three broad residential options exist in the continuum of care: home care, ALFs, and nursing homes.

A fourth emerging residential option is the independent living community. An **independent living community (ILC)** is a place for senior citizens who desire to live independently, prefer to reside near peers, have a need for additional security, and/or no longer wish to maintain a household or home. The ILC bridges the gap between maintaining a household independently and needing home care or assisted living (Tom, 2011). ILCs are sometimes referred to as retirement communities.

An alternative to residential options, adult day services centers provide care for adults with cognitive impairments or functional performance challenges in a supportive group environment outside of the home. Adult day services centers/programs, programs that support social integration, community participation, and the highest level of independence that is safely possible for clients, are an important source of support for families and respite from the demands and responsibilities of caregiving. There are approximately 4,600 adult day services programs operating in the United States that provide a needed source of respite to family caregivers (National Adult Day Services Association [NADSA] n.d.).

Productive aging can be facilitated in a variety of contexts, including home care, adult day services centers, ILCs, ALFs, and nursing homes. All of these settings and their various levels of care are components of a broad spectrum of services called a **continuing care retirement community (CCRC);** see Figure 12.1. These settings and services will be discussed in more detail here.

Adult Day Services Programs and Home Care Agencies

Adult day services centers (ADCs) provide community-based, client-centered coordinated programs that promote social, health care–related, or rehabilitative services in a group setting to more than 260,000 participants and family caregivers in the United States (MMMI , 2009; NADSA, n.d.). ADCs vary in the specific services that they offer, but most are defined by minimally offering the following services: social activities; transportation, typically door-to-door services; provision of meals and snacks; personal care, which includes assistance with toileting, grooming, eating, and other ADLs; and therapeutic activities and exercises. Nearly 50% of adult day services centers offer comprehensive rehabilitation and therapeutic interventions including occupational, physical, and speech therapies (NADSA, n.d.).

There are three models for ADCs: the social model, the medical or health-related model, and the specialized care model. ADCs offer the spectrum of care necessary for the care recipient, which ranges from needs that are primarily psychosocial to needs that require a more medically complex and involved plan of care. The social model ADC typically provides supervised, structured programs for socialization, prevention and health promotion services, and

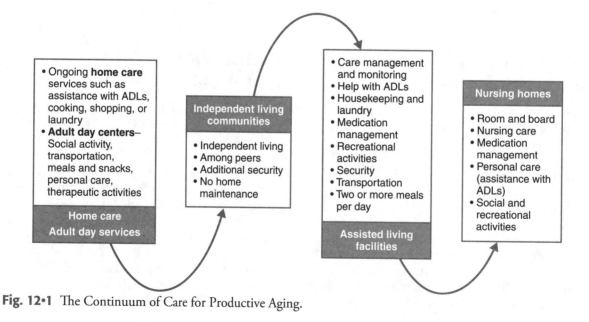

Fig. 12•1 The Continuum of Care for Productive Aging.

meals and transportation (Van Slyke, 2001). Approximately 29% of ADCs operate on the social model. The medical or health-related model ADC provides comprehensive, skilled health care and rehabilitation services (McPhee & Johnson, 2000; Van Slyke, 2001). Nearly half (48%) of the ADCs provide a combination of social and medical or health-related services. The specialized care model ADC represents 16% of ADCs and is the preferred choice for individuals who are managing chronic illnesses. The majority of specialized care model ADCs provide services for persons with Alzheimer's disease and other forms of dementia. However, the number and variety of disease-specific programs offered in specialized adult day centers is growing (MMMI, 2009; NADSA, n.d.).

Home care agencies are an increasingly popular choice for individuals who wish to age in place. Home care services may include homemaking-related tasks such as cooking, laundry, and shopping, as well as companionship and respite. Services, regulations, and licensing of home care agencies varies from state to state; however, specifications under Medicare require that Medicare-certified agencies must follow federal regulations in order to be reimbursed. As people age and acquire chronic illnesses or other conditions, independence within the home is often supplemented with home care by outside professionals.

Currently many home care services can be provided by paraprofessionals. Other home care services can be provided only by licensed health care professionals such as nurses, occupational therapists, or physical therapists under the direction of a physician. Rehabilitation services are generally required for follow-up after an acute event, or when a person requires transition services upon discharge from a hospital or rehabilitation facility. Home care is also an option for individuals who are physically healthy but require supervision for safety. This is a suitable consideration for individuals with dementia, Alzheimer's disease, significant cognitive delays, or degenerative or chronic illnesses or injuries (MMMI, 2009).

Independent Living Communities

ILCs are variations of what many recognize as retirement communities. The residents of ILCs often transition to this context when they still wish to live independently in a single dwelling situation similar to apartment living but wish to be relieved of the duties of home maintenance. Members of the community often choose this setting in order to maintain relationships with others who are similar in age or life situations. Although the time and schedules within these communities are not structured or supervised, amenities and social events are often planned and offered by committees within the residential neighborhood.

The typical resident of an ILC will not require assistance for ADLs; however, several common amenities in this context include the offering of housekeeping and laundry services. It is common for these communities to provide on-site amenities, such as dining facilities, hair salons, and small convenience stores, as well as access to transportation for off-site destinations. Caregivers and family members often cite increased monitoring and security as being an important benefit of ILCs. Some communities have a security officer on-site around the clock, promoting a sense of increased confidence in residents should an emergency occur (Tom, 2011).

Assisted Living Facilities

Residents of ALFs are provided with an array of services, including assistance with ADLs and instrumental activities of daily living (IADLs), education, play, leisure, and social participation. ALFs can also be appropriate placements for people with cognitive impairments related to disorders such as Alzheimer's disease when safety and supervision is a priority. Unlike ILCs, age is not typically a determinant when considering an ALF (MMMI, 2009).

There are more than 39,000 ALFs that offer services. Services are often determined on the basis of an individual's need, and often the cost is dependent on the level of care chosen. ALFs are categorized by the number of services included in the base-rate cost (Fig. 12.2).

Based on determined needs, many ALFs produce an **individualized services care plan** for each resident that is like a detailed map of required services. The plan is reviewed and updated collaboratively with the client and the family or caregiver. The average resident is between 75 and 84 years old, and the average length of stay is approximately 28 months (MMMI, 2009).

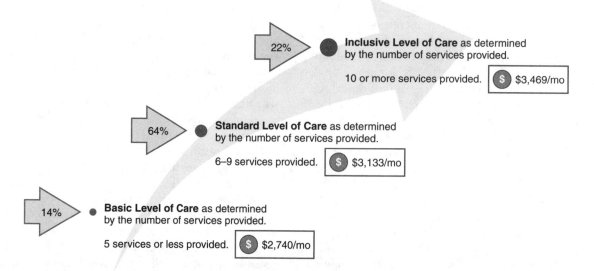

Fig. 12•2 Percentage of Assisted Living Communities Categorized by Levels of Care and Associated Base Cost. *(From MetLife Mature Market Institute. (2009).* Market survey of long-term care costs: The 2009 MetLife market survey of nursing, assisted living, adult day services, and home care costs. *Retrieved from: http://MatureMarket Institue.com)*

Unlike nursing homes, which are governed at the federal level, ALFs and ADCs are regulated by the state. Advocacy groups like the Assisted Living Federation of America (ALFA) favor state regulation, which offers more local control and allows for a greater variety of choices and cost-efficient processes to be determined locally. This flexibility of administrators and policy makers at the state level fuels industry growth, and the degree of choice is often passed along to the ALF residents (Bersani, 2011). Policy makers, care providers, and consumers are interested in overall costs, the provision of quality services, and care for individuals with increasingly complex medical needs. The overarching principles for all stakeholders, however, are outcomes that enhance and improve productive aging by producing a more satisfying quality of life for older adults and their caregivers.

Nursing Homes

Within the continuum of care, nursing homes represent the lowest level of independence for their residents. Residents of nursing homes may have chronic conditions or a cognitive impairment that requires a level of services and complex and consistent medical care that prevents the person from living in a less restrictive, and therefore more independent, secure environment. Patients of nursing homes or long-term-care facilities usually need assistance with multiple ADLs. Incontinence is a common problem, as are cognitive limitations due to Alzheimer's disease or dementia. Services provided to patients in nursing homes include room and board, nursing care, medication management, personal care (assistance with ADLs), and social and recreational activities (MMMI, 2009). Comparatively, the nursing home context is characterized by more routines and structure and less personal choice for residents than other housing and long-term-care options. The transition to a nursing home often means that limited choices are traded for supervision and increased personal safety for residents.

Most forms of care in the continuum of care are framed by the social model, which highlights independence and flexibility as well as individual choice provided in a home or home-like environment. However, nursing homes were founded based on the tenets of the medical model of practice and are therefore aligned with fewer consumer-based decisions. The medical model tends to encourage regulations, structure, fewer personal choices, and patient dependency. Nevertheless, nursing homes provide a secure environment and offer a variety of services that promote the comfort and quality of life for patients who require a more complex level of service (Golant, 2004; MMMI, 2009; Zimmerman, et al., 2005).

Occupational Therapy Roles

Occupational therapy roles and services for older adults reflect the context of care. One approach for assessing the needs of older adults that incorporates context is using the H.O.M.E.-E Principle (Box 12-1). This approach explores how occupation is meaningful to older adults when engaging in a variety of environments. By considering what occupations are meaningful to the client, and the manner in which the client currently engages in the occupations, the occupational therapist can better plan the transition to a new HOME, a new context. The natural path to successful transition to a new environment is to adapt the environment while keeping the occupations consistent and routine. In this way, a disruption of occupations is avoided, as is the potential for occupational imbalance.

Although direct care may be the role demanded most frequently in the continuing care spectrum, care planning, case coordination, and rehabilitation management are all areas in which occupational therapy can make a contribution. Research by Cruz (2006) supports the notion that "characteristics, experiences, and meanings that participants attributed to the assisted living center's structure, physical nature, sociocultural nature, and temporal-occupational nature" (p. 101) are critical to incorporate into occupation-based practice to ensure occupational balance for older adults and their caregivers. The Japanese concept of *ikigai,* a personality trait and client factor similar to having optimism or being optimistic, requires that a person have meaning in his or her life and a reason to live. If a person is to live life to the fullest, the most highly sought after outcome of occupational therapy, the occupational therapy practitioner must enable older adults and their caregivers to engage in meaningful occupations that make life worth living (Seligman, 2011).

The effect of social support, meaningful engagement, and access to community resources enhances quality of life, producing positive health outcomes. Older adults who have a more positive perception of life and a fulfilling sense of engagement are more resilient, have improved immune system functions, experience fewer depressive symptoms, and experience a better quality of life. Strong social foundations provide a sense of self-worth and self-esteem and are therefore a protective factor against stress and mental and physical illnesses (Deng, Weber, Sood, & Kemper, 2010). Best practices in occupational therapy in these contexts are informed by research evidence.

Maintaining and Maximizing Independence

It is well recognized that the broad goal of occupational therapy is to maximize the client's independence. In the past, the role of occupational therapy in ALFs relied heavily on direct interventions that focused on ADL skills, such as dressing and toileting, and IADL activities like household management, cooking, cleaning, and doing laundry. With changing client factors, and cultural and demographic demands and expectations, the occupational therapist now must integrate a more holistic approach to care. Occupational therapy practitioners also can encourage participation in leisure activities and social interactions through adaptation and facilitation of the environment or the activity to promote or enhance engagement (AOTA, 2006). Occupational therapy can also indirectly maximize or enhance the independence of older adults by providing staff training on issues that most affect the client's level of independence and participation. Often the most effective way to improve client-centered care is to provide staff education that is based on identified needs assessments

---

Box 12-1 Occupational Therapy Community Practice Implication

<u>H</u>ow is <u>O</u>ccupation <u>M</u>eaningful when <u>E</u>ngaging in one's <u>E</u>nvironment?
Remember this as the **H.O.M.E.-E.** Principle.

designed by occupational therapists with occupation-based performance indicators and outcomes in mind. Staff education can include instruction on safe transfer techniques, practical applications, and intervention strategies for individuals with cognitive or sensory impairments, or facilitation of discussion groups and focus groups determined by a thorough needs assessment (AOTA, 2006; Easton & Herge, 2011).

The elements of person-centered or client-centered care are important to consider. These elements include:

- ensuring that health care practices are ongoing and comprehensive,
- transforming organizational operations and cultures into client-centered environments,
- adopting nurturing and empowering practices,
- enabling elders and those with chronic or disabling conditions to experience meaning and purpose in their daily lives,
- offering a relationship-based culture, and
- fulfilling an obligation to make the individual feel at home (Love, 2010).

Managing Chronic Conditions

Diabetes, the seventh leading cause of death in 2007, creates a myriad of other health problems. New cases of blindness among adults younger than 75 are primarily attributed to diabetes, as are increasing cases of kidney failure, non-accidental injuries of the leg, and foot amputations. Increased consideration of prevention and health maintenance has resulted in nearly 80% of ADCs offering physical activity programs to address cardiovascular disease, diabetes, and the related constellation of symptoms (NADSA, n.d.). Occupational therapy can support successful lifestyle changes, increase functional independence, and facilitate adjustments to chronic health conditions in ADCs, ALFs, and nursing homes. When developing programs for any of the settings in the continuum of care, it is important to recognize and address the differing needs of men and women (American Association for Long-Term Care Insurance, 2010; Moss & Moss, 2007).

Interventions that incorporate dietary changes, coping skills, physical activity, social interactions, and group support are perhaps the most important

aspects of primary and secondary prevention of many chronic diseases. Diabetes, as well as coronary heart disease, obesity, chronic high blood pressure, uncontrolled cholesterol levels, arthritis, and osteoporosis can result in functional limitations and loss of independence (Centers for Disease Control and Prevention, 2001). Community-based interventions can provide a motivating source of encouraging physical activity. The successful management of disabling and chronic conditions is an integral part of providing comprehensive care.

Specialized care for chronic conditions that can be addressed by occupational therapists includes strategies for energy conservation, falls prevention, home safety, joint protection, stress management, safe driving, and community mobility. Through adaptation and education, meaningful occupations can be reintegrated into the lives of older adults with chronic conditions, which further encourage motivation to participate (AOTA, 2006). A program planning model is illustrated in Figure 12.3.

Enhancing Quality of Life

For much of the aging population, life roles and responsibilities have been chipped away until age-related dysfunction becomes self-defining. ADCs and ALFs that provide client-centered care can

Create a Balanced Calendar of Activities to Create Occupational Balance

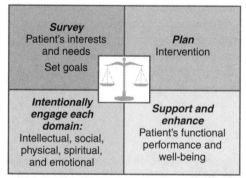

Fig. 12•3 O.T. Community Practice Implication: Program Planning. *(From McPhee, S. D., & Johnson, T. (2000). Program planning for an assisted living community. Occupational Therapy in Health Care, 12(2/3), 1–17.)*

significantly affect the quality of life of their residents. When given an opportunity to create meaning through activity, and when experiencing a sense of belonging followed by action, people feel pleasure (Cutchin, 2003). Experiences such as these provided in structured settings contribute to a sense of belonging, being a part of a community, being needed, and having a place to go. These experiences result in an individual's ability to combat depressive symptoms and manifest personal happiness. Personal happiness in turn provides a meaningful and personal definition of a life of quality.

Occupational therapy interventions in CCRSs and adult day settings have tended to be based on the underlying philosophies of the medical model of care. In a study by Horowitz and Chang (2004), evidence supported the need for occupational therapy interventions to reduce the roles of the occupational therapist in making decisions, planning, and leading groups, a perspective based on the medical model. Rather, it is recommended that the occupational therapist shift the paradigm for practice toward a social model of intervention and a more facilitative leadership style.

A social model of intervention incorporates peer support networks, group interventions led by group members, and the use of discussion and consensus building in these settings. Principles of the social model of practice align more consistently with the community-based model of practice. In addition, use of a more facilitative leadership role provides more emphasis on the five recognized domains of quality of life. These are intellectual, social, physical, spiritual, and emotional health and well-being. The Healthy Generation Model and Morningside Protocol is an example of a plan used in all LifeTrust America assisted living communities primarily in the southeastern United States (McPhee & Johnson, 2000). Careful consideration of these domains provides the fundamental foundation for improvement in the standard of care, opportunities for participation in meaningful occupations, and enhanced quality of life.

Safety, Security, and Support for Caregivers and Community

Chronic illness and productive aging interventions have historically been based on medical model principles. Current research provides evidence for the need to shift paradigms and provide a transitional bridge to support community-based health care services, which are cost-effective and focus on an increased quality of life for the individual, the caregivers, and the community. The challenge is to design interventions that promote functional performance for the older adult while considering the needs of the caregiver and the impact of the context. Providing opportunities to enjoy activities in all areas of occupations is the primary goal of occupational therapy. Nevertheless, lifestyle redesign programs that maximize functional performance and interventions that are designed to reduce functional decline in the older adult often fail to recognize the needs of those who love and care for the individual (Horowitz & Chang, 2004).

The number of caregivers for individuals who choose to age in place and for individuals with Alzheimer's disease and other related dementia is growing, yet relatively few post-acute options currently exist to support caregiver needs. It is necessary to consider the older adult holistically. The practice of integrative health care emphasizes building a relationship between the practitioner, the older adult, and the caregiver. With this principle in mind, the well-being of the older adult can only be achieved by also evaluating the stress, strain, and burden placed on the caregiver (Deng et al., 2010). Strategies for caregiver intervention can include education on advocacy for the older adult, and the provision of information about respite care for the older adult's loved ones in community-based settings, such as ADCs, ILCs, or ALFs (Perry, Dalton, & Edwards, 2010).

Conclusion

Supporting productive aging is now recognized as a philosophy of service that maintains a person's dignity in order to enhance his or her quality of life. Involvement of the community is an important element in the provision of care and can be an important contributor to the psychosocial well-being of its aging community members. Advances in medicine and technology have extended life expectancy, and much of what is to come with caring for the aging population will require a holistic, multidisciplinary, whole system intervention approach (Deng et al., 2010). The aforementioned whole system approach means that no single factor, person, or discipline will present adequate care, and it will indeed require a community approach to produce improved functional occupational performance.

With complexity comes change. The aging population is becoming increasingly complex, and occupational therapy practitioners can support change by consistently providing integrated services that improve the quality of life for clients. The successful aging process is one in which meaningful occupations are present, where dignity, respect, independence, and choice are motivating factors in choosing a place to call home. Within the community setting, occupational therapy practitioners can facilitate seamless transitions throughout the continuum of care.

CASE STUDIES

CASE STUDY 12•1 Nina and Jim

Nina and Jim left their large home on two acres where they had raised six children because they decided together that they could no longer maintain the home or property of 37 years. Jim is a retired Navy captain and the picture of health. He leads an active lifestyle, often playing golf with his sons and grandsons. At 76 years old, Jim shows little sign of slowing down. Nina, however, suffered a stroke at age 63, which affected her functional mobility. Nevertheless, as a retired librarian, she is an avid reader and active in a local book club that she attends weekly.

After Nina had her stroke, the couple received occupational therapy services at a subacute rehabilitation center. While making a home visit to prepare for Nina's discharge to home, the occupational therapist recommended the services of a home care personal attendant, who would be able to assist Nina and Jim with home care and management activities. Jim's excellent military benefits had covered much of the cost of a personal care attendant for the last 5 years. Nevertheless, the care of the home and yard had become overwhelming. Jim and Nina agreed that they were ready for less responsibility.

After careful research and consideration, Jim and Nina chose Pine Rest, a CCRC. Pine Rest serves 225 residents, with over 150 residing in independent living or assisted living apartments and about 25 residents in 1200-square-foot, two-bedroom detached cottages. The remaining residents have progressed to a skilled nursing facility located on the same campus that is affiliated with Pine Rest and a local hospital that provides constant care and emergency medical interventions.

Jim and Nina have resided at Pine Rest for 3 years and have few regrets. They made the decision to begin their residence at Pine Rest in an independent living cottage, which provided enough space to allow their grandchildren to take turns spending the weekend with them. Their contract is set up to guarantee a spot in an assisted living apartment and then in the skilled nursing facility if necessary. The CCRC has on-site amenities like a health club and wellness center, an auditorium, a convenience store, a beauty shop, two restaurants, and Nina's favorite, an on-site library, where she volunteers 3 days per week.

The cost of the CCRC is dependent upon the location (city and state), but the main goal is for the residents to not pay more to live in the CCRC than they were spending to live at home. Jim and Nina were able to sell their home and exchange the resulting amount for the entrance deposit. That is standard practice and procedure at most CCRCs. That money then returns to the residents if they decide to leave the community at any time. Monthly fees may apply as residents' care or services increase, but Jim and Nina have noted that the cost doesn't exceed their budget, which was that of an above-average middle-class retiree. The couple is satisfied with their decision. They continue to live independently without the cares and concerns of running a household. Jim comments that he feels less anxious about needing help taking care of Nina in the future.

CASE STUDY 12•1 Nina and Jim   *cont'd*

CASE STUDY 12•1 Discussion Questions

1. Do you think the home-care attendant who is helping Nina is a skilled occupational therapy practitioner? Why or why not?

2. Compare and contrast potential services offered to Nina and Jim in independent living and assisted living at Pine Rest.

3. As a community-based occupational therapy practitioner, Jim and Nina are your clients. Describe potential intervention considerations when helping them transition from their home to Pine Rest.

Learning Activities

1. Mr. S. is an 86-year-old gentleman who receives home-health services. He cares for his 82-year-old wife who has chronic obstructive pulmonary disease and dementia. His wife fell and fractured her hip, and Mr. S. is considering moving to an ALF with his wife. Research the ALFs in your area.

2. Design a handout that provides a brief description of the following agencies and resources.
- American Association of Homes and Services for the Aging
- Assisted Living Federation of America
- Center for Excellence in Assisted Living
- Consumer Consortium of Assisted Living
- National Adult Day Services Association
- National Council on Aging

REFERENCES

American Association for Long-Term Care Insurance. (2010). *Women underestimate importance of long-term care plan.* Los Angeles, CA: American Association for Long-Term Care Insurance.

American Occupational Therapy Association. (2006). *Occupational therapy's role in assisted living facilities* [Fact Sheet]. Rockville, MD: American Occupational Therapy Association.

Bersani, M. (2011). Public policy brief: Advocacy day recap 2011 ALFA fly-in makes strides. *Assisted Living Executive, March/April,* 56–57. Retrieved from http://alfapublications.org/alfapublications/20110304

Board of Scientific Counselors of the National Center for Health Statistics, Centers for Disease Control and Prevention, and the Division of Health Care Statistics. (2009). *Report of the long-term care statistics program review panel to the NCHS Board of Scientific Counselors.* Retrieved from http://cdc.gov/nchs/about/bsc/bsc_reviews.htm

Bruce, P. A. (2006). Ascendancy of assisted living: The case for federal regulation. *The Elder Law Journal, 14,* Board of Trustees of the University of Illinois.

Centers for Disease Control and Prevention. (2001). *Promoting active lifestyles among older adults.* Retrieved from http://cdc.gov/nccdphp/dnpa/physical/pdf/lifestyles.pdf

Cruz, E. D. (2006). Elders' and family caregivers' experience of place at an assisted living center. *Occupational Therapy Journal of Research, 26*(3), 97–107.

Cutchin, M. P. (2003). The process of mediated aging-in-place: a theoretically and empirically based model. *Social Science & Medicine, 57,* 1077–1090. doi: 10.1016/S0277-9536(02)00486-0

Deng, G., Weber, W., Sood, A., & Kemper, K. J. (2010). Research on integrative healthcare: Context and priorities. *Explore 6*(3), 143–158. doi:10.1016/j.explore.2010.03.007

Easton, L., & Herge, E. A. (2011). Adult day care promoting meaningful and purposeful leisure. *OT Practice, 16*(1), 20–26.

Gerson, D., & Patterson, G. (1997). Chapter 2 Productive aging: 1995 White House Conference on Aging, challenges for public policy and social work practice. Pages 9–26 in C. C. Saltz (Ed.), Social work response to the White House Conference on Aging: From issues to actions. *Journal of Gerontological Social Work, 27*(3). New York, NY: Haworth Press.

Gibson, R. C. (1995). Promoting successful and productive aging in minority populations. In L.A. Bond, S. J. Cutler, & A. Grams (Eds.), *Promoting successful and productive aging* (pp. 279–288). Thousand Oaks, CA: Sage.

Golant, S. M. (2004). Do impaired older persons with health care needs occupy U.S. assisted living facilities? An analysis of six national studies. *Journal of Gerontology: Social Sciences, 59B*(2), S68–S79.

Horowitz, B. P., & Chang, P. J. (2004). Promoting well-being and engagement in life through occupational therapy lifestyle redesign: A pilot study within adult day programs. *Topics in Geriatric Rehabilitation, 20*(1), 46–58.

Love, K. (2010). *Person-centered care in assisted living: An informational guide.* Retrieved from Center for Excellence in Assisted Living Web site: http://theceal.org

McCormack, G. L. (2011). Major accrediting organizations that influence occupational therapy practice. In Jacobs, K., & McCormack, G. L. (Eds.), *The occupational therapy manager* (5th ed.), pp. 565–575. Bethesda, MD: AOTA Press.

McPhee, S. D., & Johnson, T. (2000). Program planning for an assisted living community. *Occupational Therapy in Health Care, 12*(2/3), 1–17.

MetLife Mature Market Institute. (2009). *Market survey of long-term care costs: The 2009 MetLife market survey of nursing, assisted living, adult day services, and home care costs.* Retrieved from http://MatureMarketInstitute.com

Moss, S. Z., & Moss, M. S. (2007). Being a man in long term care. *Journal of Aging Studies, 21,* 43–45. doi: 10.1016/j.jaging.2006.05.001

National Adult Day Services Association (n.d.). *About adult day services.* Retrieved from http://nadsa.org/knowledge-base/col.php?pid=29&tpid=15&printer_friendly=1

Perry, B., Dalton, J. E., & Edwards, M. (2010). Family caregivers' compassion fatigue in long-term facilities. *Nursing Older People, 22*(4), 26–31.

Seligman, M. E. (2011). *Flourish.* New York, NY: Free Press.

Tom, J. (2011). *Independent living.* Retrieved from http://seniorhomes.com/p/independent-living/

Ullman, Samuel (n.d.). *Aging Quotes.* Retrieved from http://effective-antiaging-tips.com/aging-quotes.html

United States Department of Health and Human Services. (2011). Definition of assisted living. Retrieved from http://longtermcareeducation.com/learn_about_the_field/definition_of_assisted_living.asp

Van Slyke, N. (2001). Adult day-care programs. In M. Scaffa (Ed.), *Occupational therapy in community-based practice settings* (pp. 163–172). Philadelphia, PA: F.A. Davis.

Zimmerman, S., Sloane, P. D., Eckert, K. J., Gruber-Baldini, A. L., Morgan, L. A., Hebel, J. R.,...Chen, C. K. (2005). How good is assisted living? Findings and implications from an outcomes study. *Journal of Gerontology: Social Sciences, 60B*(4), S195–S204.

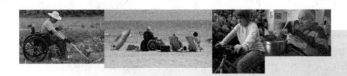

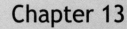

Chapter 13

Low Vision Services in the Community

Theresa Marie Smith, PhD, OTR/L, CLVT

It's not what you look at that matters, it's what you see.

—Henry David Thoreau

Learning Objectives

This chapter is designed to enable the reader to:
- Articulate the reasons for the growing population of persons with low vision.
- Identify the four major causes of low vision and available medical treatment.
- Describe how low vision affects occupational performance.
- Identify low vision team members and the services provided for this population.
- Describe occupational therapy services for clients with low vision.
- Discuss psychosocial aspects of low vision.
- Evaluate local services for clients with low vision.

Key Terms

Age-related macular degeneration (AMD)
Cataract
Certified Low Vision Therapist (CLVT)
Diabetic retinopathy
Glaucoma

Low vision
Ophthalmologist
Optometrist
Specialty Certification in Low Vision (SCLV)

Introduction

In the United States, 2.4 million people have low vision, and by 2020, this number is expected to increase by nearly 70% as the population ages (Eye Diseases Prevalence Research Group [EDPRG], 2004). One in eight persons age 65 and older in the United States has an eye disease resulting in low vision (National Eye Institute [NEI], 2006), and the prevalence of visual impairment increases with age (EDPRG, 2004). The most common eye diseases for those age 40 and over include cataract, glaucoma, diabetic retinopathy, and macular degeneration.

Etiology, prevalence, and medical treatment for the common eye diseases vary. **Cataract,** or clouding of the eye lens, is the most frequently reported condition in individuals with low vision and accounts for up to 50% of the cases among African American, Caucasian, and Hispanic individuals (EDPRG, 2004). Cataracts cause low vision, and there is a surgical procedure that can correct this problem. Cataract removal surgery has an estimated 97%–98% chance of an excellent result and only a 1% chance of achieving no improvement and/or worsening vision (Laser Surgery for Eyes, 2000). **Glaucoma,** damage to the eye's optic nerve, occurs when the normal fluid pressure inside the eyes rises, resulting in vision loss and blindness (NEI, n.d.). Treatment to save remaining vision may include eyedrops, laser trabeculoplasty, and/or conventional

191

surgery. **Diabetic retinopathy** develops secondary to diabetes and results from a change in the blood vessels of the retina. It is the most frequent cause of new cases of blindness among adults age 20–74 years (NEI, n.d.). Diabetic retinopathy can occur as non-proliferative or proliferative retinopathy. Proliferative retinopathy is treated with laser surgery or with a vitrectomy (Johns Hopkins Medicine, n.d.). Lastly, **age-related macular degeneration** (AMD), damage to the central part of the retina, occurs in one of two forms, wet or dry. It is the leading cause of vision loss in the United States for persons age 60 and older (NEI, 2007) and is more common in women and Caucasians than in other groups (American Society of Retina Specialists, 2009). There is no medical treatment for dry macular degeneration, but treatment for wet macular degeneration includes laser surgery, photodynamic therapy, and eye injections (NEI, n.d.).

Low Vision and Occupational Performance

Vision provides approximately 80% of what individuals perceive through their senses (Protect-your-sight.com, 2008). Using the ICD-9-CM threshold criteria, an individual is considered as having **low vision** if he or she has an uncorrectable and irreversible visual acuity of less than 20/60 in the better eye or a visual field of 20 degrees or less in the better eye (U.S. Department of Health and Human Services [USDHHS], 2004). Levels of impairment are assigned to ranges of acuity and/or visual fields

(Table 13-1). Low vision is irreversible and may be hereditary, congenital, or acquired.

Low vision adversely affects an individual's ability to perform everyday activities (American Academy of Ophthalmology Vision Rehabilitation Committee, 2001). Compared to individuals without disabilities (Burmedi, Becker, Heyl, Wahl, & Himmelsbach, 2002), individuals with low vision demonstrate a 15%–30% higher dependence on others to perform activities of daily living (ADLs). Despite their decreased ability to perform ADLs and instrumental activities of daily living (IADLs), persons with low vision still have the need and desire to perform everyday activities that support their life roles (Crews & Campbell, 2001; Heyl & Wahl, 2001; Horowitz, 2004; Raina, Wong, & Massfeller, 2004; Travis, Boerner, Reinhardt, & Horowitz, 2004).

The eye diseases that result in low vision affect different areas of occupational performance. Clients with cataracts may have difficulty with recognizing faces, reading, and mobility (Lundström, Fregell, & Thomas, 1994). Those with glaucoma are likely to experience problems with glare or with changes in light levels as well as outdoor mobility (Burmedi, Becker, Heyl, Wahl, & Himmelsbach, 2002). Diabetic retinopathy at all levels of severity results in difficulty in reading and driving (Coyne, Margolis, Kennedy-Martin, Baker, Klein, Paul, Revicki, et al., 2004). Persons more severely affected have difficulty with diabetic care routines, mobility issues, and increased fear of accidents leading to decreased social participation (Coyne et al., 2004). AMD adversely affects the individual's ability to read standard print and can limit his or her independence in preparing meals, using a telephone, taking care of

Table 13-1	ICD-9-CM Definitions of Low Vision and Blindness	
Definition	**Visual Acuity**	**Visual Field**
Moderate visual impairment	<20/60 to 20/160	Not considered
Severe visual impairment	≤20/200 to 20/400 visual field	≤20 degrees
Profound visual impairment	<20/400 to 20/1000 visual field	≤10 degrees
Near-total vision loss	≤20/1250	
Total blindness	No perception of light	

Data from: "Vision rehabilitation for elderly individuals with low vision or blindness," by U.S. Department of Health and Human Services, Agency for Healthcare Research and Quality, 2004, p. 20.

finances, traveling, shopping, taking medications, and washing laundry (Ryan, Anas, Beamer, & Bajorek, 2003).

Low Vision Rehabilitation Team

A number of team members in addition to occupational therapy practitioners work with clients with low vision. **Ophthalmologists** are medical doctors (MDs) who diagnose and treat eye diseases, prescribe medications, and perform surgery. **Optometrists** are doctors of optometry (ODs) and treat refractive error with glasses, contacts, and magnifiers. Vision rehabilitation therapists receive referrals from state or non-profit agencies to provide training in the home for adaptive techniques to perform everyday activities and modify the environment. Orientation and mobility (O&M) specialists are consulted for difficulties in mobility and provide training for people to travel safely using such devices as canes, guide dogs, and/or electronic devices. They teach people to take public transportation on their own and also receive referrals through the state or a nonprofit agency. Mental health service providers such as psychiatrists, psychologists, and/or social workers may be consulted to assist with psychosocial difficulties in coping and adjusting to low vision. They may address such issues as anxiety, frustration, fear, anger, and depression. Finally, family members often transport the client to appointments, may perform home modifications for the client, and assist in follow-through with home programs. Family members of the visually impaired are often more involved than are family members of other populations with functional deficits.

Occupational Therapy for Clients With Low Vision

Participating in occupational therapy may help people with low vision maintain independent and meaningful lives (American Occupational Therapy Association [AOTA], 2003). Although occupational therapy practitioners have worked with persons with low vision for decades, it was not until 1990

that physicians could refer clients for occupational therapy with a sole diagnosis of low vision. At that time the Health Care Financing Administration expanded the meaning of "physical impairment" to include low vision (Warren, 1995). The Balanced Budget Refinement Act of 1999 allowed optometrists to refer Medicare Part B patients to occupational therapy for low vision rehabilitation (Johansson, 2000). In 2002, Congress created a program memorandum to enforce Medicare coverage for beneficiaries with low vision for rehabilitation services (USDHHS, Centers for Medicare & Medicaid Services, 2002). The AOTA considers low vision services to be an emerging practice area for occupational therapy practitioners and important for productive aging (Johansson, 2000).

Two certifications are available in low vision rehabilitation for occupational therapists. In 2000, the Academy for Certification of Vision Rehabilitation and Education Professionals (ACVREP) developed several certifications for low vision providers, including the **Certified Low Vision Therapist** (**CLVT**) (Watson, Qillman, Flax, & Gerritsen, 1999). To date, there are 31 occupational therapists who hold this certification through ACVREP (J. Treviño, personal communication, April 8, 2010). To better meet the growing need for occupational therapy services, in 2006 the AOTA established a **Specialty Certification in Low Vision** (**SCLV**). The SCLV credential provides a formal recognition to occupational therapists and occupational therapy assistants for their specialized knowledge and practice expertise with the low vision population.

Low Vision Practice Settings

Occupational therapy practitioners may provide services for clients with low vision in a variety of settings, using different business models, and on vision rehabilitation teams with various service members (Table 13-2). Familiar settings for occupational therapy practitioners include outpatient clinics, low vision centers associated with universities, or private practices. In these settings, clients with low vision are scheduled and billed for their care in a manner consistent with clients in similar settings. Occupational therapy practitioners working in physicians' offices or eye clinics may need to see clients on the same day they see the physician. The Veterans

Table 13-2 Low Vision Rehabilitation Team Members

Team Member	Referral Source	Team Function
Low Vision Optometrists	Self, physician, and/or ophthalmologist	Diagnose and treat refractive errors with optical devices
Occupational Therapy Practitioner	Physician and in some states optometrists, and nonprofit agencies	Teach optical and non-optical device use, visual skills, and adaptive techniques, and modify the environment
Certified Low Vision Therapist	Optometrists and nonprofit agencies	Teach optical device use and visual skills
Vision Rehabilitation Therapists	State or nonprofit agencies	Train in the home for adaptive techniques to perform everyday activities and modify the environment
Orientation & Mobility Specialists	State or nonprofit agencies	Train in safe travel using canes, guide dogs, and/or electronic devices, and public transportation
Psychiatrists, Psychologists, and/or Social Workers	Physician, self, other team members	Assist with difficulties coping and adjusting
Family Members	Not applicable	Transport the client to appointments, perform home modifications, and assist in home program

Health Administration (VA) offers outpatient services in Vision Impairment Services in Outpatient Rehabilitation (VISOR) programs and inpatient services in Inpatient Blind Rehabilitation Centers (U.S. Department of Veterans Affairs, 2009). Veterans are placed in the program most consistent with their needs. In the VA system, veterans are provided with the technology they need to become independent at no cost.

Occupational therapy practitioners also work in community agencies serving the blind and visually impaired. In this type of setting, clients are considered consumers of the agency's services. Their care may be covered through grant funding or reimbursed by the state. Interventions may be provided one-to-one or in a group setting. In this model, funding may be available not only for therapy but also for some assistive devices. Community agencies frequently provide a continuum of care for their consumers. They usually offer services that include diagnosis, instruction in visual efficiency skills and optical device use, classes in ADL and IADL, support groups for coping with and adjusting to visual impairments, referrals

for O&M specialists, and home safety evaluations and modifications. Occupational therapy practitioners can provide many of these services for the community agency. Intervention for those with visual impairment also includes home therapy. Home visits may be provided in other settings or occur solely in the home.

Referrals for Occupational Therapy

As in any other area of occupational therapy practice, a referral for occupational therapy is required for reimbursement from Medicare or private insurance companies. Exactly what type of low vision professional (e.g., physician, optometrist) is able to refer for occupational therapy depends on state law. Because best practice requires specialized skills by all team members, and occupational therapy requires a referral source, an occupational therapist should try to partner with an existing low vision provider. The low vision referral for occupational therapy should state that an evaluation is required and what areas of occupation are impacted by the individual's low vision.

Interventions for Clients With Low Vision

Occupational therapy service needs are determined by a comprehensive evaluation. Relevant background information to collect includes: the client's diagnosis and treatment received, prior level of function, living situation, and social support system. The evaluation should then focus on the client's current level of function. The therapist should determine which areas of occupation are impacted by low vision. This may be accomplished with a self-report questionnaire and supplemented with functional tasks. Specific skills may be assessed, such as reading with the Pepper Visual Skills for Reading Test (Watson, Whittaker, Steciw, Baldasare, & Miller-Shaffer, 1995) or writing with the Low Vision Writing Assessment (Watson, Wright, Wyse, & De l'Aune, 2004). Depending on test results provided by the referral source, the occupational therapy practitioner may also assess visual acuity, tracking, and visual fields. Once the client's current level of function is determined, the therapist works with the client to develop an intervention plan to prioritize and establish his or her goals. Intervention for clients with low vision involves person, environment, and occupation factors.

Person

First, clients need to improve their visual efficiency skills, including eccentric viewing and visual scanning. Clients with macular diseases affecting their central vision need to be taught eccentric viewing, or how to use the area of the retina that has not been damaged (Stelmack, Massof, & Stelmack, 2004). Eccentric viewing is particularly useful in reading and writing tasks, and for viewing people's faces. Visual scanning, eye movements designed to locate an object of interest in the environment, is needed to complete most tasks (Warren, 1990). Clients with low vision need to be taught efficient visual scanning skills to compensate for their decreased visual fields. As with all new skills, eccentric viewing and visual scanning need to be incorporated into the performance of preferred occupations by clients as a means of adaptation.

When clients' vision cannot be improved, they can learn to use their residual vision more efficiently and adopt the use of optical devices to help in task completion. As in the selection of any type of assistive device, it is important to know the client's abilities, heed client preference, work within any financial restraints, understand the purpose of the device, and have extensive knowledge on optics. Due to the many variables affecting assistive device use by persons with low vision, most low vision clinics allow clients the opportunity to test different types of equipment before purchasing.

Several optical devices can aid near-vision tasks. Head-mounted devices such as spectacles free both hands for bilateral activities. However, learning the working distance or focal distance for spectacles can be difficult for the client. Handheld magnifiers can have the added advantage of a built-in light. However, one hand is required to hold the magnifier, and finding and maintaining the focal distance with handheld magnifiers may also be difficult. Stand magnifiers provide the correct focal distance for the client, but handheld magnifiers are easier to manipulate and transport. In addition, electronic devices such as closed-circuit televisions (CCTVs) or computer programs can enlarge print so that it is legible to the client. However, CCTVs and computers with low vision software are expensive.

Other optical devices are available for distance viewing and driving. Clients who need devices for distance viewing, such as watching sports, can use telescopes. Although telescopes provide greater acuity, they significantly limit the size of the visual field. Clients with visual field deficits may be prescribed field enhancement devices, although these devices may be difficult for some to use due to the perceptual adjustment. Bioptic telescopes that are used for driving require training, and their use is dependent on state laws.

In addition to optical devices that allow clients to participate in their preferred occupations, there are many non-optical devices. Some of these devices are dependent on the client's use of other senses such as auditory. There are talking clocks and watches, liquid indicators, books on tape, talking blood glucose meters, and scales. Clients can use their tactile sense by marking personal care products with rubber bands and different-colored clothing with safety pins.

Other devices utilize the concept of enlargement, such as large print address books, calendars, date books, or fonts on computers. There are personal care devices that have large print, including pillboxes and syringes. Grooming activities, such as applying makeup or shaving, are much easier to perform using a lighted magnification mirror. Devices with large print to aid with cooking include kitchen timers and measuring cups and spoons. Clients can participate in leisure activities by using large print playing cards, bingo cards, or a big button television remote.

Still other devices improve occupational performance using high contrast. Print is much easier to read if a client uses a black felt pen on bold lined paper. Signature guides provide an outlined area within which to sign as check templates do to fill out a check.

Environment

In general, an older person needs two to three times more light than a younger person, but people with some eye diseases may be sensitive to glare (Watson, 2001). Therefore, it is important to increase lighting without causing glare, which can be accomplished with lighting placement, choice of lighting, and glare elimination. Light can be aimed to illuminate the task at hand by using a gooseneck lamp. The type of lighting used is important. Incandescent light is commonly used in desk lamps but may not provide good contrast or color perception. Halogen provides a bright white light but generates a lot of heat. Fluorescent light is energy efficient but may be harsh and flicker annoyingly (Watson, 2001). Full-spectrum lighting is the closest to sunlight but is high on the blue light spectrum, which may result in glare. Glare can be controlled by covering high glare surfaces such as tabletops with tablecloths, and windows with sheer drapes (Cole, 2003).

Tactile markings on appliances can be very effective in facilitating occupational performance. For example, frequently used settings on the microwave, washer, and dryer can be marked with bump dots.

The concepts of enlargement and/or contrast can also be utilized in modifying the environment. Those with low vision can select clocks with large numbers on sharp contrast backgrounds. Dark bath mats can be placed over white tub edges or contrasting placemats chosen for the table. To improve contrast throughout the home, walls can be painted a lighter color and dark furniture selected.

Creating a system of organization can be very helpful for those with low vision. Inexpensive high-contrast baskets can be used to store like items, including: cleaning supplies, personal care items, medications, and/or leisure activity equipment.

Occupation

Many tasks may need modification for a person with low vision to be able to complete them in a timely and efficient manner. For example, instead of attempting to apply low-contrast toothpaste to a white toothbrush, a more efficient means is to put the toothpaste in a small cup and drag the brush in the cup, or to simply put the toothpaste in the mouth. Locating one's food on a plate can be difficult, but if food is always placed using the clock method, it is easy to find. Writing can be problematic, but letters and cards can be printed more easily. Reading, a leisure activity enjoyed by many, may become too difficult for those with low vision. In addition to books on tape available through the Library for the Blind, many books are now available as audio books. Clients can "read" while performing other activities like doing the dishes or taking a bath.

Social participation is an important area of occupation (AOTA, 2008). Unfortunately, people with low vision often become socially isolated secondary to difficulties with transportation. People can and do engage socially through virtual means. In a study by Smith, Ludwig, Andersen, and Copolillo (2009), several participants mentioned that social participation was achieved on the telephone. Today even more virtual means exist, such as communicating via e-mail or with webcams.

Psychosocial Issues Associated With Low Vision

Psychosocial issues are inherent for those diagnosed with low vision due to loss of independence and relinquishing of desired occupations. High levels of depression have been found to be correlated with severe visual impairment (Brody,

Gamst, Williams, Smith, Lau, Dolnak, et al., 2001), and AMD is a significant risk factor for depressive disorders. Studies have shown that up to 32%–33% of patients with AMD meet criteria for major depressive disorder (Brody et al., 2001; Rovner, Casten, & Tasman, 2002). In addition, visual impairment has been shown to adversely affect health-related quality of life (Margolis, Coyne, Kennedy-Martin, Baker, Schein, & Revicki, 2002). It is important for occupational therapy practitioners to be vigilant for the signs of emotional distress and to facilitate the client's ability to cope. They must also be ready to refer clients to appropriate mental health professionals (see Table 13-2). Casten and Rovner (2006) suggest that intervention for depression begin early to prevent severe depression and disability.

In interviews of persons with visual impairments, Teitelman and Copolillo (2005) noted three main themes related to the psychosocial aspects of low vision: emotional challenges, negative emotional outcomes, and indicators of emotional adaptation. Some of the emotional challenges identified by interviewees were lost independence, relinquishing of desired activities, lost spontaneity, and impact on social interactions. In addition, the participants reported distressing emotional reactions such as depression, stigma and embarrassment, frustration, and resignation. The most commonly used emotional adaptation strategies were cognitive restructuring, social support, making a contribution to family and friends, and faith. The greater the number of favorite activities that could be retained even with adaptations, the easier the emotional adjustment appeared to be. Attending to the psychosocial issues related to low vision is an important aspect of occupational therapy services.

Low vision rehabilitation services are important in combating psychological effects of visual disability. Horowitz, Reinhardt, and Boerner (2005) found that counseling services, low vision clinical services, and participants' use of optical devices were significant contributors in reducing participants' depressive symptoms. Unfortunately, people with AMD tend to underutilize available rehabilitation services shown to improve their visual function and quality of life (Casten, Maloney, & Rovner, 2005).

Low Vision Community Support

It is important for occupational therapy practitioners to be aware of community resources available for their clients with visual impairments. Is there a radio station that reads the daily newspaper or offers other interesting programming? What are the public and private transportation options? Is there a low vision support group? Are there organizations that provide social support, reading to the visually impaired, or light housekeeping duties? Where can low vision non-optical devices be obtained? Knowing where to refer clients who need these services is imperative. Keeping on hand forms qualifying clients for services and catalogs featuring low vision assistive devices can facilitate acquisition of these resources.

Funding and Billing Issues for Low Vision Occupational Therapy Services

The primary funder for occupational therapy services in low vision is Medicare Part B. However, low vision services are also covered by many private insurance companies and some state or nonprofit agencies serving the blind and visually impaired. When billing Medicare for clients with low vision, practitioners must follow the same regulations as for any client receiving Medicare services (AOTA, n.d.; USDHHS, n.d.). Medicare Part B currently pays 80% of total occupational therapy outpatient charges up to $1860 per year, and clients must make up the 20% difference unless they have a Medicare Part B supplement policy. It is possible that a client with low vision has already used the $1860 charges for one year depending on other health conditions requiring occupational therapy outpatient services. Occupational therapists providing outpatient services to clients with low vision must also be cognizant that other occupational therapy outpatient services may be needed by clients later in the year.

Necessary optical and non-optical devices for clients with low vision are not covered by Medicare or private insurance companies. Most state or non-profit agencies serving the blind and visually impaired are able to provide some optical and non-optical devices. They may have loaner programs for CCTVs or used CCTVs for resale. These agencies also may have donated equipment that can be distributed.

Conclusion

The population of persons with low vision is growing and will increase dramatically with the aging of the baby boomers. Occupational therapy practitioners have the skills to facilitate participation in all areas of occupation for this expanding population. The profession of occupational therapy should meet the needs of individuals with low vision to maintain their independence and health. Most of these services are provided in the community, and there is ample opportunity for occupational therapists to expand low vision services through the development of new programs. Occupational therapy is one of the disciplines identified as a low vision provider by Medicare and by optometrists and ophthalmologists.

Occupational therapists are uniquely qualified to address the psychosocial and physical rehabilitation needs of persons with low vision through the provision of meaningful engagement in occupations. Research has shown that "occupational therapists working in low vision can support clients by facilitating development of a social network, acting as liaisons between clients and other health practitioners, especially ophthalmologists, and encouraging policy development that supports barrier-free LVAD (low vision assistive device) acquisition and use" (Copolillo & Teitelman, 2005, p. 305). The introduction of new models of low vision occupational therapy service provision can expand the network of services currently available in the community for persons of all ages who have visual impairments.

CASE STUDIES

CASE STUDY 13•1 Mrs. Kindred

Mrs. Kindred is a 72-year-old widow who has dry macular degeneration in her right eye with a visual acuity of 20/200. She lives in a senior apartment building with an elevator within a half mile from her only child, Celia. Mrs. Kindred is a grandmother to Celia and her husband's two children: David, who is away at college, and Jennifer, who is a junior in high school. Although she spends most major holidays with Celia and her family, she maintains an active social calendar with her peer group.

During an occupational therapy evaluation, Mrs. Kindred reports difficulties in a number of areas that she would like to address. Self-care issues for Mrs. Kindred include minimal difficulty styling her hair and applying her lipstick. Meal preparation for Mrs. Kindred consists primarily of reheating food prepared by Celia or cooking with a microwave. However, she has minimal difficulty distinguishing cans of food and operating her microwave. Mrs. Kindred admits to great difficulty locating her friends' phone numbers and more frequently dialing wrong numbers. She also would like to be able to communicate via e-mail with both of her grandchildren. Celia has managed Mrs. Kindred's finances for some time, and both women are happy with this arrangement. However, Mrs. Kindred would like to be able to sign her name independently and is self-conscious as to the level of legibility of her current signature. Mrs. Kindred's problems with reading small print have adversely affected engagement in her leisure activities in a number of ways. Every 2 weeks, she goes out to dinner with a small group of friends to different restaurants. Transportation is not an issue, as several members of the group still drive. However, she has great difficulty reading the menu and would prefer not to constantly have to ask that a friend read the menu to her. Mrs. Kindred is a petite lady interested in maintaining her weight as well as staying within a monthly budget. She also loves to read and wants to keep up with current releases of her favorite authors. The occupational therapist reports to Mrs. Kindred's insurance carrier that she has good potential for rehabilitation and would benefit from occupational therapy services.

CASE STUDY 13•1 Discussion Questions

1. What areas of occupation are affected by Mrs. Kindred's low vision?
2. How might you improve her occupational performance in those areas?
3. What optical and non-optical devices would you suggest to Mrs. Kindred to improve her occupational performance?

Learning Activities

1. Develop a resource list of transportation sources available in your community that serve the blind or visually impaired.
2. What are some virtual means that people with low vision might use to engage in social participation? What accommodations might you anticipate to facilitate social engagement through virtual means?
3. Choose one room or work area in a home and design and depict environmental modifications for a client with low vision.

REFERENCES

American Academy of Ophthalmology Vision Rehabilitation Committee. (2001). *Preferred practice pattern: Visual rehabilitation for adults.* San Francisco, CA: American Academy of Ophthalmology.

American Occupational Therapy Association. (2003). *Maintaining quality of life with low vision.* Retrieved from http://aota.org/Consumers/Tips/Adults/LowVision/35135.aspx

American Occupational Therapy Association. (2006). AOTA Board Certification & Specialty Certification. Retrieved from http://aota.org/nonmembers/area15/index.asp

American Occupational Therapy Association. (2008). Occupational therapy practice framework: Domain and process (2nd ed.). *American Journal of Occupational Therapy, 62*(6), 625–683.

American Occupational Therapy Association. (n.d.). *Medicare.* Retrieved from http://aota.org/Practitioners/Reimb/Pay/Medicare.aspx

American Society of Retina Specialists. (2009). *What are your risk factors?* Retrieved from http://amdawareness.org/asrs/learn.html

Brody, B. L., Gamst, A. C., Williams, R. A., Smith, A. R., Lau, P. W., Dolnak, D., et al. (2001) Depression, visual acuity, comorbidity, and disability associated with age-related macular degeneration. *Ophthalmology, 108,* 1893–1900.

Burmedi, D., Becker, S., Heyl, V., Wahl, H., & Himmelsbach, I. (2002). Behavioral consequences of age-related low vision: A narrative review. *Visual Impairment Research, 4*(1), 15–45.

Casten, R. J., Maloney, E. K, & Rovner, B. W. (2005). Knowledge and use of low vision services among persons with age-related macular degeneration. *Journal of Visual Impairment and Blindness, 99*(11), 720–724.

Casten, R. J., & Rovner, B. W. (2006). Vision loss and depression in the elderly. *Psychiatric Times, 23*(13), 52–60.

Cole, R. (2003). *Lighting for low vision.* Retrieved from http://mdsupport.org/library/lighting.html

Copolillo, A., & Teitelman, J. L. (2005). Acquisition and integration of low vision assistive devices: Understanding the decision-making process of older adults with low vision. *American Journal of Occupational Therapy, 59*(3), 305–313.

Coyne, K. S., Margolis, M. K., Kennedy-Martin, T., Baker, T. M., Klein, R., Paul, M. D., Revicki, D. A., et al. (2004). The impact of diabetic retinopathy: Perspectives from patient focus groups. *Family Practice, 21*(4), 447–453.

Crews, J., & Campbell, V. (2001). Health conditions, activity limitations, and participation restrictions among older people with visual impairments. *Journal of Visual Impairment & Blindness, 95,* 453–467.

Eye Diseases Prevalence Research Group. (2004). Causes and prevalence of visual impairment among adults in the United States. *Archives of Ophthalmology, 122*(4), 477–485.

Heyl, V., & Wahl, H. (2001). Psychosocial adaptation to age-related vision loss: A six-year perspective. *Journal of Visual Impairment& Blindness, 95,* 739–748.

Horowitz, A. (2004). The prevalence and consequences of vision impairment in later life. *Topics in Geriatric Rehabilitation, 20,* 185–195.

Horowitz, A., Reinhardt, J. P., & Boerner, K. (2005). The effect of rehabilitation on depression among visually disabled older adults. *Aging Mental Health, 9,* 563–570.

Johansson, C. (2000). *Top 10 emerging practice areas to watch in the new millennium.* Retrieved from http://aota.org/nonmembers/area1/links/link61.asp

Johns Hopkins Medicine. (n.d.). *Diabetic retinopathy.* Retrieved from http://hopkinsmedicine.org/wilmer/Conditions/diabetic_retinopathy.html

Laser Surgery for Eyes. (2000). *Cataract removal surgery.* Retrieved from http://lasersurgeryforeyes.com/cataractsurgery.html

Lundström, M., Fregell, G., & Thomas, D. M. (1994). Vision related daily life problems in patients waiting for a cataract extraction. *British Journal of Ophthalmology, 78*(8), 608–611.

Margolis, M. K., Coyne, K., Kennedy-Martin, T., Baker, T., Schein, O., & Revicki, D. A. (2002). Vision-specific instruments for the assessment of health-related quality of life and visual functioning. *Pharmacoeconomics, 20*(12), 791–812.

National Eye Institute. (n.d.). Eye Health Information. Retrieved from http://nei.nih.gov/health/

National Eye Institute. (2006). *National plan for eye and vision research.* Retrieved from http://nei.nih.gov/strategicplanning/np_low.asp

National Eye Institute. (2007). *Age-related macular degeneration.* Retrieved from http://nei.nih.gov/health/maculardegen/armd_facts.asp

Protect-your-sight.com. (2008). *Do you know how to protect your eyesight?* Retrieved from http://protect-your-eyesight.com/

Raina, P., Wong, M., & Massfeller, H. (2004). The relationship between sensory impairment and functional independence among elderly. *BMC Geriatrics, 4,* 3.

Rovner, B. W., Casten, R. J., & Tasman, T. S. (2002). Effects of depression on vision function in age-related macular degeneration. *Archives of Ophthalmology, 120,* 1041–1044.

Ryan, E. B., Anas, A. P., Beamer, M., & Bajorek, S. (2003). Coping with age-related vision loss in everyday reading activities. *Educational Gerontology, 29*(1), 37–54.

Smith, T., Ludwig, F., Andersen, L., & Copolillo, A. (2009). Engagement in occupation and adaptation to low vision. *Occupational Therapy in Healthcare, 23*(2), 119–133.

Stelmack, J. A., Massof, R. W., & Stelmack, T. R. (2004). Is there a standard of care for eccentric viewing? *Journal of Rehabilitation Research & Development, 41*(5), 729–738.

Teitelman, J., & Copolillo, A. (2005). Psychosocial issues in older adults' adjustment to vision loss: Findings from qualitative interviews and focus groups. *American Journal of Occupational Therapy, 59*(4), 409–417.

Travis, L. A., Boerner, K., Reinhardt, J. P., & Horowitz, A. (2004). Exploring functional disability in older adults with low vision. *Journal of Visual Impairment & Blindness, 98*(9), 534–546.

U.S. Department of Health & Human Services. (n.d.). *Centers for Medicare & Medicaid Services.* Retrieved from http://cms.gov/default.asp

U.S. Department of Health and Human Services. (2004). *Vision rehabilitation for elderly individuals with low vision or blindness.* Rockville, MD: Agency for Healthcare Research and Quality. Retrieved from http://cms.hhs.gov/InfoExchange/Downloads/RTCvisionrehab.pdf

U.S. Department of Health and Human Services Centers for Medicare and Medicaid Services. (2002). *Program memorandum intermediaries/carriers.* Transmittal AB-02078. Baltimore, MD: Centers for Medicare and Medicare Services.

U.S. Department of Veterans Affairs. (2009). Coordinated Services for Veterans Who Are Blind or Visually Impaired. Retrieved from http://va.gov/blindrehab/page.cfm?pg=60

Warren, M. (1990). Identification of visual scanning deficits in adults after cerebrovascular accident. *American Journal of Occupational Therapy, 44*(5), 391–399.

Warren, M. (1995). Including occupational therapy in low vision rehabilitation. *American Journal of Occupational Therapy, 49*(9), 857–860.

Watson, G. R., Quillman, R. D., Flax, M., & Gerritsen, B. (1999). The development of low vision therapist certification. *Journal of Visual Impairment & Blindness, 93,* 451–456.

Watson, G. R. (2001). Low vision in the geriatric population. *Journal of American Geriatrics Society, 49*(3), 317–330.

Watson, G. R., Whittaker, S. G., Steciw, M., Baldasare, J., & Miller-Shapper, H. (1995). *Pepper test instruction manual.* Elkins Park, PA: Pennsylvania College of Optometry.

Watson, G. R., Wright, V., Wyse, E., & De l'Aune, W. (2004). A writing assessment for persons with age-related vision loss. *Journal of Visual Impairment & Blindness, 98*(3), 160–167.

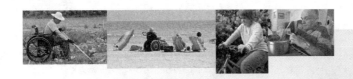

Chapter 14

Fall Prevention

Kimberly Mansfield Caldeira, MS, and Mary Becker-Omvig, MS, OTR/L

Safe and full participation in activities and control over one's ability to remain with the home and community are priorities for older adults.

—American Occupational Therapy Association (AOTA), 2004, p. 1

Learning Objectives

This chapter is designed to enable the reader to:

• Apply the evidence on fall prevention interventions to occupation-based interventions.
• Explain the role of occupational therapy in an interdisciplinary, health promotion approach to fall prevention.
• Evaluate the advantages and disadvantages of various fall prevention interventions in different community settings.
• Synthesize fall prevention guidelines to design a locally relevant falls prevention program.

Key Term

Area Health Education Centers

Introduction

According to the AOTA *Practice Framework,* the primary outcome of occupational therapy is the support of "health and participation in life through engagement in occupation" (AOTA, 2008, p. 660). In this chapter, the authors present two examples of successful community-based fall prevention programs designed and implemented by occupational therapy personnel to provide this outcome. The first example describes a brief student-led program, and the second is an ongoing program integrated within a local office on aging in suburban Maryland. Readers are challenged to identify their own local opportunities for new falls prevention programs in which to implement customized programs based on the latest available evidence (Caldeira & Reitz, 2010; Centers for Disease Control and Prevention, 2003; Moreland et al., 2003).

Fall Prevention in a Rural Senior Center

For this example, an overview of Area Health Education Centers and the project setting is provided. This is followed by a description of the needs assessment, program planning, program implementation, and program evaluation for a fall prevention initiative at a senior center in rural Maryland.

Overview of the Project

Area Health Education Centers (AHECs) were established by Congress in 1971 for the purpose of recruiting, training, and retaining health professionals in rural and urban health care professional shortage areas. The current mission of the AHECs is "to enhance access to quality health care, particularly primary and preventive care, by improving the supply and distribution of health care professionals through community/academic educational partnerships" (National AHEC Organization [NAO], n.d., ¶ 1). There are currently more than 54 programs with over 200 centers located in nearly all states and the District of Columbia. Information is regularly shared between AHECs through conferences, the Internet, and informal networking (NAO, 2009). AHECs are potential partners for fall prevention and other community-based prevention programming to serve vulnerable populations.

In 1999, the Western Maryland Area Health Education Center (WMAHEC) hosted a group of students from a variety of health professions for a service-learning opportunity in a course entitled "Interdisciplinary Prevention in Rural Communities." This prevention course was followed by a second course focusing on evaluation methods, entitled "Interdisciplinary Team Research: Applied Outcomes Research by Interdisciplinary Teams." Students and faculty from schools of social work, nursing, occupational therapy, physical therapy, and respiratory therapy were represented in these two interdisciplinary courses. The efforts of the collaborative, interdisciplinary faculty-student-community teams were coordinated by the WMAHEC's coordinator of community education and supported by a series of federal grants funded by the Quentin N. Burdick Program for Rural Interdisciplinary Training, Bureau of Health Professions, Health Resources and Services Administration, U.S. Department of Health and Human Services.

What follows is a brief description of a fall prevention program that was designed, implemented, and evaluated by students enrolled in one or both of these courses at WMAHEC in 1999. The program, entitled *STEADY As You Go,* was designed and implemented by Caldeira, Gurka, and VanSickel (1999) and subsequently evaluated by Becker-Omvig, Caldeira, Hockman, and de los Santos (1999).

The design and implementation of *STEADY As You Go* was completed on a rapid time line. The interdisciplinary planning team consisted of one student each from occupational therapy, physical therapy, and respiratory therapy. A needs assessment was conducted during the first class in early June, and program planning occurred over the next 6 weeks. The project then culminated in a pilot of

the program in mid-July. The evaluation team comprised two occupational therapy students plus one student each from nursing and social work. Evaluation data were collected on the day of the pilot and later during the formal program evaluation phase in November. Thus, the entire process, from needs assessment through evaluation, was completed in fewer than 6 months (Becker-Omvig et al., 1999).

Needs Assessment

During the needs assessment phase, the team researched the sociodemographic, cultural, and geographic characteristics of the target population and setting. A senior center located in rural western Maryland agreed to host the program. Senior center administrators provided valuable background on their clients: the majority had low incomes, most were over 70 years old, and a substantial minority had chronic conditions such as arthritis, visual impairments, and hypertension. Other data sources, such as the Maryland State Office on Rural Health, supplied descriptive data about the county of interest, such as the disproportionate numbers of residents who had low incomes and no health insurance, and the underutilization of preventive health services. Literature reviews on rural health and Appalachian culture, particularly as they relate to health behaviors, supplied the team with further insight into the possible needs and interests of the target population. Finally, the team distributed a brief questionnaire to senior center clients to assess their attitudes and beliefs about falling. The team discovered that many clients were concerned about falling and interested in reducing their risks (Caldeira et al., 1999).

Program Planning

The program-planning phase was guided by several theoretical frameworks relevant for health promotion, which were selected by the students from descriptions in the textbook for the course by McKenzie and Smeltzer (1997). The team relied heavily on constructs from the Health Belief Model (HBM), especially as related to fear of falling. Recognizing that fear of falling can contribute to falls, the team chose to design an intervention that would avoid increasing perceived risk and focus instead on promoting self-efficacy to reduce fear of falling and decreasing any perceived barriers to risk-reduction activities. Principles from Ajzen's Theory of Planned Behavior (McKenzie & Smeltzer, 1997), such as perceived behavioral control and subjective norms, were also instrumental in the planning process. The transtheoretical model developed by Prochaska and DiClemente (1983; 1992) was used by the team to incorporate messages aimed at participants in precontemplation and contemplation who might not be ready to adopt new behaviors for risk reduction (Caldeira et al., 1999). Further information on the HBM and transtheoretical model and their applicability to occupational therapy can be found in Chapter 3 of this book and other sources (Reitz & Scaffa, 2010).

Another relevant theoretical framework tapped was one from the occupational therapy literature, the ecology of human performance (EHP). The developers of the EHP (Dunn, Brown, & McGuigan, 1994) emphasize the person-environment interactions that are fundamental to occupational performance. This is very apparent in fall prevention, where in most cases it is the interaction of intrinsic and extrinsic risk factors, rather than the individual risk factors themselves, that determine a person's likelihood of falling. The EHP was especially helpful to the team in their interpretation of the evaluation results in terms of the physical, cultural, and social contexts of the participants, the administrators, and the interdisciplinary student team, all of which affected the program's success (Caldeira, 1999).

One of the first steps in program planning is to establish goals and objectives. The planning team set the following four major goals:

- To raise awareness among seniors regarding strategies to prevent falling.
- To alter dangerous behaviors in the everyday life of seniors
- To promote seniors' safety in homes and activities
- To minimize the risk of seniors falling indoors and outdoors (Caldeira et al., 1999, p. 6)

The goals were to be accomplished on multiple levels in terms of administrative objectives, learning objectives, behavioral and environmental objectives, and program objectives. Administrative objectives included specific tasks to be accomplished in preparation for the pilot, such as sending program materials to the site administrator and completing a rehearsal of the program module. Learning objectives were written to describe the new skills, knowledge, and attitudes the participants were expected to acquire. The team also set behavioral, environmental, and program objectives to be attained if the falls prevention program were implemented on an ongoing basis after the pilot and expanded to include multiple modules and sites. The behavioral objectives outlined specific behaviors expected to be observed in participants, such as physical activity, home modifications, and requesting further information. The environmental objectives specified how the program could be expanded to other sites over time. Lastly, program objectives included community-level outcomes to be measured over several years, such as reduced incidence of falls and rates of fall-related disability (Caldeira et al., 1999).

While the challenges and benefits of an interdisciplinary team experience were part of the learning experience for students in the WMAHEC courses, the interdisciplinary nature of the intervention enhanced the program's potential to benefit the participants at the senior center. The students were challenged to distinguish the areas of overlap and areas of unique expertise among their respective disciplines. The result was a program module presented as a series of complementary segments, each segment focusing on a different area of expertise from one of the three disciplines. Physical therapy's contribution pertained to exercises designed to improve balance, sensory awareness, and lower extremity strength and flexibility. A respiratory therapist presented breathing exercises designed to promote relaxation and focus, drawing in part on a Tai Chi instructional video. The occupational therapy student provided an overview of behavioral strategies to reduce the risk of falling and specific home safety recommendations for falls prevention (Caldeira et al., 1999).

Cultural barriers were another consideration in the planning of this program. In addition to generational differences that factor into many health promotion interventions with older adults, other cultural issues also were evident. The planning team reviewed the literature on the health promotion needs and barriers that characterize many rural populations. Certain features of Appalachian culture also were relevant in planning this program. For example, the team attempted to anticipate the cultural traits of self-reliance and low care-seeking by incorporating many strategies for self-help into the program, while also encouraging participants to consult with physicians and other resource persons for additional information (Caldeira, 1999).

Program Implementation

The *STEADY As You Go* program was piloted as scheduled in mid-July at the senior center. A total of 17 participants attended the one-hour module, which was followed by lunch. The module proceeded according to the agenda shown in Table 14-1. Each segment of the module was interactive with demonstrations, visual aids, and as many opportunities for discussion as possible. The participants reacted to the program with enthusiasm, which contributed significantly to the program's success. In a very brief amount of time, the program presented a multidisciplinary approach to falls prevention, including practical suggestions for maintaining balance and physical fitness, choosing simple home modifications to enhance safety, and adopting deliberate behavioral strategies to avoid falls. The team incorporated a wide variety of interactive presentation methods to accommodate diverse learning styles and maximize participants' enjoyment. Some portions were didactic with visual aids, others were participatory with opportunities to practice demonstrated exercises, while the bingo game was competitive and interactive and reinforced concepts covered throughout the module. Illustrated handouts were provided to facilitate individual performance of the breathing and balance exercises at home. Finally, the team prepared a falls prevention resource guide for the staff of the senior center, which included recommendations for program enhancements at the senior center and copies of various informational resources on falls prevention (Caldeira et al., 1999).

The STEADY acronym provided a unifying theme for much of the program. This acronym is displayed in Box 14-1. The acronym was designed to be a catchy mnemonic device that could be applied to a more expanded and comprehensive falls prevention program at the site, possibly incorporating home evaluations, ongoing group exercise sessions, and other interventions. As part of the pilot curriculum, the acronym functioned as a simplified framework for an occupation-based educational component. To reinforce carry-over of the theme and its principles into the home, all participants received a refrigerator magnet as a thank-you gift for participating in the program. The acronym appeared on the magnet along with an attractive logo designed by the team.

Program Evaluation

An interdisciplinary student team conducted the program evaluation, beginning approximately 1 month after the program's pilot implementation. The evaluation team first established that the evaluation's purpose was to determine the program's impact on three outcomes: "consumer satisfaction, participants' fall prevention behaviors, and senior center program enhancements" (Becker-Omvig et al., 1999, p. 46). The evaluation plan utilized a combined goal-based

Table 14-1	STEADY As You Go Pilot Module	
Segment	**Time**	**Student Leader(s)**
Introduction	5 minutes	Occupational Therapy
STEADY theme	5 minutes	Occupational Therapy
Sensory awareness	5 minutes	Physical Therapy
Breathing exercises	5 minutes	Respiratory Therapy
Postural exercises	5 minutes	Physical Therapy
Tai Chi video	5 minutes	Respiratory Therapy
Home safety devices	10 minutes	Occupational Therapy
Bingo	15 minutes	All
Wrap-up	5 minutes	Physical Therapy
Total Time	60 minutes	

Box 14-1	Description of STEADY Acronym
S	Safe Footing
T	Take Your Time
E	Energy Conservation
A	Active
D	Devices
Y	You're in Charge!

and goal-free model (McKenzie & Smeltzer, 1997), which allowed the team to determine whether the program had achieved its specified goals and assess any unanticipated outcomes in an open-ended way.

Evaluation data were collected in a variety of ways during a single visit to the site approximately 4 months after the intervention. Qualitative data were collected in a brief focus group with 14 of the original participants and in two 30-minute individual interviews with two members of the senior center's staff. A schedule of questions for the interviews and the focus group were developed in advance. Quantitative data were collected via a written questionnaire administered to the same 14 participants (Becker-Omvig et al., 1999).

The questionnaire was developed to capture the attitudes, beliefs, and behaviors according to the theoretical constructs of the HBM and Social Cognitive Theory (SCT). It consisted of 20 items with a combination of both Likert items and yes/no response formats. For example, to measure perceived self-efficacy, participants were asked to respond to the statements "I learned ways to prevent falls from the *STEADY As You Go* program" and "The *STEADY As You Go* program has helped me to be more steady and safe" from five levels ranging from "strongly disagree" to "strongly agree." In this way, data from the 20-item questionnaire were compiled into five HBM subscales: perceived self-efficacy, perceived susceptibility, knowledge, likelihood of taking action, and actions taken (Becker-Omvig et al., 1999).

All four members of the evaluation team participated in theme coding the qualitative data from the interviews and focus group. Coded data were analyzed according to the same five HBM subscales used in the questionnaire. The team met to discuss emergent themes and identify areas of agreement and discrepancy between the three data sources (Becker-Omvig et al., 1999).

Results of the evaluation were analyzed in each of the three main outcome areas. First, consumer satisfaction was determined to be high, based on qualitative data from the interviews and focus group. Second, the impact on participants' behavior was evaluated in terms of the five HBM subscales using data from the focus group and questionnaire. Respondents scored highly on every subscale except actions taken and provided favorable feedback in the focus group, indicating a positive impact on many

constructs related to behavior. The data were mixed on actions taken, given that the majority said they had started participating in physical activity to reduce their risk of falls, but very few had sought out advice and information on fall prevention from providers or other sources. Finally, the program's impact on enhancements to the senior center was less favorable. Data from the focus group and interviews indicated that no environmental changes had been made at the senior center to enhance safety, and the only program enhancements had been related to exercise (Becker-Omvig et al., 1999).

Ultimately, the lessons learned from the implementation and evaluation of *STEADY As You Go* led to the development of recommendations for other similar programs in the future. First, the importance of "buy-in" among the facility staff is critical in creating momentum from the program. This could be facilitated through close collaboration with staff during the program planning phase, and periodic follow-up to monitor compliance with recommendations and offer resources and support, possibly including an on-site environmental evaluation. Second, many older adults are highly motivated to adopt simple behavior changes to reduce their risk of falling and are eager to learn new strategies. Moreover, while the program might be more effective in an expanded multi-session format, the pilot program alone still produced favorable outcomes among a small group of individuals, providing the senior center with a model for replication and future expansion, and the student teams with valuable experience in program development and evaluation.

Aging in Place Initiative

Many of the lessons learned from the *STEADY As You Go* program were transferred to the development of an occupational therapist-led health promotion program for older adults in Howard County, Maryland. The Howard County Office on Aging (HCOOA) originally funded one full-time occupational therapist through a 3-year grant from the Horizon Foundation. Following the grant cycle, two full-time positions were permanently funded by local government. The program, entitled the Aging in Place Initiative, was intended to build capacity in a variety of community agencies to provide gap-filling services for older adults. At the HCOOA, the occupational therapist spearheaded the development of a new fall prevention program as part of the countywide Aging in Place Initiative.

Aging in Place programs and initiatives have been growing in recent years and are supported by older adults and a variety of stakeholders, including occupational therapy. In the following aging in place example, the occupational therapist was responsible for fostering agency collaborations with a comprehensive geriatric assessment team, conducting home evaluations and direct client interventions, providing staff education to facilitate collaborative interdisciplinary efforts, and educating the public in multiple community venues. With the goal of enabling older adults to continue living in the community for as long as possible, the program addressed falls prevention in a multifactorial way as part of a larger health promotion strategy.

The HCOOA is the local agency that plans, advocates, develops, and coordinates programs and services for seniors and their family members. The HCOOA provides a variety of services and resources to the county's growing population of older adults, often at no cost to the county resident. Multiple funding sources provide subsidized services for eligible residents, including chore services to assist with homemaking and personal care services to assist with bathing and other activities of daily living.

One of the unique contributions of the occupational therapist in the Fall Prevention Program was to initiate a paradigm shift in the overarching strategies of various HCOOA programs. The occupational therapist's influence led various HCOOA programs to begin focusing on maximizing clients' ability to function as independently as possible. This approach gradually replaced the former strategy of providing as many service hours as could be justified by the client's current level of disability. The occupational therapist discovered many opportunities for clients to reduce their need for supportive services by increasing their functional performance through appropriate interventions. Clients were provided with assistive devices and trained in their proper use; home modifications were performed to enhance safety and functional mobility; and referrals for more intensive rehabilitation were made where appropriate. Furthermore, by maximizing functional independence and safety, clients enjoyed a higher quality of life and autonomy.

The paradigm shift introduced by the occupational therapist began with the in-home evaluation and service plan provided to new clients. In the past, during the initial service evaluation, once the client's eligibility was established the client and staff would select an appropriate combination of supportive services. Later, under the *Aging in Place Initiative,* clients began receiving follow-up evaluations by the occupational therapist. In these occupational therapy evaluations, clients were often found to be capable of functioning at a higher level of independence with appropriate interventions, and therefore needed fewer supportive services. On the other hand, some clients who had been prescribed many hours of service were found to be fundamentally unsafe in their current living situation due to severe cognitive deficits or other irreversible functional limitations. For these clients, the *Aging in Place Initiative* provided counseling, referrals, and support to the family and client to facilitate the transition into a new living situation. In either case, the occupational therapy evaluation and intervention provided through the *Aging in Place Initiative* aimed to optimize the match between the client and his/her environment by modifying both the environment and the person, in order to maximize functional independence and minimize the need for supportive services.

In addition to anecdotal improvements in clients' quality of life and consumer satisfaction, the occupational therapist's presence contributed to significant improvements in the program's cost-effectiveness. A program pilot demonstrated a 40% reduction in the cost of chore and personal care services. Unfortunately, despite the favorable outcomes of the program pilot, institutional barriers prohibited the full adoption of the occupational therapy recommendations. Therefore, leveraging her prior experiences with program development and outcome measurement, the therapist initiated a more rigorous method of evaluation to promote future "buy-in" from agency administration. This evaluation study used a random experimental design to collect more data on the occupational-therapy-based model of service delivery in an attempt to quantify the value of this new model.

The influence of occupational therapy within a social service agency has challenged the traditional idea of aging in place, consistent with a shift from a literal interpretation of staying in the "home" to a much broader perspective of aging in the community with a focus on a better person-environment fit. Often disparity exists between the support costs necessary to keep individuals in an environment with a poor match to their needs and the ever-decreasing resources available to provide such services. Through the unique lens of occupational therapy evaluation and interventions incorporated into social service agencies, public resources in the future may be allocated with greater efficiency and better outcomes.

Multiple opportunities continue to emerge at the HCOOA and in other agencies as the value of occupational therapy is realized. The program continues to grow as new occupational therapy positions are created to provide direct services and contribute to overall program development. The occupational therapist's approach of maximizing clients' independence offers both personal and fiscal advantages that have proved to be desirable for both community agencies and the clientele they serve.

Conclusion

Opportunities abound in the community for occupational therapists to provide community-based health promotion services for older adults.

Because falls prevention is widely recognized as a serious concern for older adults, their families, and providers, it may serve as an effective lead-in to comprehensive health promotion programs addressing the multifactorial causes of falls. Complex programs such as the Aging in Place Initiative provide linkages to a wide range of services, and therefore offer maximum flexibility to tailor services to the values, interests, and needs of their clients. On the other hand, even a simple one-day program in a senior center, like *STEADY As You Go*, can successfully raise awareness and capitalize on the positive attitudes of participants. Readers are encouraged to cultivate their own opportunities for program development by conducting community needs assessments and networking with local public and private stakeholders (e.g., government agencies, private foundations, consumer groups, health care facilities). Often an initial investment of volunteered time and expertise (e.g., in the form of a demonstration program) can be enough to stimulate a demand for broader programs with sustainable funding streams.

CASE STUDIES

CASE STUDY 14•1 Ms. Fay

Ms. Fay is a 75-year-old female diagnosed with macular degeneration, rheumatoid arthritis, diabetes, and neuropathy in both feet. Ms. Fay was widowed 2 years ago and now lives by herself. She was admitted to the hospital for a right hip replacement 1 year ago. She was discharged from rehabilitation and home health following 3 months of physical and occupational therapy. Ms. Fay has had two falls over the past few months while getting up in the middle of the night to use the bathroom. She acknowledges having a fear of falling that has resulted in a decreased level of daily activity.

Living Situation: She lives in a two-story home with attached garage. The home is located on a quiet cul-de-sac near a park and local shopping area.

Mobility: She ambulates with a single-prong cane and is able to walk for about 10 minutes without rest. She can transfer sit to stand with moderate effort. Stairs are difficult for her, which is problematic because the only bedroom and bathroom are located on the second floor of her home. The home has five steps at the entrance with one handrail.

Household: Ms. Fay can prepare her own meals. However, she does not drive and requires transportation for shopping. She manages her own finances, and most bills are managed by direct payment. Neighbors help her with yard work and household maintenance. She has one son who lives 60 miles away, and she sees him once a month.

Bathroom: Ms. Fay showers independently. She transfers in/out of the tub by holding on to a towel bar outside the bathtub/shower unit. She stands during showering. There are no grab bars or non-slip mats in the tub.

Continued

CASE STUDY 14•1 Ms. Fay   *cont'd*

Medications: She can read large print and has been prepared for total blindness within 2 years. She struggles with managing six different medications taken twice a day. She currently keeps her medications in the bathroom and identifies them by the size of the bottle and the number of rubber bands she has placed around each bottle. Ms. Fay occasionally drinks socially with friends.

Communication: There is only one phone in the home. She remembers her friend's phone number and emergency numbers only.

Leisure: Ms. Fay enjoys reading and socializing with friends and family. She participates in faith-based activities and plays cards at the local senior center weekly.

CASE STUDY 14•1 Discussion Questions

1. Identify and prioritize fall risk factors.
2. What environmental adaptations would you suggest?
3. Identify community resources you could recommend for fall prevention.
4. Identify barriers that might exist for Ms. Fay as she considers changing her behavior and/or environment to reduce her risk of falling.
5. Prepare a list of recommendations for Ms. Fay and her son.
6. Evaluate the pros and cons of your recommendations and how they may increase/decrease the likelihood of Ms. Fay adopting a behavior and/or environmental change.

Learning Activities

1. Visit www.stopfalls.org and identify a fall prevention program you could implement in your local community. Write a one-page rationale as to why you selected the program, addressing the advantages and disadvantages of the program.
2. Identify at least 5 community agencies for a first-time meeting to propose the implementation of a fall prevention program. For one of these agencies:
   a. Prepare an action list outlining the steps you will take prior to the meeting.
   b. Identify specific information will you want to gather prior to and during your first meeting.
   c. Identify and prioritize goals for the meeting. What do you hope to accomplish?
   d. List critical points you will want to communicate during the meeting.
   e. Role-play the meeting for the class.
3. A peer-led support group for older adults with arthritis contacts you to present a 1-hour session on fall prevention. Prepare a two-page outline of your presentation incorporating experiential activities for participants.

Acknowledgments: The authors wishes to thank Phyllis Madachy of the Howard County Office on Aging for providing readers with the example of its Aging in Place program, which has been a national model for community-based health promotion for older adults.

Example one was part of a Quentin N. Burdick Program for Rural Interdisciplinary Training project of the Western Maryland Area Health Education Center in collaboration with the University of Maryland, Baltimore; University of Pittsburgh; Towson University; Frostburg State University; and Allegany College of Maryland. This project was supported by funds from the Department of Health and Human Services, Health Resources and Services Administration, Bureau of Health Professions, and Quentin N. Burdick Program for Rural Interdisciplinary Training. The conclusions are those of the authors and should not be construed as the official position or policy of, and endorsements should not be inferred by, the Department of Health and Human Services, Health Resources and Services Administration, Bureau of Health Professions, or the U.S. government.

REFERENCES

American Occupational Therapy Association. (2004). *Occupational therapy and prevention of falls: Education for older adults, families, caregivers, and healthcare providers.* [AOTA Fact Sheet]. Bethesda, MD: Author.

American Occupational Therapy Association. (2008). Occupational therapy practice framework: Domain and process (2nd ed.). *American Journal of Occupational Therapy, 62,* 625–683.

Becker-Omvig, M., Caldeira, K., Hockman, L., & de los Santos, L. (1999). *Evaluation of the STEADY As You Go fall prevention program.* Unpublished manuscript. Cumberland, MD: Western Maryland Area Health Education Center.

Caldeira, K. (1999). *Interdisciplinary prevention in rural communities: Outcome evaluation of the STEADY As You Go fall prevention program.* Unpublished manuscript. Towson, MD: Towson University.

Caldeira, K. M., & Reitz, S. M. (2010). Preventing falls among community-dwelling older adults. In M. E. Scaffa, S. M. Reitz, & M. A. Pizzi (Eds.), *Occupational therapy in the promotion of health and wellness* (pp. 470–492). Philadelphia, PA: F.A. Davis.

Caldeira, K., Gurka, J., & VanSickel, T. (1999). STEADY As You Go: A community-based program for fall prevention among older adults in Garrett County, Maryland. Unpublished manuscript. Cumberland, MD: Western Maryland Area Health Education Center.

Centers for Disease Control and Prevention. (2003). Fatalities and injuries from falls among older adults—United States, 1993–2003 and 2001–2005. *Morbidity and Mortality Weekly Report, 55*(45), 1221–1224.

Dunn, W., Brown, C., & McGuigan, A. (1994). The ecology of human performance: A framework for considering the effect of context. *American Journal of Occupational Therapy, 48*(7), 595–607.

McKenzie, J. F., & Smeltzer, J. L. (1997). *Planning, implementing, and evaluating health promotion programs: A primer* (2nd ed.). Boston, MA: Allyn & Bacon.

Moreland, J., Richardson, J., Chan, D. H., O'Neill, J., Bellissimo, A., Grum, R. M., & Shanks, L. (2003). Evidence-based guidelines for the secondary prevention of falls in older adults. *Gerontology, 49*(2), 93–116.

National AHEC Organization. (n.d.). *About Us: AHEC Mission.* Retrieved from http://nationalahec.org/About/AHECMission.asp

National AHEC Organization. (2009). *NAO 2009 brochure.* Retrieved from http://nationalahec.org/Publications/NAOBrochure.asp

Prochaska, J. O., & DiClemente, C. C. (1983). Stages and processes of self-change of smoking: Toward an integrative model of change. *Journal of Counseling and Clinical Psychology, 51*(3), 390–395.

Prochaska, J. O., & DiClemente, C. C. (1992). Stages of change in the modification of behavior problems. In M. Hersen, R. M. Eisler, & P. M. Miller (Eds.), *Progress in behavior modification* (pp. 184–214). Sycamore, IL: Sycamore Press.

Reitz, S. M., Scaffa, M. E., Campbell, R. M., & Rhynders, P. A. (2010). Health behavior frameworks for health promotion practice. In M. E. Scaffa, S. M. Reitz, & M. A. Pizzi (Eds.), *Occupational therapy in the promotion of health and wellness* (pp. 46–69). Philadelphia: F.A. Davis.

Chapter 15

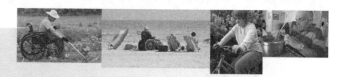

Aging in Place and Naturally Occurring Retirement Communities

Peggy Strecker Neufeld, PhD, OTR/L, FAOTA

Nobody grows old merely by living a number of years. We grow old by deserting our ideals. Years may wrinkle the skin, but to give up enthusiasm wrinkles the soul.

—Samuel Ullman

Learning Objectives

This chapter is designed to enable the reader to:

- Define aging in place and livable communities.
- Identify aging trends, societal issues, and key policies related to aging in place.
- Describe the concept of Naturally Occurring Retirement Community (NORC), NORC-Supportive Service Program, and the common elements and differences across NORCs.
- Discuss evidence for benefits to older adults for living in an active senior community or a NORC.
- Discuss roles for occupational therapy practitioners in aging in place communities and NORCs.

Key Terms

Aging-friendly communities
Aging in place
Capacity building
Longevity revolution
Naturally Occurring Retirement Community (NORC)

NORC-Supportive Service Program (NORC-SSP)
Productive aging
Self-management
Social capital

Introduction

With a rapidly growing population of older adults in the United States, aging in place has become a societal concern (National Association of Area Agencies on Aging [NAAAA], 2006). National agencies concerned about "livable" communities for all ages define **aging in place** as continued living in one's own home and having needed services to be safe, independent, and comfortable while growing older. Settings that promote aging in place not only provide supportive services for health but also offer lifestyle opportunities for productive aging.

Productive aging may be defined as activities such as volunteering, caregiving, and employment (Hinterlong, Morrow-Howell, & Sherradan, 2001), but it also refers to living life fully, socially engaged with a positive zest for life and expressing oneself creatively with the ability to achieve positive outcomes (National Center for Creative Aging, n.d.). To provide for aging in place, occupational therapy practitioners, along with other professionals, are called upon to respond to critical concerns for proactive planning. Communities across the nation are experimenting with ways to assist older adults to age in place. One approach is through supporting neighborhoods with a high concentration of seniors who have been living in their own homes for decades. A geographic area identified as having a higher percentage of older adult residents than typical is a **naturally occurring retirement community (NORC)** (Hunt & Gunter-Hunt, 1985; Hunt & Ross, 1990). NORCs have the capacity to support aging in place through a low-cost neighborhood approach of social networking, meaningful activity options, and informal caring to maintain health and wellness (Masotti, Fick, Johnson-Masotti, & MacLeod, 2006). NORCs and related service models (NORC-Supportive Service Programs [NORC-SSPs]) are emerging areas for occupational therapy practice.

Societal trends and issues related to aging in place are explored in this chapter along with the potential roles for occupational therapy practitioners. NORCs are described as an innovative setting to support successful aging. A review of research evidence linking health, occupations, networks, and aging has significant implications for practice in aging in place settings. Examples from a specific NORC-SSP demonstrate integrated occupational therapy practice at individual, interpersonal, and community levels.

Societal Trends Impacting Aging in Place and Implications

Today's changing demographics are striking and have led to a **longevity revolution** (Butler, 2008; Centers for Disease Control and Prevention [CDC], 2008), which is the remarkable gain in life expectancies and the significant impact anticipated on society overall. In the United States, people are living longer, with the number of older adults expected to increase to 72.1 million by the year 2030 (one older adult in every five), which is more than twice the number than in 2000. Seniors at 85 years and older are the fastest growing segment of the aging population and are expected to increase from 4.6 million in year 2000 to 9.6 million in 2030 (Ortman & Guarneri, 2010). The increased numbers of seniors will be more racially and ethnically diverse than the current older adult population given predictions that by the

year 2050 there will be no single majority racial group in the United States.

One effect of the increased older adult population in the United States will be a bigger demand on medical and social services, public health services, and the related budgets. The CDC (2009) predicts that, due to changes in demographics, disease, and behavioral conditions, health care expenditures will increase 25% by 2030. Current chronic diseases that are leading causes of death include heart disease, cancer, stroke, respiratory diseases, and diabetes. Poor health behaviors add to the concerns, with leading behavioral causes of death and poor health due to smoking, obesity, physical inactivity, and falls. The health of the growing senior population is of great concern for the potential for successful aging in place.

Due to increasing numbers of seniors with incurable diseases, they will find it essential to use a self-management approach in which they manage their long-term conditions through making healthy lifestyle changes and partnering with medical professionals (Lorig & Holman, 2003). **Self-management** is defined by Lorig and colleagues as having or obtaining the ability to manage the consequences of disease. Others recognize that a community approach with its potential social support and networking can further enhance self-management knowledge, skills, and confidence (Community Preventive Services, 2001). Occupational therapy practitioners can play crucial roles in assisting older adults manage aging conditions such as transitions from change or loss in employment, spouse, and friends, and maintaining one's home. To address older adults' chronic health conditions, practitioners can teach self-management skills and promote successful aging.

Another societal concern from the increased number of baby boomer retirees leaving the U.S. work force in the coming decade is the large number of seniors who will be facing this significant life transition at the same time. Many may go through a loss of roles and productivity upon leaving full-time work responsibilities and may find it challenging to adopt new lifestyles that are rewarding and meaningful. Studies show that retirees experiencing instability during the retirement transition or a lack of control may be at risk for adverse health effects (Marshall, Clarke, & Ballantyne, 2001; Solinge,

2007). One way to ease the transition into a retirement lifestyle is for retirees to become professional and leadership volunteers (National Council on Aging [NCOA], 2008). Professional volunteers assume leadership roles and contribute skills from their past work into new life roles, such as sharing skills from prior experiences in business, marketing, education, technology, and their networking connections.

In light of the increasing number of baby boomer retirees, the NCOA, a national non-profit organization, asserts that many agencies are poorly prepared to take advantage of the boom of older adults as professional volunteer resources (Endres, 2006). Professional volunteers can significantly benefit non-profit agencies and businesses in retiree civic engagement roles (Martinson & Minkler, 2006). Civic engagement involves volunteering but also includes civic life activities such as community activism, keeping well informed about current events, voting, and caregiving. The NCOA acted on these concerns by launching the RespectAbililty Initiative to promote older Americans as "untapped resources" to help renew communities. The initiative has fostered new community models through establishing innovative partnerships that successfully recruit and train "mature adult" volunteers—especially capturing the interests and skills of baby boomer retirees as professional volunteers for civic engagement.

Aging-friendly communities is an initiative related to the worldwide concerns of increased numbers of seniors. In a global online conference on creating aging-friendly communities, additional important factors were recognized for promoting the health and well-being of older adults—factors that apply to countries across the world. In his keynote presentation, Scharlach (2008) points out the importance of communities offering continuity, compensation, and opportunity for healthy aging. Specifically, these are the continuity of continued engagement in life and community, the compensation for any supports or accommodations needed for functional limitations due to aging, and opportunities for familiar and new activities for enhanced quality of life.

Occupational therapy practitioners are good partners for communities of active aging adults due to shared interests in enhancing productive aging. The potential to assist capacity building in organizations with similar interests positions occupational therapy practitioners as critical players in addressing societal concerns. **Capacity building** refers to strategies and actions carried out by an agency to continue growth toward its goals and mission and to achieve sustainability (DeVita & Fleming, 2001).

NORC: A Solution for Successful Aging in Place

Aging in place in a NORC occurs naturally when a person lives in a home for decades that was not originally designed for seniors. Living in a NORC means not relocating to a retirement home or a continuing care retirement community. NORCs have a substantially higher percentage of older adult residents than the national average of 12%–14% of residents aged 60 and over in typical communities (Jewish Federations of North America [JFNA], 2010a). Others define a NORC as an area with a density of older adults that is more than typical in their state, or simply that the area is a NORC if it feels like a NORC.

As NORCs are identified throughout the country, **NORC-Supportive Service Programs (NORC-SSPs)** are created as structures to maximize opportunities and services to enhance aging in place in one's own home instead of moving to a senior-designed and seniors-only setting. In 1996, the first professionally staffed NORC-SSP was created at Penn South in New York City. Currently in the state of New York more than 50 NORCs have been established (United Hospital Fund, 2010). In 2001, the United Jewish Communities (UJC) developed a federally funded initiative of NORC-SSP and more than 40 were established across the United States (2006) with funding from the Administration on Aging and assistance from state and local funders.

NORCs differ considerably based on geographic and housing characteristics, neighborhood cultures, and available services. By virtue of the dense senior population in the United States, many NORCs exist but are not identified as such and do not offer supportive services. Vertical NORCs, which are typical of populous cities such as New York City or Los Angeles, consist of large apartments or condominiums. These urban

NORCs often comprise one or more city blocks, with a number of NORCs existing within the city. Suburban and rural areas have horizontal NORCs, consisting of houses, condominiums, and apartments that can stretch over a few miles, although not often beyond 3 miles. NORC-SSPs vary depending on the partnerships available with community agencies, health care professionals, and existing services.

There is a consensus that a NORC-SSP's five key defining elements critical to their growth and sustainability are partnerships, programs, resident participation, communication/outreach, and evaluation (JFNA, 2010b). Initial development of a NORC benefits from coalescing potential community partners and stakeholders for purposes of determining needs, strengths, and resources. Potential NORC partnerships include health care agencies and professionals, social service agencies, government agencies (e.g., Area Agencies on Aging, AOA, CDC, National Institute on Aging), universities, businesses, housing complexes, religious organizations, libraries, and the local residents.

NORC-SSPs promote older adults' health by using a comprehensive perspective that addresses physical, social, cognitive, environment, and participation factors. This community level of intervention is consistent with the societal trend toward using preventative approaches to health. NORC programs are designed for either individuals or a neighborhood-wide population or for specific groups of residents, such as those tailored for different age groups (Haight, Schmidt, & Burnside, 2005).

Typically, a NORC offers an assortment of services and programs for socialization, community engagement, physical activity, other health concerns, lifelong learning, home management, and safety (JFNA, 2010b). Resident participation is critical to the success of a NORC, although many seniors who do not participate in the NORC state they feel comforted that the services will be there whenever needed (Neufeld, 2005). Seniors are encouraged to become active participants, linking with neighbors to enrich lives and make connections to decrease social isolation and increase awareness of resources. Home services include finding trustworthy services, help with home repair and yard work (through volunteer services), assistance in making the home safe, and assessing and implementing home modifications as needed. Health education activities assist seniors in learning and adopting proactive health behaviors such as effective decision making, problem solving, and finding resources. NORC group educational opportunities can heighten awareness for fall prevention, driver safety, and self-management strategies to prevent disabilities. Meaningful volunteer opportunities also help strengthen the community and provide direct benefits to the volunteers and to those receiving assistance.

Outreach within a NORC-SSP includes communication with its residents and the organizations and businesses in its larger community. A successful NORC will identify shared interests and mutual benefits with potential partners for continued growth. The NORC model typically offers professional staff telephone outreach to older adults who are frailer and less active to connect them with needed support and enable them to participate as possible in programs. Communication with adult children, who live either within the NORC or at a distance, also helps meet family needs of those who are providing "long-distance caregiving."

The fifth common element in a NORC is routine program evaluation to determine impact on residents, to inform ongoing program development, and to provide accountability to residents and funders. The NORC Blueprint Web page (United Hospital Fund, 2006) recommends that NORCs need sufficient resources allocated for evaluation from the start and emphasizes making evaluations practical. It also recommends sharing findings with partners for assistance in analyzing the program's impact on residents and communities and in translating findings to action.

The costs to older adult residents for NORC-SSPs vary considerably and are important to consider in developing a cost-effective model. Some neighborhood models, with professional staff coordination, have annual individual membership fees of $30 to $120 per year for a variety of programs including education and activity sessions for health and socialization, volunteer services, and assistance in finding community resources. In contrast, the village concept, which is a self-governing NORC, charges members up to $1,000 per year (Moeller, 2009) primarily for concierge services to assist residents in finding needed home services and business discounts.

Research Evidence Linking Healthy Aging, Community Characteristics, and Occupations

Communities for active aging take note of growing research evidence that links health, everyday life occupations, networks, and positive aging. The research suggests that communities with increased numbers of senior residents (such as NORCs) may have great potential to be an untapped resource for productive aging, health, and wellness in older adults (Masotti et al., 2006) by virtue of the concentration of older adults in a specific neighborhood. The potential exists within active aging communities for increased social engagement (i.e., participation in social and community activities) and civic engagement (Callahan & Lanspery, 1997). Enhancing social engagement in older adults can significantly improve function in daily living activities, decrease disability, and increase life satisfaction (Bassuk, Glass, & Berkman, 1999; Mendes de Leon, 2005). The concentration of older adults also suggests increased possibilities for **social capital**, which are collective social networks with trustworthy and reciprocal relations (Putnam, 2001). Current research can inform occupational therapy interventions (see Table 15-1).

Although a community concentration of older adults suggests that aging in place in a NORC would promote health and productive aging, not all NORCs automatically promote social engagement and social capital. A healthy NORC is one in which a "healthy NORC resident feels drawn into a vibrant active community" (Masotti et al., 2006, p. 1167). Masotti et al. asserts "a NORC can be made healthier by changing [community] characteristics to increase activity, decrease stress and provide a sense of community and well-being" (p. 1167). In this way NORCs can become a low-cost approach to healthy aging. The potential cost-effectiveness of a NORC-SSP is apparent when compared to fees for alternative senior living.

Research on NORCs is beginning to demonstrate evidence for positive benefits to its older adult residents. An IRB-approved national study explored the impact of the United Jewish Council–initiated (UJC) NORC-SSPs on older adult participants (Bedney, Schimmel, & Goldberg, 2007). The variables selected for the UJC impact study were social isolation, awareness and use of community services, volunteerism, and self-reported health because prior research supported these as key factors for healthy aging and aging in place. Social isolation has shown to highly correlate with mortality, morbidity, and dementia occurrence (Hawkley, Burleson, Bernston, & Cacioppo, 2003; Wilson, Krueger, Arnold, Schneider, Kelly, Barnes, Tang, & Bennett, 2007). Studies on perceptions of available help showed older adults who are aware that help is available report fewer "physically unhealthy days" than do those who are unaware of available help (Keyes et al., 2005). Research documented that providing assistance to the oldest-old decreases the need for their placement in high-cost care settings (Stewart, 2004). Volunteerism has been shown to have a positive relationship with older adults' sense of well-being and mortality (Lum & Lightfoot, 2005). Also, self-reported poor health has correlated with increased occurrence of hospitalization and nursing home placement (Weinberger et al., 1986).

Findings from the UJC 2007 study, which involved 461 older adult participants from 24 NORC-SSP sites, support NORCs as having a positive impact on socialization, use of community services, volunteerism, and perceived health. Responses included participants' strong agreement (72% to 95%) with statements indicating that since participating in the NORC they know and talk with more people, participate in more activities, and are more aware of and use available community services. They also report to more likely continue living in their community (88%), feel healthier (70%), and volunteer more (48%).

Occupational Therapy Roles in Aging in Place Communities and NORCs

Occupational therapy community practice is a good fit with aging in place programs, including NORCs. The occupation-based, context-driven, and client-centered interventions of occupational therapy bring an added benefit and unique perspective when working in a multidisciplinary community team. Wilcock (2010) urges occupational therapy practitioners to apply their occupation focus to population health, defining five occupational therapy

Table 15-1   Evidence-Based Implications for Occupational Therapy Interventions

Sample Evidence Linking Health, Occupations, Networks, and Aging	Implications for Occupational Therapy
Environmental support enabling occupations promotes health and prevents functional decline associated with aging (Everard, Lac, Fisher, & Baum, 2000; Lawton & Nahemow, 1973).	• Include assessments of the physical and social environment to investigate enablers and barriers that will inform programming. • Assist development of policies and programs that enhance active participation, safety, and accessibility in homes, buildings, and outdoor areas (e.g., neighborhood walkability survey, accessibility survey of buildings, education in self-management for social support needs, etc.).
Increased physical, social, and productive activity is linked to decreased morbidity (Glass, Mendes de Leon, Marottoli, & Berkman, 1999).	• Assist the design and implementation of programs that *integrate* physical, social, and productive actions (e.g., bus outings to educational and cultural events, new group dance step lessons, community activism projects, etc.).
Social engagement related to physical health modifies and protects against cognitive aging and reduces risk for disabilities (Bassuk et al., 1999; Everard et al., 2000; Menec, 2003).	• Design and teach educational sessions that include participatory learning and provide opportunities for seniors to interact with others with similar interests. • Assist in planning and implementing events that include opportunities that facilitate socialization.
Social capital in housing areas relates to positive self-rated health (Cannuscio, Block, & Kawachi, 2003; Kim, Subramanian, & Kawachi, 2006).	• Promote gatherings in housing complexes that encourage socialization and information exchange. • Foster senior support organizations' collaborative partnerships with community (e.g., condo management, realtor agency, tenant councils, etc.).
Older adults' meaningful social and community occupations are linked to self-rated positive health and participation (Clark, et al., 1997).	• Identify seniors' occupational interests and the community's occupational profile to foster program choices that match interests. • Foster volunteer opportunities that recognize and use seniors' skills to strengthen the organization's capacities.
Wellness courses promote confidence for self-management skills, proactive behaviors, lifestyle changes, and volunteerism (Clark et al., 1997; Neufeld & Kniepmann, 2001).	• Design and teach educational and support classes or programs for small groups of older adults.

approaches of wellness, preventive medicine, community development, occupational justice, and ecological sustainability. Her approach suggests occupational therapy practitioners can contribute at the individual, group, community, societal, and global-political levels. Similarly, according to the American Occupational Therapy Association (AOTA) guiding professional document (AOTA, 2008), occupational therapy attends to the complex factors that enable and empower client engagement and participation in occupations.

To begin a relationship with an aging in place community, initially occupational therapy practitioners can reach out to a community organization to learn about its services, strengths, and challenges. Often a relationship develops when shared interests are identified and the practitioner gives advice as a "professional volunteer"; offers an educational group session on a health, wellness, and senior living topic; or becomes an advocate by facilitating partnerships among agencies and professionals. Once they form a relationship with an agency, occupational therapy practitioners may negotiate reimbursement for services as a consultant, program developer, evaluator, research team member, or grant writer.

The occupational therapy process in aging in place communities involves the steps of assessment, intervention, monitoring, outcome assessment, and collaboration, similar to individual direct practice and as outlined by AOTA (2008). An occupational therapy practitioner's initial assessment may be part of a team's comprehensive needs assessment to identify enablers and barriers for aging in place related to the particular community environment and cultural contexts. An occupational profile can be conducted to evaluate a community and its residents, looking for occupational routines, opportunities, and gaps as well as interests and strengths. Possible primary sources of information for use in a needs assessment include interviews; written or mailed surveys; focus groups with residents, family members, and agency staff; and observation of seniors' activities in different community contexts. Secondary sources include policies, brochures, and flyers specific to the community, as well as research literature on evidence, models, and policies that promote aging in place in related communities.

Community occupational therapy interventions foster healthy lifestyle patterns through activities offered on multiple levels. With goals of promoting aging in place and building aging-friendly communities, practitioners may draw from theories aimed at the individual, interpersonal, and community levels. Numerous community theories are available as tools for capacity building on the community and organization level (see Chapter 3).

Respecting older adults' variation in capacities (from those who are less active, frail, and need support services to others who are more active and interested in education, prevention, and socialization) is a driving factor for occupational therapy practice in aging in place. Customizing interventions for work with non-profit organizations assists in developing aging-friendly organizational policies. For example, agencies could benefit from occupational therapy practitioners' fresh perspectives on ways to involve seniors in models of "significant" volunteer service; that is, fostering residents' volunteerism and leadership in planning and bringing

resources to the programs. Other examples of possibly needed community policies include bus transportation to programs, use of meeting spaces, routine programming, newsletter articles, program flyers, systems for phone reminders to seniors, and referral methods for occupational therapy in-home services that assess needs for home modifications for increased independence. Community partners should be able to count on occupational therapy practitioners emphasizing residents' perspectives and occupational concerns when planning policies and activities.

Program evaluation, another occupational therapy role in aging in place communities, includes performing process and outcome evaluations. A process evaluation describes the elements, strategies, and challenges in implementing a program over a specified time to see if it was carried out as intended. A process evaluation in a new NORC could capture the first year changes in policies, programs, partnerships, and residents' responses. A more focused process evaluation could examine a specific aspect of a program, such as one carried out recently in a suburban NORC to examine the process of using theoretically based recruitment strategies to encourage older adults' enrollment in a physical activity promotion program (Hildebrand & Neufeld, 2009).

Outcome evaluations are used to determine the impact of programs. Possible outcomes could include residents' positive self-reports on physical and mental health, supportive relationships and networks, and adoption of healthy lifestyle activities. Other desired outcomes in a NORC could include residents' awareness of and satisfaction with opportunities for occupational engagement, services, and resources; and community participation. Another occupation-based indicator of success in a NORC would be evidence of residents assuming leadership in planning, promoting, and/or delivering programs and assuming advocate roles for the community.

Positive outcomes on the organizational level could include enhancing organizational capacities (e.g., finding resources, recruiting volunteers, strategic planning) and integrated organizational services and relationships with agencies and businesses for sustaining services and programs. For example, a successful NORC would look for community partners requesting NORC information and forwarding it to their clients or consumers. Also, NORC-SSPs would aim for community partners to offer services, space, staff support, and/or funds for benefits to the residents and for the operation of the NORC.

Determining outcomes for a healthy community is best as a collaborative process with its stakeholders identifying intermediate as well as long-term outcomes (Anderson, Scrimshaw, Fullilove, & Fielding, 2003; Bauer, 2003). In the example of a NORC-SSP, the ultimate outcome is healthy aging and residents able to live in their own homes as long as desired. Because there is no "gold standard" for measuring the impact of a NORC, establishing multiple intermediate goals or outcomes will be important to assess ongoing changes. Some steps toward achieving a healthy NORC include a neighborhood with safe, aging-friendly environments (e.g., policies; physical and social environment); residents' increased access to opportunities for social engagement, civic engagement, health promotion, and supportive resources; and residents' participation and control in decision making related to their community.

Occupational therapy students in a St. Louis NORC, with faculty supervision, offer additional services to aging in place communities. A NORC may serve as a "living laboratory" for students as they benefit from direct experiences with community-residing older adults while practicing professional skills and exploring research questions. Occupational therapy students at Washington University School of Medicine appreciate learning from direct interactions with well seniors (that is, older adults living in their own homes) and completing assignments within the authentic contexts of the NORC. While NORC residents are eager to be involved with university students, enjoying their energy and learning contemporary perspectives and knowledge, the residents also enjoy participating in research activities because they view it as a form of volunteerism and civic engagement. For examples of occupational therapy student activities, see Table 15-2.

Conclusion

Societal concerns for healthy aging and aging in place call for occupational therapy practitioners

Table 15-2 Student Experiences in the St. Louis NORC	
Research Experiences (on master's and doctoral levels or research course assignments)	• Interview older adults within a community-wide needs assessment • Assist with focus groups to assess occupational profiles of older adults residing in the NORC • Case study research to assess impact of initial NORC residents' participation • Assess recruitment for and participation in an 'Active Living Every Day' course within the NORC • Process evaluation of a mailed version of an OT created NORC wellness course for older adults • Participatory action research with OT students and residents creating a storytelling Web site and using a digital voice recorder to collect stories • Participant-observation in NORC programs and follow-up field notes

Fieldwork Level I and II	• Assist as co-leader to implement health and wellness courses or sessions within the NORC
	• Design, teach, and evaluate health, wellness, and senior living educational sessions; e.g.:
	  • Friendships—As Times Change
	  • Cooking Nutritiously for One
	  • Film Analysis Promoting Self-Management of Home
	  • Music Reminiscing—Tune Up and Tune In
	• Assist in NORC program evaluation (data entry and analysis)
	• "Ask the OT student" monthly resource sessions for drop-in visits by NORC seniors (topics such as seeking work, finding a companion/dating, aging pets, helping adult children with their health problems, etc.)

Continued

Table 15-2 Student Experiences in the St. Louis NORC—cont'd	

Course Assignments	• Computer instruction to individuals and groups
	  • Searching interests in travel, recipes, etc.
	  • Searching online health information
	  • Determining validity of health information
	  • Learning e-mail skills
	  • Learning new applications (Excel, Publisher, Word)
	• Doctoral students coordinate and supervise a NORC Activity Fair with two MSOT students per booth on recreational, fitness, social, and health management activities topics determined via students' assessment of seniors interests
	  • Writing letters to legislators
	  • Grandparenting
	  • Transportation resources
	  • Driver safety
	  • Travel tips for seniors
	  • Dance demonstration
	  • Indoor gardening
	  • Fall prevention
	  • Smart gadgets—helpful strategies
	  • Resources to prevent disabilities

to envision and fulfill expanded community roles in partnership with multidisciplinary professionals. The occupation-focused and strength-based approach of occupational therapy can bring fresh perspectives to interventions that can enhance community participation and assist programs in achieving their missions for older adults. As an emerging innovative aging in place model, NORC-SSPs are one example where occupational therapy practitioners can become critical players to help build and sustain healthy communities for active and productive aging.

CASE STUDIES

CASE STUDY 15•1 Morris, Finding Purpose in Helping Others

Morris is in his early 70s and retired about 10 years ago from his work as a salesman. He and his wife have been married for 50 years and lived for a number of decades in their current home in the suburban NORC. Their lives have been full, including caring for an adult child with developmental disabilities who lives with them. Morris's son has numerous health crises and often Morris is at the hospital with him. Also, Morris supports his parents who are in their late 90s and live in their own home in another part of the city. Life became even more challenging when Morris became ill and required serious surgery.

When Morris returned home, his resilience and help from the NORC enabled him to slowly resume his multiple life roles, although he often has relapses and fatigue. He is quick to thank the NORC for helping him. He says, "In this high-tech, high-pressure, impersonal world we seem to be living in, NORC is truly a sigh of relief." By calling the NORC volunteer coordinator, he can request volunteers to help with house tasks, such as home repair, moving heavy items in the house, yard work, and computer training. A NORC referral to an occupational therapy in-home visit resulted in home modifications that increased his safety and function in the home. Morris also enjoys participating in NORC programs that meet his personal interests. He is an avid storyteller and reflective listener who meets often with other residents in monthly storytelling sessions. He and his wife enjoy NORC outings to cultural events for continued learning and engagement with others.

CASE STUDY 15•1 Morris, Finding Purpose in Helping Others   *cont'd*

Despite his busy life and family caregiving, Morris willingly assumed the additional role of being a NORC ambassador for his community. As an ambassador, he volunteers his wisdom and talents from a lifetime of work and caregiving. He gives his time willingly to help build a healthy community. He finds a sense of purpose in advocating for the NORC as he shares how he has benefited and encourages others to become dues-paying members also. He brings his business talents to meetings with other NORC ambassadors to help plan strategies for building and sustaining the NORC for the years to come in their community.

CASE STUDY 15•1 Discussion Questions

1. What type of preventive occupational therapy services may be useful to Morris?
2. How could occupational therapy support the NORC in attracting younger seniors such as Morris to share their professional skills as volunteers for enhanced productive aging and the good of the community?

Learning Activities

1. Speak to local agencies in your area to find where there is a concentration of seniors and identify the available supportive services. Determine if and how occupational therapy has been involved.
2. Contact an agency that provides senior services and programs to offer assistance in their needs assessment related to residents' aging in place or the agency's capacity building activities. Identify theories and research that would inform the issues surrounding the agency's focused concern.

REFERENCES

American Occupational Therapy Association. (2008). Occupational therapy practice framework: Domain & process (2nd ed.). *American Journal of Occupational Therapy, 6*(6), 625–683.

Anderson, L., Scrimshaw, S., Fullilove, M., & Fielding, J. (2003). The Community Guide's Model for linking the social environment to health. *American Journal of Preventative Medicine, 24*(3S), 12–20. doi: 10.1016/S0749-3797(02)00652-9

Bassuk, S. S., Glass, T. A., & Berkman, L. F. (1999). Social disengagement and incident cognitive decline in community-dwelling elderly persons. *Annuals of Internal Medicine, 131,* 165–173.

Bauer, G. F. (2003). Sample community health indicators on the neighborhood level. In M. Minkler & N. Wallerstein (Eds.), *Community-based participatory research for health* (pp. 438–445). San Francisco, CA: Jossey-Bass.

Bedney, B., Schimmel, D., & Goldberg, R. (2007). *Rethinking aging in place: Exploring the impact of NORC supportive service programs on older adult participants.* Paper presented at the 2007 Joint Conference of the American Society on Aging and the National Council on Aging. Chicago, IL.

Butler, R. N. (2008). *The longevity revolution: The benefits and challenges of living a long life.* New York, NY: PublicAffairs.

Callahan, J., & Lanspery, S. (1997, January–March). Density makes a difference: Can we tap the power of NORCs? *Perspective on Aging,* 13–20.

Cannuscio, C., Block, J., & Kawachi, I. (2003). Social capital and successful aging: The role of senior housing. *Annals of Internal Medicine, 139,* 395–399.

Centers for Disease Control and Prevention. (2008). *Older Americans 2008.* Retrieved from http://agingstats.gov/agingstatsdotnet/Main_Site/Data/Data_2008.aspx

Centers for Disease Control and Prevention. (2009). *Health, United States 2009.* Retrieved from http://cdc.gov/nchs/data/hus/hus09.pdf

Clark, F., Azem, S. P., Zemke, R., Jackson, J., Carlson, M., Mandel, D., & Lipson, L. (1997). Occupational therapy for independent-living older adults: A randomized controlled trial. *Journal of the American Medical Association, 278,* 1321–1326.

Community Preventive Services. (2001). *Behavioral and social approaches to increase physical activity: Social support interventions in community settings.* Retrieved from http://thecommunityguide.org/pa/behavioral-social/community.html

DeVita, C. J., & Fleming, C. (2001). *Building capacity in non-profit organizations.* Retrieved from http://urban.org/publications/410093.html

Endres, T. (2006). *NCOA RespectAbility in America: Guiding principles for civic engagement among adults 55+.* Retrieved from http://ncoa.org/news-ncoa-publications/publications/asa-finalversion-6-21-06.pdf

Everard, K. M., Lac, H. W., Fisher, E. B., & Baum, M. C. (2000). Relationship of activity and social support to the functional health of older adults. *Journal of Gerontology, 55B,* S208–S212.

Glass, T. A., Mendes de Leon, C., Marottoli, R. A., & Berkman, L. F. (1999). Population-based study of social and productive activities as predictors of survival among elderly Americans. *British Medical Journal, 319,* 478–483.

Haight, B., Schmidt, M. G., & Burnside, I. (2005). Demographic and psychosocial aspects of aging. In B. Haight & F. Gibson (Eds.), *Burnside's working with older adults: Group process and techniques* (pp. 7–24). Sudbury, MA: Jones and Bartlett.

Hawkley, L. C., Burleson, M. H., Bernston, G. C., & Cacioppo, J. T. (2003). Loneliness in everyday life: Cardiovascular activity, psychosocial context, and health behaviors. *Journal of Personality and Social Psychology, 85*(1), 105–120.

Hildebrand, M., & Neufeld, P. (2009). Recruiting older adults into a physical activity promotion program: 'Active Living Every Day' offered in a Naturally Occurring Retirement Community. *Gerontologist, 49*(5), 702–710.

Hinterlong, J., Morrow-Howell, N., & Sherraden, M. W. (Eds.). (2001). *Productive aging: Concepts and challenges.* Baltimore, MD: Johns Hopkins University Press.

Hunt, M. E., & Gunter-Hunt, G. (1985). Naturally occurring retirement communities. *Journal of Housing Elderly, 3,* 3–21.

Hunt, M. E., & Ross, L. E. (1990). Naturally occurring retirement communities: A multiattribute examination of desirability factors. *The Gerontologist, 30,* 667–674.

Jewish Federations of North America (2010a). *NORCS— An aging in place initiative.* Retrieved from http://norcs.com/page.aspx?id=160634

Jewish Federations of North America. (2010b). NORC public policy. Retrieved from http://norcs.ujcfedweb.org

Keyes, C. L., Michalec, B., Kobau, R., Zahran, H., Zack, M. M., & Simoes, E. J. (2005). Social support and health-related quality of life among older adults— Missouri, 2000. *Morbidity and Mortality Weekly Report, 54*(17), 433–437.

Kim, D., Subramanian, S., & Kawachi, I. (2006). Bonding versus bridging social capital and their associations with self-rated health: A multilevel analysis of 40 US communities. *Journal of Epidemiological Community Health, 60,* 116–122.

Lawton, M. P., & Nahemow, L. (1973). An ecological theory of adaptive behaviour and aging. In C. Eisdorfer & M. P. Lawton (Eds.), *The psychology of adult development and aging* (pp. 657–667). Washington, DC: American Psychological Association.

Lorig, K. R., & Holman, H. R. (2003). Self-management education: History, definition, outcomes, and mechanisms. *Annuals of Behavior Medicine, 26,* 1–7.

Lum, Y. & Lightfoot, E. (2005). Effects of volunteering on the physical and mental health of older people. *Research on Aging, 27*(1), 31–55.

Marshall, V. W., Clarke, P. J., & Ballantyne, P. J. (2001). Instability in the retirement transition: Effects on health and well-being in a Canadian study. *Research on Aging, 23*(4), 379–409.

Martinson, M., & Minkler, M. (2006). Civic engagement and older adults: A critical perspective. *Gerontologist, 46*(3), 318–324.

Masotti, P. J., Fick, R., Johnson-Masotti, A., & MacLeod, S. (2006). Healthy naturally occurring retirement communities: A low-cost approach to facilitating healthy aging. *American Journal of Public Health, 96,* 1164–1170.

Mendes de Leon, C. F. (2005). Social engagement and successful aging. Special section on Social engagement and health outcomes among older people, *European Journal of Ageing, 2*(1), 64–66.

Menec, V. (2003). The relation between everyday activities and successful aging: A 6-year longitudinal study. *Journal of Gerontology, 58B,* S74–S82.

Moeller, P. (2009, October 30). Seniors finding that it does take a village. *U.S. News & World Report.* Retrieved from http://usnews.com/money/blogs/the-best-life/2009/10/30/seniors-finding-that-it-does-take-a-village.html

National Association of Area Agencies on Aging. (2006). *Maturing of America: Getting communities on track for an aging population.* Retrieved from http://n4a.org/pdf/MOAFinalReport.pdf

National Center for Creative Aging. (n.d.). *Productive aging.* Retrieved from http://artsandaging.org/index.php?id=7

National Council on Aging. (2008, October). *The power of professional volunteers.* Retrieved from http://ncoa.org/assets/files/pdf/Respectability-IB-3-final_Power-of-Volunteers.pdf

Neufeld, P. (2005, April). *Process evaluation: The first year of programs (3/2004 to 3/2005) in the St. Louis Naturally Occurring Retirement Community (NORC) Demonstration Project.*

Neufeld, P., & Kniepmann, K. (2001). Gateway to wellness: An occupational therapy collaboration with the National Multiple Sclerosis Society. *Occupational Therapy in Health Care, 13*(3/4), 67–84.

Ortman, J. M., & Guarneri, C. E. (2010). *United States population projections: 2000 to 2050— US Census Bureau.* Retrieved from http://census.gov/population/www/projections/analytical-document09.pdf

Putnam, R. D. (2001). *Bowling alone: The collapse and revival of American community.* New York, NY: Simon & Schuster.

Scharlach, A. (2008, February 20). *Why our communities must become more aging-friendly.* Keynote address presented at Creating Aging-Friendly Communities Online Conference. Retrieved from http://icohere.com/agingfriendly/program.htm

Solinge, H. (2007). Health change in retirement: A longitudinal study among older workers in the Netherlands. *Research on Aging, 29*(3), 225–256.

Stewart, S. T. (2004). Do out-of-pocket expenditures rise with age among older Americans? *Gerontologist, 44,* 48–57.

United Hospital Fund. (2010). NORC blueprint: A guide to community action. Retrieved from http://norcblueprint.org/about/

Weinberger, M., Darnell, J. C., Tierney, W. M., Martz, B. L., Hiner, S. L., Barker, J., & Neill, P. (1986). Self-rated health as a predictor of hospital admission and nursing home placement in elderly public housing tenants. *American Journal of Public Health, 76*(4), 457–459.

Wilcock, A. (2010). Population health: An occupational rationale. In M. E. Scaffa, S. M. Reitz, & M. A. Pizzi, (Eds.), *Occupational therapy in the promotion of health and wellness* (pp. 110–121). Philadelphia, PA: F.A. Davis.

Wilson, R. S., Krueger. K. R., Arnold. S. E., Schneider. J. A., Kelly, J. F., Barnes, L. L., & Bennett, D. A. (2007). Loneliness and risk of Alzheimer disease. *Archives of General Psychiatry, 64*, 234–240.

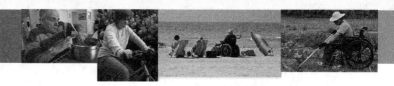

Work and Industry

Chapter 16

Ergonomics and Prevention of Work-Related Injuries

Peter Bowman, OTD, MHS, OTR/L, OT(C), Dip COT

The economic impact of work-related injury and illness has been estimated to be $171 billion annually, the same as cancer or cardiovascular disease and much greater than the burden from HIV/AIDS or Alzheimer's disease.

—National Institute for Occupational Safety and Health [NIOSH], 2009, p. 7

Learning Objectives

This chapter is designed to enable the reader to:

- Discuss the issues involved in provision of ergonomic intervention in community settings.
- Differentiate among common ergonomic interventions in work, home, and recreational settings.
- Evaluate positioning for optimal function in a variety of work tasks.
- Apply the seven basic concepts of universal design.
- Describe the implications of cognitive workload and psychosocial factors as they relate to working productively.
- Discuss the role of occupational therapy in providing ergonomic interventions to a variety of community settings.

Key Terms

Client-centered practice
Cognitive workload
Community ergonomics

Ergonomics
Transitional return to work model
Universal design

Introduction

The practice of ergonomics in occupational therapy is evolving. During entry-level education, occupational therapists should gain foundational skills in the analysis of client factors; an understanding of principles of biomechanics and ergonomics; and the ability to assess and modify home, work, and community contexts (Accreditation Council for Occupational Therapy Education [ACOTE], 2009). The intent of the chapter is to build on this knowledge and introduce the components of community ergonomic assessment as they apply to prevention and cure for clients. Clients who can benefit from ergonomic consultation include individuals, families, groups, agencies, governments, businesses, organizations, and communities. Community ergonomic assessment is specialized, and continued education is required to develop and maintain the expertise required to deliver community-based services.

In this chapter, the term "ergonomics" is defined, a brief history is provided, and injury rates are reviewed. This is followed by an exploration of occupational therapy's role in community ergonomics in the home, the workplace, and recreational venues. Next, detailed information about work-related practice, universal design, and a case study are provided.

Ergonomics Definitions and History

"Human factors (ergonomics) is a body of knowledge about human abilities, human limitations and other human characteristics that are relevant to design" (Chapanis, 1991, p. 2). The implementation of **ergonomics** "is the application of human factors information to the design of tools, machines, systems, tasks, jobs, and environments for safe, comfortable and effective human use" (Chapanis, 1991, p. 2).

The first documented recognition of the concept of ergonomics was from an Italian, Bernardino Ramazzini, who had an interest in occupational health based on his observations of workers primarily in foundries and tanneries. Although his primary focus was the relationship between workers and the diseases they contracted, Ramazzini anticipated the need for workplace analysis and identified potential and actual hazards to workers' health. He summarized his work in 1700 in a publication entitled "de Morbis Artificum," which, when translated, reads, "Disease of Workers" (Franco, 1999). Almost 150 years later, in 1857, Wojciech Jastrzebowski created the term "ergonomics." The term "ergonomics" is derived from the Greek words *ergos,* or work, and *nomos,* meaning "study of" or "law" (Ergoweb, 2011a).

During the Industrial Revolution (1750–1830), many machines and types of equipment were updated and modified as manufacturing became more sophisticated and more efficient. At this stage of industrial development, the major interest was in production, not working conditions. Frederick Taylor pioneered a method called "scientific management" to find the best method to complete a job and all of its component parts. In the early 1900s, scientific management became known as Taylorism and was very popular as a method to improve worker efficiency. Taylor also addressed the issues of human capabilities and limitations relative to the demands of work (Internet Center for Management and Business Administration, 2010). The current practice of requiring screening tests after job offers is influenced by Taylorism.

The Second World War prompted a major interest in ensuring the best interaction between human and machine to ensure efficiency of increasingly sophisticated technology, especially fighter aircraft (Ergoweb, 2011b). Design concepts were implemented that focused on fitting the human to the machine and ensuring that controls were logical and understandable. After the Second World War, the focus of ergonomics expanded to include worker safety as well as productivity. Research began to be conducted to examine the factors involved in ergonomics, such as the following:

- Muscular strength required for a task
- Intervertebral disc force on the low back
- Cardiovascular response to manual labor
- Maximum weights that can be pushed, pulled, and carried

Proponents of ergonomics and human-factor concepts include individuals from diverse groups comprised of industrial engineers, industrial psychologists, occupational medicine physicians, industrial hygienists, and safety engineers, among others. Professions that use ergonomics/human factors information include architects, health and safety officers, occupational therapists, physical therapists, occupational medicine nurses, and insurance loss control specialists (Ergoweb, 2011b). A major challenge for the future is to incorporate evidence-based practice into the practice of ergonomics.

Role of Occupational Therapy in Community Ergonomics

Occupational therapy **community ergonomics** involves the utilization of knowledge of the client's community to expand potential ergonomic interventions in order to maximize the impact on occupational performance and social participation. These community interventions can include direct observations of the ergonomic aspects of the client's activities of daily living (ADLs), instrumental activities of daily living (IADLs), work, and leisure activities, as well as the contexts in which these occupations are performed. During initial evaluation of a client, occupational therapists must ascertain subjectively and objectively the future needs and goals of the client in carrying out his/her ADLs, IADLs, work, and leisure activities. In general, there are two types of community ergonomic practice. One focuses on individual work with clients, as will be detailed in the case study at the end of this chapter; the other type addresses program development through consultation with a business, agency, or other entity. The knowledge of and skills in ergonomics necessary to perform either role are similar and will be addressed throughout this chapter.

Providing ergonomic services in the community setting requires the ability to evaluate a multiplicity of environments where people work, learn, play, and recuperate. During the evaluation, occupational therapists must consider both preventative and curative intervention strategies. In addition, they have to be prepared to work with clients from a number of referring sources and agencies, including but not limited to physicians; workers' compensation; insurance companies; home health agencies; attorneys; individual clients; family members; federal, state, and local government agencies; and manufacturing and industrial companies. Funding sources for community-based ergonomic practice vary tremendously and potentially can include: health insurance, fee for service, workers' compensation, legal settlements, Medicare, Medicaid, non-profit organizations, foundations, and government agencies.

General Ergonomic Considerations

There are many aspects of ergonomics with which the occupational practitioner working in the community must be familiar. These include posture, positioning, and lifting; cognitive workload; and psychosocial factors.

Posture, Positioning, and Lifting

Positioning in relation to any type of work activity is critical to carrying out sustained activity safely and without fatigue. All specifics are based on the global rules that a good biomechanical position is required and that no one position should be adopted for excessive amounts of time. In general, a neutral joint position is best (Cornell University Human Factors Group, 1996). The Canadian Center for Occupational Health and Safety (CCOHS) provides a very good review of issues and solutions for working in a standing position (2008).

Prolonged sitting is a considerable challenge, especially for those with back injuries. Research shows that sitting places more strain on the back than standing. Chaffin, Andersson, and Martin (1984) reported increased disc pressure on the back in a variety of sitting positions when compared with standing. Although all sitting positions increase disc pressure, the position and type of chair in use does make a big difference in the amount of disc pressure. The CCOHS (1998/2010) provides a cogent overview of working in the sitting position. A poor and an improved sitting position when using a computer laptop are shown in Figure 16.1. The improved position illustrates the importance of leaning backwards slightly against the back of the chair and properly positioning the laptop. The worker's

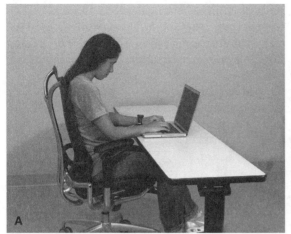 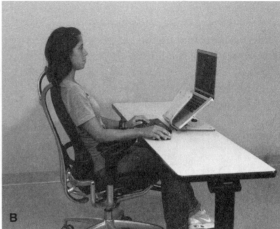

Fig. 16•1 A. Poor sitting position with laptop. **B.** Improved sitting position with laptop. *(Photos courtesy of Gary Melancon, Audio Visual Production Manager, College of Health Professions, Information and Educational Technology Team at the Medical University of South Carolina.)*

posture could be further improved by uncrossing her ankles and placing both feet flat on the floor.

Many injuries in the community result from lifting too much weight or improper positioning during lifting at home, work, and sites of recreation. In regard to work activities, the official lifting limitation set by the NIOSH is 51 pounds in the revised lifting equation (Waters, Putz-Anderson, & Garg, 1994). Using the revised NIOSH formula, Waters (2007) reports a 35-pound limitation for patient handling tasks; when weight exceeds this limit, assistive devices should be used.

Lifting technique is obviously important. Good posture must be maintained, and clients should be instructed to maximize use of the large muscles of the legs to assist in raising objects from the floor to other levels. Lifting symmetrically without twisting the spinal column is important to avoid excessive strain on the spine, and the ease with which an object can be grasped and held with the hands also must be considered. Examples of preferred and problematic lifting are shown in Figures 16.2 and 16.3. The quality of grasp that can be achieved is called "coupling" and is described as being good, fair, or poor. The rating is assigned based on the size of the object; ease with which the object can be held; the object's texture, such as rough or slippery; the presence of an asymmetrical center of mass; the

stability of the materials; the need for gloves to lift; and the presence or absence of handles or cutouts to use to lift.

Cognitive Workload

Cognitive workload is an area of work assessment and ergonomic consideration that is too often ignored. Therapists have a tendency to concentrate on the biomechanical analysis of lifting, carrying, and reaching and ignore the very important factors involved in cognition and the psychological issues involved in the workplace and home situation. The level of intensity at which an individual works is a functional outcome of cognitive workload. For effective cognitive workload processing to occur, information must be received, integrated, and remembered. The measurement of **cognitive workload** involves assessing how much mental effort is used to accomplish a task, and that measurement is based on the worker's perception of work performance and work difficulty. This information can be obtained by a number of means, including self-report of time load, mental effort, and psychological stress load.

Assessing cognitive workload is most important when a client reports being either under- or overloaded cognitively. When clients experience

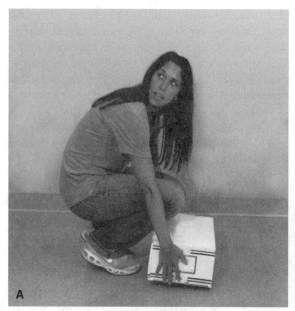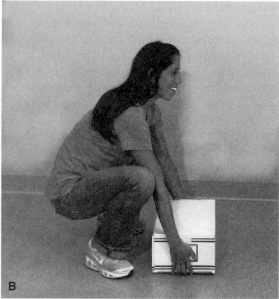

Fig. 16•2 A. Poor lift from floor. **B.** Improved lift from floor. *(Photos courtesy of Gary Melancon, Audio Visual Production Manager, College of Health Professions, Information and Educational Technology Team at the Medical University of South Carolina.)*

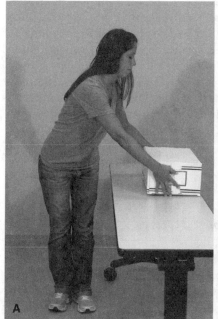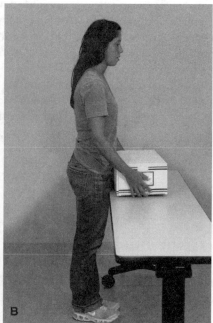

Fig. 16•3 A. Poor lift/positioning at workstation. **B.** Improved lift/positioning at workstation. *(Photos courtesy of Gary Melancon, Audio Visual Production Manager, College of Health Professions, Information and Educational Technology Team at the Medical University of South Carolina.)*

cognitive workload issues because of distractions such as noise, temperature, and vibration, they are unable to perceive and integrate the excessive information and occupational performance is affected. The result of feeling or being cognitively overloaded often results in a decrease in work capacity, increase in error rate, and an increase in a variety of physical complaints (Jacobs, 1999). To address cognitive workload in all realms of activity (e.g., home, work, education, and leisure), the occupational therapist needs to either modify the activity parameters to suit the client or modify and expand the functional limits of the client. The first of these two options is often easier to achieve.

Cognitive workload is affected by mental space and is determined by intellectual and genetic endowment, learned knowledge, social status, personality, and physical development. These factors vary from person to person; therefore, the occupational therapist must assess and address these factors in order to maximize a client's participation in life through full engagement in occupation. For example, an individual's personality type has an impact on cognitive workload (Table 16-1). Although most individuals are somewhat of a mix of the A and B personality types, these factors do have implications for individuals' self-perception or self-efficacy.

Factors such as noise, temperature, and vibration can be distracters from full participation in areas of occupation and affect cognitive workload. Occupations are often carried out with tools. To effectively use tools a number of skills must coalesce, such as coordination, laterality, endurance, fine and gross motor coordination, strength, and visual integration. To ensure a maximum level of achievement in occupations in all community settings, the therapist needs to observe and measure the actual and perceived client workload; offer strategies that enable the client to eliminate, reduce, or ignore extraneous factors; and move the worker from a negative overwhelmed state to one of recognition and familiarity.

Psychosocial Factors

The NIOSH (1997) reports three types of psychosocial factors or characteristics that have implications for the client. These include:

- Factors associated with the job and work environment
- Factors associated with the extra-work environment (outside of the work environment)
- Characteristics of the individual worker

Interactions of factors constitute what is referred to as a "stress process," the results of which are thought to affect both health status and job performance (Sauter & Swanson, 1996). Psychological factors are influenced by the physical environment, factors intrinsic to the job (e.g., workloads), arrangement of work time (e.g., hours of work), management of operating practices (e.g., worker roles), and technology changes. Psychological factors can affect work performance through reactions to job and work environment factors, such as intensified workload, monotonous work, levels of job control, level of job clarity, availability and use of social support, and general level of job satisfaction or dissatisfaction.

Sites for Community Ergonomics

The overall goal of community ergonomic practice is to enhance occupational performance in home, recreation, and work environments. Occupational therapists are trained in the evaluation of human abilities; this training provides the foundation for an occupational therapy ergonomic practice. The focus of this practice is to fit the work or occupation of the individual to conditions at the home, recreation site, or

Table 16-1	Type A and Type B Personality Types	
Type A Personality	**Type B Personality**
Urgency	Less urgency
Striving	Less striving
High activity level	Lower level of activity
Potential to overload capacity	Expectations can seem impossible
Less likely to report cognitive overload	More likely to report cognitive overload
More stressed out	Less stressed out

Data from: Ergonomics for Therapists, 2nd ed. (pp. 112–113), by K. Jacobs, 1999, Boston: Butterworth-Heinemann. Copyright 1999.

workplace, thus enabling the individual to safely, efficiently, and consistently produce a quality product or outcome. Enhanced occupational performance is consistent with the broad outcomes identified in the *Occupational Therapy Practice Framework: Domain and Process* (American Occupational Therapy Association [AOTA], 2008). However, other outcomes listed in the *Framework* may also result from community ergonomic practice, such as adaptation, health and wellness, participation, prevention, quality of life, role competence, self-advocacy, and occupational justice (AOTA, 2008, pp. 662–663).

Client-centered practice, also supported by the *Framework,* requires that clients be involved in the process of decision making. Therapists should advocate both for and with clients to meet their needs in terms of modifications to environments, tools, or processes. Client-centered practice ensures respect for clients, their families, and the choices they make. The clients have the ultimate responsibility for decisions about daily occupations and occupational therapy services. The interventions should be flexible and individualized to enable clients to solve occupational performance issues, with a focus on the transaction between person-environment-occupation (Law et al., 1996). Examples of modifications to each of three environments, home, recreation site, and the workplace, follow.

Home

Ensuring safe interaction with all everyday tasks at home in an effective, efficient manner is one of the major goals of occupational therapy intervention. Ideally, evaluation of the home would cover a number of the areas of occupation from the *Framework* including: ADLs, IADLs, rest and sleep, education, work, play, and social participation (AOTA, 2008, pp. 631–633). Occupational therapists need to enable clients to be independent in their daily activities and routines with utilization of good biomechanical positioning, while accounting for psychosocial and cognitive factors. Whereas occupational therapists ensure that basic ADLs can be achieved, they may not be as focused on technology tasks, such as computer use in the home. Access to e-mail and Internet resources is very important to a large percentage of the population, and knowledge of ergonomics is essential when trying to ensure efficient use of such technology.

Ergonomics is very important in the kitchen; positioning of kitchen equipment and a review of tools used in the kitchen is essential. Use of electrical kitchen devices, such as can openers and carving knives, can decrease stress on joints in the hands and wrists. Knife safety is also important; knives with large and/or ergonomically shaped handles and protective blade guards are very useful. Food processors can be used to reduce the pressure on hands for intensive chopping, shredding, slicing, and dicing. Products such as the OXO Good Grips line (OXO International, 2006) offer universally designed kitchen implements that have large cushioned handles to minimize the strain on the hands while preparing foods. The old adages to keep frequently used items within easy reach and to avoid heavy lifting remain pertinent. Simple hints, for instance sliding heavy pots and pans along the kitchen counter surface, can save lifting. Successful transfers of tools and food from one surface to another are an obvious practical concern for many occupational therapy clients to avoid slips and falls due to spills. Preferably, these issues should be addressed in the natural context of the client's home. All rooms used by the client need to be fully assessed for accessibility and safety, including rooms for leisure and education.

Advanced community-based ergonomics in the home environment necessitates gaining additional knowledge regarding home environment modifications to ensure safe, efficient access to all locations in the home at a simple level, which may involve the provision of assistive technologies such as raised toilet seats, bath boards, and grab rails. At a more advanced level and following mentoring and training, consultation with architects might be appropriate. Consultations with architects should be sought for major alterations to kitchens and bathrooms, as for wheelchair access, using the concepts of universal design.

Recreation Sites

Ergonomics in the community is often about access for all; able-bodied and disabled populations should be able to access community activities regardless of social class, ethnicity, or physical ability. Many sports and recreational activities can be adapted to allow participation for all. Games such as softball can be adapted. Access to equipment and recreational facilities by individuals with varying abilities and ages is possible if adaptations are made. Because occupational justice is a desirable outcome of occupational therapy intervention (AOTA, 2008), occupational therapists should advocate for clients' abilities to fully integrate in every environment in their communities, including recreation sites.

When occupational therapists or occupational therapy assistants discover community locations lacking accessibility, they should notify the local regulatory agency, which may include town, city, or county officials. Occupational therapy student projects, such as access studies, have identified issues that can then be addressed to improve access. Input from occupational therapists regarding accessibility issues is not commonly funded, so participation in this important role is often on a volunteer basis. Occupational therapists can provide input on specific projects, such as the Miracle League programs that provide baseball fields where children with disabilities can play baseball on rubberized surfaces (Miracle League, 2008) and other community projects such as the adaptation of playgrounds.

Workplace

A workplace can be any number of environments in which work activities take place, including space for paid employment, volunteer work, and even recreational activities that are thought of as work, such as gardening. The focus should be matching capabilities of the person to work demands through an understanding and use of occupational biomechanics to decrease the risks of mechanical trauma. The approach needs to be functional and occupational when examining the ability of the worker in relation to the job demands. Utilization of the systems approach that examines satisfaction in relation to work systems and equipment can be useful. The ergonomic tool kit (Jacobs, 1999) can be helpful, as it offers the opportunity to examine the many dimensions of the work environment (e.g., the organization's culture, motivational factors, and problems identified by the facility worker). The tool kit addresses stress levels, comfort, and safety.

Use of the Person-Environment-Occupation Model (Law et al., 1996) enables occupational therapists to examine not only the broader work environment but also the person and the occupations being carried out by the person, as well as the relationship between these three elements. Whenever occupational therapists examine the work situation, they should do so at three levels:

1. Micro—worker level; interaction between the person and the product
2. Meso—task level; environment worked in by the worker
3. Macro—corporate; impact of the organization on the worker.

There are a variety of interventions that can be used in community ergonomics. In order to provide ergonomic interventions, an understanding of terms used in this practice area is needed. Definitions of terms used in ergonomics are provided by Ergoweb (2011a). Interventions at the workplace can include a number of options:

- Assessment of the work site, observing another employee doing the work tasks of the client
- Assessment of the work site of/with an injured worker
- Consultation on work site–based prevention of injury plans
- Education of management and workers about risk conditions
- Facilitation of recommendations from engineers and administration to reduce the identified risk conditions
- Identification and control of work site risk factors
- Performance of clinic-based worker assessment
- Provision of early work return program
- Provision of work return preparation/work hardening programs

Potential goals for these interventions are identified in Box 16-1. Regardless of the site of community-based ergonomic practice, universal design principles are relevant and useful.

Universal Design

Many industrialized countries provide infrastructure to implement universal access. There are excellent positive examples of universal design where locations have been created to allow a lived-leisure experience for all, such as the sensory garden in Japan (Sensory

Box 16-1 Goals of Workplace Community Ergonomics

- Reduction of occupational injury and illness
- Containment of workers' compensation costs
- Improvement in productivity
- Improvement in work quality
- Reduction in absenteeism
- Compliance with government regulations

Trust, n.d.). **Universal design** as defined by Mace is the purposeful design of products and environments to ensure they can be used by all people no matter their ability level or age (Center for Universal Design, 2010). These types of initiatives are very useful for accessibility and injury prevention. The seven principles of universal design (Connell et al., 1997), which are the gold standard for ensuring maximum access for all, appear in Table 16-2.

Table 16-2 Principles of Universal Design

Principle	Guidelines
PRINCIPLE ONE: Equitable Use The design is useful and marketable to people with diverse abilities.	1a. Provide the same means of use for all users: identical whenever possible; equivalent when not. 1b. Avoid segregating or stigmatizing any users. 1c. Provisions for privacy, security, and safety should be equally available to all users. 1d. Make the design appealing to all users.
PRINCIPLE TWO: Flexibility in Use The design accommodates a wide range of individual preferences and abilities.	2a. Provide choice in methods of use. 2b. Accommodate right- or left-handed access and use. 2c. Facilitate the user's accuracy and precision. 2d. Provide adaptability to the user's pace.
PRINCIPLE THREE: Simple and Intuitive Use Use of the design is easy to understand, regardless of the user's experience, knowledge, language skills, or current concentration level.	3a. Eliminate unnecessary complexity. 3b. Be consistent with user expectations and intuition. 3c. Accommodate a wide range of literacy and language skills. 3d. Arrange information consistent with its importance. 3e. Provide effective prompting and feedback during and after task completion.
PRINCIPLE FOUR: Perceptible Information The design communicates necessary information effectively to the user, regardless of ambient conditions or the user's sensory abilities.	4a. Use different modes (pictorial, verbal, tactile) for redundant presentation of essential information. 4b. Provide adequate contrast between essential information and its surroundings. 4c. Maximize "legibility" of essential information. 4d. Differentiate elements in ways that can be described (i.e., make it easy to give instructions or directions). 4e. Provide compatibility with a variety of techniques or devices used by people with sensory limitations.
PRINCIPLE FIVE: Tolerance for Error The design minimizes hazards and the adverse consequences of accidental or unintended actions.	5a. Arrange elements to minimize hazards and errors: most used elements, most accessible; hazardous elements eliminated, isolated, or shielded. 5b. Provide warnings of hazards and errors. 5c. Provide fail safe features. 5d. Discourage unconscious action in tasks that require vigilance.
PRINCIPLE SIX: Low Physical Effort The design can be used efficiently and comfortably and with a minimum of fatigue.	6a. Allow user to maintain a neutral body position. 6b. Use reasonable operating forces. 6c. Minimize repetitive actions. 6d. Minimize sustained physical effort.

Continued

Table 16-2   Principles of Universal Design—cont'd

Principle	Guidelines
PRINCIPLE SEVEN: Size and Space for Approach and Use Appropriate size and space is provided for approach, reach, manipulation, and use regardless of user's body size, posture, or mobility.	7a. Provide a clear line of sight to important elements for any seated or standing user. 7b. Make reach to all components comfortable for any seated or standing user. 7c. Accommodate variations in hand and grip size. 7d. Provide adequate space for the use of assistive devices or personal assistance.

Data from: Developed by the Center for Universal Design by B. R. Connell, M. Jones, R. Mace, J. Mueller, J. Mullick, E. Ostroff, J. Sanford, J. Steinfeld, E. M. Story, & G. Vanderheiden. (1997). The Principles of Universal Design, Version 2.0. Raleigh, NC: North Carolina State University. Copyright © 1997 NC State University, The Center for Universal Design.

The Principles of Universal Design were conceived and developed by The Center for Universal Design at North Carolina State University. Use or application of the Principles in any form by an individual or organization is separate and distinct from the Principles and does not constitute or imply acceptance or endorsement by The Center for Universal Design of the use or application.

Occupational Risks and Common Work Injuries

A review of injury statistics can assist in recognizing where both prevention and rehabilitation efforts need to be targeted. The U.S. Department of Labor, Bureau of Labor Statistics (USDL, BLS) reports that the 2009 injury rate was 3.7 per 100 full-time workers, a decrease from 4.0 per 100 in 2008 (USDL, BLS, 2010a). The total number of incidents requiring days away from work decreased in 2009 by 9% to 1,238,490 cases (USDL, BLS, 2010b). One way to determine severity of injury or illness, median days away from work, was 8 days in 2009, which was unchanged from the previous year (USDL, BLS, 2010b). Tables 16-3 and 16-4 provide additional data for days away from work by injury and type of injury event or exposure.

Positive findings in the decreased accident rates for 2009 are noted; however, the alarming fact is that injuries caused by repetitive strain, such as carpal tunnel syndrome (CTS), caused more lost work days than amputations. Therefore, CTS and other repetitive motion injuries are of paramount importance in terms of prevention as well as intervention. Occupational therapy assistants and occupational therapists can have a major impact, not only post-injury but also in the correction of poorly designed work sites and work procedures to prevent injuries.

A number of occupations have higher risk of injury. Certain types of work have risks for particular disorders. Table 16-5 provides a list of job types, disorders that commonly occur in each job, and activity demands of the job. Injuries that occur commonly at work are CTS, Repetitive Strain Injuries (RSI), and Low Back Pain (LBP). These common diagnoses first need to be treated to resolve symptoms. Once symptoms have been resolved, the next important step is

Table 16-3   Missed Work Days by Event or Exposure

Event or Exposure	Median Number of Days Away from Work
Contact With Objects	5
Fall to Lower Level	13
Fall on Same Level	9
Slips or Trips Without Fall	8
Overexertion	10
Repetitive Motion Injuries	21
Exposure to Harmful Substances	3
Transportation Accidents	10
Fires and Explosions	9
Assaults and Violent Acts	7
All Other	10

Data from: "Table 4: Number, incidence rate, and median days away from work for nonfatal occupational injuries and illnesses involving days away from work by selected injury or illness characteristics and private industry, state government, and local government," 2009, by U.S. Department of Labor, Bureau of Labor Statistics, 2010a.

Table 16-4 Missed Work Days by Injury

Nature of Injury	Median Number of Days Away from Work
Carpal Tunnel Syndrome	21
Fractures	30
Amputations	20
Tendonitis	14
Multiple Traumatic Injuries	8
Sprains, Strains, Tears	10
Heat Burns	5
Bruises, Contusions	4
Cuts, Lacerations, Punctures	4
Chemical Burns	3

Data from: "Table 4: Number, incidence rate, and median days away from work for nonfatal occupational injuries and illnesses involving days away from work by selected injury or illness characteristics and private industry, state government, and local government," 2009, by U S. Department of Labor, Bureau of Labor Statistics, 2010a.

ensuring that the work location that caused the injury is evaluated and appropriate changes are made to factors such as positioning, lifting, repetition, sitting and standing posture, and any other factor that places the client at risk of re-injury.

A number of online ergonomics assessment tools that are useful to assess risk factors for common upper extremity injuries are provided by NexGen Ergonomics. NexGen's tool is called the ErgoIntelligence Upper Extremity Assessment (UEA) and includes the Rapid Upper Limb Assessment (RULA), Rapid Entire Body Assessment (REBA), Strain Index (SI), Occupational Repetitive Actions Index (OCRA), and the Cumulative Trauma Disorders (CTD) Risk Index. Trial versions of these assessments can be obtained online (NexGen Ergonomics, 2008).

Injury Prevention

Prevention of injuries in the community should address all aspects of participation in all of areas of occupation, including ADLs, IADLs, rest and sleep,

Table 16-5 Job Identified Disorders and Occupational Risk Factors

Type of job	Disorders	Activity Demands
1. Buffing, Grinding	Tenosynovitis Thoracic Outlet Carpal Tunnel De Quervain's Pronator Teres Tendinitis of the Wrist and Shoulder	Repetitive wrist motions, prolonged flexed shoulders, vibration, forced ulnar deviation, repetitive forearm pronation.
2. Punch Press Operators	Tendinitis of the Wrist and Shoulder De Quervain's	Repetitive forceful wrist extension/flexion. Repetitive shoulder abduction/flexion, forearm supination. Repetitive ulnar deviation in pushing controls.
3. Overhead Assembly (Welders, car mechanics, painters	Thoracic Outlet Shoulder Tendinitis	Sustained hyperextension of arms. Hands above shoulders.
4. Belt Conveyor Assembly	Tendonitis of Shoulder and Wrist Carpal Tunnel Thoracic Outlet	Arms extended, abducted, or flexed more than 60°, repetitive forceful wrist motions.
5. Typing, Keypunch, Cashier	Tension in Neck Thoracic Outlet Carpal Tunnel	Static restricted posture, arms abducted/flexed, high-speed finger movement, palmar base pressure, ulnar deviation.

Continued

Table 16-5 Job Identified Disorders and Occupational Risk Factors—cont'd		
Type of job	**Disorders**	**Activity Demands**
6. Sewers and Cutters	Thoracic Outlet De Quervain's Carpal Tunnel	Repetitive shoulder flexion, repetitive ulnar deviation. Repetitive wrist flexion/palmar base pressure.
7. Small Parts Assembly (Wiring, bandaging wrap)	Tension in Neck Thoracic Outlet Wrist tendinitis Epicondylitis	Prolonged restricted posture, forceful ulnar deviation and thumb pressure, repetitive wrist motion, forceful wrist extension and pronation.
8. Musicians	Wrist Tendinitis Carpal Tunnel Epicondylitis Thoracic Outlet	Repetitive forceful wrist motions, palmar base pressure, prolonged shoulder abduction/flexion, forceful wrist extension with forearm pronation.
9. Bench Work (Glass cutters phone operators)	Ulnar Nerve Entrapment	Sustained elbow flexion with pressure on ulnar groove.
10. Operating room personnel	Thoracic Outlet Carpal Tunnel De Quervain's	Prolonged shoulder flexion, repetitive wrist flexion, ulnar deviation (holding retractors).
11. Packing	Tendinitis of Shoulder and Wrist Tension in Neck Carpal Tunnel De Quervain's	Prolonged load on shoulders, repetitive wrist motions, over-exertion, forceful ulnar deviation.
12. Truck Drivers	Thoracic Outlet	Prolonged shoulder abduction and flexion.
13. Housekeepers, Cooks	De Quervain's Carpal Tunnel	Scrubbing, washing, rapid wrist rotational movements.
14. Carpenters, Bricklayers	Carpal Tunnel Guyon's Tunnel	Hammering, pressure on palm base.
15. Stockroom, Shipping	Thoracic Outlet Shoulder Tendinitis	Reaching overhead. Prolonged load on shoulder in unnatural position.
16. Materials Handling	Thoracic Outlet Shoulder Tendinitis	Carrying heavy loads on shoulders.
17. Lumber/Construction	Shoulder Tendinitis Epicondylitis	Repetitive throwing of heavy load.
18. Butcher/Meat packing	De Quervain's Carpal Tunnel	Ulnar deviation, flexed wrist with exertion.
19. Letter carriers (most especially if carrying mail)	Shoulder Problems Thoracic Outlet	Carrying heavy load with shoulder strap.

education, work, play, leisure, and social participation. In addition to ensuring individuals are performing work within their safe limitations, injury prevention has been demonstrated to provide savings in a number of workers' compensation claims (Littleton, 2003). Injury prevention should include education in many environments but especially in the work environment. Education regarding not only basic safety but also to address the position of work, work tools, and equipment in the work environment is vital. In general, a neutral joint position is one of less strain, and placing items closer to a person is preferable to having to reach excess distances. The role of the therapist is to ensure that efficiency and safety are incorporated into work or tasks, and that safety is not viewed as just avoidance of hazards. Guidelines for safety positioning for work activities are provided by the CCOHS (n.d., 1998/2010, 2008) and the NIOSH (Cohen, Gjessing, Fine, Bernard, & McGlothlin, 1997).

Another aspect of injury prevention is ongoing ergonomic education of workers. This entails making employers aware of issues and ensuring that they initiate and continue staff training about appropriate positioning and methodologies for safe, efficient work activity in their particular industry. In this role therapists can either be employed by an industry or act as consultants to industry. Occupational therapists can conduct pre-employment screens, which have been shown to be effective in preventing injuries (Isernhagen, 2009), and they can perform functional capacity assessments that have been effective in indicating work activity limitations. In addition, occupational therapists may recommend what is described as ergonomic equipment. This equipment is useful but should be recommended only after carefully considering the potential benefits and adverse effects of using the equipment, furniture, device, or tool. Evidence shows that many items labeled as "ergonomic" either have proved to be ineffective or are contraindicated, and even the most highly recommended items can be used incorrectly, be the wrong size, or be adjusted inappropriately. An example of poor ergonomics is the provision of computer keyboard wrist pads. If keyboard operators press down on the wrist pad, then they are actually at increased risk for developing CTS (Hedge, 2011).

Occupational therapists in the community should be promoting prevention of injuries by offering educational programs at area businesses and to various industries covering various topics:

- General ergonomics
- Office ergonomics for the computer workstation
- On-site exercise and stretching programs for workers before, during, and after a work shift
- Prevention of cumulative trauma disorders
- Proper body mechanics and prevention of low back pain

Comprehensive Work-Related Ergonomic Evaluation: Worker Assessment

The assessment of the client who needs to return to work is critical. Initially the occupational therapist should conduct an occupational profile (AOTA, 2008). The Canadian Occupational Performance Measure (COPM) is useful to discover the client's perspective on important issues, performance ratings, and satisfaction with performance (Law et al., 2005). Assessment should include the use of an evidence-based functional capacity assessment. Evaluating the areas of occupation identified in the *Framework* (AOTA, 2008) can also be useful. Many practitioners also include lists of activities they deem relevant to the client's functional status. While conducting an occupational profile, it is important to elicit the client's perception about his or her occupational performance. A list of activity demands and occupations that can be helpful to review in this process is presented in Table 16-6.

Objective Assessment

The objective assessment needs to include observations of items reported by the client as issues in ADLs, IADLs, and work-related activities. An occupational therapist should evaluate the problem area to identify which activity demands and performance skills are deficient. An evidence-based functional capacity assessment should be used to gather accurate, objective assessment data. A number of functional capacity assessment systems claim to be accurate, valid, and have good inter-rater reliability; however, the operational definitions in these assessments use many terms interchangeably (Soer, van der Schans, Groothoff, Geertzen, & Reneman, 2008).

The Physical Work Performance Evaluation (PWPE) and the West-Epic (lifting-capacity section only) systems have been evaluated for inter-rater reliability with results published in peer-reviewed journals (King, Tuckwell, & Barret, 1998). Other systems frequently used (Matheson, 2003) include:

- Blankenship System Functional Capacity Evaluation©

Table 16-6	**Activity Demands and Occupations to Review with an Ergonomic Client During an Occupational Profile**
Activity Demands and Occupations	**Occupational Performance (client's self-report)**
Lift	
Carry	
Push/Pull	
Stand	
Walk	
Cook	
Clean	
Vacuum	
Wash and Dry Laundry	
Garden	
Use Stairs	
Dress	
Reach Up	
Reach Down	
Sit	
Other Information	
Work History	
Other Medical Problems	
Additional Information	

- Ergo Science Physical Work Performance Evaluation©
- ERGOS Work Simulator©
- Isenhagen Functional Capacity Assessment©
- Key Method Functional Capacity Assessment©
- LIDO WorkSET Work Simulator©
- Matheson Work Capacity Evaluation©
- Work Hab©

Analysis of occupational performance is completed during a functional capacity assessment to identify the client's assets, establish goals, and implement an intervention plan. Occupational therapists should ensure that they have the needed training or certification to use an assessment in any practice area, including community ergonomics.

Work Location Assessment

Review of the work environment, physical demands, task factors, perceptual requirements, and mental demands at the jobsite is important. The work environment includes the following factors: purpose of work, layout of work area, dimensions, seating, displays and dials, controls, handheld equipment, climate, lighting, noise, vibration, hazardous exposure, protective clothing requirements, floors, stairs, ramps, time of day, social interaction, training, and distractions. The potential physical demands include standing, walking, sitting, lifting, carrying, pushing, pulling, climbing, balancing, stooping, crouching, kneeling, twisting, turning, crawling, handling/manipulating, and reaching to a variety of heights. Task factors include the required postures, required mobility, frequency of activity, duration of activity, workload, work/rest pattern, range of motion requirements, and force requirements. The perceptual requirements include vision, sensation, audition, balance, smell, and taste. The mental demands include information processing, decision making, maintaining or enhancing knowledge and skills, and the potentially draining impact if the job is monotonous. A work assessment should be structured to provide an evaluation of all activity factors within the work location being assessed. An example of items for standing, sitting, driving, lifting, and carrying is provided in Box 16-2.

Occupational Therapy Intervention Evidence

Interventions for work-related injuries have not been well researched; thus evidence of effectiveness is limited. However, efforts have begun to address this issue. For example, Guzelkucuk et al. (2007) reported that the use of simulated ADL activities was more effective in treating acute hand injuries than traditional exercise alone. However, Amini (2011) reports gaps in evidence for the use of techniques such as physical agent modalities, splints, and workplace modifications. Bohr (2011, p. 27), when reporting evidence on elbow injury intervention, states, "the findings support the need for OT practitioners to collect and analyze data related to all aspects of occupational therapy, particularly as interventions affect functional outcomes."

| Box 16-2 | Work Assessment, Jobsite Analysis |

1. Standing:
   a. Required: *Either yes or no to do the job safely and normally. If no, put "not applicable."*
   b. Frequency: *How much time or percentage of shift.*
   c. Rest periods: *How many? And when?*
   d. Type of floor: *Surface such as vinyl, concrete, carpet, etc.*
   e. Work task(s): *The tasks actually performed in the standing position.*
2. Sitting:
   a. Required: *Either yes or no to do the job safely and normally. If no, put "not applicable."*
   b. Duration: *The amount of time before a break is taken.*
   c. Location: *Place the person is sitting. Sitting height and proximity to other work equipment. If the prime role is at a computer workstation, a more detailed evaluation, such as the computer workstation evaluation, should be carried out.*
3. Driving:
   a. Required: *Either yes or no to do the job safely and normally. If no, put "not applicable."*
   b. Duration at work: *The amount of time before a break is taken. Do note if much stop-start driving is done, such as by a delivery driver. Time and approximate distance driven.*
   c. Duration to get to work: *Time and approximate distance driven.*
   d. Type of vehicle: *Size and type of vehicle driven.*
4. Lifting:
   a. Required: *Either yes or no to do the job safely and normally. If no, put "not applicable."*
   b. Maximum weight: *The most lifted during normal work routine measured with a bathroom scale, spring scale, or exertional scale.*
   c. Frequency: *How much time or percentage of shift.*
   d. Average weight: *Routine amount of weight lifted measured with a bathroom scale, spring scale, or exertional scale, if possible; if not, ask how much items weigh or, as a last resort, estimate the weight.*
   e. Bilateral lifting: *Lifting using both hands together to lift, such as in lifting a box; weight measured with a bathroom scale, spring scale, or exertional scale.*
   f. Body mechanics required: *Note if normal good upright positioning can be used and also if there are any awkward work positions required to carry out the job. Include the horizontal distance away from the body as a measurement from between the ankles to the object, and also the vertical measurement either with a tape measure or the body as a guide so vertical reaching may be from knee level to shoulder, or shoulder to above head height.*
   g. Work task(s): *Tasks actually performed naming the object being lifted.*
5. Carrying: *Walking with an object such as a bucket.*
   a. Required: *Either yes or no to do the job safely and normally. If no, put "not applicable."*
   b. Duration: *The amount of time before a break is taken.*
   c. Frequency: *How much time or percentage of shift.*
   d. Type of object(s): *Name and or describe object(s).*
   e. Weight of object(s): *Actually weigh the object(s) with a bathroom scale, spring scale, or exertional scale if possible; if not, ask how much they weigh or, as a last resort, estimate the weight.*
   f. Distance: *Vertical height of lift and horizontal distance.*
   g. Work task(s): *Tasks actually performed, naming the object being carried.*

Return to Work and Work Modification

Returning an injured worker to the job should be done as soon as possible. Research has shown that after 12 weeks of disability only 50% of workers return to the job and after one year of disability 85% do not return to work (Basich, Driscoll, & Wickstrom, 2007). Ergonomic intervention and work site accommodations make it possible for a worker to return to the job sooner and be productive. If a client has been injured or sick, a successful return to work is dependent upon multiple factors to ensure that the individual is able to work safely and productively in the workplace. If at all possible, an early return to work is most beneficial to keep the client in the habit of going to work. The work may have to be reduced to part time or modified to light work duties. The worker's initial activity tolerance would be ascertained from a work assessment by the occupational therapist, and if needed, some clinic-based work hardening activity should be instituted. Work modifications could include the initial alteration in hours at work with a program to progressively increase them. Duties at work may be altered or the equipment used may be adapted to better fit the client. Issues of cognitive challenges and psychosocial stress also must be addressed at this time.

According to Basich et al. (2007), the transitional model of return to work has significant advantages over the traditional medical/clinical model of return to work programs. The **transitional return to work model** is a job-specific intervention approach that increases the worker's functional capacities, teaches safe work methods to prevent reinjury, and provides and modifies job accommodations as needed. When this model is used, injured workers go back to work to get well. Services are provided at the jobsite instead of in medical facilities. The transitional return to work model involves a job analysis and thorough evaluation of the worker. Job tasks are then assigned based on what the worker is capable of performing safely and productively. Safe performance means that the work will not cause re-injury, so work activities are assessed in light of the specific injury. Productive work duties are those that contribute to the needs of the employer and the purpose of the job position. Some job tasks are also therapeutic and may improve strength, endurance, and flexibility. Identification of the job tasks that the worker is not capable of performing also is important. This information can be used to guide intervention planning. An effective intervention usually consists of three elements: therapy services provided at the jobsite, participation in work tasks that have therapeutic benefit, and job accommodations.

An important component of successfully carrying out work activity is ensuring that work space reach can be accomplished with ease and without excess repetition. For example, work done in a standing position should use these guidelines (CCOHS, 2008, "What is an Example of a Workstation," ¶ 2):

- Precision work, such as writing or electronic assembly, should be positioned approximately 5 cm above elbow height and elbow support should be provided.
- Light work, such as assembly line or mechanical jobs, requires that the work be positioned about 5–10 cm below elbow height.
- Heavy work that demands downward force should be positioned from 20–40 cm below elbow height.

Computer Equipment and Accessories

Computers have become such an integral part of time spent at work and at home that safe use of them is key for the health of a large proportion of the population. The use of the computer workstation is about much more than the computer alone; the use of all of the accessories present in a work or home office context affects function and comfort. Therefore, the positioning and accessibility of the document holder, telephone, stapler, hole puncher, tape dispenser, and any other frequently used tool are just as important as the aspects of computer ergonomics. Those individuals using a phone frequently should use a lightweight phone headset to avoid poor head and neck positioning. The traditional computer workstation can be adjusted to fit well to the client to ensure good positioning. There are numerous Web sites that provide ergonomic recommendations, such as the USDL, OSHA (n.d.), and CCOHS (1998/2010, 2008).

Laptop/Notebook Computer Issues

Marked increase in use of laptop/notebook computers has created a major problem, because the vast majority of laptop/notebook computer screens and keyboards are not able to be separated. This means that either the keyboard or the screen is being used in an inappropriate position unless a docking station or separate keyboard is used to address this issue. University of California at Berkeley

(2007) provides some very good information through its Ergonomics@Work program.

Program Development and Business Consultation

As noted earlier in this chapter, community ergonomic practice is situated in the community. It can include interventions with individuals and consultations with groups, agencies, governments, businesses, organizations, and communities. Whereas occupational therapy ergonomic practice often focuses on the individual worker, growing numbers of practitioners are using this expertise to provide services at the community level. Examples include providing ergonomic consultative services at a university (Scaffa et al., 2010) and for an engineering firm (Goodman et al., 2005). Using the steps outlined in Chapters 5–7 in this text, together with knowledge of the specific mission and needs of a community business (or other institutions) as well as current and sufficient expertise in ergonomics, occupational therapists can provide community ergonomic consultation that improves productivity and social participation.

Conclusion

Community ergonomics can positively affect clients at work or at home during ADLs, IADLs, and leisure activities. The ergonomics movement primarily grew out of increased knowledge of human factors and physical limitations in the workplace. Although these characteristics are important, occupational therapists must have knowledge of factors other than physical limitations, such as psychosocial and cognitive dimensions of work. As modern technology continues to change not only the work environment but also the tools used to accomplish that work, the role of ergonomics and the use of ergonomic principles will become even more significant. Advances in health care and life expectancy make it possible for older adults to continue to work at advanced ages, either by choice or because of economic conditions, and underscores the increasing need for occupational therapy ergonomic practitioners. The future for community occupational therapy practice absolutely must include knowledge and application of ergonomics to individuals, businesses, government agencies, and other institutions.

CASE STUDIES

CASE STUDY 16•1 Sandy

Sandy, a 35-year-old woman, was diagnosed with CTS in her right, dominant hand. For the 10 years prior to this diagnosis she had worked in a variety of clerical positions, using a computer for the majority of the workday. Approximately one year before her diagnosis, she received a promotion that she reported increased her workload considerably, making it essential for her to take work home to complete the work her employer expected her to perform.

Sandy described her workstation and reported that she would like her work situation to be evaluated because she was sure it was not set up correctly for her small stature. At work she used a laptop/notebook computer in a docking station, which she stated is set up like a regular computer workstation. She reported that her computer workstation has a nice chair, but the chair seems not to fit her well. She also indicated that nobody has instructed her in how to adjust the chair correctly. At home she uses the laptop/notebook computer placed on a dining room table.

Sandy reported that she had seen a hand surgeon, who remarked that if her current symptoms worsen, it would be necessary to carry out a surgical release of the flexor retinaculum to remove pressure from the median nerve, which is causing considerable pain on the palmer surface of her right hand. The client stated that she told the doctor she did not want surgery unless it was absolutely essential. Her hand surgeon gave her a cortisone injection and referred her to occupational therapy. He also referred her for nerve conduction studies. The occupational therapy referral requested an evaluation of her symptoms; wrist cock-up splinting; a computer workstation evaluation, specific to CTS; therapeutic exercises; and precautionary and preventative education.

Continued

Sandy completed the COPM with her occupational therapist. She reported that the pain was worst at night and at work; she also reported having difficulty sleeping, feeling overwhelmed at work, and feeling inadequate to perform her current job. She had missed work on three separate occasions due to her symptoms in the recent past, had been absent from work for the last two days, and was in the process of submitting a claim for workers' compensation. Her COPM importance scores were all high, and her performance and satisfaction scores were all relatively low. During the completion of the COPM, she reported her major problems to be difficulty sleeping and completing work tasks; she noted that she was bothered by feelings of inadequacy at work and difficulties carrying out routine ADLs due to pain in her right wrist. Cognitively, she reported she could not cope with the complexity of her work since her promotion and believed she was less than competent at her job. She could not see a way of overcoming her work performance deficits.

In addition to the COPM, her physical function was assessed, and education and a splint were provided. Active range of motion was within normal limits in the right hand, wrist, and elbow. Tinel's test and Phalen's test were both positive. Her sensation testing had positive finding in the right median nerve distribution, and she had stereognosis deficits. Her grip and pinch strengths were slightly lower in the right hand than the left. A right wrist splint was fabricated and fitted; a schedule for splint wearing and positioning information to enable her to sleep more comfortably were also provided. In addition, Sandy was instructed in tendon gliding and median nerve gliding exercises.

A computer work assessment was carried out at her work location, and her chair and other workstation devices were adjusted to fit well. In addition, the following items were requested to ensure a good fit at her workstation:

- Foot rest
- Back support filler (Obus-Forme cushion)
- Document holder
- Phone headset

The computer wrist pad in front of her keyboard was removed because she was pressing down on it very firmly. She was educated about the importance of positioning the whole upper extremity to gain as good a position as possible without placing excess pressure on the palmer surface of her hand in the region of the flexor retinaculum.

Education was provided with handouts to reinforce the importance of proper positioning at work and home. Educational materials were also provided regarding easy adaptations to make at home to correct the screen height of her laptop/notebook computer and on the use of a separate keyboard and mouse. A consultation with her work supervisor occurred, and he reported that he was not aware of the client's concerns. He noted that he would provide instruction to the client and intended to send her to two training courses to enable her to feel more competent in her new role. He reported that she was a good worker and capable of carrying out the work in her new job role. The occupational therapist discussed with Sandy the difficulties with routine ADLs by reviewing the tasks she reported to be difficult or those that caused pain. The tasks reported as most difficult were opening cans with a manual can opener and lifting heavy pots and pans. Ways to avoid aggravating her injury were discussed, and it was suggested she use an electric can opener and avoid lifting heavy pans when cooking.

After 3 weeks of intervention, the client was reassessed and her COPM findings were much improved, so intervention was discontinued. She had returned to work one week prior to discharge and was managing much better at work using her modified workstation location. She reported that she was pleased that she was scheduled to complete training courses at work. She had tried using her laptop at home on a box with a separate keyboard and mouse and had found this much better than using the laptop/notebook alone. After doing her exercises at home, she had completed some of her routine ADLs and was now managing all routine ADL and IADL tasks without difficulty when using the suggested modified methods and electronic equipment.

CASE STUDY 16•1 Discussion Questions

1. What was the impact of ergonomic interventions on Sandy's work, leisure, ADL, and IADL performance?
2. How do the overall framework, constructs, and principles of a theoretical model match the interventions provided?

Learning Activities

1. Compare and contrast how ergonomics could affect a work situation from biomechanical, cognitive, and psychosocial perspectives.
2. Identify the work sites at your college, university, or institution that could benefit from an ergonomic consultation.
3. Review the safety and ergonomic concerns of a significant local industry to become aware of possible injuries in this industry and prevention methods.

REFERENCES

Accreditation Council for Occupational Therapy Education. (2009). *Accreditation council for occupational therapy education standards (ACOTE ®) and interpretative guidelines.* Retrieved from http://aota.org/Educate/Accredit/StandardsReview/guide/42369.aspx

American Occupational Therapy Association. (2008). Occupational therapy practiceframework: Domain and process (2nd ed.). *American Journal of Occupational Therapy, 62,* 625–683.

Amini, D. (2011). Occupational therapy interventions for work-related injuries of the forearm, wrist and hand: A systematic review. *American Journal of Occupational therapy, 65*(1), 29–36.

Basich, M., Driscoll, T., & Wickstrom, R. (2007). Transitional work therapy on site: Work is therapy. *Professional Case Management, 12*(6), 351–355.

Bohr, P. C. (2011). Systemic review and analysis of work-related injuries to and conditions of the elbow. *American Journal of Occupational Therapy, 65*(1), 24–28.

Canadian Center for Occupational Health and Safety. (n.d.). *Office ergonomics.* Retrieved from http://oshcanada.com/oshanswers/ergonomics/office/#tphp

Canadian Center for Occupational Health and Safety. (1998/2010). *Working in a sitting position: Basic information.* Retrieved from http://ccohs.ca/oshanswers/ergonomics/sitting/sitting_overview.html

Canadian Center for Occupational Health and Safety. (2008). *Working from a standing position: Basic information.* Retrieved from http://ccohs.ca/oshanswers/ergonomics/standing/standing_basic.html

Center for Universal Design. (2010). *Ronald L. Mace.* Retrieved from North Carolina State University, College of Design Web Site: http://ncsu.edu/project/design-projects/udi/cente-for-universal-design/ron-mace/

Chaffin, D. B., Andersson, G., & Martin, B. J. (1984). *Occupational biomechanics* (4th ed.). New York, NY: Wiley.

Chapanis, A. (1991). To communicate the human factors message, you have to know what the message is and how to communicate it. *Human Factors Society Bulletin, 34*(11), 1–4.

Cohen, A. L., Gjessing, C. C., Fine, L. J., Bernard, B. P., & McGlothlin, J. D. (1997). Toolbox tray 6-A: Recommended workstation measurements. In *Elements of ergonomics programs: A primer based on workplace evaluations of musculoskeletal disorders.* National Institute for Occupational Safety and Health: Atlanta, GA. Retrieved from http://cdc.gov/niosh/docs/97-117/eptbtr6a.html

Connell, B. R., Jones, M., Mace, R., Mueller, J., Mullick, A., Ostroff, E., Sanford, J., Steinfeld, E., Story, M., & Vanderheiden, G. (1997). *The principles of universal design.* Retrieved from http://ncsu.edu/www/ncsu/design/sod5/cud/about_ud/udprinciplestext.htm

Cornell University Human Factors Group. (1996). *Performance oriented ergonomic checklist for computer (VDT) workstations.* Retrieved from http://ergo.human.cornell.edu/CUVDTChecklist.html

Ergoweb Inc. (2011a). *Concepts.* Retrieved from http://ergoweb.com/resources/faq/concepts.cfm

Ergoweb Inc. (2011b). *History of ergonomics.* Retrieved from http://ergoweb.com/resources/reference/history.cfm

Franco, G. (1999). Ramazzini and workers' health. *Lancet, 354,* 858–61.

Goodman, G., Landis, J., George, C., McGuire, S., Shorter, C., Sieminski, M., & Wilson, T. (2005). Effectiveness of computer ergonomics interventions for an engineering company: A program evaluation. *Work, 24,* 53–62.

Guzelkucuk, U., Duman, I., Taskaynaynatan, M. A., & Dincer, K. (2007). Comparison of therapeutic activities with therapeutic exercises in the rehabilitation of young adult patients with hand injuries. *Journal of Hand Surgery, 32(a)*, 1429–1435.

Hedge, A. (2011). *Cornell University: Ergonomic guidelines for arranging a computer workstation—10 steps for users.* Retrieved from http://ergo.human.cornell.edu/ergoguide.html

Internet Center for Management and Business Administration. (2010) *Frederick Taylor and scientific management.* Retrieved from http://netmba.com/mgmt/scientific/

Isernhagen, S. J. (2009). Functional capacity testing: What's new? What's different? *Rehab Management: The Interdisciplinary Journal of Rehabilitation, 22*(9), 20–23.

Jacobs, K. (1999). *Ergonomics for therapists* (2nd ed.). Boston, MA: Butterworth-Heinemann.

King, P. M., Tuckwell, N., & Barret, T. E. (1998). A critical review of functional capacity evaluations. *Physical Therapy, 78*(8), 852–866.

Law, M., Cooper, B., Strong, S., Stewart, D., Rigby, P., & Letts, L. (1996). The person-environment-occupation model: A transactive approach to occupational performance. *Canadian Journal of Occupational Therapy, 63*(1), 9–23.

Law, M., Baptiste, S., Carswell, A., McColl, M. A., Polatajko, H., & Pollock, N. (2005). *Canadian Occupational Performance Measure* (4th ed., pp. 1–5). Ottawa, ON: CAOT Publications ACE.

Littleton, M. (2003). Cost effectiveness of a prework screening program for the University of Illinois: Chicago physical plant. *Work 21*(3), 243–50.

Matheson, L. (2003). The functional capacity evaluation. In G. Andersson, S. Demeter, & G. Smith (Eds.), *Disability evaluation* (2nd ed., pp. 18–22). Chicago, IL: Mosby Yearbook.

Miracle League. (2008). *Home.* Retrieved from http://miracleleague.com/

National Institute for Occupational Safety and Health. (1997). *Chapter 7: Work-related musculoskeletal disorders and psychosocial factors.* Retrieved from http://cdc.gov/niosh/docs/97-141/pdfs/97-141g.pdf

National Institute for Occupational Safety and Health. (2009). *Delivering on the nation's investment in worker safety and health.* Retrieved from http://cdc.gov/niosh/docs/2009-144/pdfs/2009-144.pdf

NexGen Ergonomics. (2008). *Ergointelligence Upper Extremity Assessment.* Retrieved from http://nexgenergo.com/ergonomics/ergointeluea.html

OXO International. (2006). *Our roots.* Retrieved from http://oxo.com/oxo/about_roots.htm

Sauter, S. L., & Swanson, N. G. (1996). Psychological aspects of musculoskeletal disorders in office work. In S. Moon & S. Sauter (Eds.), *Psychosocial factors and musculoskeletal disorders* (pp. 3–21). London: Taylor and Francis.

Scaffa, M. E., Chromiak, S. B., Reitz, S. M., Blair-Newton, A., Murphy, L., & Wallis, C. B. (2010). Unintentional injury and violence prevention. In M. E. Scaffa, S. M. Reitz, & M. A. Pizzi (Eds.), *Occupational therapy in the promotion of health and wellness* (pp. 350–375). Philadelphia, PA: F.A. Davis.

Sensory Trust. (n.d.). *Oizumi Ryokuchi Park, Osaka, Japan.* Retrieved from http://sensorytrust.org.uk/information/greenspace/japan.html

Soer, R., van der Schans, C. P., Groothoff, J. W., Geertzen, J. H., & Reneman, M. F. (2008).Towards consensus in operational definitions in functional capacity evaluation: A Delphi study. *Journal of Occupational Rehabilitation, 18(4)*, 389–400.

University of California at Berkeley, University Health Services, Tang Center, Ergonomics Program for Faculty and Staff. (2007). *Ergonomic tips for laptop users.* Retrieved from http://uhs.berkeley.edu/facstaff/pdf/ergonomics/laptop.pdf

U. S. Department of Labor, Bureau of Labor Statistics. (2010a). *Injuries, illnesses, and fatalities.* Retrieved from http://bls.gov/iif/oshsum.htm

U. S. Department of Labor, Bureau of Labor Statistics. (2010b). *Nonfatal occupational injuries and illnesses requiring days away from work, 2009* [Press release]. Retrieved from http://bls.gov/news.release/osh2.htm

U. S. Department of Labor, Occupational Safety and Health Administration. (n d.). Computer workstations: Good working positions. Retrieved from http://osha.gov/SLTC/etools/computerworkstations/positions.html

Waters, T. R. (2007). When is it safe to manually lift a patient? *American Journal of Nursing, 107*(8), 53–58.

Waters, T. R., Putz-Anderson, V., & Garg, A. (1994). *Application manual for revised NIOSH lifting equation.* Retrieved from http://cdc.gov/niosh/docs/94-110/pdfs/94-110.pdf

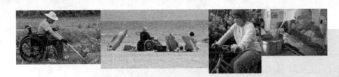

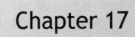

Chapter 17

Work and Career Transitions

Susan M. Nochajski, PhD, OTR/L, and S. Maggie Reitz, PhD, OTR/L, FAOTA

Real success is finding your lifework in the work that you love.

—David McCullough

Learning Objectives

This chapter is designed to enable the reader to:
- Describe the role of federal legislation in the employment of persons with disabilities.
- Identify trends within occupational therapy that influence work transitions.
- Formulate plans to address issues related to transition to work by students with disabilities.
- Identify issues related to return to work by persons with disabilities, including those of returning warriors.
- Facilitate individual and group transition to partial employment and retirement.
- Describe the role of the occupational therapy practitioner in various aspects of work transition and work transition programs.

Key Terms

Americans with Disabilities Act (ADA)
Individuals with Disabilities Education Act
School to Work Opportunities Act
Secretaries Commission on Achieving Necessary Skills (SCANS)
Self-determination

Ticket to Work and Work Incentives Improvement Act of 1999
Transition
Warrior Transition Unit
Work and Careers Opportunities Program (WCOP)

Introduction

All individuals experience transitions in a variety of areas throughout their life span. **Transition** can be described as a process of change or movement from one place, situation, or context to another. Work transitions include transitioning into and out of the workplace. It can include the transition of youth with disabilities from school to employment or the transition of people returning to or starting work following a disability, injury, or illness. Other types of work transition include wounded warriors returning to post-military service employment as well as older adults transitioning from the workforce to retirement.

The transition of persons with disabilities into or out of community employment is an important societal issue that can be addressed by occupational therapy. Data indicate that approximately 78% of adults between 18 and 64 years of age are employed, compared with only 37% of persons with disabilities; employment rates are even lower for individuals with severe disabilities (Long-Bellil & Henry, 2009; Wehman, 2001). Current economic conditions exacerbate the problem for students with disabilities transitioning into work roles and for persons with disabilities who want to return to work. Potential lifetime costs due to a lack of vocational skills and subsequent unemployment or low employment rates include lower wages and increased dependence on social programs (Lehr, 2004; Wagner & Cameto, 2004).

The American Occupational Therapy Association (AOTA) *Occupational Therapy Practice Framework* (AOTA, 2008) guides both the domain and process of occupational therapy practice. Within the context of the *Framework,* work is identified as a primary domain of occupational therapy practice. In conjunction with the *Framework,* several pieces of federal legislation, such as the Individuals with Disabilities Education Act (IDEA), provide a basis for the vital role occupational therapy practitioners can play in facilitating various work transitions. In this chapter, information on key issues related to various types of work transition and the relevance or connection to community-based occupational therapy practice is provided.

Transitioning From School to Employment

For adolescents and young adults, the transition from high school to employment or post-secondary education is very significant (Orentlicher & Michaels, 2000). However, transitioning from secondary schools to adult roles remains problematic for many students with disabilities; school to work transitioning has been far from optimal for many of these students. Statistics indicate that students with disabilities have significantly less successful outcomes related to employment rates and retention, advancement in employment, independent living, and community participation than students without disabilities (Kohler & Field, 2003; Wagner & Davis; 2006; Wagner, Newman, Cameto, Levine, & Garza, 2006). Growing numbers of students with disabilities are exiting the public school system without the occupational skills needed to succeed in entry-level jobs. Due to an increase in high-performance businesses across the nation, there is also an increasing demand for employees with a combination of academic and occupational skills (Benz, Yovanoff, & Doren, 1997).

Federal legislation has been enacted in an effort to improve the school to work transition outcomes of students with disabilities. Aspects of the **Individuals with Disabilities Education Act** and its subsequent amendments (IDEA 1990, 1997, 2004) that have a relationship to school to work transition are briefly discussed.

The Education for All Handicapped Children Act of 1975 (PL 94-142) was the first enacted federal legislation mandating educational services, particularly a free and appropriate public education, for all children regardless of their disability status. However, it was not until 1990 with the passage of the IDEA (PL 101-476) that transition services were mandated. With its subsequent amendments (IDEA 1997, 2004), there has been a greater emphasis placed on transition planning and services for students with disabilities and the utilization of related service providers, including occupational therapists. Transition from secondary education was a particularly strong component of the IDEA 1997, which mandated that transition planning in the Individualized Education Program (IEP) process was to begin at the time of the student's 14th birthday; this has since been changed to age 16 in IDEA 2004.

Role of Occupational Therapy in School to Work Transition

Occupational therapists are related service personnel who possess skills and knowledge that can be very beneficial to the secondary transition process. Although occupational therapy practitioners have the skills necessary to support their involvement in school to work transition programs, a relatively small percentage are involved in the actual provision of transition services (Kardos & White, 2005; Spencer, Emery, & Schneck, 2003; Swinth, Chandler, Hanft, Jackson, & Shepard, 2003). Spencer and colleagues (2003) reported that occupational therapists provided only about 3.3% to 11.7 % of the services for school to work transition. Two reasons provided for the lack of involvement of occupational therapy in transition planning and delivery included a lack of demand from parents or teachers and a lack of understanding of the role that occupational therapists could play. This lack of understanding was demonstrated by educators and related service personnel, including occupational therapists.

The potential role of occupational therapy in school to work transition appears to be poorly understood by a majority of school-based occupational therapists. Kardos and White (2005) surveyed 80 occupational therapists who worked in secondary transition on their knowledge of and degree of participation in secondary transition planning. The majority of respondents indicated that they understood the terminology of the 1990 and 1997 IDEA amendments but reported minimal participation in secondary transition planning, assessment, and intervention. Their involvement in secondary transition was more frequent in relation to working with students pursuing post-secondary education (20%) than with those students pursuing post-secondary employment (16%). Overall, only 30% of the respondents indicated that they thought their involvement with transition service maximized their professional skills and abilities in any area of secondary transition.

Spencer et al. (2003) noted that occupational therapists need to explore expansion of their current roles to more fully utilize their skills and qualifications to improve secondary transitioning. Students with disabilities require more than a transition program focusing on work skills to enable them to have successful transition outcomes. They may need assistance with activities of daily living, instrumental activities of daily living, communication and social skills, emotional regulation skills, and cognitive skills, all of which are areas within the domain of occupational therapy practice (AOTA, 2008). A community-based school to work transition program developed by occupational therapists is discussed below.

Community-Based School to Work Transition Programs

Several model programs have been developed to assist schools in the development and implementation of transition programs and services for students with disabilities. However, relatively few of these programs have had occupational therapy practitioners as primary program developers or an occupation-based focus on school to work transition.

School to Work Transitions Program

The School to Work Transitions Program was developed through a 4-year model demonstration project funded by the U.S. Department of Education (Nochajski, Schweitzer, & Chelluri, 2003). This program was developed by occupational therapists and included a significant role for occupational therapy in a transition program for students classified as having emotional and behavioral disabilities (EBD). The program ensured that children with EBD had educational and vocational training opportunities to obtain necessary skills for work and adult roles. Three components of the **School to Work Opportunities Act** of 1994 provided the

foundation for the program: school-based learning and activities, community-based learning and activities, and linking or connecting activities. The program was also based on self-determination and identified best practices related to school to work transition.

Self-determination can be described as a set of behaviors that includes skills such as decision making, problem solving, goal setting and attainment, self-observation and awareness, self-instruction, self-advocacy and leadership, positive attitudes about outcomes, and internal self-control (Blancher, 2004; Browder, Wood, Test, Karvonen, & Algozzine, 2001; Wehmeyer, Agran, & Hughes, 2000). Activities incorporating these characteristics of self-determination were embedded within the program.

The program also was based on best practices suggested by Sample (1998) and Kohler's Taxonomy for Transition Planning (1996). Sample (1998) identified six best practices that were correlated with positive post-school employment outcomes for youth with disabilities. These practices included:

1. vocational intervention;
2. paid work experience;
3. social skills training;
4. interagency collaboration;
5. parent involvement; and
6. individualized planning.

Kohler's taxonomy was used to provide a conceptual framework for the program model. Similar to Sample's best practices, the conceptual framework used includes the following four components: student development, student-focused planning, family involvement, and interagency collaboration.

Student-focused planning and student development are primary features of the program. Successful transition outcomes for students with disabilities, particularly employment in an area related to students' interests, is the paramount theme toward which all program activities were directed. School-based and work activities were developed taking the interests and needs of the students into account. Student development is a core feature of the model and is exemplified in all phases of the project. Likewise, family involvement must be viewed as an important aspect of the transition process (Chadsey-Rusch & Rusch, 1996) and is another important component of the program.

Collaboration, both interagency and interdisciplinary, is essential in order to facilitate successful transition outcomes. This program had a strong focus on collaboration between the university, school personnel, and community businesses as well as between students, families, and program personnel.

The program consisted of four sequential phases of training and work-related experiences, which are depicted in Table 17-1. Each phase was approximately 10 weeks in length with weekly activities totaling approximately 10 hours. Students were expected to use and generalize the skills learned in previous phases. In the last phase, the on-site role of the job coach faded as the student gained self-respect by performing the job independently. In place of the job coach, the student now took direction from an employed supervisor (i.e., boss). However, if the student was not ready for independent work, he or she could continue with the supported work experience and utilize the assistance of a job coach while making gains toward the goal of competitive employment.

Overall, the program was highly effective in helping students with EBD obtain employment. Over 70% of the participants were employed in a variety of positions after completing the program. They reported satisfaction with the program, and employers were extremely satisfied with their productivity. This program was developed and implemented with students with EBDs who attended an educational day program. After the grant funding ended, the agency hired an occupational therapist to continue the program.

Subsequent federal funding was received to revise and evaluate the effectiveness of the program with students with a variety of disabilities who were attending regular education programs in an urban school district. The "new" program was called the **Work and Careers Opportunities Program (WCOP).** The conceptual foundation and overall structure of the WCOP remained the same.

Table 17-1 Phases of the School to Work Transitions Program

Phase	Focus/Activities
Phase 1: School-Based Learning Strategies	Job Acquisition Skills • Completing job applications • Interviewing • Developing community-access strategies • Identifying job interests and aptitudes Identification with Worker Role • Temporal organization • Organization of space and objects Bi-weekly individual and small-group instruction
Phase 2: Volunteer Experience in Community-Based Agency	Assuming Responsibility for Initiation, Continuation, and Termination of Volunteer Tasks Agencies Involved • Community theater • Day-care center • Nursing home • Refugee agency • Habitat for humanity • Retail agencies
Phase 3: Paid, Supported-Work Experience	Supervised by job coach
Phase 4: Acquisition of Paid, Competitive Employment	Supervised by employer

However, skills identified by the **Secretaries Commission on Achieving Necessary Skills (SCANS)** were included as part of the program.

The SCANS has been the leading force in the improvement of work-related skills over the past decade (Packard & Brainard, 2003). The foundation skills and competencies that are necessary for these entry-level positions (Nash & Korte, 1997) were identified by the SCANS. The SCANS initiative was designed to assist students in a successful transition from school to work (Nash & Korte, 1997). Stone and Jossaim (2000) reported that positive work attitudes were consistently linked to participation in jobs where SCANS skills were being developed. The SCANS skills have been successfully incorporated into several vocational exploration programs with excellent results and were included in the WCOP. The SCANS skills include basic skills, thinking skills, personal qualities, identification and appropriate use of resources, interpersonal skills development, information processing, understanding of systems, and using technology.

The effectiveness of the WCOP was evaluated using a randomized control trial. Students in three schools were randomly assigned to either the WCOP intervention group (n=56) or a control group (n=55). The students in the control group did not participate in any specialized transition programs and received general information about transition and transition services from special education personnel. The majority of students in both the WCOP group and the control group had a learning disability. The WCOP was found to be highly effective. Seventy five-percent of the students in the WCOP group were competitively employed post-WCOP versus 9% in the control group. Additionally, 51% of the students in the WCOP group obtained employment within the first 3 months after completion of the program, 19% within 3–6 months, and 3% within 6–9 months. In the WCOP group, 33% of the students sustained their competitive part-time and/or full-time jobs compared with 18% of the students in the control group 6 months after completion of the program. The school district was very satisfied with and interested in continuing the program.

Outcomes from the WCOP Evaluation Study have shown the program to be effective in fostering independence, self-advocacy, self-determination, and post-secondary school and work opportunities for students with disabilities (Nochajski, Nerber, & Patterson, 2008). Similarly, the WCOP is a very good example of the positive role that occupational therapy can play in providing school to work transition services to students with disabilities. However, the WCOP is not readily replicable due to the intensive resources needed for implementation. The WCOP needs to be revised to make it more time and cost-effective and to better address student needs. The program had a paid work experience whereby students were paid a minimum wage stipend through the grant for a total of 80 hours. In order to be sustainable in a school district, the paid work experience might be replaced with additional volunteer activities. However, the stipend was a very strong extrinsic motivator and might be difficult to replace. A focus on health promotion also should be included in the program activities. Students need information related to health and wellness and a better understanding of the impact that health and lifestyle choices made today have on their future employability. These are areas that are within the scope of practice of occupational therapy.

The current economic environment and the potential for layoffs is another topic that needs to be discussed with students in the program. Two students who completed the WCOP were hired in local businesses. They were able to complete the requirements of the job, and the employer was very satisfied with their performance. However, the business needed to downsize, and those employees with the least seniority were laid off. The students had considerable difficulty understanding why they were being let go. This type of situation would be better addressed proactively rather than reactively.

Employers value teamwork, interpersonal skills, and behavior more than traditional work-related skills addressed by high school occupational education curriculums (Allred & Baker, 1997). Transition planning and services must focus on students' strengths and abilities that they will one day try to market to prospective employers (McKenna, 2000). Occupational therapists have the skills and knowledge to do this and can become vital members of the transition team. The case study that appears at the end of this chapter describes a student's experience in the WCOP.

Transitioning to Work Following a Disability

Similar to school to work transition, federal legislation has also been enacted in an effort to facilitate and enable persons with disabilities to return to work. The **Americans with Disabilities Act** (ADA) and its 2008 Amendments and the **Ticket to Work and Work Incentives Improvement Act (TWWIIA) of 1999** have important implications for individuals transitioning to work following a disability.

Stapleton and Burkhauser (2003) view the ADA of 1990 as a driving force in changing disability policy so that individuals with disabilities can become competitively employed rather than relying on various types of disability benefits. The ADA and its reauthorization in 2008 and 2010 protect the civil rights of and prohibit discrimination against workers with disabilities. The ADA also mandates the provision of reasonable accommodations to enable workers with disabilities to be successful in the workplace. The 2010 amendment also clarifies the use of service animals; wheelchairs; manual mobility devices, which include canes, crutches, and walkers; and other types of power-driven mobility devices, such as Segways, which are not designed for the exclusive use of persons with disabilities (Resource Centers on Independent Living, n.d.). Although the purpose of the ADA was well intended, research has suggested that employment rates of persons with disabilities did not increase significantly after the passage of this legislation. One potential reason suggested was that many persons with disabilities were concerned about the loss of benefits, particularly health benefits. Many persons with disabilities, because of the nature of their disability, are able to work only on a part-time basis. However, in many situations, a person must be employed full-time in order to be covered by health insurance plans offered by the employer. The TWWIIA legislation, discussed in greater detail in Chapter 18, was an attempt to address this issue. Under this legislation, persons with disabilities could return to work and continue to receive health care coverage from programs such as Medicaid.

Historically, occupational therapy practitioners have been involved in return to work programs by performing functional capacity evaluations and implementing work hardening programs.

These activities, while focusing on occupation, are typically more rehabilitation center–based than community-based.

In community-based practice focusing on the transition to work by persons with disabilities, there are numerous roles for occupational therapy practitioners, including:

- completing ergonomic evaluations and interventions in the workplace;
- consulting on community and transportation accessibility;
- making recommendations for reasonable accommodations; and
- providing direct service with the individual focusing on the occupational performance areas related to activities of daily living and instrumental activities of daily living.

An increasing number of occupational therapy practitioners are involved in workplace ergonomic evaluations and interventions (AOTA, 2004), which are described in detail in Chapter 16 of this text. Evaluations might include the identification and minimization of factors that contribute to accidents or injury in the workplace. Interventions might focus on modification of tools and equipment, and the provision of education and training on injury prevention.

An accessible community and transportation are necessary in order for a person with a disability to return to work. Although still relatively uncommon, consulting on community and transportation accessibility is an emerging role for occupational therapy practitioners (Iwarsson, Stahl, & Carlsson, 2003).

Occupational therapy practitioners frequently are called upon to make recommendations for workplace accommodations. The Job Accommodation Network (JAN, 2009) is a program under the auspices of the Office of Disability Employment Policy in the U.S. Department of Labor whose major purpose is to facilitate the employment and retention of workers with disabilities. The JAN provides a valuable resource that can be used by occupational therapy practitioners for their own information or to share with persons with disabilities or employers. Through its Web site, JAN addresses physical, cognitive, sensory, and mental conditions and disabilities, including etiology, symptoms, and treatment. Whether or not the disability or condition is covered under the

ADA, numerous examples of accommodations for a variety of disabilities or conditions are included on this Web site. Extensive resources and references are also provided.

Occupational therapy practitioners continue to have a crucial role in providing direct service to persons with disabilities in order to enable them to return to work. Depending on the nature of their disability, people may need assistance or suggestions for activities of daily living (ADLs) related to getting ready for work or instrumental activities of daily living (IADLs) related to getting to work. They might also need assistance with assertiveness and self-advocacy in asking for reasonable accommodations or information on what accommodations might be reasonable to request. These tasks are all within the domain of occupational therapy.

Transitioning to Active Duty or Civilian Employment

Occupational therapy has been actively involved in providing services to military personnel since the early years of the profession (McDaniel, 1968). Beginning in World War I, its practitioners have responded to the reconstruction and rehabilitation needs of injured soldiers, both stateside and abroad. The goal of the reconstruction work in World War I was to enable soldiers to return to either active service or paid employment following discharge from the military. While the majority of occupational therapy practitioners worked in the United States, 55 occupational therapy reconstruction aides were stationed in France and Germany by May 1919 with the American Expeditionary Forces. Their duty was to work with those soldiers most likely to be enabled to transition back to battle or other support roles near but behind the battle lines. The most common injuries of these soldiers included orthopedic cases and neuropsychiatric disorders (McDaniel, 1968). In addition to the services provide at the base hospitals, occupational therapy was carried out experimentally in a neuropsychiatric hospital in the forward area. The experiment lasted only 2 weeks but the medical officer in charge indicated that, through the assistance of workshop treatment, men were returned to duty who had previously been listed for evacuation to base hospitals for further treatment (McDaniel, 1968, p. 90).

A trial program somewhat similar to the one mentioned above in World War I was implemented in Afghanistan in 2010 to provide occupational therapy evaluation and intervention services to military personnel immediately following a mild head injury (Johnson, n.d.). The goals of this program were to facilitate the quick return to action for those soldiers who were medically fit and the evacuation of those in need of a higher level of care (E. Johnson, personal communication, November 21, 2009; Barth, Whitney, & Johnson, 2011).

Increasing attention is being placed on facilitating the transition of military service personnel back to active service or civilian life. Based on the results of a 2007 congressionally mandated review of care for "warriors in transition," 35 **warrior transition units (WTUs)** were developed by the Army to better meet the rehabilitation and vocational training needs of injured soldiers. The WTUs were designed for soldiers who required more than 6 months of medical care and were located close to medical treatment facilities across the United States as well as in a few international locations. The philosophy of the WTUs was to band together in units, a traditional organizational structure in the military, soldiers who have the same duty, to train them in order to return to active military duty or to gain civilian employment (Erickson, Secrest, & Gray, 2008).

Active and reserve duty troops, whether they are deployed in areas of conflict or are based within the United States, are eligible for services provided through WTUs. In 2008, the most common injuries for which soldiers were assigned to a WTU included orthopedic conditions, mainly injuries to the back and knees, "followed by internal and neurological conditions. About 1% of the soldiers have sustained some of the most devastating conditions, such as burns or amputations" (Erickson et al., 2008, p. 11).

Injury rates for traumatic brain injury (TBI) and post-traumatic stress disorder (PTSD) are increasing among soldiers, as are suicide rates, according to U.S. Army data (Table 17-2). These increases have been observed for 5 consecutive years (Starr, 2010; U.S. Army, 2009). There were 115 suicide deaths in 2007 and at least 128 in 2008. In 2009 there were 249 suicides and 1,713 attempted suicides (Starr, 2010; U.S. Army, 2009). Injury rates from TBI and PTSD and the continuing rise in suicides among military personnel indicate an increasing need for transitional services before and during deployment, as well as prior to and following return stateside. While the army has increased its efforts in this area in recent years, civilian occupational therapy practitioners need to be aware of the possibility of groups of wounded warriors in their communities who may no longer be receiving services from the military.

Although occupational therapy interventions for wounded warriors, regardless of their diagnoses, may be similar to those for their civilian counterparts, these individuals also need access to specialized transitional services. Occupational therapy practitioners who wish to seek funding and support for developing such programs in their community must ensure they have an understanding of military lifestyle and culture as well as of resources such as Pets to Vets. This knowledge can be gained through a variety of ways, including:

- communicating via e-mail (e.g., Johnson, n.d.) or Facebook with occupational therapists in the military
- seeking evidence-based articles on interventions with military personnel
- reviewing military Web sites, such as www.army.mil
- reading current related literature
- attending state and national conferences sessions on this population
- volunteering with organizations that provide assistance to veterans

Jimmy Childers, who sustained a leg amputation while serving as a marine in Afghanistan, noted "the toughest thing is not the physical, it's the mental assimilation into society" (quoted by Hendrix, 2011, p. B1). Childers credits his dog, Tidus, with facilitating his assimilation. He received this shelter dog through a program called P2V.org (Pets to Vets). A retired airman named Sharpe established the non-profit program to reduce the time and cost for veterans to access trained service dogs. He thought each could assist the other; "Eighteen vets commit suicide every day in this country, and one animal is put to sleep every eight seconds. They can help save each other" (Sharpe quoted by Hendrix, 2011, p. B1). Programs such as this can be a first step in the transition back to life and work, and could benefit from the skills of occupational therapy practitioners as volunteers.

A variety of initiatives are being developed to meet the needs of wounded warriors. A review of the *Conference Guide* from the 2011 AOTA Conference and Exposition (AOTA, 2011) revealed that at least 10 education sessions or posters were presented at that conference regarding initiatives for wounded warriors. Examples of topics of sessions included post-combat driving anxiety, vision impairments, community reintegration programs, warrior transition units, and outcome measures development for the military population. Articles are also appearing in the occupational therapy literature. Hofmann (2008) reviewed the needs of veterans, and Sheffield (2009) described a joint venture between Scripps Memorial Hospital and Camp Pendleton in California to provide specialized driving services and community mobility services as well as a day treatment program for wounded warriors. The potential to facilitate transitions of military personnel to civilian paid work or volunteer positions is being partially realized but requires expansion; occupational therapy practitioners are well equipped to meet this growing need.

Table 17-2 **TBI and PTSD Rates**		
Reporting Period	**Number of Soldiers in Army Wounded Warrior Program**	**Percentage Diagnosed with TBI or PTSD**
Fall 2008	3,800	38%
Fall 2009	5,200	52%
Spring 2010	6,500	58%

Data from: "Invisible Wounds," by C. Rivero, in "Diagnosis: Battle Wound," by G. Jaffe, 2010, July 18. *Washington Post,* pp. A1, A6–A7.

Transitioning to Retirement

The movie *The Bucket List* (Reiner & Zackham, 2007) drew attention to the need for retirement planning with an eye toward eventual death via a humorous but poignant tale of two strangers' joint exploration of new occupations. The characters, both with terminal illnesses, embarked on a quest to complete as many items on their bucket lists (i.e., "to do" lists before they "kick the bucket") as possible. They gained a sense of mastery and fulfillment through mutually explored occupations. Occupational therapy practitioners are equipped to assist individuals in designing their unique bucket list as part of a comprehensive, occupation-based retirement strategy. In addition, these practitioners can provide strategies for engagement in the chosen occupations where and when adaptations or an alteration of the occupation itself is required. There is no need to await a terminal illness diagnosis to begin preparing a bucket list. In fact, the earlier people start their list, the more likely they are to complete some of the occupations. While there are many possible reasons for individuals or couples to postpone retirement discussions, such as an irrational fear that planning for the future will hasten their death or a desire to ignore the process of aging, a bucket list–style approach may be used as an occupation-based method to introduce the topic. This strategy also could be used by occupational therapy practitioners themselves, to ensure they too "live like you ... [are] dying" (Nichols & Wiseman, 2004). In this section of the chapter, occupation-based retirement will be further discussed, along with the ideas of bridge employment and legacy planning at the employment site.

Occupation-Based Retirement Planning

The need for comprehensive pre-retirement (Cantor, 1981) and retirement planning (Broderick & Glazer, 1983) beyond solely financial planning has been appreciated by occupational therapists for some time. While financial planning is essential for a quality retirement, an activity or occupation engagement plan also is needed. However, the financial planning portion of retirement planning must occur first, as occupation planning will be constrained by the projected financial resources for retirement. The Tactical Activity Planning (TAP) developed by Cantor (1981) can serve as a basis for an updated process based on the occupational profile as outlined in the AOTA *Framework* (2008), Canadian Occupational Performance Measure (Law et al., 2005), or similar client-centered assessment.

Bridge Employment

A phased or graded approach to retirement, known as bridge employment, can aid in the transition to the retirement role. Bridge employment is less than full-time employment in which people engage prior to their full retirement (Feldman, 1994). Zhan, Wang, Liu, and Shultz (2009) found that bridge employees had improved mental health if they continued their employment in the same career and decreased functional limitations if they worked either in their original career or a new career. An occupational therapist may recommend a graded approach to bridge employment, where a person progressively decreases his or her work hours until full retirement. Bridge employment can be a planned reduction in both work hours and responsibility in order to provide for increased time with family, volunteer activities, or other desired occupations.

Individuals may wish to retire but due to unplanned circumstances, such as a disadvantageous financial situation, need to continue bridge employment or full-time work. Given the current and recurring recessions, often employees find themselves continuing to work beyond their planned retirement date due to the impact on retirement savings from financial downturns or the illness or loss of a partner or spouse. While these are painful possibilities, they need to be addressed in both financial and occupation retirement planning. In reality, more than one plan is needed. The first plan is based on the individual or the individual and his or her partner remaining healthy and able to work until their desired time frame for full retirement or bridge employment. The second is a plan that accounts for the possibility that one becomes ill and needs care.

Occupational therapy practitioners can offer community-based retirement planning that comprises both types of plans. In the "ideal" plan, a decision to decrease work hours gradually versus stopping work suddenly might help with the adjustment to the retirement role and allow old habits to support self-identity as new habits or a resumption of old habits is formalized. In the second or "contingency" plan, having a relationship with an employer as a successful part-time employee or being known as someone who is available to fill in for others' vacations may be helpful if a return to work for financial reasons is needed.

In both plans, the possibility of future limitations should be taken into consideration. After a bucket list or occupation "to do" list is formed, the occupations should be ranked in order of desired performance based on financial cost, time needed, available resources, and energy expenditure. Possible questions to help prioritize the list include the following:

- Which occupations may be better to complete while having employer provided health insurance or when you can afford travel insurance?
- Which occupations can be done while working part-time?
- Which occupations are likely to experience a future increase in financial cost to the point where they become cost prohibitive?
- Which occupations can be graded, with the more strenuous options completed at an earlier age?

For example, if hiking is a favorite lifetime occupation, list all the hikes the person wants to undertake and their associated costs. Then, place those hikes that require more physical effort (and possibly more money) earlier on the list. Also ask questions such as "Are any of the hikes close to places where you may attend a business meeting or a conference in the future?" This type of questioning helps fiscal decision making. This activity analysis can be very helpful in assisting people in being strategic in their pre-retirement and retirement occupation planning.

Legacy Planning in Employment and Volunteer Settings

In many ways, legacy planning is a type of phased retirement. It is simply projecting when one wants to no longer be responsible for specific roles or tasks, and then working with the appropriate people in the organization proactively to ensure a smooth transition. The eventual transition can be eased by ensuring that the individuals who will be assigned the work tasks in the future are oriented to them while the expert is still available for questions and guidance. This type of planning may make it easier for individuals to leave roles and not feel they need to stay to protect the work or volunteer unit. Erickson's developmental stage of older adults referred to as generativity has been shown to be met through bridge employment (Dendinger, Adams, & Jacobson, 2005); legacy planning might be fashioned in a manner that also meets this developmental task. Legacy planning is another situation where activity analysis can assist in work transitions by helping to determine when and how to initiate the legacy plan.

With the projected workforce needs in the near future, individuals, including occupational therapy practitioners, will have many options regarding when and how they choose to transition to retirement. Community-based retirement programs can be developed that focus on individuals with similar financial and occupation plans. While individuals with upper-middle incomes and above may have funds to pay for these services, others may not. Seeking grant funding to ensure that people in other economic brackets also can benefit from such planning and support programs would be an important contribution of the profession based on the values of its founders. Occupational profiles, occupation-based assessments, and activity analysis are useful tools for occupational therapy practitioners in facilitating transitions to work in both their personal and professional lives.

Conclusion

"Work can offer a person a sense of mastery over the environment, as well as a sense of accomplishment and competence leading to an improved quality of life" (Siporin, 1999, p. 23). Quality of life, participation, prevention, and other outcomes of the occupational therapy process (AOTA, 2008) are well matched to outcomes of transitional work programs. Whether it is focusing on school to work transition, transition into employment, or transition into partial or complete retirement, occupational therapy practitioners can play an important role in facilitating positive outcomes. However, the services of occupational therapy practitioners often are not used to the fullest potential, especially in school systems where occupational therapy practitioners are already present. Increasing the visibility of the profession in the provision of occupational therapy transitional work services and programs is supported by the profession's commitment to social and occupational justice and the prevention of occupational imbalance (AOTA, 2008, 2010; Scaffa, Van Slyke, & Brownson, 2008). Increasing access to transitional work services, collecting data on results of these services, and disseminating outcome data from such efforts is one very important step along the road to fulfilling the Centennial Vision of the AOTA.

CASE STUDIES

CASE STUDY 17•1 Carol

The following case study describes the experiences of a student participant in the Work and Careers Opportunities Program (WCOP) discussed earlier in this chapter. Carol (pseudonym) was a 17-year-old woman who was classified as having a mild intellectual disability and attention deficit disorder. She was in 11th grade at an urban area school that was participating in the WCOP program. Carol attended regular education classes and received special education services in the school's resource room. At the time the WCOP started in her school, she was not receiving occupational therapy services and had not since the fifth grade. Her transition plan indicated that she would receive "traditional" transition services, including meeting monthly with a guidance counselor. Carol had difficulty focusing on activities and maintaining attention to detail. Her handwriting was not legible, and she read at approximately the sixth-grade level. She generally had positive social interactions with peers and adults.

As part of the work interest profile completed by Carol during Phase 1 of the WCOP, she discovered and expressed an interest in becoming an elementary school teacher. As is seen with the career goals of many youth, Carol's career goal of becoming a teacher was not currently realistic for her as she would most likely not be accepted at a college or university based on her academic performance. However, it was important not to "squash" her career aspirations. The occupational therapist working with the program discussed several options with Carol. Field trips were used during Phase 1 to explore different job possibilities, and Carol visited several day-care centers and after-school programs for children.

During Phase 2 of the WCOP, Carol completed a volunteer experience at a local day-care center. She worked with preschool children at the center and involved them in several games and activities under the supervision of her job coach and an aide. Over the course of the 10-week volunteer experience, Carol was able to function with greater independence and less direct supervision. She related very well with the children and the children with her.

The director of the day-care center was very satisfied with Carol's performance and agreed to let her complete the internship associated with Phase 3 of the WCOP at the center. During this time, the occupational therapist also worked with Carol on computer skills so she could use word processing to complete job applications, develop a resume, and perform other work-related tasks. Carol and the occupational therapist also worked on using public transportation to and from her home to the day-care center.

When she completed the WCOP, Carol was hired as a part-time day-care aide; she worked 3 hours a day after school, 3 days a week and 4 hours on Saturday mornings. After she graduated from high school, she was hired in a full-time position at the center and is investigating the possibility of attending a community college to earn an associate's degree in human services with a focus on early childhood education.

Continued

CASE STUDY 17•1 Carol   *cont'd*

CASE STUDY 17•1 Discussion Questions

1. How can the role of occupational therapy in providing school to work transition services to high school students with and without disabilities be expanded?
2. What skill sets and competencies do occupational therapy practitioners have that enable them to provide community-based work transition services and programs?
3. What skill sets and competencies do occupational therapy practitioners need in order to enable them to provide community-based work transition services and programs?

Learning Activities

1. Investigate your community or county and determine what work transition programs are available for youth, retirees, returning warriors, parents re-entering the work force, and retirees exiting the work force. Summarize your findings in a table.
2. Develop an interview protocol and then conduct an interview with a manager or director of one of the programs.
3. Based on the interview, develop an outline for a potential proposal to describe occupational therapy's contribution to the program.

REFERENCES

Allred, K., & Baker, E. L. (1997). Review of workforce readiness theoretical frameworks. In H. F. O'Neil (Ed.), *Workforce readiness: Competencies and assessment* (pp. 3–25). Mahwah, NJ: Lawrence Erlbaum Associates.

American Occupational Therapy Association. (2004). *Ergonomics: Occupational therapy in the workplace.* Retrieved from http://promoteot.org/docs/Ergonomics.pdf

American Occupational Therapy Association. (2008). Occupational therapy practice framework: Domain and process (2nd ed.). *American Journal of Occupational Therapy, 62*(6), 625–683.

American Occupational Therapy Association. (2010). *Occupational Therapy Code of Ethics and Ethics Standards.* Retrieved from http://aota.org/Practitioners/Ethics/Docs/Standards/38527.aspx

American Occupational Therapy Association. (2011). *Occupational therapy in high definition.* [Conference program guide]. American Occupational Therapy Association: Bethesda, MD.

Americans with Disabilities Act (ADA) of 1990, PL 101-336, 42 U.S.C. §§12101 *et seq.*

Americans with Disabilities Amendments Act (ADAA) of 2008, PL 110-325.

Barth, J., Whitney, R., & Johnson, E. (2011, April). *Lead with your heart and spirit: People will follow.* Short course presented at the American Occupational Therapy Association 91st Annual Conference & Expo, Philadelphia, PA.

Benz, M. R., Yovanoff, P., & Doren, B. (1997). School-to-work components that predict post-school success for students with and without disabilities. *Exceptional Children, 63*(2), 151–165.

Blancher, J. (2004). Self-determination: Why is it important for your child? *Exceptional Parent, 34*(3), 80–82.

Broderisk, T., & Glazer, B. (1983). Lesiure participation and the retirement process. *American Journal of Occupational Therapy, 37*(1), 15–22.

Browder, D. M., Wood, W. M., Test, D. W., Karvonen, M., & Algozzine, B. (2001). Reviewing resources on self-determination: A map for teachers. *Remedial and Special Education, 22*(4), 233–244.

Cantor, S. G. (1981). Occupational therapists as members of pre-retirement resource teams. *American Journal of Occupational Therapy, 35*(10), 638–643.

Chadsey-Rusch, J., & Rusch, F. R. (1996). Promising transition practices for youth with disabilities. *Contemporary Education, 68,* 9–12.

Dendinger, V. M., Adams, G. A., & Jacobson, J. D. (2005). Reasons for working and their relationship to retirement attitudes, job satisfaction and occupational self-efficacy of bridge employees. *Aging and Human Development, 61*(1), 21–35.

Education for All Handicapped Children Act of 1975, PL 94-142, 20 U.S.C. §§ 1401 *et seq.*

Erickson, M. W., Secrest, D. S., & Gray, A. L. (2008, July 28). Army occupational therapy in the Warrior Transition Unit, *OT Practice, 13*(13), pp. 10–14.

Feldman, D. C. (1994). The decision to retire early: A review and conceptualization. *Academy of Management Review, 19,* 285–311.

Hendrix, S. (2011, June 23). Dogs' devotion helps heal vets' inner wounds. *Washington Post,* pp. B1, B10.

Hofmann, A. O. (2008, September 8). Veterans affairs. *OT Practice, 13*(6), 12–15.

Individuals with Disabilities Education Act (IDEA) of 2004, PL 108-446.

Individuals with Disabilities Education Act (IDEA) Amendments of 1997, PL 105-17, 20 U.S.C. §§ 1400 *et seq.*

Individuals with Disabilities Education Act (IDEA) of 1990, PL 101-476, 20 U.S.C. §§1400 *et seq.*

Iwarsson, S., Stahl, A., & Carlsson, G. (2003). Accessible transportation: Novel occupational therapy perspectives. In L. Letts, P. Rigby, & D. Stewart (Eds.), *Using environments to enable occupational performance* (pp. 235–251). Thorofare, NJ: SLACK.

Job Accommodation Network. (2009). *Accommodation information by disability: From A to Z.* Retrieved from http://jan.wvu.edu/media/atoz.htm

Johnson, E. (n.d.). *About me.* Retrieved from http://web.me.com/johnsonvillemelee/armyOTguy.com/About_Me.html

Kardos, M., & White, B. (2005). Evaluating options for secondary transition planning. *American Journal of Occupational Therapy, 60*(3), 333–339.

Kohler, P. D. (1996). Preparing youth with disabilities for future challenges: A taxonomy for transition planning. In P. D. Kohler (Ed.), *Taxonomy for transition programming: Linking research and practice* (pp. 1–62). Champaign, IL: Transition Research Institute.

Kohler, P. D., & Field, S. (2003). Transition-focused education: Foundation for the future. *Journal of Special Education, 37(3),* 174–183.

Law, M., Baptiste, S., Carswell, A., McColl, M. A., Polatajko, H., & Pollock, N. (2005). *Canadian Occupational Performance Measure (COPM)©* (4th ed.). Ottawa, CA: Canadian Association of Occupational Therapists.

Lehr, C. (2004). Alternative schools and students with disabilities: Identifying and understanding the issues. *Information Brief, 3*(6), 1–5. Retrieved from http://ncset.org/publications/viewdesc.asp?id=1748

Long-Bellil, L., & Henry, A. D. (2009). Promoting employment for people with disabilities. *OT Practice, 14*(7), CE1–CE8.

McDaniel, M. L. (1968). Occupational therapists before World War II (1917–40). In H. S. Lee & M. L. McDaniel (Eds.), *Army Medical Specialist Corps* (pp. 69–97). Washington, DC: Office of the Surgeon General, Department of the Army. Retrieved from http://history.amedd.army.mil/corps/medical_spec/chapteriv.html

McKenna, K. (2000). The transition journey. *The Exceptional Parent, 30*(7), 56–58.

Nash, B. E., & Korte, R. C. (1997). Validation of SCANS competencies by a national job analysis study. In H. F. O'Neil (Ed.), *Workforce readiness: Competencies and assessment* (pp. 77–101). Mahwah, NJ: Lawrence Erlbaum Associates.

Nichols, T., & Wiseman, C. (2004). Live like you were dying [Recorded by Tim McGraw]. On *Live like you were dying* [CD]. United States: Curb.

Nochajski, S. M., Nerber, C., & Patterson, M. (2008). *Evaluation of the Work and Careers Opportunities Program, Final Report Grant # H324C040156,* United States Department of Education.

Nochajski, S. M., Schweitzer, J. A., & Chelluri, C. (2003, November 3). Learn to earn: A job development program

for students with emotional and behavioral disorders. *OT Practice, 8*(20), 16–21.

Orentlicher, M., & Michaels, C. (2000). Some thoughts on the role of occupational therapy in the transition from school to adult life: Part I. *American Occupational Therapy Association: School System Special Interest Section Quarterly, 7*(2), 1–4.

Packard, A. C., & Brainard, S. (2003). *Implementing SCANS. Highlight Zone: Research @ Work.* Washington, DC: Office of Vocational and Adult Education. Eric Document 474 319.

Reiner, R. (Director), & Zackham, J. (Writer). (2007). *The bucket list* [Motion picture]. United States: Warner Brothers Pictures.

Resource Centers on Independent Living. (n.d.). Highlights of the final rule to amend the Department of Justice's regulation implementing Title II of the ADA. Retrieved from http://reachcils.org/home/disability_info/2011-ada-changes.php4

Rivero, C. (2010, July 18). Invisible wounds. In G. Jaffe, Diagnosis: Battle wound. *Washington Post*, pp. A1, A6–A7.

Sample, P. L. (1998). Post-school outcomes for students with significant emotional disturbance following best-practice transition services. *Behavioral Disorders, 23*(4), 231–242.

Scaffa, M. E., Van Slyke, N., & Brownson, C. A. (2008). Occupational therapy in the promotion of health and the prevention of disease and disability. *American Journal of Occupational Therapy, 62*(6), 694–703.

School to Work Opportunities Act of 1994, P.L. 103-239, 20 U.S.C. §§6101–6235.

Sheffield, F. (2009, October 26). Driving rehab for wounded warriors. *OT Practice, 14*(19), 14–18.

Siporin, S. (1999). Help wanted: Supporting workers with developmental disabilities. *OT Practice, 4,* 19–24.

Spencer, J., Emery, L., & Schneck, C. (2003). Occupational therapy in transitioning adolescents to post-secondary activities. *American Journal of Occupational Therapy, 57*(4), 435–441.

Stapleton, D. C., & Burkhauser, R. V. (Eds.). (2003). *The decline in employment of people with disabilities: A policy puzzle.* Kalamazoo, MI: W. E. Upjohn Institute for Employment Research.

Starr, B. (2010, July 29). Report: 'High-risk behavior' contributes to rising Army suicide rate. *CNN U.S.* Retrieved from http://cnn.com/2010/US/07/29/army.suicides/index.html?section=cnn_latest

Stone, J. R., & Jossaim, B. (2000). The impact of school supervision on work and job quality on adolescent work attitudes and job behaviors. *Journal of Vocational Education Research, 25*(4), 532–574.

Swinth, Y., Chandler, B., Hanft, Jackson, B., & Shepard, J. (2003). Personnel issues in school-based occupational therapy. Retrieved from http://coe.ufl.edu/copsse/docs/IB-1/1/IB-1.pdf

Ticket to Work and Work Incentive Improvement Act (TWWIIA) of 1999, PL 106-170, 42 U.S.C. §§1305 *et seq.*

U.S. Army, Office of the Chief of Public Affairs, Media Division. (2009, January 1). U.S. Army releases 2008 suicide data, highlights efforts to prevent suicide. Retrieved from http://army.mil/-newsreleases/2009/01/29/16219-us-army-releases-2008-suicide-data-highlights-efforts-to-prevent-suicide/

Wagner, M., & Cameto, R. (2004). The characteristics, experiences, and outcomes of youth with emotional disturbances. *NLTS2 Data Brief, 3*(2), Minneapolis, MN: University of Minnesota, Institute on Community Integration. Retrieved from http://ncset.org/publications/viewdesc.asp?id=1687

Wagner, M., & Davis, R. (2006). How are we preparing students with emotional disturbances for the transition to young adulthood? Findings from the National Longitudinal Transition Study—2. *Journal of Emotional and Behavioral Disorders, 14*(2), 86–98.

Wagner, M., Newman, L., Cameto, R., Levine, P., & Garza, N. (2006). An overview of findings from wave 2 of the National Longitudinal Transition Study—2. Menlo Park, CA: SRI International. Retrieved from http://nlts2.org/reports/2006_08/

Wehman, P. (2001). *Life beyond the classroom: Transition strategies for young people with disabilities.* Baltimore, MD: Paul H. Brookes.

Wehmeyer, M. L., Agran, M., & Hughes, C. (2000). A national survey of teacher's promotion of self-determination and student-directed learning. *Journal of Special Education, 34*(2), 56–68.

Zhan, Y., Wang, M., Liu, S., & Shultz, K. S. (2009). Bridge employment and retirees' health: A longitudinal investigation. *Journal of Occupational Health Psychology, 14*(4), 374–389.

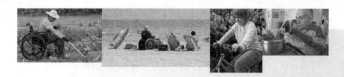

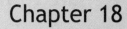

Chapter 18

Welfare to Work and Ticket to Work Programs

Emily Wilson Mowrey, MS, OTR/L, and Lauren Ashley Riels, MS, OTR/L

Give a man a fish and you feed him for a day. Teach a man to fish and you feed him for a lifetime.

—Chinese Proverb

Learning Objectives

This chapter is designed to enable the reader to:

* Discuss issues relating to Welfare to Work reform, causes of low job retention, and possible solutions for improving return to work.
* Identify potential roles of and implications for occupational therapists and occupational therapy assistants within Welfare to Work and Ticket to Work Programs.
* Describe the five main focus areas of the Ticket to Work Program.
* Discuss the different payment system options associated with the Ticket to Work Program.
* Identify the benefits and limitations of the Ticket to Work Program.

Key Terms

Continuing Disability Reviews (CDRs)
Employment Networks (ENs)
Individual Work Plan (IWP)
Milestones-Outcomes payment system
Outcomes-Only payment system
Personal Responsibility and Work Opportunity
    Reconciliation Act (PRWORA)

Substantial Gainful Activity (SGA)
Temporary Assistance for Needy Families (TANF)
Ticket
Ticket holder

Introduction

Poverty is one of the major social issues in the United States today. As of 2009, about 14.3% of the population (42.9 million individuals) lived below the poverty line (Bishaw & Macartney, 2010). This social problem has afforded new opportunities for occupational therapists and occupational therapy assistants to come to the service of the disenfranchised. Two such disenfranchised populations

are individuals and families on welfare and persons with disabilities. The Welfare to Work program is designed to help persons receiving government aid to find and secure long-term employment, and the Ticket to Work Program has the same goal for persons with disabilities. The history of welfare reform, characteristics of the Welfare to Work and Ticket to Work programs, and potential roles for occupational therapy practitioners in these programs will be discussed in this chapter.

Welfare to Work

History of Welfare Reform

The welfare system was created in 1935 as the government offered Aid for Families with Dependent Children (AFDC) for children who experienced poverty after the absence or death of their father, or if their father could no longer work (Blank & Blum, 1997). Over time, AFDC provided needy families with food stamps, Medicaid health coverage, and assistance for other essential needs such as housing expenses. As a pattern of dependency on federal assistance developed, taxpayers expressed concerns that the welfare system was not assisting people to gain financial independence but rather was creating a population of families who could not live without this support.

Reform of the welfare system was spurred by Governor Thompson in Wisconsin, who began a program called Work Not Welfare in 1995. This Welfare to Work program was the first to require recipients to work in order to receive benefits, and its success encouraged the U.S. Congress to consider welfare reform.

In 1996, the most significant welfare reform bill to date was passed. Under the **Personal Responsibility and Work Opportunity Reconciliation Act (PRWORA),** former benefit programs such as AFDC and the welfare-to-work program called Job Opportunities and Basic Skills (JOBS) were eliminated. These were replaced with a grant to each state to establish **Temporary Assistance for Needy Families (TANF)** (Pavetti, 1997). Each state was now responsible for distributing benefits and offering employment services. Other changes included time limits on the receipt of benefits. A family could not exceed 2 years of receiving benefits at one time or a total of 5 years of benefits in a lifetime (Gittleman, 1999). These caps on welfare assistance were meant to encourage recipients to enter the workforce and become financially independent without eliminating the temporary assistance families needed during a crisis.

The new guidelines outlined in PRWORA required federally funded state programs to have 50% of their welfare recipients participate in work activities for 30 hours per week by the year 2002 (Pavetti, 1997). Training programs could only be paid for after the recipient had begun work activities, which

meant that federal Welfare to Work funds could not be used for education and job skills training prior to job placement (Trutko, Nightingale, & Barnow, 1999).

Statistically speaking, PRWORA has been one of the most successful pieces of legislation in history. Between August 1996 and September 2003, the number of families receiving welfare benefits decreased by 54% (U.S. Department of Health and Human Services [USDHHS], 2004). There is much debate, however, about how much of that decline was due to the welfare reform legislation and how much was due to a booming economy and healthy labor markets during that time (Lichter & Jayakody, 2002).

In 2010, the 108th Congress approved the Personal Responsibility and Individual Development for Everyone (PRIDE) Act, which reauthorized the PRWORA. Some changes that occurred from this reauthorization included extending the time that rehabilitation counts as work from 3 to 6 months, allowing states to include child care or caregiving for other family members as work, and requiring states to make an attempt to contact the family before imposing sanctions (National Association of Social Workers, 2005). These changes to the original legislation decreased the fear that the requirements would force welfare offices to push recipients into jobs that are not appropriate matches to their skills (Fonte, 2002).

Recipient and Participant Demographics

Recipients of TANF services are families. Of the families who received TANF during fiscal year (FY) 2008, only 3.6% had two or more adult recipients in the household, and only 6% of the adult recipients were men. Thirteen percent of the adult recipients were exempt from the mandatory work requirement. In addition, another 30% of adults who were required to participate in mandatory work did not. The remaining 40% of all adults participated in work activities for an average of 25 hours per week (USDHHS, 2009). Other demographics are outlined in Box 18-1.

In FY 2009, the average number of families receiving TANF each month was 4.3 million (although the number of actual recipients is estimated at 1.0 million adults and 3.3 million children) (USDHHS, 2011). Of the families receiving TANF benefits, 29.4%

Box 18-1 Demographics of Recipients of Welfare

- Family: 90% female heads of household
- Average number of children: 1.8
- Average age of children: 7.8 years
- Ethnicity: 37% black adults, 38% white adults, 20% Hispanic or Latino adults, 1.5% Native American, 1.7% Asian
- Work: 45% participated in work activities for average of 25 hours per week

Data from: USDHHS (2009b). *Characteristics and Financial Circumstances of TANF Recipients Report 2006.* Retrieved from http://acf.hhs.gov/programs/ofa/character/FY2008/indexfy08.htm

were participating in work activities. Of those participating, 66% were involved in unsubsidized employment, 8% were gaining work experience, and another 11% were receiving vocational education. The remaining participants are involved in either job search or other waiver activities. Averages vary greatly among states, as do caseloads. For example, California and New York combined make up one-third of the total recipients of TANF and almost half of the total cash payments made by the U.S. government (USDHHS, 2010).

According to the National Evaluation of Welfare to Work Strategies, the average participant was a 30-year-old single woman with two children. Most of these women had one child less than 6 years of age. They were of varied racial/ethnic backgrounds depending on location. The average number of years of school completed was fewer than 10. The barriers to employment that most of the women in these programs faced were having no high school diploma, being unemployed for 5 or more years, or receiving welfare for 5 or more years. One fourth of the women had health or emotional problems in the family, and one fourth of the women also had a reluctance to leave their children to go to work (Hamilton, 2002).

Assessment of Welfare to Work Programs

This distribution of funds created a two-sided debate among Welfare to Work professionals. One side, the Human Capital Development (HCD) approach,

argued that education and skills training should take place before the recipient enters the workforce, in order to prepare the recipient for increased success. The U.S. government preferred a WorkFirst approach, however, which placed recipients into jobs immediately. Any training and education under these programs was to occur after the recipient was participating in "work activities." Work activities are clearly defined in welfare policy as a certain number of hours that must be spent in paid employment, skills training, or educational activities (Cohen, 1998).

Throughout the 1990s, the Manpower Demonstration Research Corporation (MDRC) conducted a 5-year study of 11 Welfare to Work programs across the country to examine their effectiveness in removing individuals from welfare and increasing their overall income. This National Evaluation of Welfare to Work Strategies (NEWWS) compared the programs that used the WorkFirst strategy and the HCD strategy. The studies indicated that although the programs had a positive effect on individuals moving from welfare to work, the employment-based programs were more effective than the education-based programs in increasing income and maintaining employment. These employment-focused programs were also cheaper to operate, while the more expensive programs did not necessarily produce better results (Hamilton, 2002).

Issues Related to Welfare to Work Transition

Causes of Low Job Retention

It is important to examine how Welfare to Work programs can be successful at increasing job retention, or the ability of a person to maintain employment after placement. Rangarajan (1996) summarized the challenges that a person moving from welfare to work commonly experiences, including difficulties with budgeting, adjusting to a work environment and demands that come with full-time employment, and a lack of a strong emotional support system. These challenges, unfortunately, often result in a loss of employment and a return to welfare. This life change can be a dramatic adjustment for families, and many welfare recipients do not have the personal or social resources that facilitate success.

Another group of barriers that are prevalent within the welfare community may be hidden. Hidden barriers include mental health impairments, domestic violence, and substance abuse, all of which have a significant impact on an individual's ability to transition to the workforce (East, 1999; Pavetti, 1997). Mental health problems, especially undiagnosed, can have a negative impact on a recipient's employability. These clients may experience depression, anxiety, severe stress, substance abuse, or posttraumatic stress disorder (East, 1999). Lack of diagnosis and treatment, combined with the stressors of returning to work, could result in difficulties in the workplace.

Enhancing Success in Welfare to Work Programs

The literature indicates that many programs have taken the quickest route to decrease caseloads rather than examining needs of recipients and providing appropriate services. According to Meckstroth, Pavetti, and Johnson (2000), Welfare to Work programs should have a screening process to identify recipients' barriers to employment. For example, trained practitioners could screen clients for learning disabilities, domestic violence, substance abuse, and mental health disorders, all of which are prominent concerns for a person's employability. Once identified, welfare offices could provide support for clients in three ways. First is with intensive case management that would connect each individual to the support services that would best fit his or her needs. Next, direct intervention could be used to provide treatment for substance abuse, learning disabilities, or mental health impairments, utilizing professionals with expertise outside the welfare office. Finally, the system could provide supported and transitional work programs. These include a gradual support system to move a person into independent work, with the use of a job coach or supervised work experience.

Occupational Therapy in Welfare to Work Programs

Wilson (2000) identified services currently offered in 23 Welfare to Work programs and examined the role of occupational therapy. Programs were selected from Welfare to Work literature and studied from materials provided by the programs upon request. The services provided were categorized into themes and analyzed for frequency and relation to occupational therapy domain. The 22 services are described in Box 18-2.

Of the services offered, many are occupational therapy–related, including: job skills, case management, assessment, job coaching, career planning, job

Box 18-2	Services Offered by Welfare to Work Programs
Job skills:	Training in technical skills that are specifically designed to be used on the job.
Soft skills:	Training in the skills needed to be an employee at any job, such as customer service skills, conflict management, interpersonal communication with co-workers, time management, and promptness.
Counseling:	Personal and professional advice about the decisions that the recipient makes regarding work.
Case management:	One-on-one assistance in organizing the recipient's job search, placement, training, financial assistance, or other services.
Assessment:	Evaluation of the recipient's skills, education, interests, or abilities.
Job coaching:	Assistance for the recipient from a program staff person while he or she is actually on the job.
Career planning:	Creation of goals and a plan for long-term employment and self-sufficiency.
Job seeking:	Assistance in searching for an appropriate job, as well as training in the skills that are needed to acquire a job, such as searching the classified ads, creating a resume, and interviewing techniques.
Self-esteem:	Counseling provided either individually or in a group that focuses primarily on increasing the recipient's self-esteem.

Box 18-2	Services Offered by Welfare to Work Programs—cont'd
Life skills:	Training in the areas that are essential to self-sufficiency but not directly related to performance at the workplace. For example, some life skills training may include budgeting, home management, family planning, and crisis prevention.
Support group:	Personal support and counseling provided by a group of peers that may or may not be accompanied by a professional.
Parenting:	Classes or support groups that specifically focus on improving the recipient's parenting skills.
Child care:	Assistance in seeking child care or placing a child in care, financial subsidies for use in child care, or direct care for children while the recipient is working.
Mentoring:	Providing contact with a person in the community, a volunteer, or another member of the Welfare to Work program who gives the recipient advice, counseling, support, or other assistance.
Basic education:	Classroom training in basic reading and math skills, including preparation for the General Education Development (GED) exam.
Job placement:	Assistance in not only searching for a job but also helping the recipient secure the job.
Transportation:	Assistance in finding transportation to and from work.
Job development:	Generation of jobs for which welfare recipient can apply by collaborating with employers in the community.
Work experience:	Opportunity to practice skills in a work environment within the security of the program.
Health care:	Direct health care provided for recipients and their families, or financial assistance that is intended for health care.
Apprenticeship:	Work experience that is supported by an individual co-worker or supervisor who trains the recipient in the skills needed for the job for a certain period of time.
Financial assistance:	Direct financial benefits for the recipient during the time he or she is in the program, including tax credits, financial crisis assistance, clothing, payment for legal expenses, and opportunities for investment.

Data from: Wilson (2000). *The role of occupational therapy in Welfare to Work.* (Unpublished master's thesis). Ithaca College, Ithaca, NY.

seeking, life skills, community mobility, and parenting. Based on a frequency analysis to determine how often the services are currently used in Welfare to Work programs, it was determined that 55.6% of the services provided by these programs were considered to be occupational therapy–related and 44.4% were considered to be not occupational therapy–related (Wilson, 2000). Occupational therapy practitioners could provide many of the services offered by Welfare to Work programs. Therefore, it seems appropriate to utilize occupational therapists and occupational therapy assistants to develop effective services for the Welfare to Work population (Wilson, 2000).

Occupational Therapy Roles

An increasing number of occupational therapists have been attracted to this innovative setting. Some are working under federal grants to identify mental health impairments or other hidden barriers to employment as discussed above. Others are helping to educate employers and staff on the needs of employees with learning disabilities or limited previous work experience. Recently, some programs have discovered the benefits of hiring an occupational therapist full-time to cover a wide variety of needs in the program.

There are several roles that an occupational therapist could potentially fulfill in Welfare to Work programs. These include direct care provider, consultant-educator, and broker-advocate (Box 18-3).

Direct Care Provider Role

As a direct care provider, the occupational therapist would work directly with participants in the Welfare to Work program to develop performance skills in order to improve occupational performance in the area of work. An occupational therapist may use

Box 18-3 Potential Roles for Occupational Therapists in Welfare to Work

- *Direct care provider:* create and carry out an intervention plan in order to improve client's ability to transition from welfare to successful employment.
- *Consultant-educator:* consult on individual client dysfunction or on program development. Also directly educate welfare recipients and program staff.
- *Broker-advocate:* act as liaison between client and employer or case manager to advocate for the client's needs in the workplace.

Data from: Wilson (2000). *The role of occupational therapy in Welfare to Work.* (Unpublished master's thesis). Ithaca College, Ithaca, NY.

therapeutic occupations and activities to develop a welfare recipient's job skills, such as organizing work space in order to efficiently complete tasks. Other strategies to manage work stress may include having the client practice appropriate interactions with a supervisor or work colleagues through role-playing and learning stress management and coping skills. Occupational therapists could also develop a client's life skills, such as family planning, budgeting, or job seeking skills, which can include searching classified ads for potential jobs, and may serve as a job coach, assessing job sites for potential challenges and modifying environments for competent occupational performance.

The role of direct care provider also includes the occupational therapist assessing the welfare recipient's skills, abilities, priorities, interests, and limitations and developing an occupational profile. Some of the client's limitations may be due to past experiences or lack of opportunities, for which occupational therapists could identify appropriate training needs. However, the occupational therapist may discover an underlying cause of work difficulty, such as a mental health disorder, past or present history of domestic abuse, or a learning disability. In this case, the occupational therapist would consider these underlying client factors and implement interventions for successful Welfare to Work transition.

Consultant-Educator Role

The consultant-educator role encompasses both an indirect model of intervention through consultation and a more direct form of intervention through education. The educator role could involve both direct education of welfare recipients and staff education. Some examples may include developing parenting groups to teach welfare recipients about child care and child development, or implementing support groups to increase self-esteem and coping skills in newly working welfare recipients so that they may better meet the challenges of the worker role. This may also include helping a welfare recipient develop short-term and long-term goals, a career development strategy, and techniques to successfully complete the plan.

In the consultant role, the occupational therapist can assist with program development. Staff persons could identify workers' training adjustment difficulties and refer to an occupational therapist for evaluation. The occupational therapist may perform an evaluation, determine appropriate goals and interventions for the client, and make recommendations to the client's case manager.

Broker-Advocate Role

In the broker-advocate role, the occupational therapist acts as an advocate for the recipient's needs. For example, a client in a work apprenticeship program may have difficulty completing work because the supervisor refuses to make accommodations for a learning disability. The occupational therapist may communicate with the supervisor to assist in developing proper modifications to the environment to compensate for the client's impairment. The occupational therapist may also act as a case manager for a client. If a client needed to find reliable child-care service in order to participate in the work program, the occupational therapist could give the client a list of child-care resources and instruction on how to set up an interview with the child-care providers.

Barriers to Occupational Therapy Practice in Welfare to Work Programs

One of the most prominent barriers to developing occupational therapy in Welfare to Work programs is the lack of awareness of occupational therapy services by Welfare to Work staff persons. Active marketing of the benefits of occupational therapy interventions to the directors of Welfare to Work programs can increase occupational therapy's visibility and promote awareness. This increased awareness comes when occupational therapy practitioners publish their research, market their services, increase their visibility, and get involved in government issues and policy. Occupational therapists may need to offer consultative interventions because many programs will not be able to afford a full-time occupational therapist on staff.

Another obstacle to occupational therapists working with Welfare to Work programs is funding. Many programs are on a tight state budget, often operating under a federal grant. They may not be able to afford occupational therapy interventions. Occupational therapists may need to create ways to decrease the cost of their services, such as leading groups instead of seeing participants individually, or hiring occupational therapy assistants to provide direct intervention.

Finally, it is important to consider the barriers that occupational therapists may have in adjusting to the Welfare to Work setting. First, occupational therapists in many settings focus on persons with disabilities and may need to adjust skills appropriately to work with individuals who are not labeled "sick" or "disabled." Also, occupational therapists may need to increase professional knowledge on the public welfare system since this is a different setting from traditional occupational therapy practice. As with every new setting, a different set of assessment and intervention approaches would be used with this population.

The Future of Occupational Therapy in Welfare to Work Programs

Research has shown that welfare recipients will be most successful in the transition to work if skill training is specific to their employment and is combined with a quick employment strategy (Trutko et al., 1999). This is consistent with the occupational therapy philosophy that clients learn most effectively in their own natural environments. Rangarajan and Novak (1999) noted that case management services are most effective when they are individualized, recognizing that each person needs a different combination of services. This is consistent with occupational therapy's client-centered and context-specific approach.

Occupational therapists are well trained to work with individuals with hidden barriers, such as domestic violence, substance abuse, and mental health problems (East, 1999). Occupational therapists focus on positive occupational engagement and implement interventions to develop appropriate skills and coping strategies related to employment and socialization. These skills can be used to transition from reliance on welfare to self-sufficiency through work.

Occupational therapy practitioners can also provide services to the children of mothers on welfare. As Page (2002) found, daughters of welfare-dependent parents were three times more likely than other daughters to become welfare recipients themselves. Occupational therapy practitioners can develop intervention programs for children of welfare recipients to prepare them for a working role in the future and prevent them from becoming welfare dependent themselves. Research has also demonstrated that children raised in conditions of poverty are at higher risk for health problems, poor school performance, abuse and neglect, emotional distress, and victimization of violent crime (Duncan & Gunn, 2000). Many factors contribute to these negative outcomes, including the quality of the child's home environment, the quality of care children receive outside of the home, family economic pressure that leads to conflict, parental health and parent-child interactions, and the neighborhoods in which these children reside (Duncan & Gunn, 2000). Occupational therapists may address some of these risk factors by providing parent education and training, home and educational enrichment services, and mental health support for parents and children. In addition, occupational therapists may empower recipients to locate and use child-care resources that are more dependable so that the client can then develop occupational routines and habits that support the worker role.

Ticket to Work Programs

Providing opportunities for employment for persons with disabilities has long been a priority in U.S. federal policies. Examples of policy initiatives promoting work include the Americans with Disabilities Act of 1990, vocational rehabilitation services, the Work Incentive Tax Credit, and the Ticket to Work Program (Barnow, 2008).

Background

Individuals with disabilities have a much lower employment rate than individuals without disabilities of the same age. According to the Bureau of Labor Statistics (BLS) (2009), 29.7% of non-institutionalized individuals with disabilities who were classified as working age were employed either part-time or full-time as compared to 70.7% of individuals of working age without disabilities. For individuals diagnosed with mental disorders, the unemployment rate is 60%–80%, whereas the general population experiences a rate of 9% (BLS, 2009; National Alliance on Mental Illness, 2010). In addition, the poverty rates for individuals with disabilities are twice as high as those for individuals without disabilities. Over the past 30 years, legislation and incentives have combined to increase the employment rates of individuals with disabilities. One of the most significant is the 1999 Ticket to Work and Work Incentives Improvement Act (Hernandez, Cometa, Velcoff, Rosen, Schober, & Luna, 2007; Stapleton, O'Day, Livermore, & Imparato, 2006).

The Ticket to Work (TTW) and Work Incentives Improvement Act of 1999 was originally implemented in February of 2002 in 13 states, and the program was in full operation in all states by September of 2004. The five main focus areas of the TTW Program are to provide beneficiaries with:

1. Access to more rehabilitation service provider options,
2. Better quality of rehabilitation services,
3. Paid employment,
4. Access to services for an extended period of time in order to maintain paid employment, and
5. Support from Employment Networks (ENs) and State Vocational Rehabilitation Agencies (SVRAs) (Ticket to Work and Work Incentives Advisory Panel, 2004).

Employment Networks

Employment Networks (ENs) are "public or private organizations that provide ticket holders with vocational training, job placement, and employment support/retention services" (Hernandez et al., 2007, p. 192). **Ticket holders** are beneficiaries who are eligible to participate in the TTW Program (Hernandez et al., 2007). The implementation and participation of ENs has greatly altered the ways in which Social Security Administration beneficiaries receive vocational rehabilitation services (VRS). Prior to the implementation of ENs, each state had a Disability Determination Service that identified persons who were eligible to receive VRS. The eligible beneficiaries were then referred to SVRAs and mandated to participate or potentially lose all current benefits. In addition, SVRAs were the only source of VRS for the beneficiaries.

The implementation of TTW and the participation of ENs have provided beneficiaries with an alternative to SVRAs and ended the Disability Determination Services (Silva, 2007). The TTW Program allows almost any public or private association to sign up as an EN, which essentially gives beneficiaries endless options when selecting a provider of VRS (Silva, 2007).

Employment networks assist beneficiaries with problems affecting employment that are not directly related to their disabilities. These problems may include little or no work history, low education levels, older age, English as a second language, and the need for child care. In addition, beneficiaries who participated in tickets to ENs rather than SVRAs worked more hours, had higher hourly wages, and earned more each month (Stapleton, Livermore, & Gregory, 2007).

Implementation Process

The TTW Program consists of a process that the beneficiaries must follow in order to receive services under the program. Eligible beneficiaries with disabilities who are receiving social security disability insurance (SSDI) payments or supplemental security income (SSI) payments receive a ticket by mail that can be redeemed with an EN or SVRA for vocational rehabilitation services (Capella-McDonnall, 2008; Hernandez et al., 2007). The **ticket** is a document that shows the EN or SVRA that the Commissioner of the Social Security Administration has agreed to pay for services provided. Eligibility for this program is based on many factors, including age (18–64 years) and the receipt of payments under a Title II or Title XVI disability (Social Security Administration, 2008).

Once the ticket is submitted, the agency must set goals that focus on the individual's return to work.

Together, the beneficiary and EN or SVRA form an **Individual Work Plan (IWP)** that states the goals for the beneficiary and the services to be provided by the EN or SVRA. In addition to the goal of returning to work, the TTW Program also focuses on decreasing barriers to employment (Hernandez et al., 2007).

Payment Systems

The TTW Program allows ENs and SVRAs to receive compensation for their services through one of two payment methods: Outcomes-Only or Milestones-Outcomes. The **Outcomes-Only payment system** "allows for up to 60 monthly payments, to begin only after the beneficiary has left the disability program rolls due to earnings" (Silva, 2007, p. 118). In addition, providers receive 40% of the nationwide average monthly SSI or SSDI payments every month that a beneficiary receives no SSA benefits due to earnings above the substantial gainful activity (SGA) level (Cook et al., 2006; Silva, 2007). **Substantial Gainful Activity (SGA)** level refers to a set earnings level at which SSA benefits stop entirely once the beneficiary has earned more than this set amount for 9 months. The SGA for 2011 was set at $1,000 per month (Social Security Administration, 2011).

Under the **Milestones-Outcomes payment system,** providers receive payments for the first, third, seventh, and twelfth month that the beneficiary earnings exceed the SGA level. Once these milestones have passed, the providers receive smaller payments for up to the next 60 months (Cook et al., 2006; Silva, 2007). The smaller payments, referred to as outcome payments, are set to equal 34% of the nationwide average monthly SSI or SSDI payments (Silva, 2007).

Benefits and Limitations of the Ticket to Work Program

Benefits of the TTW Program

The TTW Program has many positive aspects and implications for individuals with disabilities related to attaining and maintaining employment. Many of the benefits that came from the TTW Program stem from the changing of SSI and SSDI programs so that there are fewer disincentives and more incentives for employment. The five major benefits are listed in Box 18-4.

Box 18-4 Benefits for Beneficiaries

Five major benefits for TTW beneficiaries include:
- Beneficiaries are no longer subject to continuing disability reviews
- New, faster reinstatement policy
- Addition of Work Incentives Planning Assistance (WIPA) providers
- Extension of Medicare coverage from 39 months to 93 months for beneficiaries who maintain employment and are forced to leave the rolls due to SGA
- Permission of beneficiaries to purchase Medicaid insurance coverage on an income-based scale

Data from: Thornton & O'Leary (2007). Slow change in the employment services market: The early years of Ticket to Work. *Journal of Vocational Rehabilitation, 27,* 73–83.

The first benefit is that beneficiaries who are actively using their tickets to attain or maintain employment are no longer subject to continuing disability reviews (CDRs). **Continuing Disability Reviews (CDRs)** are reviews that decide if an individual is unable to work due to a medical disability (Capella-McDonnall, 2008; Thornton & O'Leary, 2007). This means that beneficiaries can work without worrying about losing their current disability status due to a CDR.

The second benefit is that the TTW Program set up a new, faster reinstatement policy for beneficiaries. If a beneficiary needs to return to SSI or SSDI benefits within 5 years of beginning the TTW Program, he or she no longer has to complete a new application process (Thornton & O'Leary, 2007). This gives beneficiaries who leave the SSA rolls while employed the assurance that they can easily regain benefits if they are unable to continue working.

The third benefit is the addition of Work Incentives Planning Assistance (WIPA) providers. These providers explain the process of the TTW Program to beneficiaries to ensure that they have a full understanding of the incentives offered. In addition, groups of advocacy and protection providers were created to assist beneficiaries with any negotiations related to the program (Thornton & O'Leary, 2007). The beneficiaries can now use WIPA providers to ensure that beneficiaries are knowledgeable about the process and employers are treating them fairly.

The fourth benefit is the extension of Medicare coverage from 39 months to 93 months for beneficiaries who maintain employment and are forced to leave the SSA rolls due to SGA. In addition, the TTW Program made it simpler for state agencies to create programs or services that permit beneficiaries to purchase Medicaid insurance coverage on an income-based scale. This is beneficial, because beneficiaries are able to purchase Medicaid insurance even if they are no longer covered under Medicare (Thornton & O'Leary, 2007). This ensures beneficiaries will be able to retain insurance even if their employers do not offer health-care benefits.

In addition to the changes listed above, other aspects and policies of the TTW Program offer benefits to the beneficiaries. With the addition of ENs, TTW increased the options that beneficiaries have when choosing a VR provider. The creation of IWPs gives the beneficiary a wide array of choices in the services that he or she will receive. It also gives the beneficiaries control over their individual programs and allows them to choose the options that are most significant to them. This, and the fact that beneficiaries have the ultimate choice of whether or not to use their tickets, ensures a consumer-driven program (Thornton & O'Leary, 2007).

All of these factors combined contribute to the fact that beneficiaries in the TTW Program are three times more likely to be employed than other beneficiaries are. TTW participants also had higher mean wages, higher monthly wages, and worked more hours per week than beneficiaries who were employed but were not TTW participants (Stapleton et al., 2007). Thus, the TTW Program gives states flexibility in the resources that they use to serve the beneficiaries, and it provides beneficiaries with better outcomes related to attaining and maintaining employment (Thornton & O'Leary, 2007).

Limitations of the TTW Program

Even though the TTW Program has many benefits for the beneficiaries and the providers, participation rates have been low. While many beneficiaries state that they want to work, few participate in the TTW Program. As of March 2007, only 2% of beneficiaries who received tickets had assigned them to an EN or SVRA (Thornton & O'Leary, 2007). Specifically, 12 million tickets were mailed by February 2007 but only 159,411 had ever been assigned, and

the majority of the tickets assigned were still being assigned to SVRAs under the traditional payment system (Hernandez et al., 2007).

These low numbers have been attributed to a lack of knowledge among beneficiaries, misperceptions, and a lack of understanding of the program as a whole. A study based on beneficiaries' perceptions of the TTW Program found that "some participants thought the program was a job bank because of its name" (Hernandez et al., 2007 p. 197). Many beneficiaries perceived the tickets as junk mail and threw them away without opening the package. This same study found that beneficiaries also had the misperception that any medical benefits would cease once they opted to participate in the program and that it would take a long time to reinstate the benefits if they were to lose their jobs while participating in the program (Hernandez et al., 2007).

In addition to low participation rates from beneficiaries, ENs and SVRAs have been skeptical about the TTW Program. Several studies have found that ENs and SVRAs have been reluctant to participate in the TTW Program due to:

- increased perceived financial risk,
- burdensome paperwork and managerial procedures and costs, and
- low volume of ticket assignments among beneficiaries (O'Day & Revell, 2007; Silva, 2007; Thornton & O'Leary, 2007; Wehman & Revell, 2006).

ENs and SVRAs that elect to participate in the TTW Program must use their own money to buy equipment and tools needed for training to ensure that the beneficiaries are employable (Stapleton et al., 2006). SVRAs have reported that monies are already limited, and this has forced these providers to place some beneficiaries on waiting lists even though they could potentially receive reimbursement through the TTW Program (Thornton & O'Leary, 2007). One study found that ENs were spending two to three times more on program implementation than they were receiving from the program (Silva, 2007). These factors have contributed to the view among ENs and SVRAs that the TTW Program is more economically burdensome than beneficial; therefore, these providers have been very selective of beneficiaries to whom they provide services (Silva, 2007).

In addition to the perceived economic burden of the TTW Program, the extended waiting periods and extensive paperwork associated with funding decrease the likelihood of participation among providers. The first major issue is the fact that providers must submit beneficiaries' check stubs as a form of documentation. This is extremely difficult due to the limited compliance of beneficiaries. The second major managerial burden faced by ENs is the fact that they must wait for extended periods, as long as 6 to 8 months, to receive payments under this program. Moreover, many ENs complained that the time they spent waiting to get accurate information from Program Managers was excessive (Silva, 2007).

The low volume of ticket assignments among beneficiaries results in a decreased need or demand for ENs. In August of 2005, 98,000 tickets had been assigned to ENs, but only 7,800 of these ENs were not SVRAs. As a result, ENs are reluctant to participate in the program (Wehman & Revell, 2006). Since SVRAs are receiving most of the tickets, and most SVRAs assign the tickets under the traditional payment system, nothing has changed significantly for the beneficiaries participating in this program (O'Day & Revell, 2007).

Implications for Occupational Therapy

The implementation of the TTW Program has several implications for occupational therapists, particularly those working in community-based practice. One study found that beneficiaries who have limitations in activities of daily living (ADL) and instrumental activities of daily living (IADL) performance were 50% less likely to participate in the TTW program compared with those who displayed independence in these areas (Stapleton et al., 2007). Occupational therapists could play a crucial role in helping beneficiaries gain independence and improve their ADL and IADL performance. These occupational therapy interventions have the potential to increase overall participation in the program.

Another characteristic that was found to greatly affect participation in the TTW Program was the age of disability onset. Beneficiaries who obtained a disabled status before age 18 were most likely to

participate, and those who obtained a disabled status after age 55 were the least likely to participate (Capella-McDonnall, 2008; Stapleton et al., 2007). Younger individuals have less experience in performing tasks and routines in a set method than older individuals do; therefore, the younger individuals are better able to adapt to a change in conditions. Occupational therapists could help older individuals with recently acquired disabilities adapt to different circumstances and engage in occupations within the limitations of their disability. This could potentially lead to greater participation not only in the TTW Program but also in other areas of occupation.

Research has found that eligible beneficiaries are often uninterested in TTW and unmotivated to learn more about the program because they do not understand how it is different from previous programs that emphasized return to work (Hernandez et al., 2007). Occupational therapists working with eligible beneficiaries should be knowledgeable about the TTW Program in order to appropriately refer individuals with disabilities who want to begin working or return to work. If occupational therapists build rapport and earn the trust of these beneficiaries, they can offer a reliable and trustworthy source of knowledge about the TTW Program. Moreover, if occupational therapists become knowledgeable and are able to explain the program effectively to the beneficiaries, they could become an invaluable member of the TTW process.

The overall goal of the TTW Program, to enable eligible beneficiaries to become employed by reducing barriers and disincentives associated with employment, is perfectly compatible with occupational therapy philosophy. Occupational therapists can play a vital role in the community by training beneficiaries to become employable.

Conclusion

Changes in welfare legislation in recent years have led thousands of people in the United States to transition from welfare to work. This trend provides a new opportunity to explore potential roles for occupational therapists and occupational therapy assistants in Welfare to Work and Ticket to Work programs. Literature suggests many potential reasons why some individuals have difficulty attaining and maintaining employment. Barriers to success, such as low skill level, lack of support for work, or mental health impairments, have been identified. Many of the services already provided by Welfare to Work and TTW programs fit within the occupational therapy domain. Occupational therapy practitioners could provide services in three roles to improve success in the workplace for these individuals, as direct care provider, consultant-educator, or broker-advocate. Some Welfare to Work programs have already experienced the benefits of hiring an occupational therapist, particularly for the participants considered "hardest to employ." Moreover, occupational therapy is one of the most utilized services by TTW participants. Occupational therapy practitioners have a unique set of skills that are useful to both populations. Further research, increased awareness, and demonstration of efficacy are needed in order to maximize occupational therapy participation in these programs.

CASE STUDIES

CASE STUDY 18•1 Aundria

Aundria is a single 30-year-old Caucasian female with two children, ages 4 and 6. She has been unemployed since her first child was born, and she receives welfare benefits monthly. Her work history includes working as a cashier at a convenience store for 6 months and as a cashier at a doughnut shop for 2 weeks. Aundria also worked as a customer service representative for 1 year before her first child was born. Aundria completed 10 years of school before quitting due to heavy drug and alcohol use. Aundria is interested in attaining employment but is concerned about leaving her children when she goes to work.

Aundria enrolled in the Welfare to Work program and as a result was assigned a case manager who referred her to the occupational therapist on staff. The therapist completed an initial evaluation and developed an occupational profile on Aundria. As a result of this assessment and profile, the therapist implemented a plan for Aundria that included:

- therapeutic activities to increase specific job skills (i.e., role-play scenarios);
- connecting Aundria with community resources to assist with child care;
- identifying community resources to help Aundria work toward obtaining her GED;
- guiding Aundria through the process of searching for employment opportunities and applying for these opportunities; and
- meeting with potential employers to assess potential barriers to employment.

Aundria was compliant with the occupational therapy plan, and she had several positive outcomes as a result. She was attending GED classes and was planning to graduate in the next 2 months. Moreover, she had attained employment as a part-time customer service representative at a local retail store. Aundria found a babysitter with a flexible schedule to attend to her children while she is at work or in classes. Aundria had the ultimate goals of obtaining her GED, becoming a full-time employee, and possibly attending college to obtain a degree that would make her eligible for a management position with her current employer.

CASE STUDY 18•1 Discussion Questions

1. What are two methods of evaluation that would be appropriate for this case?
2. Identify three appropriate community resources for Aundria to help address her specific needs.
3. What are three specific interventions that can help Aundria meet her goals?
4. Use your available resources (i.e., Internet, journals, etc.) to find evidence to support the interventions chosen in question #3.

CASE STUDY 18•2 Austin

Austin is a 23-year-old male who suffered a T12 spinal cord injury 4 years ago as a result of a car crash. The injury resulted in paraplegia. Austin began receiving SSDI benefits 2 years ago and was classified as an eligible beneficiary for the Ticket to Work Program. He received his ticket in the mail 2 months ago, but he had some concerns. Austin had limited work skills and did not understand the program. After contacting an employment network in his area, the coordinator gave him the contact information for an occupational therapist who was contracted as a consultant for the program. After contacting the consultant, Austin decided to meet with the therapist. During the consultation session, the occupational therapist:

- explained the TTW Program so that Austin had the knowledge to make informed decisions regarding his rights and employment opportunities;
- contacted the employment network to discuss potential modifications and adaptations that could be made to allow Austin to be successful as an employee; and
- initiated the process to offer Austin occupational therapy services to increase work skills and employment training.

Austin began receiving occupational therapy services, and, after a workplace evaluation, his prospective employer agreed to make some simple adaptations to allow Austin to be successful on the job. Austin's work skills increased dramatically, and he was successfully employed part-time after 4 weeks of therapy. Austin maintained employment throughout the next 6 weeks of therapy, and he had the ultimate goal of increasing his employment status to full-time.

CASE STUDY 18•2 Discussion Questions

1. Create an explanation of the TTW Program that would be appropriate for and understandable by Austin.
2. Identify three intervention strategies that the occupational therapist can implement to address Austin's primary areas of need.
3. Identify three appropriate community resources for Austin to help address his specific needs.
4. Identify five potential modifications that could be made to the workplace to help Austin to be successful.

Learning Activities

1. Use the Internet to find the current welfare participant statistics related to employment for your state. Create a proposal to present to administrators at your local Welfare to Work program recommending the integration of occupational therapy services into the existing program.
2. Identify one Employment Network (EN) in your geographic area. Contact the EN and gather information regarding the process of placing Ticket to Work participants into employment positions.
3. Contact one SVRA in your geographic area. Find out if an occupational therapist is currently working for the agency. Ask questions related to the roles and responsibilities of SVRA employees related to the Ticket to Work Program. Write a summary of these roles and responsibilities, and discuss how occupational therapy services might be integrated into this program.
4. Write a summary that describes the Ticket to Work Program as if you were describing the program to clients. Make sure that the wording used describes the program effectively enough for the clients to make informed decisions regarding their potential participation. Create an attractive information sheet or brochure about the program.

REFERENCES

Barnow, B. S. (2008, November). The employment rate of people with disabilities. *Monthly Labor Review*, 44–50.

Bishaw, A., & Macartney, S. (2010). *Poverty: 2008 and 2009. U.S. Census Bureau American Community Survey Briefs.* Retrieved from http:// census.gov/prod/2010pubs/ acsbr09-1.pdf

Blank, S. W., & Blum, B. B. (1997). A brief history of work expectations for welfare mothers. *Future of Children, 7*(1), 28–38.

Bureau of Labor Statistics (BLS). (2009). *Persons with a disability: Labor force characteristics-2009.* Retrieved from http:// bls.gov/news.release/pdf/disabl.pdf

Capella-McDonnall, M. (2008). The Ticket to Work program and beneficiaries with blindness or low vision: Characteristics of beneficiaries who assign their tickets and preliminary outcomes. *Rehabilitation Counseling Bulletin, 51*(2), 85–95.

Cohen, M. (1998). Education and training under welfare reform. *Welfare Information Network Issue Notes, 2*(2). Retrieved from http://welfareinfo.org/edissue.htm

Cook, J. A., Leff, H. S., Blyler, C. R., Gold, P. B., Goldberg, R. W., Clark, R. E.,...Burke-Miller, J. K. (2006). Estimated payments to employment service providers for persons with mental illness in the Ticket to Work program. *Psychiatric Services, 57*(4), 465–471.

Duncan, G. J., & Gunn, J. B. (2000). Family poverty, welfare reform and child development. *Child Development, 71*(1), 188–196.

East, J. (1999). Hidden barriers to success for women in welfare reform. *Families in Society, 80*(3), 295–304.

Fonte, R. (2002). A modest welfare reform proposal: Compromise. *Community College Week, 15*(5), 5–6.

Gittleman, M. (1999). Time limits on welfare receipt. *Contemporary Economic Policy, 17*(2), 199–209.

Hamilton, G. (2002, July). *Moving people from Welfare to Work: Lessons from the National Evaluation of Welfare-to-Work Strategies.* New York: Manpower Research Demonstration Corporation. Retrieved from http://mdrc. org/Reports2002/NEWWS_synthesis.htm

Hernandez, B., Cometa, M. J., Velcoff, J., Rosen, J., Schober, D., & Luna, R. D. (2007). Perspectives of people with disabilities on employment, vocational rehabilitation, and the Ticket to Work program. *Journal of Vocational Rehabilitation, 27,* 191–201.

Lichter, D., & Jayakody, R. (2002). Welfare reform: How do we measure success? *Annual Review of Sociology,* 117–141.

Meckstroth, A., Pavetti, L., & Johnson, A. (2000). The future is now: Transforming the welfare system to identify and address chronic barriers. *Policy and Practice of Public Human Services, 58*(3), 8–12.

National Alliance on Mental Illness. (2010). *The high cost of cutting mental health: Unemployment.* Retrieved from http://nami.org/Template.cfm?Section=About_the_Issue &Template=/ContentManagement/ContentDisplay.cfm &ContentID=114540

National Association of Social Workers. (2005). *Senate Finance Committee Approves Bipartisan TANF Bill.* Retrieved from http://socialworkers.org/advocacy/updates/2005 /031105.asp

O'Day, B., & Revell, G. (2007). Experiences of state vocational rehabilitation agencies with the Ticket to Work program. *Journal of Vocational Rehabilitation, 27,* 107–116.

Page, M. E. (2002). New evidence on intergenerational correlations in welfare participation. Retrieved from http://econ.ucdavis.edu/Faculty/mepage/w-corrapr02.pdf

Pavetti, L. (1997). *Against the odds: Steady employment among low-skilled women.* Washington, DC: Urban Institute.

Rangarajan, A. (1996). *Taking the first steps: Helping welfare recipients who get jobs keep them.* Princeton, NJ: Mathematica Policy Research. Retrieved from http:// mathematica-mpr.com

Rangarajan, A., & Novak, T. (1999). *The struggle to sustain employment: The effectiveness of Postemployment Services Demonstration.* Princeton, NJ: Mathematica Policy Research, Inc.

Silva, T. (2007). The involvement of employment networks in Ticket to Work. *Journal of Vocational Rehabilitation, 27,* 117–127.

Social Security Administration. (2008). *Code of Federal Regulations.* Retrieved from http://socialsecurity.gov/OP_ Home/cfr20/411/411-0125.htm

Social Security Administration. (2011). *The Red Book.* Retrieved from http://www.ssa.gov/redbook/eng/ whatsnew.htm#1

Stapleton, D., Livermore, G., & Gregory, J. (2007). Beneficiary participation in Ticket to Work. *Journal of Vocational Rehabilitation, 27,* 95–106.

Stapleton, D. C., O'Day, B. L., Livermore, G. A., & Imparato, A. J. (2006). Dismantling the poverty trap: Disability police for the twenty-first century. *The Milbank Quarterly, 84*(4), 701–732.

Thornton, C., & O'Leary, P. (2007). Slow change in the employment services market: The early years of Ticket to Work. *Journal of Vocational Rehabilitation, 27,* 73–83.

Ticket to Work and Work Incentives Advisory Panel. (2004). *Advice Report to Congress and the Commissioner of the Social Security Administration: The Crisis in EN Participation.* Retrieved from http://www.ssa.gov/work/panel/panel_ documents/panel_documents_main.html

Trutko, J., Nightingale, D., & Barnow, B. (1999). *Post-employment education and training models in the welfare-to-work grants program.* Washington, DC: The Urban Institute. Retrieved from http://icesa.org/articles/temp. results_art_filename=postemploy.htm

U.S. Department of Health and Human Services. (2004). *HHS news: Welfare rolls drop again.* Retrieved from http://acf.hhs.gov/news/press/2004/TanfCaseloads.htm

U.S. Department of Health and Human Services. (2009). *Characteristics and Financial Circumstances of TANF Recipients: Fiscal Year 2008.* Retrieved from http://acf.hhs. gov/programs/ofa/character/FY2008/indexfy08.htm

U.S. Department of Health and Human Services. (2010). *Work Participation Rates: Fiscal Year 2008.* Retrieved from http://acf.hhs.gov/programs/ofa/particip/2008/ index2008.htm

U.S. Department of Health and Human Services. (2011). *Caseload Data 2010.* Retrieved from http://acf.hhs.gov/ programs/ofa/data- reports/caseload/caseload_current. htm#2010

Wehman, P., & Revell, W. G. (2006). The Ticket to Work program: Marketing strategies and techniques to enhance implementation. *Journal of Vocational Rehabilitation, 24,* 45–63.

Wilson, E. (2000). *The role of occupational therapy in Welfare to Work.* (Unpublished master's thesis). Ithaca College, Ithaca, NY.

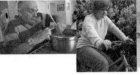
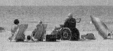
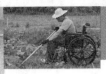

Mental Health

Chapter 19

Community Mental Health Programs*

Ruth Ramsey, EdD, OTR/L

Recovery is a process, a way of life, an attitude, and a way of approaching the day's challenges.... The need is to meet the challenge of the disability and to re-establish a new and valued sense of integrity and purpose within and beyond the limits of the disability; the aspiration is to live, work, and love in a community in which one makes a significant contribution.

—P. E. Deegan (1988)

Learning Objectives

This chapter is designed to enable the reader to:

• Describe the evolution of community-based mental health services.
• Discuss the relevance of various psychological and occupational therapy theories to community mental health practice.
• Describe different types of community mental health programs.
• Discuss the role of occupational therapists in community-based mental health settings.
• Understand the supports and services needed for successful community integration of persons with serious mental illness.
• Identify and describe major evidence-based mental health community interventions.

Acknowledgments: Many thanks to Marian Scheinholtz, MS, OT, for her input and feedback on this chapter.

271

Key Terms

Assertive Community Treatment (ACT)
Community integration
Partial hospitalization program
Peer support/peer-run programs
Permanent supportive housing
Psychiatric rehabilitation

Reasonable accommodation
Recovery
Supported education programs
Supported employment
WRAP (Wellness Recovery Action Plan)

Introduction

Occupational therapy has had a long and meaningful history of providing services for persons with serious mental illness (SMI) since the inception of the profession in 1917. Early occupational therapists promoted habits of healthy living and meaningful occupations for their patients using modalities such as crafts, woodworking, basketry, gardening, and work activities. They were influenced by the work of social worker and reformer Jane Addams and the settlement house movement, which sought to teach recent immigrants how to adapt to life in a new country through the use of occupations. Their work was community-based and would today be considered primary prevention. It focused on creating safe, clean communities; promoting child health and welfare; and providing educational courses on topics such as nutrition, adult literacy, and sewing at the settlement houses (Addams, 1910).

In the 1960s, as abuses in mental health hospitals were exposed and new psychotropic medications more effectively controlled symptoms of SMI, mental health advocates and experts demanded treatment focused on recovery, not maintenance or custodial care. During the deinstitutionalization movement, state hospitals downsized and many patients were discharged to non-existent or ill-prepared community treatment services and programs. The Community Mental Health Act of 1963 greatly influenced the shift of treatment of persons with SMI from the hospital to the community. However, funding for the legislation was inadequate and the infrastructure for a system of integrated medical, rehabilitative, and supportive services never materialized (President's New Freedom Commission, 2003). This resulted in a nearly complete failure of deinstitutionalization and led to the present situation where many individuals with SMI receive little to no community support services and are homeless, imprisoned, and/or marginalized by society.

In the late 1970s, the National Institute of Mental Health introduced Community Support Programs (CSPs), which were designed to create a framework that would support people with SMI to live successfully outside of institutions. Elements of these programs included 24-hour crisis assistance, psychosocial rehabilitation, long-term supportive services, case management, and employment services. As funding for community supports is often inadequate, people with SMI have higher rates of homelessness, poverty, and incarceration, and lower rates of employment and stable housing than the general population. Action was taken to reverse these trends in 2001 when President George W. Bush signed the *President's New Freedom Initiative for Mental Health,* a policy statement affirming the nation's commitment to help people with mental illness live and work in integrated community settings (U.S. Department of Health and Human Services, 2003).

In California, the passage of Proposition 63, known as the Mental Health Services Act (MHSA), in November 2004 provided the first opportunity in many years for increased funding, personnel, and other resources to support new public mental health programs and monitor progress toward statewide mental health service and outcome goals for children, transition-age youth, adults, older adults, and families. The Act addresses a broad continuum of prevention, early intervention, and service needs, and the necessary infrastructure, technology, and training elements that effectively support this system. This Act is funded by a 1% income tax on personal income in excess of $1 million, and so far has generated over $900 million dollars (California State Department of Mental Health, 2011). Similar legislation enacted in other states focused on the need to develop community-based programs may create new career opportunities for occupational therapy practitioners.

More recently, community mental health programs focused on rehabilitation and recovery have been developed. These programs, staffed by multidisciplinary teams of health professionals, provide individuals with SMI the practical skills they need for working and living in the community and avoiding cycles of re-hospitalizations (Anthony, 1993). As treatment programs and services moved into the community, goals shifted to enhancing wellness, promoting independent living, facilitating employment, and community integration. **Community integration** refers to the ability of persons with disabilities to live in housing of their choice and participate in home, family, school, work, and community settings with or without supports and services (Bond, Salyers Rollins, Rapp, & Zipple, 2004).

While some occupational therapists moved with these programs into the community, the profession as a whole did not respond effectively or dynamically to this new practice paradigm (Kielhofner, 2009). As a result, the numbers of occupational therapists practicing in mental health fell dramatically. In 2010, fewer than 3% of all occupational therapists described themselves as practicing in primary mental health settings (American Occupational Therapy Association [AOTA], 2010). Most of those are working in institutional settings such as hospitals, providing treatment that is based on a medical model of practice rather than on a recovery model of practice. However, the shift toward strengths-based approaches, such as psychiatric rehabilitation, provides an excellent fit with the theoretical knowledge and skills of occupational therapists, provided they are educated and trained in the use of recovery-based models of practice.

In this chapter, the role of occupational therapists in community-based programs for persons with SMI will be described, focusing on how occupational therapy practitioners can function within established or emerging service systems. Mental disorders addressed are those illnesses and disorders, other than substance abuse and addictive disorders, defined in the *Diagnostic and Statistical Manual of Mental Disorders, Fourth Edition-TR* (American Psychiatric Association [APA], 2000). Epidemiological studies indicate that approximately one out of four persons in the United States experiences a mental health disorder in his or her lifetime. Nearly 5% of the U.S. population, or 11 million adults, live with serious mental illnesses such as schizophrenia, major depression, or bipolar disorder (U.S. Department of Health and Human Services, 2010).

Mental health disorders co-occur at a significant rate with physical medical conditions such as traumatic brain injury, rheumatoid arthritis, diabetes, and chronic pain. Individuals with mental health disorders have shorter life spans and worse overall health than non-disabled individuals, possibly due to poor self-care, self-injury, lower socioeconomic status, and significantly higher rates of smoking than the overall population. According to the Parks Report, persons with SMI are dying 25 years earlier than the general population (Parks, Svendsen, Singer, Foti, & Mauer, 2006). This increased morbidity and mortality is due in part to treatable medical conditions that are caused by modifiable risk factors such as smoking, obesity, substance abuse, and inadequate access to medical care (Hyman, 2000; Hyman & Rudorfer, 2000). Many individuals with a primary mental health disorder carry two or more additional diagnoses that may complicate their ongoing care and functional capacity.

The primary focus of this chapter is on adults with serious mental illness or serious and persistent mental illness (SPMI). As a result of cognitive limitations associated with these disorders, persons with SMI often have impairments in one or more areas of daily living, and need assistance to achieve and maintain community function. Services for children, youth, seniors, and persons with substance abuse disorders are covered elsewhere in the text (see Chapter 20).

The chapter begins with a review of theoretical and conceptual models of community-based mental health, describes programs and services offered in community settings, and discusses roles for occupational therapists in those settings. A brief discussion of payment, reimbursement, and advocacy is also presented. The chapter concludes with a case example and a discussion of challenges and opportunities for occupational therapists working in community mental health settings.

Theoretical and Conceptual Models

Several theoretical and conceptual models used in community-based mental health practice are presented here, including the stress-vulnerability theoretical model, the psychiatric/psychosocial rehabilitation models, the recovery model, and an occupation-based approach to the provision of services to people with SMI in community settings.

Stress-Vulnerability Model

The stress-vulnerability model was originally proposed to explain the occurrence of the symptoms of SMI through an understanding of the interaction of environmental "stressors" and personal "vulnerabilities" inherent in individuals diagnosed with this disorder (Birchwood, Hallet, & Preston, 1989; Neuchterlein, 1987). While originally conceptualized to explain schizophrenia, this model is particularly helpful in understanding the exacerbation and remission of symptoms in individuals with mental health disorders living in a community setting. Episodes of symptom exacerbation are usually accompanied by a decrease in the individual's ability to perform in functional tasks and occupational roles. According to the stress-vulnerability model, these episodes can be prompted by environmental stress in vulnerable individuals (Neuchterlein, 1987). Individual vulnerabilities may result from abnormal brain functioning, physical illnesses, or disorders such as addiction or developmental disability. The degree of intrinsic vulnerability is inversely related to the level of stress that provokes acute episodes of mental disorder (Birchwood et al., 1989).

As an individual becomes more stressed, the condition is further impacted, resulting in deterioration of skills, narrowing of environmental parameters where the individual is able to function, and decrease the ability to perform responsibilities associated with his or her occupational roles. Each relapse directly increases vulnerability and the likelihood of future relapse and is associated with progression of the illness. Subsequent entry into institutions such as hospitals further isolates the individual and reinforces the life role of patient, increasing dependency, negativity, and hopelessness.

Some believe the stress-vulnerability model contains some inherently flawed assumptions about the amount of stress that persons with mental illness can handle, especially related to employment (Marrone, Gandolfo, Gold, & Hoff, 1998). Rather than avoid stressful situations, the focus should be on helping the client develop personal and environmental protective factors that prevent or diminish the intensity of symptom recurrence (Birchwood et al., 1989). Community-based programs for people with SMI are designed to teach individuals how to cope with life stressors, develop increased resilience in the face of adversity, and reverse the negative cycle of symptom recurrence and re-hospitalization. In this context, "resilience" is defined as the ability to recover from adversity through the development of a positive mind-set and the support of social networks (Edward, Welch, & Chater, 2009).

Psychiatric/Psychosocial Rehabilitation Models

Psychiatric/psychosocial rehabilitation models were developed to help persons in recovery gain the skills they need to function at their highest level, despite their mental illness, and were based on the rehabilitation of persons with physical disabilities. **Psychiatric Rehabilitation** "promotes recovery, full community integration, and improved quality of life for persons who have been diagnosed with any mental health condition that seriously impairs their ability to lead meaningful lives. Psychiatric rehabilitation services are collaborative, person directed, and individualized. These services are an essential element of the health care and human services spectrum, and should be evidence-based. *They focus on helping individuals develop skills and access resources needed to increase their capacity to be successful and satisfied in the living, working, learning, and social environments of their choice*" (emphasis added) (Anthony & Farkas, 2009, p. 9).

The focus of psychiatric rehabilitation programs is on the development of community living, employment, and social interaction skills. This includes housing in the least restrictive environment, competitive employment with supports as needed, and any other resources that are required. Individuals receiving services are referred to as clients or consumers, and interventions are individualized, client-centered, and focused on functional outcomes.

Psychiatric rehabilitation programs start with an extensive evaluation of client strengths and weaknesses determined from detailed history taking and personal review. Then the individual is assisted in setting personal goals for optimal community function. Community supports are identified, and the need for environmental modification is determined.

Restoration or development of skills is desired and can be set as a goal. If skills cannot be acquired or improved, goals are modified and/or environmental supports are utilized. Practical techniques are used to directly address vocational, social, housing, and recreational needs. Every individual is perceived as having the ability and need to be productive through paid or unpaid employment or another productive social role, such as homemaker or volunteer (Anthony & Blanch, 1987).

This model has much in common with the occupational therapy principles that contributed to its development (Munich & Lang, 1993). The similarities include a focus on function rather than intrapsychic processes, the belief that health is achieved through meaningful occupation, and the understanding that change can be effected through client choice and engaging in activities that promote skill building, exploration, education, and community role development (Auerbach & Jeong, 2004).

Recovery Model

Recovery is viewed as a process, and it is recognized that symptoms may linger or last indefinitely and that function may never be fully restored. **Recovery** is "a deeply personal, unique process of changing one's attitudes, values, feelings, goals, skills, and/or roles. It is a way of living a satisfying, hopeful, and contributing life, even with limitations caused by illness" (Anthony, 1993, p. 528). The key components of a recovery-oriented program are listed in Box 19-1.

Ragins (2002) asserts that recovery is a process that can occur without professional intervention, can occur

Box 19-1 Components of Recovery

- Individualized and Person-Centered
- Self-Direction
- Hope
- Responsibility
- Empowerment
- Respect
- Peer Support
- Strengths-Based
- Non-Linear
- Holistic

Retrieved from www.samhsa.gov/pubs/mhc/MHC_recovery.htm

even though symptoms reoccur, and does not usually follow a linear path. According to proponents of the model, recovery has four stages: hope, empowerment, self-responsibility, and finding a meaningful role in life. As the clients move through these stages, it is the job of the professional staff to support the process through an emphasis on mutual respect, client choice, and promoting quality of life (Ragins, n.d.b.).

One process that has been widely used to assist persons recovering from mental illness to manage their own health is the WRAP®, which stands for Wellness Recovery Action Plan. A **WRAP** "is a structured system for monitoring uncomfortable and distressing symptoms and, through planned responses, reducing, modifying or eliminating those symptoms" (Copeland, 2001, p. 129). The focus of a WRAP is to help the person develop a wellness plan that includes establishing and maintaining healthy routines and habits. Occupational therapists are well trained to support people in recovery by helping them with this process. The WRAP is designed to help people with SMI successfully integrate into their communities and receive assistance as needed. Persons with SMI need supported housing, supported employment, active case/care management, and effective strategies for symptom management in order to achieve meaningful community integration (Carling, 1995; Provencher, Gregg, Mead, & Mueser, 2002).

Occupation-Based Approach

Occupational therapists believe that intentional and supported engagement in occupation is necessary for the health and well-being of all people, including those with SMI (AOTA, 2008). Occupational therapy models typically look at the interaction between the person, the environment, and the occupation (AOTA, 2008). Occupational therapists seek to minimize barriers to engagement through person-focused interventions that increase self-awareness and skill competence, occupation-focused interventions that restructure or modify characteristics of the tasks themselves, and environment-focused interventions that modify or adapt the environment so the client can experience success. Recovery and psychiatric rehabilitation models of service are highly compatible with core occupational therapy constructs of meaningful occupation and engagement.

Community-Based Services for People With Serious Mental Illness

A variety of program models are used when serving people with SMI in community settings. These include partial hospitalization programs, intensive outpatient programs, home health services, peer support programs, supported education programs, transitional housing, and programs designed specifically for military veterans. Occupational therapists can serve in a variety of roles in these programs as shown in Table 19-1.

Partial Hospitalization/Intensive Outpatient Programs

Partial hospitalization and intensive outpatient programs are forms of ambulatory behavioral health care services. These programs typically use a medical model approach to the provision of services and are associated with a hospital or established health care center. Ambulatory services are designed for people

Table 19-1 Community-Based Services for People with Serious Mental Illness		
Setting	**Model**	**Role of Occupational Therapy**
Partial Hospitalization	Medical	Individual assessment and intervention, group development and leadership, case management, community reintegration
Intensive Outpatient	Medical	Individual assessment and intervention, group development and leadership, case management, community reintegration
Home Health	Medical	Individual assessment and intervention for psychiatrically homebound individuals
ACT/PACT Programs	Social/Recovery	WRAP development, skill building, case management, group interventions as requested
Supported Housing	Social/Recovery	Helping clients secure and maintain permanent housing through skill building, case management, assessment of functional strengths and limitations, implementing of environmental modifications as needed. Assessment and development of community living skills, home management skills, conflict management related to living with roommates.
Peer Support / Peer-Run Programs	Social	Social, educational, and/or recreational groups; staff/peer development and training; individual support and training as requested by clients
Supported Employment	Social/Recovery	Assisting clients to identify job skills and interests, help securing and keeping jobs, job development
Supported Education	Social/Recovery	Assisting clients to identify educational/skills and interests, help entering the educational setting, referral to additional resources such as financial aid and tutoring as needed
Veterans Services	Medical and/or social	All of the above, plus coping with re-entry to civilian life, symptoms of post-traumatic stress disorder (PTSD), accessing services through the Veterans Administration
Transitional Housing	Social	Helping residents develop skills needed for employment, independent living, money management, parenting. Working with children and families on developmentally appropriate play, normalizing routines of daily life.

of all ages who do not require 24-hour care but do need psychiatric care that is more intense than can be provided by outpatient visits. Services include a comprehensive evaluation of client needs and a coordinated array of active treatment components. Services are delivered in a manner that is least disruptive to and/or simulates daily functioning, and community and family are involved in the treatment process. The nature of these services makes them cost effective because they are delivered in the least restrictive environment, with reliance on client strengths and the utilization of existing resources and family/community support systems (Association for Ambulatory Behavioral Healthcare, 2010).

Partial hospitalization programs are intended to divert the person from hospitalization or serve as an intermediary step toward community living after an acute inpatient course of treatment. As an alternative to the hospital, the goal is to reduce acute symptoms and provide crisis intervention. Persons at this level exhibit severe symptoms that cause significant functional disability, possibly resulting from an acute illness/episode or the exacerbation of a chronic illness. Services are usually provided on a full-time basis with attendance in a daylong program at least four days per week. Occupational therapy is specifically listed as a covered service by Medicare in partial hospitalization programs. Occupational therapy practitioners play a significant role in partial hospitalization programs due to the extremely short lengths of stay in acute care hospital settings and the need for intense aftercare services upon discharge.

Occupational therapy practitioners in this setting focus on comprehensive and accurate assessment of function; preparation for community reintegration; and teaching of coping, stress management, and community living skills. Intensive outpatient programs are designed as a step-down from partial hospitalization programs. Persons at this level may be functioning adequately in one or more of their occupational roles but need more support or therapy than that offered by traditional outpatient treatment.

Home Health Services

Occupational therapy practitioners can provide home health services to persons with psychiatric disorders following the same general guidelines for services provided to persons with a physical illness. Home health care is a Medicare covered benefit for both physical and mental health disorders and may be covered by third-party payers and managed-care companies. However, psychiatric home health services are less common, especially those utilizing occupational therapy services. Psychiatric home health services are provided to individuals with acute symptoms, who are unable to leave their homes except for short periods and/or must be accompanied by a caregiver. Diagnoses include, but are not limited to, major depressive episode, agoraphobia, obsessive-compulsive disorder, schizophrenia, and dementia.

Psychiatric nurses are most commonly the first professionals involved with homebound clients diagnosed with mental illnesses. The nurse's role is to assess mental status and home safety and to administer and monitor medications. Social workers address legal and financial issues, family dynamics, and use of community resources (Earle-Grimes, 1996). The occupational therapy practitioner's primary focus is rehabilitative, evaluating the functional impact of "severe anxiety, immobilizing depression, memory impairments, agoraphobia, impaired judgment, impaired safety awareness and paranoid delusions" on function (Azok & Tomlinson, 1994, p. 1).

Occupational therapy intervention focuses on how clients manage daily activities, meet social needs, cope with stress, and resolve problems in daily living (Earle-Grimes, 1996). The occupational therapy practitioner identifies meaningful and purposeful activities, assesses cognitive functioning, instructs family and caregivers about cognitive deficits, and teaches adaptive techniques for enhancing self-care and home-care management (Earle-Grimes, 1996). Time management, compensatory strategies for sensory-motor deficits, and community re-entry skills may be other areas of therapeutic intervention.

Home health services allows the professional to observe the actual environment in which consumers perform their daily living activities and make suggestions to improve safety and effective performance. For example, living space may be extremely chaotic and disorganized, leading to frustration, lack of motivation, and increased risk for falls. In addition, home health services provide direct access to family and caregivers who can significantly impact consumers' ability to function. Therapeutic collaboration with families can result in problem solving and adaptation to make the consumer more independent, and the occupational therapy practitioner can model more effective responses and interventions for the family (Azok & Tomlinson, 1994).

Peer Support and Peer-Run Programs

Peer support or peer-run programs are developed and run by clients as drop-in centers or day programs, and were originally modeled after the Fountain House program. Participants are called members or consumers, and everyone is expected to participate fully in the day-to-day operations of the program. Roles for occupational therapists vary in these programs and typically focus on vocational and prevocational services, as well as providing opportunities for socialization and peer support (Kavanagh, 1990; Urbaniak, 1995).

In peer-run programs, occupational therapy roles range from direct care to administrative. Direct care roles include member evaluation, usually done using naturalistic observation and interview techniques; interaction using modeling and coaching with members in work units or social programs; clinical case management; and the development, monitoring, and revision of members' individual service plans. Administrative roles include managing the program, supervising staff in the implementation of the service plan, and managing and developing vocational programs. The transitional employment concept that originated with Fountain House continues to be used in many peer-run programs. Job coaching and other types of supported employment models are also used to expand the range of employment opportunities for consumers.

Consumer-run businesses are part of many programs and allow members to earn salaries of varying amounts. Staff facilitates the business by assisting members with community contacts, preparing for work assignments, and supporting clients to be successful on the job. Examples of these types of businesses include food carts, gardening services, newspaper delivery services, thrift shops, recycling operations, and courier services. Some businesses are run solely by consumers, subsidized by grants and contracts with state departments of vocational rehabilitation. Others are run by professional staff that trains and supervise consumers while also preparing them for competitive employment. Some of these businesses are partnerships with private individuals or corporations. Other peer-run programs use a social enterprise model to provide competitive employment apart from agency-sponsored work programs (Herron, Gioia, & Dohrn, 2009). In this model, the goal of the business is to generate earned income while employing people with and without psychiatric disabilities, thus accomplishing its social mission. Employees are permanent, receive benefits, and are allowed to continue as employees through difficulties and relapses. One such program offers a daily morning meeting with a brief check-in that creates an opportunity to offer support to employees as needed and monitor individuals who may be displaying early signs of relapse (Herron, Gioia, & Dohrn, 2009).

Volunteer work can be used for work adjustment or as a final outcome by establishing a productive life role for a person living with a mental illness. A successful group volunteer project in one peer-run program involved having members take animals to a local nursing home for regular visits and pet therapy. Members participated in other activities with the elders, including helping with simple craft activities and holiday events (Tryssenar, 1998). Volunteer work is a way for consumers who are unable or unwilling to seek paid employment to be altruistic and contribute to society. Further, consumers can choose their own hours and type of activity. Volunteer job matching, education of the volunteer agency/workplace, and volunteer job accommodations improve the effectiveness of placement. Volunteer work placements throughout the Clinical Center at the National Institutes of Health (NIH) have been utilized by occupational therapists for many years as work therapy for persons with affective disorders, schizophrenia, and Alzheimer's disease (NIH Clinical Center, 2011).

Supported Education Programs

Supported education programs help individuals with psychiatric disabilities start, continue, or complete post-secondary education (Chandler, 2008). The purpose of **supported education programs** is to address barriers to education, develop strategies for success, and provide resources and accommodations as needed. Post-secondary education is seen by many as a developmentally appropriate activity that enables individuals to gain access to meaningful employment, achieve community integration, and fulfill life goals. Supported education programs have been developed in community colleges, adult education programs, and universities throughout the country. Supports offered in these programs include educational and vocational exploration, educational assessment, educational goal planning, assistance in securing financial aid, stress and time management skills, talking through performance problems and developing solutions, and collaborating with campus and community resources.

Occupational therapists have been involved in many supported education programs. In one such program, occupational therapy students and faculty work with clients over a 6-week period, meeting with them twice weekly to help them with study skills, time management skills, reading and writing skills, and basic computer and Internet skills, among other skills. Participants also are partnered with an educational mentor/occupational therapy student who helps them find educational and job-training programs, complete application forms for specific programs, and use compensatory strategies as needed (Gutman, 2008).

Veterans Support Services

The U.S. Department of Veterans Affairs (USDVA) is becoming a leader in psychosocial rehabilitation and implementation of evidence-based practices for persons with SMI (Goldberg & Resnick, 2010). Due to the wars in Iraq and Afghanistan, more veterans than ever before are returning from combat situations with a variety of psychiatric and mental health needs. In response to this, the Veterans Administration has developed programs such as the Federal Recovery Coordination Program. In these programs, a Local Recovery Coordinator (LRC) develops a Federal Individualized Recovery Plan with input from the service member or veteran's multidisciplinary heath care team, the service member or veteran, and his or her family or caregiver. The LRC tracks the care, management, and transition of a service member or veteran through recovery, rehabilitation, and reintegration.

The Psychosocial Rehabilitation and Recovery Center (PRRC) at the San Francisco VA Hospital supports veterans who have mental illnesses in developing skills, support systems, and wellness strategies to help improve their quality of life. Veterans participate in classes aimed at promoting community integration through effective symptom management, communication, coping, and computer skills (San Francisco VA Medical Center, 2010). Classes also are held on topics such as anger management, stress management, health and wellness, maximizing cognitive function, and social skills. Clients also participate in community outings designed to facilitate community reintegration and receive intensive case management services. The VA has long recognized and valued the contributions of occupational therapy in mental health practice.

Transitional Housing

Persons who are experiencing homelessness often need to spend time living in temporary housing or homeless shelters before securing permanent housing. These individuals can benefit from the specialized knowledge and skills of occupational therapists. Facilitating the development of skills such as managing money and time, developing leisure skills, finding affordable housing, and gaining employment are all important areas of need. Occupational therapists lead individual and group sessions on topics such as assertive communication, cognition, independent living skills, stress management, and wellness (Griner, 2006).

Many people experiencing homelessness are mothers with children. Schultz-Krohn (2004) found that lack of daily routines and decreased parental authority are often issues for these families. Occupational therapists can help children through the facilitation of developmentally appropriate play. Teaching appropriate parenting skills such as establishing healthy routines, helping with homework, managing challenging behaviors, and supporting healthy eating habits is also an area that occupational therapists can address in these settings. Helfrich, Chan, and Sabol (2011) investigated the effectiveness of an occupational therapy life skills intervention program for people with mental illness who have been homeless. They found that participants in the program made gains in the areas of food management, money management, and safe community participation.

Evidence-Based Practices

Research on the relative effectiveness of interventions for people with SMI has been designed to establish evidence in support of these interventions through well-designed clinical trials. Although much of the research is focused on medications, research has also been done on the relative effectiveness of interventions used by occupational therapists and other mental health professionals. Third-party payers and consumers are increasingly demanding evidence that interventions work. Several systematic review articles are available that examine the effectiveness of occupational therapy interventions for employment and education of persons with SMI (Arbesman & Logsdon, 2011), community re-integration (Gibson, D'Amico, Jaffe, & Arbesman, 2011), and activity-based work groups (Bullock & Bannigan, 2011).

In the following section, several evidence-based practices used by occupational therapists and other mental health professionals in community-based mental health are reviewed, including: assertive community treatment, supported employment, permanent supportive housing, illness management, and family psychoeducation.

Assertive Community Treatment (ACT)

Programs for assertive community treatment (PACT), also known as **assertive community treatment** (ACT) programs, are comprehensive community-based intervention models for persons with severe mental illness. ACT programs began in 1972 in Madison, Wisconsin, during the closing of some state psychiatric hospital units and provide intensive treatment, rehabilitation, and support services to clients in their homes, at their jobs, and in social settings (Allness & Knoedler, 1998).

In this approach, a multidisciplinary mental health team is organized as a type of mobile mental health agency. The members function as a transdisciplinary team, each fulfilling his or her unique role (e.g., physician, psychiatric nurse, psychologist, occupational therapist, social worker, counselor, vocational specialist) and also taking on other roles to provide seamless, uninterrupted services that are available when and where clients need them. The team is the primary provider of services and the "fixed point of responsibility" for the client. Based on a comprehensive evaluation, services are highly individualized. The manner of delivery is based on the individual client's current needs and preferences.

ACT services are delivered continuously and over a long term. The occupational therapist contributes to the initial comprehensive evaluation in the areas of occupational and social functioning and to the ongoing assessment of effectiveness of interventions on impaired areas of functioning. As members of the team, occupational therapy practitioners provide rehabilitation services to clients and rehabilitative expertise to the team (Scheinholtz, 2001).

The ACT team assists clients in structuring their time on a day-to-day basis in normal daily activities, rather than referring them to other day-treatment programs or sheltered workshops. Clients are helped to establish a daily plan of what needs to be accomplished and how it is to be done. The ACT team provides support to varying degrees and at varying levels, based on the client's needs and goals. This includes assistance with employment, personal and instrumental daily living activities (IADLs), social participation, and use of leisure time.

Helping clients find and keep a job is central to the ACT model. All clients are involved in the vocational rehabilitation process. Employment-related services are delivered in a community-based setting, emphasizing real jobs. Once employment is attained, the team provides support and assistance to clients and their employers. Rather than disincentives, entitlements are viewed as financial support while the client is preparing for competitive employment. The methods used by the ACT team in providing rehabilitation services are congruent with occupational therapy theory and values and have been proven to be effective in accomplishing client goals. This approach can be applied in many of the community settings and programs where occupational therapy practitioners work (Scheinholtz, 2001). For examples of how occupational therapists can use PACT methods, see Box 19-2.

Research on ACT programs has demonstrated effectiveness in producing successful outcomes (Santos, Henggeler, Burns, Arana, & Meisler, 1995). These positive outcomes include:

- significantly fewer hospitalizations and significantly shorter stays for those who are hospitalized,

Box 19-2 · Occupational Therapy Use of PACT Methods

- *Helping clients establish and maintain normal daily routines.* Clients are assisted in scheduling activities of daily living, employment, and social leisure time activities. The team schedules are developed after the client's schedule is established, based on the client's need for assistance to engage in the activities. Clients are then informed as to when to expect to see team members.
- *Lending side-by-side assistance to establish or re-establish adult role activities.* Team members actively participate with the client in planning and carrying out living, working, and social activities. The team member may initially do the bulk of the activity, but service intensity decreases when routines are established and client stamina and ability to concentrate are increased. This is especially important with home maintenance, money management, dealing with social service providers such as public welfare or social security, and structuring leisure time.
- *Modeling (demonstration), rehearsal (practice), coaching (prompts), and feedback.* Strategies are provided individually or in groups with clients and in real-life situations in the community. Feedback from families, roommates, employers, landlords, and others is regularly scheduled with team members to provide valuable information to both the client and the team.
- *Providing environmental adaptations to meet client needs.* Environmental adaptations are based on assessment of clients and their surroundings to determine when the environment is creating an obstacle to clients' successful performance of life activities. These adaptations may include limiting the length of holiday visits with family when a full-day visit is too long, scheduling frequent breaks during work hours for a client with a short attention span, and helping a client who is experiencing paranoia while riding a bus to work to find housing within walking distance.

- more time employed and more earnings from competitive employment,
- overall greater time in independent living situations,
- fewer symptoms,
- greater satisfaction with life, and
- modestly increased social functioning.

However, studies indicate that when clients are discharged from the program, their gains are not always sustained. This indicates a need for ongoing support services for persons with SMI (Allness & Knoedler, 1998). Recent funding challenges have led to a decrease in the number of ACT programs nationally. While successful, ACT programs are extremely expensive to staff and maintain. Many communities have significantly altered their programs from the original model, reduced the number of persons eligible for ACT services, or shifted to less-intensive programs.

Supported Employment

Persons with mental disorders have identified that work is extremely important in the process of recovery and the ability to live a normal, satisfying life (National Council for Community Behavioral Healthcare, 2009). According to Iannelli and Wilding (2007), work provides a sense of responsibility, self-worth, and identity. Work helps participants build a positive sense of their own future (Leufstadius, Erlandsson, & Eklund, 2006) and has a stabilizing effect, reducing the chance of relapse and promoting improved health and well-being (Marrone, Gandolfo, Gold, & Hoff, 1998).

Supported employment was initially developed to assist persons with developmental disabilities to work in places of competitive employment instead of sheltered workshops. Currently, supported employment is used extensively in the field of psychosocial rehabilitation, in peer-run programs, and in programs providing primarily vocational services (Cook & O'Day, 2006).

According to Arbesman and Logsdon (2011), there is strong evidence of the effectiveness of supported employment using individual placement and support (IPS) to result in competitive employment. These two occupational therapists conducted a systematic review of 46 articles describing work-related interventions within the scope of occupational therapy practice. The evidence supported a role for occupational therapists in supported employment and education programs, providing goal setting, skill development, and cognitive training. Using IPS models, which focus on first placing a client in a job and then providing needed supports to maintain employment, occupational therapists and other mental health professionals can help facilitate positive work outcomes for their clients.

Interventions in supported employment programs start with an initial evaluation, after which the person is matched to a job. The job coach works with the employer to train the individual to perform the job and makes recommendations for appropriate accommodations. The job coach or agency provides education to employers about mental illness, focusing on the abilities and reliability of workers. The job coach is available to help the employee with difficulties encountered on the job or by supporting daily living functions. The job coach works in conjunction with a case manager to assist the consumer with recurring symptoms, medication changes, or other issues that might interfere with successful job performance. Occupational therapy practitioners can play a role in supported employment during the initial evaluation of the consumer, during the job matching process, and in the development of necessary accommodations. Because salaries for job coaches are generally modest, this might be an appropriate role for an occupational therapy assistant who would be supervised by an occupational therapist. The evidence-based toolkit on supported employment available from the Substance Abuse and Mental Health Services Administration (SAMHSA) is an excellent resource (SAMHSA, 2010a).

Reasonable Accommodations

The Americans with Disabilities Act (ADA) (1990) guarantees workers the right to reasonable accommodations on the job, provided they can perform its essential functions. Essential job functions are those tasks that an individual who holds the job would be required to perform on a regular basis. **Reasonable accommodations** are modifications or adjustments made in a system to enable a person with a disability to successfully perform the duties required of a specific job (U.S. Office of Personnel Management, n.d.).

The business community is required to comply with the ADA for workers with physical and psychiatric impairments. While the interpretation of the law for persons with psychiatric impairments is extensive, employers still need assistance to understand the appropriate types of accommodations and the standards with which they must comply. Occupational therapy practitioners have worked with employers prior to and since the passage of the ADA to address accommodations for persons with physical disabilities. The same opportunity exists to recommend accommodations for persons with psychiatric disabilities. Advocacy is an integral part of this work, initially to educate employers about the causes and treatment of mental illness, then to help dispel the stigma of mental illness, and finally to support employee success.

Some specific accommodations include structuring the work environment to eliminate distraction; providing frequent supervision, flexible work hours, and breaks; job coaching; and time off for doctor or therapy appointments. Assessing the work environment prior to the client beginning work may be helpful to determine whether the job is a good match and if accommodations can be made. For accommodations to occur, the employee must disclose that he or she has a psychiatric disability sometime after being hired. Occupational therapists can help consumers determine the positive and negative aspects of disclosure and educate them regarding their rights under the ADA.

Permanent Supportive Housing

When people with SMI were discharged from large institutional settings in the 1960s, they were often placed in board-and-care facilities. Often these facilities were located in economically disadvantaged and/or undesirable urban centers, creating new problems as the clients were victimized or shunned by society. In time, it was recognized that a better long-term solution was to help the clients develop independent living skills, place them into subsidized housing units, and provide ongoing support as needed to help them remain housed. Because people with psychiatric disabilities are often unable to work full-time, their primary source of income is supplemental security income (SSI). This low level of income typically makes it impossible for them to afford market rate housing. In response to this situation, a variety of federally funded programs have been created, including public housing units, Section 8 housing vouchers that enable people to obtain private rental apartments, and housing units maintained by community programs serving persons with SMI (SAMHSA, 2005).

Permanent supportive housing refers to a private and secure place for persons with mental disorders to live, with the same rights and responsibilities as other tenants, and access to support services as needed (SAMHSA, 2010b). Evidence has shown the overwhelming majority of people with SMI desire to and are able to live independently in their own homes, without 24-hour supervision (SAMHSA, 2005). However, some supports have been shown to increase success in community housing programs. These include assistance in learning household management skills such as budgeting, meal preparation, and basic home care. Case managers also assist with resolving conflicts that may arise between roommates and can be helpful in teaching and modeling effective communication skills.

Occupational therapists in these settings may provide care management or case management services. A care manager is described as "a broker of service, skill instructor, conflict mediator, and cheerleader" for the person with mental illness (Gray, 2010, p. 293). Occupational therapists have a strong skill set to bring to care management work, including an understanding of both person and environment issues that may be impacting occupational performance, the ability to administer functional assessments to determine the strengths and needs of the client, and the ability to analyze and grade tasks.

SAMHSA (2010b) has published an evidence-based toolkit for the development of permanent supportive housing for people with serious mental illness. This resource is intended to serve as a guide for consumers, policy makers, practitioners, funders, and government agencies in developing and implementing supportive housing programs in their communities. Included is an extensive bibliography of research articles that identify characteristics and outcomes of effective supportive housing programs.

Gibson, D'Amico, Jaffe, and Arbesman (2011) have conducted a systematic review of research on occupational therapy interventions for recovery in community reintegration and normative life roles. They found moderate support for the effectiveness of life skills, IADL, and neurocognitive training; limited but positive evidence in support

of client-centered and intensive training; and inconclusive support for providing interventions in natural contexts. Their findings can be used to guide occupational therapists in developing interventions and also indicate a need for more research in this area.

Illness Management and Recovery

Illness Management and Recovery (IMR) is a curriculum that a mental health professional, such as an occupational therapist, can implement to help people develop personal strategies for managing their mental illness and moving forward with their recovery (SAMHSA, 2010c). IMR practitioners use a combination of motivational, educational, and cognitive-behavioral techniques. IMR includes education about mental illness but emphasizes helping people set and pursue personal goals, select strategies, and implement them in their everyday lives. This action-oriented approach to recovery is a good fit with the knowledge, skills, and philosophy of occupational therapy practitioners.

The IMR program can be provided in an individual or group format. IMR participants are asked to do home practice/homework, and families and other supportive people are included if desired. The following subjects are typically covered in educational handouts: recovery strategies, practical facts about mental illness, the stress vulnerability model and treatment strategies, building social support, reducing relapses, using medication effectively, coping with stress, coping with problems and symptoms, and getting their needs met in the mental health system (SAMHSA, 2010c).

Family Support and Education

Families of people with mental illness often struggle with a variety of issues. They need help to cope with their complex emotional responses to their family member, which often include sadness, anger, loss, frustration, embarrassment, shame, and bewilderment. Urish and Jacobs (2011) suggest that occupational therapists can offer support to families of people with SMI in a variety of ways, including leading family support groups and offering family psychoeducation groups on topics such as symptom management, medication management, and living with a mentally ill family member. It is important to help family members understand the reality of mental illness, the need to support their family member to stay on prescribed medications, and the fact that their mentally ill family member can still achieve many standard and desired life goals, including independent living, meaningful adult relationships, and meaningful employment.

SAMHSA (2010d) offers a free evidence-based toolkit on family psychoeducation, available on its Web site. Occupational therapists can also help plan and implement programs that bring together clients and families for enjoyable activities such as picnics, hikes, and community outings.

Occupational Therapy in Community Mental Health Settings

For occupational therapists to be successful in community mental health settings, they should embrace the basic values of recovery and wellness; be skilled in functional assessment, intervention planning, and implementing group and individual interventions that are designed to remediate areas of functional deficit; have or develop case management skills; be aware of neurocognitive and sensorimotor impairments that often affect people with SMI; and be able to design and offer a variety of groups and programs that help people with SMI improve and maintain basic health, such as nutrition, smoking cessation, exercise, and sleep hygiene (Pitts & Ingersoll, 2009). Consumers of mental health services also want care providers who are committed, hold positive attitudes toward clients, work well in teams, adjust well to change, and are able to act independently (Aubry, Flynn, Gerber, & Dostaler, 2005) as well as interact positively with family members.

Role of Occupational Therapists

Limited research has been conducted on the role of occupational therapists in community mental health settings. Wollenberg (2001) described a process of creating an occupational therapy program in a community mental health setting, defining the relationship with clients as a partnership that involves accompanying the client on the recovery journey. Teaching skills, modifying the environment, and adapting tasks to the skill level of the client are examples of ways in which occupational therapists can be effective. Clients with physical disabilities or conditions are also referred to the occupational therapist as the team member with the most expertise in that area.

As Wollenberg described, occupational therapists can be important members of the team in community mental health settings. Typically, occupational therapists work with other mental health professionals, including counselors, social workers, psychologists, and nurses. Psychiatrists often work on a consultation basis with community mental health programs, and many teams also include unlicensed paraprofessionals who serve in case management or community support positions.

The occupational therapy practitioner may work as a direct general service provider or serve in a variety of specialized roles (Table 19-2). The occupational therapist may also provide evaluation and intervention with consumers, serve as a program or project manager, be a consultant to a program or system of care, and train and supervise paraprofessional and professional staff. While some occupational therapists have expressed a preference for more of a rehabilitation specialist role on the team (Lloyd, King, & Bassett, 2002), most value working as part of an interdisciplinary team (Eklund & Rahm, 2000).

Occupational Therapy Evaluation and Interventions

Evaluation

A variety of standardized functional assessments are used by occupational therapists when working with clients with SMI in community settings (Brown, 2011). ADL and IADL evaluations include the:

- Katz Index of Independence in Activities of Daily Living Scale (Katz, 1983),
- Independent Living Skills Survey (Wallace, Liberman, Tauber, & Wallace, 2000),
- Kohlman Evaluation of Daily Living Skills (Thompson, 1992),

Table 19-2 Occupational Therapy Roles in Community Mental Health

Roles	Functions
Direct Service Provider	• Functional evaluation of client • Home and job site analysis to determine environmental supports and barriers to success • Work with client, employer, and housing staff to facilitate function and optimal occupational engagement
Employment Specialist	• Work with clients to identify vocational interests, abilities, and limitations • Develop employment plan and supports • Seek employment opportunities for clients • Consult with employers on job site modifications for people with serious mental illness
Consultant	• Conduct needs assessments of individuals and/or systems of care • Develop and deliver services for individual • Plan and implement program changes • Train staff, develop resource materials
Supervisor	• Train and evaluate multidisciplinary staff and students • Develop and review treatment plans and progress updates • Solve problems as needed • Contribute to budget and program development
Program Director	• Provide day-to-day program direction • Assume overall budget responsibility • Supervise midlevel staff • Participate in grant development • Participate in program development • Perform public relations
Case Manager	• Coordinate client service delivery • Collaborate with community providers • Manage entitlements and finances as needed • Interact with families and significant others regarding client's services
Community Integration Specialist	• Work with clients to achieve independent living • Develop skills for successful community integration • Community mobility; management of daily living; identification and utilization of community resources for leisure, education, social engagement, and employment

- Milwaukee Evaluation of Daily Living Skills (Leonardelli, 1988), and
- Test of Grocery Shopping Skills (Hamera, Brown, Rempfer, & Davis, 2002; Hamera & Brown, 2000).

Work assessments include the Occupational Performance History Interview (Kielhofner et al., 2004), the Work Environment Impact Scale (Moore-Corner, Kielhofner, & Olsen, 1998), and the Occupational Self-Assessment (Baron, Kielhofner, Iyenger, Goldhammer, & Wolenski, 2002).

It is beyond the scope of this book to fully explore all these assessments; the reader is referred to the references for a full explanation of their uses.

Interventions

Because the focus of community-based programs for people with SMI is on work, housing, and community integration, occupational therapy interventions should also be focused in these areas. The use of WRAPs is common, so occupational therapists should be knowledgeable about how to develop these plans in collaboration with their clients. Clients often need help learning or relearning basic IADLs to maintain independent living, including meal preparation, household management, budgeting, and clothing care. Clients who wish to work may need assistance in seeking and maintaining employment, managing psychiatric symptoms at work, developing positive working relationships, and managing workplace stress. With an increased focus on health and wellness for people with SMI, occupational therapists can help clients with nutrition, exercise, weight loss, symptom management, smoking cessation, sleep hygiene, and avoidance of drugs and alcohol (Swarbrick, 2011).

Clients living in the community also desire to have meaningful leisure occupations and social relationships, so occupational therapists can be of assistance in these areas. One important difference between community-based and hospital-based occupational therapy interventions is that community-based programs typically use more individual interventions in naturalistic settings rather than group interventions. For example, rather than having a cooking group on an in-patient unit, a community-based occupational therapy practitioner might help a client plan a week's work of menus, develop a shopping list, take public transportation to the grocery store, make healthy choices at the store, and safely transport and store the groceries. Teaching basic cooking and kitchen safety skills might be the focus of a second visit. Examples of potential occupational therapy interventions in community mental health settings are listed in Table 19-3.

Funding for Community-Based Mental Health

Several sources of funding for community mental health programs incorporating occupational therapy services are available. These include the federal entitlements, Medicare and Medicaid, state funds for persons with SMI, private insurance, grant funding, and state block grants. Partial hospitalization programs (PHPs) and intensive outpatient programs are based in hospitals as outpatient services or in community mental health programs. Medicare and private insurers pay for these programs. Occupational therapy is specified as an included, but not mandated, service in the Medicare partial hospitalization benefit. In 2000, PHPs came under a prospective payment system. Unlike the prospective payment system for skilled nursing facilities, there are no categories that account for patient severity. The daily rate is an average of all patients, and occupational therapy is bundled into the daily rate for PHPs (Centers for Medicare and Medicaid Services, 2012).

Community rehabilitation programs usually receive funds from a variety of sources. These can include Medicaid, state block grants, and other grant funding. In addition, some receive funds from departments of vocational rehabilitation if they have an approved work adjustment and placement program. Medicaid definitions as to what constitutes

Table 19-3 Occupational Therapy Interventions in Community Mental Health

Intervention	Examples
Activities of daily living	Grooming, bathing, oral hygiene, medication management
Instrumental activities of daily living	Money management, meal preparation, community mobility, household management
Work-related skill building	Seeking and maintaining employment, managing workplace stress, work relationships
Social interaction/leisure	Leisure time management, community resources, relationship skill building
Health and wellness	Diet, smoking cessation, exercise, weight loss, symptom management, stress management, sleep management
Environmental modification	Workplace adjustments, supported housing

required and optional benefits vary from state to state. For example, in California, occupational therapists are eligible providers under the Medicaid Mental Health Rehabilitation option and can provide case management and mental health rehabilitation services (Pitts & Ingersoll, 2009). Many states contract with managed-care companies to manage the Medicaid benefit program, and mental health benefits may be "carved out" and managed by behavioral health care companies. Third-party payers may cover occupational therapy services for "parity" diagnoses, most often through the beneficiary's medical benefit rather than his or her mental health benefit. Occupational therapists have had some success in obtaining reimbursement for outpatient services provided to persons with psychiatric disorders (Pitts & Ingersoll, 2009). Veterans Administration programs are funded through the federal government.

Each state receives about 10% of its state mental health budget from the federal government through the SAMHSA. A requirement of this funding is that each state has a mental health advisory planning council that provides input on how the money is spent. The membership of these councils must be composed of at least 50% consumers and their families, with the remainder consisting of other stakeholders. Occupational therapy practitioners can volunteer to serve on these planning councils, and advocate for the inclusion of occupational therapy in community programs for persons with SMI.

Recent federal and state health care reform legislation creates challenges and opportunities for occupational therapy. The Mental Health Parity and Addiction Equity Act of 2008 is a federal law that provides participants who already have benefits under mental health and substance use disorder coverage parity with benefits limitations under their medical/surgical coverage (U.S. Department of Labor, n.d.). Through demonstrating the cost effectiveness of occupational therapy interventions, occupational therapists may be able to secure a place among other mental health professionals as mandated service providers.

Conclusion

People with SMI want and deserve to live in communities of their choice and be provided with the necessary supports for them to flourish. Community-based programs for people with psychiatric disabilities focus on recovery; rehabilitation; wellness; and the provision of jobs, housing, and support. Occupational therapists use their understanding about the value of meaningful occupation and skills in functional assessment, planning, and intervention to help persons in their process of recovery and rehabilitation. Occupational therapists also serve as team members, focusing on promoting overall physical health and wellness in persons with SMI, in a variety of roles, including case manager, specialist, and program director. With the advent of health care reform, more opportunities than ever before are available for occupational therapists to make meaningful contributions to the lives of people with serious mental illness.

CASE STUDIES

CASE STUDY 19•1 Antonio

Contributed by Karen Leigh, MS, OTR/L, San Francisco Veterans Administration Homeless Mentally Ill Outreach Program

Antonio is a 63-year-old male who emigrated from Nicaragua at the age of 11 with both parents and an older brother. He reports he developed symptoms of schizophrenia following an automobile accident shortly after high school graduation, and that his symptoms were exacerbated by his service in the U.S. Navy and worsened following a breakup with his girlfriend. Antonio had been hospitalized five times prior to seeking treatment at the Veterans Administration (VA) hospital and was primarily living on the street, in shelters, or in single-room-occupancy hotels. He self-medicated with cocaine, amphetamines, marijuana, and alcohol, and initially presented to the VA for substance abuse treatment in 2001. Following an acute hospitalization and a 3-year stay in a locked facility, Antonio has been living in a

Continued

CASE STUDY 19•1 Antonio *cont'd*

board-and-care home and receiving intensive case management services at an out patient VA clinic for the past 2 years, where he has remained abstinent from all substances and regularly attends AA meetings.

Antonio began attending an outpatient Psychosocial Rehabilitation program where he completed an initial evaluation with the occupational therapist. The evaluation revealed that Antonio's most important goal was "to shave more often," and together he and the occupational therapist determined this would be every other day. He was currently shaving about once a week and typically only when reminded by board-and-care staff. Further evaluation using the Allen Cognitive Level Assessment demonstrated that Antonio's cognitive level of functioning was consistent with the need for striking visual cues to initiate ADLs. An evaluation of his living environment revealed that some shaving supplies were kept in a closed cabinet in his room and others were kept locked up by the board-and-care operator and provided upon request.

Antonio's intervention plan included the purchase of an electric razor that he would be allowed to keep in his room. The occupational therapist and client reviewed use and proper care of the razor, and together determined a place near the sink where the razor would be visible to maximize the likelihood of its use. A can of shaving cream was also placed with the razor. The occupational therapist educated the board-and-care operator on the need for these items to be left where they had been placed in order to maximize their use.

CASE STUDY 19•1 Discussion Questions

1. What other types of functional difficulty might Antonio be having?
2. What other interventions might the occupational therapist provide?
3. Which community supports might the occupational therapist refer Antonio to?

Learning Activities

1. Visit one of the following Web sites to obtain more information about community-based mental health services:

www.iapsrs.org:	International Association of Psychosocial Rehabilitation
www.nami.org:	National Association for Mental Illness
www.mha.org:	National Mental Health Association
www.samhsa.org:	Substance Abuse and Mental Health Association
www.potac.org:	Psychiatric Occupational Therapy Coalition
www.vinfen.org:	VinFen Services, Boston, MA
www.buckelew.org:	Buckelew Services, Marin County, CA
www.ottp.org:	Occupational Therapy Training Program

2. Identify an occupational therapist in your community who works with people with SMI. Interview this individual and explore what he or she does in the course of a typical workday.
3. Read a first-person account of a person recovering from a SMI. Consider the challenges he or she experiences on a daily basis while engaging in valued occupations. What gives meaning and purpose to this person's life? How could you as an occupational therapist engage with this person in his or her recovery process?

REFERENCES

Addams, J. (1910). *Twenty years at Hull House.* New York, NY: Signet Classics.
Allness, D. J., & Knoedler, W. H. (1998). *The PACT model of community-based treatment for persons with severe and*

persistent mental illnesses: A manual for PACT start-up. Arlington, VA: National Alliance on Mental Illness.

American Occupational Therapy Association. (2008). Occupational therapy practice framework: Domain and process (2nd ed.). *American Journal of Occupational Therapy, 62,* 625–683.

American Occupational Therapy Association. (2010). *AOTA 2010 compensation and workforce report.* Bethesda, MD: Author.

American Psychiatric Association. (2000). *Diagnostic and statistical manual of mental disorders* (4th ed.-TR). Washington, DC: American Psychiatric Association Press.

Americans with Disabilities Act (ADA) of 1990, P.L. 101-336, §2,104 Stat. 328 (1991). Retrieved from http://www.ada.gov/

Anthony, W. (1993). Recovery from mental illness: The guiding vision of the mental health service system in the 1990's. *Psychosocial Rehabilitation Journal, 16*(4), 11–23.

Anthony, W. A., & Blanch, A. (1987). Supported employment for persons who are psychiatrically disabled: A historical and conceptual perspective. *Psychosocial Rehabilitation Journal, 11*(2), 5–23.

Anthony, W., & Farkas, M. (2009). *A primer on the psychiatric rehabilitation process.* Boston University Center for Psychiatric Rehabilitation, Boston, MA.

Arbesman, M., & Logsdon, D. (2011). Occupational therapy interventions for employment and education for adults with serious mental illness: A systematic review. *American Journal of Occupational Therapy, 65*(3), 238–246.

Association for Ambulatory Behavioral Healthcare. (2010). *Fast facts about partial hospitalization.* Retrieved from: http://www.aabh.org/content/fast-facts-php

Aubry, T. D., Flynn, R. J., Gerber, G., & Dostaler, T. (2005). Identifying the core competencies of community support providers working with people with psychiatric disabilities. *Psychiatric Rehabilitation Journal, 28*(4), 346–353.

Auerbach, E., & Jeong, G. (2004). Vocational programming. In E. Cara & A. MacRae, (Eds.), *Psychosocial occupational therapy: A clinical practice* (2nd ed., pp. 591–619). Albany, NY: Delmar.

Azok, S. D., & Tomlinson, J. (1994). Occupational therapy in a multidisciplinary psychiatric home health care service. *Mental Health Special Interest Newsletter, 17*(2), 1–3.

Baron, K., Kielhofner, G., Iyenger, A., Goldhammer, V., & Wolenski, J. (2002). *The Occupational Self Assessment (OSA) Version 1.2.* Chicago: Model of Human Occupational Clearinghouse, Department of Occupational Therapy, College of Applied Health Sciences, University of Illinois at Chicago.

Birchwood, M. J., Hallet, S. E., & Preston, M. C. (1989). *Schizophrenia: An integrated approach to research and treatment.* New York, NY: New York University Press.

Bonder, G. R., Salyers, M. P., Rollins, A. L., Rapp, C. A. & Zipple, A. M. (2004). How evidence-based practices contribute to community integration. *Community Mental Health Journal, 40*(6), 569–588.

Brown, C. (2011). Activities of daily living and instrumental activities of daily living. In C. Brown & V. Stoffel (Eds.),

Occupational therapy in mental health: A vision for participation. Philadelphia, PA: F.A. Davis.

Bullock, A., & Bannigan, K. (2011). Effectiveness of activity-based group work in community mental health: A systematic review. *American Journal of Occupational Therapy, 64*(3), 257–261.

California Department of Mental Health. (2011). Mental Health Services Act (Proposition 63). Retrieved from http://www.dmh.ca.gov/prop_63/MHSA

Carling, P. J. (1995). *Return to community: Building support-systems for people with psychiatric disabilities.* New York, NY: Guilford Press.

Centers for Medicare and Medicaid Services. (2012). *Medicare & Your Mental Health Benefits.* Retrieved from www.medicare.gov/pubs/pdf/10184.pdf

Chandler, D. (2008). *Supported education for persons with psychiatric disabilities.* Retrieved from: http://www.cimh.org

Cook, J., & O'Day, B. (2006). *Supported employment: A best practice for people with psychiatric disabilities.* Washington, DC: Cornell University Institute for Policy Research.

Copeland, M. (2001). Wellness recovery action plan: A system for monitoring, reducing, and eliminating uncomfortable or dangerous physical symptoms and emotional feelings. *Occupational Therapy in Mental Health, 17*(3/4), 127–150.

Deegan, P. (1988). Recovery: The lived experience of rehabilitation. *Psychosocial Rehabilitation Journal, 11,* 11–19.

Earle-Grimes, G. (1996). Psychiatric home health care: New horizons for occupational therapy. *Mental Health Special Interest Newsletter, 17*(2), 3–4.

Edward, K., Welch, A., & Chater, K. (2009). The phenomenon of resilience as described by adults who have experienced mental illness. *Journal of Advanced Nursing, 65*(3), 587–595.

Eklund, M., & Rahm, I. (2000). Factors influencing job satisfaction among Swedish occupational therapists in psychiatric care. *Scandinavian Journal of Caring Sciences, 14* (3), 162–171.

Gibson, R., D'Amico, M., Jaffe, L., & Arbesman, M. (2011). Occupational therapy interventions for recovery in community integration and normative life roles for adults with serious mental illness: A systematic review. *American Journal of Occupational Therapy, 65*(3), 247–256.

Goldberg, R. W., & Resnick, S. G. (2010). United States Department of Veterans Affairs efforts to promote psychosocial rehabilitation and recovery. *Journal of Psychiatric Rehabilitation, 33*(4), 255–258.

Gray, K. (2010). Community resources and care management, In K. Scheinholtz (Ed.), *Occupational therapy and mental health: Considerations for advanced practice* (pp. 281–308). Bethesda, MD: AOTA Press.

Griner, K. (2006). Helping the homeless: An occupational therapy perspective. *Occupational Therapy in Mental Health, 22*(1), 49–61.

Gutman, S. (2008). Supported education for adults with psychiatric disabilities. *Psychiatric Services, 59*(3), 326–327.

Hamera, E., Brown, C., Rempfer, M., & Davis, N. (2002). Test of grocery shopping skills: discrimination of people with and without mental illness. *Psychiatric Rehabilitation Skills, 6,* 296–311.

Hamera, E., & Brown, C. (2000). Developing a context-based performance measure for persons with schizophrenia: The test of grocery shopping skills. *American Journal of Occupational Therapy, 54,* 20–25.

Helfrich, C., Chan, D., & Sabol, P. (2011). Cognitive predictors of life skill intervention outcomes for adults with mental illness at risk for homelessness. *American Journal of Occupational Therapy, 65*(3), 277–286.

Herron, J., Gioia, D., & Dohrn, B. (2009). A social enterprise model for employment. *Psychiatric Services, 60*(8), 1140.

Hyman, S. E. (2000). Schizophrenia. In D. C. Dale and D. D. Federman (Eds.), *Scientific American Medicine* (Section VII, pp. 1–5). New York: Healtheon.

Hyman, S. E., & Rudorfer, M. V. (2000). Depressive and bipolar mood disorders. In D. C. Dale and D. D. Federman (Eds.), *Scientific American Medicine* (Section II, pp. 1–19). New York: Healtheon.

Iannelli, S., &Wilding, C. (2007). Health-enhancing effects of engaging in productive occupation: Experiences of young people with mental illness. *Australian Occupational Therapy Journal, 54,* 285–293.

Katz, S. (1983). Assessing self-maintenance: Activities of daily living, mobility, and instrumental activities of daily living. *Journal of the American Geriatrics Society, 31,* 721–726.

Kavanagh, M. R. (1990). Way station: A model community support program for persons with serious mental illness. *Mental Health Special Interest Newsletter, 13*(1), 68.

Kielhofner, G. (2009). *Conceptual foundations of occupational therapy practice.* Philadelphia, PA: F.A. Davis.

Kielhofner, G., Mallinson, T., Crawford, C., Nowak, M., Rigby, M., Henry, A., & Walens, A. (2004). *A User's Manual for the Occupational Performance History Interview (Version 2.1) OPHI-II.* Chicago: Model of Human Occupational Clearinghouse, University of Illinois at Chicago.

Leonardelli, C. A. (1988). *The Milwaukee evaluation of daily living skills: Evaluation in long term psychiatric care.* Thorofare, NJ: SLACK.

Leufstadius, C., Erlandsson, L.-K., & Eklund, M. (2006). Time use and daily activities in people with persistent mental illness. *Occupational Therapy International, 13,* 123–141.

Lloyd, C., King, R., & Bassett, H. (2002). A survey of Australian mental health occupational therapists. *British Journal of Occupational Therapy, 65*(2), 88–96.

Marrone, J., Gandolfo, C., Gold, M., & Hoff, D. (1998). Just doing it: Helping people with mental illness get good jobs. *Journal of Applied Rehabilitation Counseling, 29*(1), 37–48.

Moore-Corner, R. A., Kielhofner, G., & Olson, L. (1998). *A user's manual for Work Environment Impact Scale, Version 2.0.* Chicago, IL: Model of Human Occupation Clearinghouse, University of Illinois at Chicago.

Munich, R., & Lang, M. (1993). The boundaries of psychiatric rehabilitation. *Hospital and Community Psychiatry, 44*(7), 661–665.

National Council for Community Behavioral HealthCare. (2009). *Policy issues and resources: Employment and housing.* Retrieved from http://www.thenationalcouncil.org/cs/employment_housing

National Institutes of Health Clinical Center. (2011). *Volunteering at the NIH Clinical Center.* Retrieved from http://clinicalcenter.nih.gov/volunteers/index.html

Neuchterlein, K. H. (1987). Vulnerability models for schizophrenia: State of the art. In J. Haffner, W. F. Gattaz, & W. Janzarik (Eds.), *Search for the causes of schizophrenia.* Heidelberg: Springer-Verlag.

Parks, J., Svendsen, D., Singer, P., Foti, M. E., & Mauer, B. (2006, October). *Morbidity and mortality in people with serious mental illness* (Tech rep 13). Alexandria, VA: National Association of State Mental Health Directors, Medical Director's Council. Retrieved from http://www.nasmhpd.org/general_files/publications/med_directors_pubs/Mortality%20and%20Morbidity%20Final%20Report%208.18.08.pdf

Pitts, D., & Ingersoll, B. (2009). *Occupational Therapy Practitioners: Role and Importance in Public Mental Health* [White Paper]. Sacramento, CA: Occupational Therapy Association of California.

President's New Freedom Commission on Mental Health. (2003). *Achieving the promise: Transforming mental health care in America* (Final Report, DHHS Pub. No.SMA-03-3832). Rockville, MD: Author.

Provencher, H., Gregg, R., Mead, S., & Mueser, K. (2002). The role of work in the recovery of persons with psychiatric disabilities. *Psychiatric Rehabilitation Journal, 26*(2), 132–145.

Ragins, M. (n.d.a.). *Recovery with severe mental illness: Changing from a medical model to a psychosocial rehabilitation model.* Retrieved from http://www.village-isa.org/Ragin's%20Papers/recov.%20with%20severe%20MI.htm

Ragins, M. (2002). *Road to recovery.* Retrieved from http://mhavillage.squarespace.com/storage/08ARoadtoRecovery.pdf

San Francisco VA Medical Center. (2010). Psychosocial Rehabilitation and Recovery Center. Retrieved from http://www.SANFRANCISCO.va.gov/SANFRANCISCO/services/prrc.asp

Santos, A. B., Henggeler, S. W., Burns, B. J., Arana, G. W., & Meisler, N. (1995). Research on field based services: Models for reform in the delivery of mental health care to populations with complex clinical medical problems. *American Journal of Psychiatry, 152,* 1111–1123.

Scheinholtz, M. K. (2001). Community-based mental health services. In M. E. Scaffa, *Occupational therapy in community-based practice settings.* Philadelphia: F.A. Davis.

Schultz-Krohn, W. (2004). The meaning of family routines in a homeless shelter. *American Journal of Occupational Therapy, 58*(5), 531–542.

Substance Abuse and Mental Health Services Administration. (2005). *Transforming mental health care in America: The federal action agenda: first steps.* Retrieved from http://www.samhsa.gov/Federalactionagenda/NFC_FMHAA.aspx

Substance Abuse and Mental Health Services Administration. (2010a). *Supported employment evidence-based practices toolkit.* Washington, DC: Author.

Substance Abuse and Mental Health Services Administration. (2010b). *Permanent supportive housing evidence-based practices kit.* Washington, DC: Author.

Substance Abuse and Mental Health Services Administration (2010c). *Illness management and recovery evidence-based practices toolkit.* Washington, DC: Author.

Substance Abuse and Mental Health Services Administration (2010d). *Family psychoeducation evidence-based practices toolkit.* Washington, DC: Author.

Swarbrick, M. (2011). Occupation-focused community health and wellness programs. In M. Scheinholtz (Ed.), *Occupational therapy and mental health: Considerations for advanced practice*, pp. 27–44. Bethesda, MD: AOTA Press.

Thompson, L. (1992). *The Kohlman Evaluation of Living Skills* (3rd ed.). Bethesda, MD: American Occupational Therapy Association.

Tryssenar, J. (1998). Vocational exploration and employment and psychosocial disabilities. In F. Stein & S. K. Cutler (Eds.), *Psychosocial occupational therapy: A holistic approach.* San Diego, CA: Singular Publishing Group.

Urbaniak, M. A. (1995). Yahara House: A community-based program using the Fountain House model. *Mental Health Special Interest Newsletter, 18*(1), 1–3.

Urish, C., & Jacobs, B. (2011). Families living with mental illness. In C. Brown & V. Stoffel, (Eds.), *Occupational therapy in mental health: A vision for participation* (pp. 415–432). Philadelphia, PA: F.A. Davis.

U.S. Department of Health and Human Services (2003). *New Freedom Initiative.* Retrieved from http://www.hhs.gov/newfreedom/init.html

U.S. Department of Health and Human Services. (2010). *Results from the 2009 national survey on drug use and health: Mental health findings.* Retrieved from http://www.oas.samhsa.gov/NSDUH/2k9NSDUH/MH/2K9MHResults.pdf

U.S. Department of Labor. (n.d.). *Fact sheet: The Mental Health Parity and Equity Act of 2008 (MHPAEA).* Retrieved from http://www.dol.gov/ebsa/newsroom/fsmhpaea.html

U.S. Office of Personnel Management. (n.d.). *Federal employment of people with disabilities: Reasonable accommodation.* Retrieved from http://www.opm.gov/disability/reasonableaccommodation.asp

Wallace, C., Liberman, R., Tauber, R., & Wallace, J. (2000). The independent living skills survey: A comprehensive measure of the community functioning of severely and persistently mentally ill individuals. *Schizophrenia Bulletin, 26,* 631–658.

Wollenberg, J. (2001). Recovery and occupational therapy in the community mental health setting. *Occupational Therapy in Mental Health, 17*(3/4), 97–114.

Chapter 20

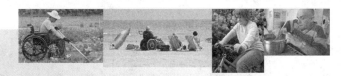

Community-Based Approaches for Substance Use Disorders

Marjorie E. Scaffa, PhD, OTR/L, FAOTA, Lauren Ashley Riels, MS, OTR/L, Penelope A. Moyers, EdD, OTR, FAOTA, and Virginia C. Stoffel, PhD, OT, BCMH, FAOTA

If you treat an individual as he is, he will stay as he is, but if you treat him as if he were what he ought to be and could be, he will become what he ought to be and could be.

—Johann Wolfgang von Goethe

Learning Objectives

This chapter is designed to enable the reader to:

- Describe the impact of substance use disorders on the community.
- Discuss the effects of substance use disorders on occupational behavior.
- Describe a variety of types of community-based services for substance use disorders.
- Identify and describe evidence-based interventions for substance abuse treatment.
- Discuss the role of occupational therapy in community-based programs for substance use disorders.

Key Terms

Aftercare program
Behavioral rehearsal
Brief intervention
CAGE
Crisis intervention
Employee assistance program (EAP)
FRAMES

Intensive outpatient program (IOP)
Motivational enhancement therapy (MET)
Motivational interviewing
Mutual support programs
Substance use disorder

Introduction

Substance abuse is an escalating problem in the United States that often results in increased risk of dysfunction at work, in marriages, in families, and in the health of the user (O'Day, 2009). In addition to being a mental health problem, substance use disorders are a major factor in many medical, public health, social, and safety issues within a community. As a medical problem, substance use, including alcohol use, contributes to diseases of the liver, pancreas, and digestive tract. Depending on the drug of choice, the respiratory, nervous,

and cardiovascular systems also may be affected (Mertens, Weisner, Ray, Fireman, & Walsh, 2005). High rates of comorbidity of substance abuse with other psychiatric diagnoses complicate and increase the cost of treating schizophrenia and other mental disorders (Ziedonis, Smelson, Rosenthal, Batki, et al., 2005).

As a community public health problem, substance use disorders have been linked to AIDS, tuberculosis, and neonatal defects. Community social problems, such as unemployment and homelessness, are also strongly associated with substance use disorders. In terms of safety issues within a community, the relationships of substance use with crime, industrial accidents, burns, spinal cord injury, and traumatic brain injury are well established (Levy, Mallonee, Miller, Smith, Spicer, Romano, & Fisher, 2004; Weisner, 1995).

The impact of substance use on the family cannot be underestimated. Persons with substance abuse or dependence typically have extensive marital and family problems. Children of parents with substance dependence are considered to be at high risk for experiencing a variety of difficulties, including cognitive, emotional, social, and academic problems. The home environments for the children are characterized by more marital conflict, parent-child conflict, and family violence when compared to the environments of children with parents who do not use substances. In addition, negative consequences, such as separation and divorce, are much more common in marriages containing an addicted partner in comparison with couples in the general population (Saatcioglu, Erim, & Cakmak, 2006).

In this chapter, substance use terms are defined, the influence of substance use disorders on occupational performance is discussed, community-based treatment programs are described, evidence-based interventions that can be used by occupational therapists are highlighted, and the relationship between these interventions and the Stages of Change model are illustrated. In addition, the potential contributions of occupational therapy to these community programs to better support recovery behaviors are reviewed.

Substance Use Terminology

The *Diagnostic and Statistical Manual of Mental Disorders, Fifth Edition (DSM V)* (American Psychiatric Association [APA], 2013) defines various substance use disorders according to groups of substances of 10 classes of drugs. These include:

1. alcohol
2. stimulants
3. caffeine
4. cannabis
5. hallucinogens
6. inhalants
7. tobacco
8. opioids
9. sedatives, and
10. other (or unknown)

Substance abuse and dependence disorders can be applied to nearly every class of substance. Therefore, the characteristics of these two diagnoses are similar across the various drug classes. However, saliency of a symptom may vary, and some symptoms are not present in a given drug class. Some symptoms are more or less pronounced, depending on the drug involved. For example, withdrawal symptoms typically are not present for hallucinogen dependence.

The chief feature of **substance use disorder** is continued use of a substance despite significant, persistent, and adverse substance-related consequences that usually results in tolerance, withdrawal, and compulsive drug-taking behavior (APA, 2013). Compulsive substance use behavior typically includes the following:

- Drinking or using the substance for a longer time period or in greater quantity than originally planned,
- Unsuccessful attempts to decrease or discontinue use of the substance,
- Spending an inordinate amount of time seeking, using, and recovering from substance use, and
- Giving up or reducing important social, occupational, and recreational activities (APA, 2013).

Substance use disorder is characterized by failure to fulfill major role obligations at work, school, or home; repeated legal troubles related to substance use; and recurrent social and interpersonal problems as a result of intoxication (APA, 2013). Other primary features are tolerance, withdrawal, and a pattern of compulsive use. Occupational therapists are in an excellent position to evaluate occupational roles and to detect the impact that substance abuse or dependence may have on an individual's performance.

Substance Use Disorders and Occupation

Occupations are the day-to-day activities or goal-directed pursuits that typically extend over time, have meaning to the performer, and involve multiple tasks (Christiansen, Clark, Kielhofner, & Rogers, 1995). Usually occupations are considered to be health enhancing, positively valued by the culture, and necessary for daily survival. However, occupations that lead to negative consequences or are considered to be deviant from socially acceptable norms need to be taken into account. Substance use can be thought of as an occupation because of its many associated tasks and activities, which may include:

- Raising money for the drugs
- Purchasing or making the deal to obtain the drug supply
- Protecting the supply from others, or hiding drug use
- Removing barriers to using, such as ignoring family members who object to the person's behavior
- Creating situations for using
- Seeking persons with whom to use
- Spending time using
- Recovering from the effects of using
- Resuming the drug use process all over again (Moyers, 1997).

As performance in occupations other than drinking or using substances progressively deteriorates, the individual becomes more and more alienated from normal occupations and becomes deprived of their healthy effects. Further engagement in non-using occupations becomes devoid of usual meanings, meaningful only to the extent that these occupations serve as barriers or facilitators to drinking or using drugs, thus perpetuating the negative cycle of occupational alienation and deprivation.

Occupational therapists should consider including substance use questions in the initial interview as a routine component of the development of an occupational profile regardless of the practice setting. When this screening indicates a possible alcohol or other drug use problem, the occupational therapist attempts to ascertain the client's readiness to change and uses motivational strategies to encourage the client to seek additional evaluation and treatment as necessary (Stoffel & Moyers, 2004). In addition, the occupational therapy evaluation can determine whether the person's activities of daily living, work, leisure, and other productive activities have been affected by substance use (Fig. 20.1). The occupational therapist thus

Occupational Performance	Performance Skills	Performance Context
Are ADLs/IADLs affected?	***Cognitive***	***Temporal***
• Promiscuity • Poor eating habits • Drunk driving • Unsafe sexual practices	• Rigid thinking • Uses familiar strategies even though proven ineffective • Blackouts/memory lapses	• Temporary reaction to a major life change? • Rite of passage in a young adult? • Experimental use in adolescence?
Are work/education activities affected?	***Sensory, Motor and Praxis***	***Physical***
• Late for work/school • Unexcused absences/ too many sick days • Argumentative behavior • Not meeting deadlines	• Peripheral neuropathy • Overall lack of conditioning/fitness	• Physical cues for drinking/using, such as places, objects, sounds, smells
Are leisure activities affected?	***Communication, Social, and Emotional Regulation***	***Social/Cultural***
• Choosing only activities involving drinking/using • No time for leisure • Uninhibited dangerous behavior during leisure pursuits (boating, skiing, hunting while under the influence)	• Difficulty establishing and maintaining close/intimate relationships • Aggressive and hostile • Copes with stress by increasing use of substances	• Friends who drink/use • Prevalence of alcohol at social/ recreational/sports events • Holiday celebrations • Family rituals

Fig. 20•1 Analyzing the Impact of Substance Abuse on Occupational Performance and Participation.

evaluates the impact of substance use on occupational performance and occupational participation. More specifically, impairments of a sensorimotor, cognitive, or psychosocial/psychological nature attributed to a substance use disorder are identified.

Community-Based Substance Abuse Services

Community-based substance abuse services include outpatient and partial hospitalization programs, dual-diagnoses programs, and aftercare programs. These programs equip the person with the skills and strategies to stop drinking and using, and develop the behavioral flexibility necessary for maintaining abstinence. People who seek formal addiction intervention programs have often tried other methods (e.g., personal contracting to reduce or stop their alcohol/drug use or seeking support through church or self-help groups) but have been unsuccessful. The most effective intervention programs include a full continuum of services, which typically include: programs for groups, individuals, and families, and support and self-help groups. Substance abuse and addiction intervention services can occur in a variety of medical and community settings (Box 20-1). Crisis intervention, intensive outpatient, aftercare, and employee assistance programs will be discussed here.

Crisis Intervention

Crisis intervention refers to the management of alcohol or other drug emergencies due to overdose, adverse drug reactions, or catastrophic psychological responses. Similar to those services provided to persons with other mental health diagnoses, such as depression, crisis intervention often occurs as the result of suicide gestures made while the individual is intoxicated or experiencing a severe withdrawal syndrome. Persons in crisis are believed to be negatively acting out their desire to change. Thus, family members, community officials, and professionals must take advantage of this momentary opportunity for change by offering specific and structured forms of help.

However, it is now recognized that a crisis or "hitting bottom" is not necessary for motivating

---

Box 20-1   Substance Abuse and Addiction Service Delivery Sites

Institutions
- Addictions and dual-diagnoses inpatient units
- Detoxification units
- Partial hospitalization programs
- Prisons

Outpatient
- Intensive outpatient programs
- Aftercare programs
- Outpatient office visits

Community
- Community mental health centers
- Schools, colleges, universities
- Halfway houses
- Employee assistance programs
- Wellness centers and programs
- Homeless shelters
- Community centers
- Sheltered workshops
- Battered women shelters
- Mobile crisis units/crisis intervention programs
- Public health departments
- Church ministry programs

---

change as was once believed. Through the use of the Stages of Change model, "motivation is now understood to be the result of an interaction between the drinker [or drug user] and those around him or her. This means that there are things a therapist can do to increase motivation for change" (Miller, 1995, p. 91). In crisis intervention, the goal is to address the immediate psychological, criminal, or medical dangers. Once out of danger, the goal changes to treatment for the substance use disorder.

Intervention by the police may be necessary when substance use produces violent and unpredictable behavior, particularly when overly high doses of the drug are ingested or when the content of the drug is laced with some other unknown mixture. For instance, amphetamine abuse and dependence may lead to a psychosis with a close resemblance to paranoid schizophrenia (Sadock & Sadock, 2008).

Medical crises may result when an individual takes lethal mixtures of alcohol and barbiturates, when a person with alcohol dependence experiences delirium tremens as the result of an unsupervised withdrawal, or when an individual engages in self-injurious behavior (Sadock & Sadock, 2008). The specific life-threatening conditions associated with the abuse of amphetamines, including cocaine and crack, include myocardial infarction, severe hypertension, cerebrovascular disease, and ischemic colitis. Inhalant use can lead to respiratory depression, cardiac arrhythmias, irreversible hepatic or renal damage, seizures, and a decreased intelligence quotient along with other neurological signs and symptoms.

Crisis intervention thus involves evaluation of the lethality of suicidal or homicidal gestures; the potential for violence or other negative and unpredictable behaviors; the danger of medical symptoms related to overdose, withdrawal, or combinations of multiple drugs and alcohol; and the extent of injuries related to trauma sustained as the result of intoxication. This evaluation may initially occur over the telephone, with instructions to proceed to the nearest emergency room, mental health hospital or unit of a hospital, or an alcohol and drug rehabilitation hospital or unit. Paramedics and police may also provide the initial evaluation and thus may arrest the individual as being dangerous to self or others. Emergency department personnel now routinely evaluate persons with traumatic injuries for alcohol and drug problems, once medical stability has been achieved (Rumpf, Hapke, Erfurth, & John, 1998). Arrests for drunk and disorderly behavior, public intoxication, or driving while under the influence may initially trigger involvement of the legal system. However, many courts later mandate intervention in place of, or in conjunction with, incarceration.

Intensive Outpatient Programs

Intensive outpatient programs (IOPs) are independent or hospital-associated programs that serve individuals with substance abuse disorders and include partial hospitalization, or intensive treatment, for approximately 4 hours per day. Patients can be admitted into these programs at different stages of the treatment process. For example, these programs can be used as initial treatment, as a more intensive approach to regular outpatient services, or as a less intensive approach than acute inpatient treatment programs, residential programs, and day treatment programs (United Behavioral Health, 2011).

Intensive outpatient programs have been found to be effective in treating alcohol dependency, with 64% of participants being sober 6 months after treatment ended (Bottlender & Soyka, 2005). Furthermore, treatment of individuals with co-occurring mental and substance abuse disorders at intensive outpatient programs can reduce stays at inpatient treatment facilities (Wise, 2010).

In order for an individual to be considered for an intensive outpatient program, candidates must meet all of the following criteria:

- not pose a threat of serious harm to self or others;
- not be in active withdrawal, or the withdrawal symptoms can be managed in an outpatient setting;
- any co-occurring medical or mental health conditions can be effectively managed in an outpatient setting; and
- be able to understand and abide by the rules set forth by the specific program (United Behavioral Health, 2011).

The core services offered by intensive outpatient programs are listed in Box 20-2. Many IOPs, especially in more urbanized areas, also offer specialized

---

Box 20-2   Core Services Provided by Intensive Outpatient Substance Abuse Programs

- Program orientation and intake
- Comprehensive medical and mental health assessment
- Individual treatment planning
- Group and family counseling
- Psychoeducational interventions
- Case management
- Integration of patients into the community
- 24-hour crisis lines
- Drug and alcohol testing
- Vocational and educational services
- Psychiatric evaluation and psychotherapy
- Medication management
- Transition and/or discharge planning

Data from: Substance Abuse and Mental Health Services Administration (1993). SAMHSA/CSAT Treatment Improvement Protocols: Services in Intensive Outpatient Treatment Programs. Retrieved from http://www.ncbi.nlm.nih.gov/books/NBK25875/ .

services, such as HIV or AIDS counseling and education (Center for Behavioral Health Statistics and Quality, 2011).

Occupational therapists can play a major role in many of the core services offered by IOPs. By fulfilling many diverse roles, they are of value to these programs. Case management is one service for which occupational therapists are well qualified, because of their training in evaluation of individuals' cognitive status, physical condition, communication or social skills, and environmental factors (American Occupational Therapy Association [AOTA], 2008). Based on the results of the assessments, occupational therapists can assist clients to identify the best resources to meet their needs. For example, community resources related to daily living skills and vocational rehabilitation may be identified and utilized frequently in this type of setting (Chapleau, Seroczynski, Meyers, Lamb, & Haynes, 2011).

Aftercare Programs

Aftercare programs are designed to provide counseling and support to individuals who have completed a treatment program in either an inpatient residential facility or an intensive outpatient program. This counseling and support can be in the form of individual counseling, support group meetings, specialized services such as vocational rehabilitation, or a combination of the above. Most programs require that the individual has remained abstinent from alcohol and drugs for a certain period of time (Everything Addiction, 2011).

Aftercare programs have been shown to be effective in helping individuals maintain abstinence for longer periods of time than intensive treatment alone. Including self-help aspects, such as the 12-step philosophy, in the program increases the likelihood that individuals will participate in aftercare programs (Frydrych, Greene, Blondell, & Purdy, 2009). In addition, programs that emphasize relapse prevention tend to produce higher self-efficacy and confidence ratings in participants (Brown, Seraganian, Tremblay, & Annis, 2001).

Occupational therapists can serve clients participating in aftercare programs in numerous ways, facilitating clients' participation in different environments and contexts without using alcohol

or drugs. Occupational therapists can provide community reintegration and relapse prevention activities that enhance physical and mental health and increase the clients' sense of well-being.

Employee Assistance Programs

Since most adults with substance abuse problems are employed, the work site is an excellent place in which to identify persons needing intervention. **Employee assistance programs** (EAPs) are workplace-based programs designed to address problems that negatively impact employee well-being and contribute to reduced productivity in the workplace, absenteeism, injuries, and work site disruptions (Merrick, Volpe-Vartanian, Horgan, & McCann, 2007). EAPs offer services such as crisis intervention, substance abuse assessments, treatment referrals, and aftercare sessions. Employees can self-refer or be referred by employers based on observation of declines at work. The eight goals of a typical EAP are listed in Box 20-3.

Several different types of EAPs exist. Internal programs are implemented in-house, and the professionals offering services are employed by the company. External vendors are contracted individuals that the company uses to provide services at a different location. Integrated programs include features of both internal and external programs. Consortia programs include a group of employers who come together

---

Box 20-3 Goals of Employee Assistance Programs (EAPs)

- Identify problems before work is seriously affected,
- Offer an easy evaluation and referral process to motivate employees to participate,
- Provide participants with high-quality, best-fit services,
- Provide cost-effective, early intervention solutions,
- Decrease workers' compensation claims through easy contact to intervention,
- Decrease turnover rates,
- Provide employers with options other than firing employees, and
- Offer support to employees

Data from: U.S. Department of Labor (2011). Drug-Free Workplace Advisor: Employee Assistance Program. Retrieved from http://www.dol.gov/elaws/asp/drugfree/drugs/assistance/screen89.asp.

to divide the costs of providing an EAP. Finally, peer assistance EAPs utilize employees who are trained to offer peer counseling and services to identified employees who may be having problems (U.S. Department of Labor, 2011).

Research on the effectiveness of EAPs has demonstrated "improved clinical and work outcomes and positive economic effects measured in a variety of ways (Merrick, Volpe-Vartanian, Horgan, & McCann, 2007, p. 1263). Occupational therapists can play a significant role in EAPs by implementing intervention strategies that incorporate effective management of daily activities, and strategies to deal with life and work stressors that may trigger the use of alcohol or drugs.

Evidence-Based Practices

Occupational therapists in all areas of practice work with individuals who have substance use disorders. Populations that experience particularly high rates of substance abuse include persons with mental disorders, spinal cord injuries, and traumatic brain injuries due to motor vehicle crashes and other traumas (Levy, Mallonee, Miller, Smith, Spicer, Romano, & Fisher, 2004). No single treatment approach is effective for all individuals. In order to assist occupational therapy practitioners to more effectively address substance abuse problems, Stoffel and Moyers (2004) completed an interdisciplinary literature review of effective interventions as part of the AOTA Evidence-Based Literature Review Project (Lieberman & Scheer, 2002). Interventions with demonstrated efficacy to positively impact a "person's engagement in occupations and activities necessary for role functioning, health and quality of life" (Stoffel & Moyers, 2004, p. 571) that can be incorporated into occupational therapy practice will be described here. These include brief interventions, motivational strategies, cognitive-behavioral therapy, and 12-step programs.

Brief Interventions

Brief interventions "are those practices that aim to investigate a potential problem and motivate an individual to begin to do something about his substance abuse, either by natural, client-directed

means or by seeking additional substance abuse treatment" (Substance Abuse and Mental Health Services Administration [SAMHSA], 1999a, para. 10). Brief interventions typically consist of five or fewer sessions each of relatively brief duration, such as a few minutes up to one hour (SAMHSA, 2010). Brief interventions may occur face-to-face during a health care visit, via phone calls or electronic communication (e-mail), or through the use of written materials such as workbooks (Stoffel & Moyers, 2004). Because brief interventions have been found to be feasible, practical, and cost effective for implementation by a wide range of professionals, they are increasingly being used to bridge the gap between prevention efforts and more intensive treatment approaches for persons with severe substance dependence disorders (SAMHSA, 1999a). Consequently, Zweben and Rose (1999) advocate the integration of brief interventions into all medical and social service programs, including those programs staffed by occupational therapy practitioners.

The basic goal of brief intervention is to "reduce the risk of harm that could result from continued use of substances," which may include reducing amount and/or frequency of use, practicing abstinence, or attending a 12-step meeting (SAMHSA, 1999a, para. 17). Occupational therapy practitioners are able to integrate these strategies into the intervention plans of their clients in multiple settings, even though the client initially may be referred for another reason, such as a hand injury (Moyers & Stoffel, 1999).

One type of brief intervention provides information in a written format, such as self-help manuals, educational materials, pamphlets, and brief self-scoring questionnaires. These materials can be supplied in the waiting rooms of any occupational therapy setting and thus do not need to be formally discussed with the client unless the client asks specific questions. The idea is to promote client responsibility while still providing information that moves the client into the next stage of change, such as from precontemplation to contemplation or from contemplation to action. Miller and Munoz (1982) developed a self-help manual to supplement treatment that has been shown to successfully enhance intervention outcomes. Thus, occupational therapy practitioners might do well to review their client education materials for content related to prevention and treatment of substance use disorders and problem drinking. Populations for which occupational therapy practitioners provide services could each have specifically designed materials addressing the problems related to substance use, prevention strategies, and resources for intervention. When this information is presented in the context of the health condition that is of most concern to the client, it may have a greater impact.

The key to effective brief intervention strategies is to establish rapport and to use appropriate open-ended questions based on a topic that is of concern to the individual (Rollnick & Bell, 1991). A brief intervention consists of five steps:

1. Introducing substance use concerns in the context of the person's health
2. Screening and evaluation of substance use patterns
3. Providing feedback based on assessment results
4. Talking about change and setting goals
5. Summarizing concerns, goals, and plans (SAMHSA, 1999a).

Miller and Sanchez (1994) developed the FRAMES model for brief interventions. **FRAMES** is a mnemonic device that stands for feedback, responsibility, advice, menu, empathy, and self-efficacy. Throughout the interview, the professional gives clear and specific *feedback* from the assessment that supports the need for change. The information is not accusatory and the focus is not on diagnostic labeling. Instead, the emphasis is on the person's *responsibility* to interpret and act on the information. The interviewer does give *advice* in relationship to the medical consequences for continued use. The professional supplies a *menu* of change options, ranging from self-help programs or manuals to hospitalization. Throughout the interview, the professional is *empathetic* and avoids hostile confrontations, power struggles, and judgmental and paternalistic attitudes. Additionally, the professional's attitude promotes the *self-efficacy* of the client or a belief in the individual's ability to make decisions about when and how to change.

Depending on the circumstances, the occupational therapy practitioner may find that the FRAMES process rarely occurs in one session. Rather, it occurs over time. The individual may be able to absorb only some feedback, with emphasis on the client's own responsibility during a single interview. If a client, after a series of brief interventions, indicates a willingness to plan and take action about the substance use, the occupational therapy practitioner readily helps the client make specific and realistic plans, offers to initiate a referral, and provides support for implementing other change strategies on the menu of options.

Motivational Approaches

According to Miller and Rollnick (2002), motivation consists of three critical components: readiness, willingness, and ability. Motivation is multidimensional and dynamic, not static. It can be influenced and modified through interpersonal and intrapersonal factors. Motivation can be affected by critical life events, cognitive appraisal of the impact of behavior on one's life, recognition of negative consequences of one's current behavior, and external incentives, both positive and negative. Motivation increases the "probability that a person will enter into, continue, and adhere to a specific change strategy" (SAMHSA, 1999b, para. 1). Motivational approaches, such as motivational interviewing and motivational enhancement therapy, are based on the Transtheoretical or Stages of Change Model discussed in Chapter 3 of this text. Strategies inherent in the motivational approaches include:

- Focusing on the client's strengths rather than weaknesses
- Respecting the client's autonomy and decisions
- Using empathy rather than authority and power as motivators
- Individualizing treatment
- Focusing on early interventions before significant consequences occur
- Developing a therapeutic partnership
- Supporting small, incremental steps toward recovery (SAMHSA, 1999b).

Motivational approaches can be used at various phases of the intervention process. For example, motivational strategies, such as motivational interviewing, may be used in the early phases as part of a brief intervention. Motivational enhancement therapy may be used in later phases as a way of sustaining the client's ongoing commitment once change has been initiated.

Motivational Interviewing

According to Miller and Rollnick (2002), **motivational interviewing** is "a client-centered, directive method for enhancing intrinsic motivation to change by exploring and resolving ambivalence" (p. 25). The purpose of motivational interviewing is to elicit self-motivational statements and behavioral change from the client. Motivational interviewing is not a set of techniques per se but rather a way of interacting with a client. The spirit of motivational interviewing can be described by the following principles/directives:

- motivation to change is intrinsic and elicited from within the individual, not imposed from the outside;
- it is the client's task, not the counselor's, to identify, articulate, and resolve his or her ambivalence;
- the counselor uses an empathic, supportive, and collaborative style; direct persuasion or confrontation generally increases client resistance and is counterproductive;
- readiness to change is not a static trait but rather a fluctuating product of the interpersonal therapeutic interaction; and
- the professional respects and affirms the client's autonomy, freedom of choice, and self-direction (Rollnick & Miller, 1995).

Motivational interviewing occurs in two phases. The first phase is designed to resolve ambivalence and build intrinsic motivation for change. The second phase involves strengthening commitment to change and developing a plan of action (Miller & Rollnick, 2002). Motivational interviewing consists of:

- Asking open-ended questions
- Active listening and reflective responses
- Summarizing what has transpired during the session
- Affirming the client's strengths, motivation, intentions, and progress
- Eliciting self-motivational statements (SAMHSA, 1999b).

Clients can be categorized along two dimensions of intrinsic motivation. These dimensions are the client's perceptions of the importance of change and their confidence to change. The resulting four categories are:

1. low importance, low confidence,
2. high importance, low confidence,
3. low importance, high confidence, and
4. high importance, high confidence (Miller & Rollnick, 2002).

The motivational strategies needed vary depending on the category to which the client belongs (Fig. 20.2).

High Importance, High Confidence	**High Importance, Low Confidence**
These individuals believe that change is important and they also believe in their ability to succeed. Intervention: affirm the person's commitment to change and develop a plan of action	These individuals believe that change is important but they have little belief in their ability to succeed. Intervention: increase self-efficacy through encouragement, support, and feedback
Low Importance, High Confidence	**Low Importance, Low Confidence**
These individuals believe they could succeed if they desired to change, but they do not believe that change is necessary or important. Intervention: identify disadvantages of the status quo and the advantages of change	These individuals do not believe change is important nor do they believe they could succeed in making a change if they tried. Intervention: explore goals and values, identify disadvantages of the status quo and the advantages of change, elicit examples of other areas in the person's life where they were successful in making changes

Fig. 20•2 Categories of Intrinsic Motivation. (From Miller & Rollnick (2002). *Motivational interviewing: Preparing people for change, 2/e.* New York: Guilford Press.)

Motivational Enhancement Therapy

Motivational enhancement therapy (MET) is an adaptation of motivational interviewing developed by Miller, Zweben, DiClemente, and Rychtarik (1992) that consists of four highly structured sessions. The sessions include a drinker's check-up (DCU) and the FRAMES approach to interviewing for change (Miller & Sanchez, 1994). The DCU is a comprehensive assessment offered as a health check-up for persons with problem drinking. In addition to asking the individual quantity and frequency-of-use questions, other screening tools measuring the impact of problem drinking are administered, the most common tool being the CAGE (Ewing, 1984). **CAGE** stands for the following four questions:

1. Have you ever felt that you should *cut down* on drinking?
2. Have people *annoyed* you by criticizing your drinking?
3. Have you ever felt *guilty* about your drinking?
4. Have you ever had a drink first thing in the morning to steady your nerves or get rid of a hangover (*eye opener*)?

Two positive answers on the CAGE would indicate the presence of alcohol-related problems, and three or more positive answers indicate potential alcohol dependence.

The DCU would then proceed by using more specific questionnaires, such as the Michigan Alcohol Screening Test (MAST), which analyzes the social, medical, legal, and psychosocial consequences associated with problematic drinking, such as blackouts, loss of employment, and drunk driving arrests (Selzer, 1971). An occupational therapy practitioner would add an occupational history, highlighting the impact of the substance use on occupational performance to the DCU (Moyers & Stoffel, 1999). Blood testing for alcohol and urine testing for drugs may be conducted, along with medical laboratory screens that assess liver functions and other systems impacted by long-term use of chemicals. Results from the DCU are used to provide feedback so that the individual can successfully move through the successive stages of change.

Cognitive-Behavioral Approaches

Cognitive -behavioral therapy (CBT) emphasizes the impact of cognitive appraisals, attributions, and self-efficacy expectations on substance use behavior. CBT often focuses on the development of coping skills in order to reduce substance abuse and prevent relapse. CBT is equally effective when provided individually or in groups and is best used when a person demonstrates a readiness to change his or her substance use behavior. In order for cognitive-behavioral approaches to be effective, the individual must possess adequate memory, problem solving and judgment abilities, and the ability to process information and express oneself verbally (Stoffel & Moyers, 2004).

Central to the cognitive-behavioral approach is the identification of an individual's antecedents: (A) to substance use behavior (B) and the short-term and long-term consequences (C) of that use. These are referred to as the ABCs of cognitive behavioral therapy as depicted in Figure 20.3. Antecedents are those situations, conditions, locations, activities, people, cues, thoughts, or feelings that precede and lead to substance use. Cues are stimuli related to substance use, for example, the smell of a substance, a setting (such as a bar, tavern, club, or restaurant), an activity, or even certain times of day or special events (e.g., New Year's Eve). Consequences can be positive or negative and refer to the physical, emotional, and social effects that result from substance use.

A cognitive-behavioral approach was used successfully with clients with substance use disorders who had difficulty managing anger. A 12-session anger management group intervention

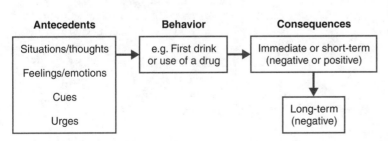

Fig. 20·3 ABCs of Cognitive-Behavioral Therapy. (From Center for Substance Abuse Treatment (2005). *Substance abuse relapse prevention for older adults: A group treatment approach.* Rockville, MD: Substance Abuse and Mental Health Services Administration.)

demonstrated effectiveness in reducing anger and improving social-emotional functioning, as well as decreasing substance use. Four types of CBT interventions are frequently used when treating persons with anger issues. These include:

- Relaxation interventions to decrease the emotional and physiological arousal associated with anger;
- Cognitive interventions to address cognitive appraisals, irrational beliefs, and hostile attributions that trigger anger responses;
- Communication skills interventions to improve assertiveness and conflict resolution skills; and
- Combined interventions that integrate multiple intervention methods and target multiple anger-related domains (Reilly & Shopshire, 2002).

Occupational therapists can incorporate cognitive-behavioral strategies through role modeling, structured opportunities to practice coping skills, and timely feedback. Clients can be helped to change their distorted thought patterns regarding substance use, develop self-efficacy, and establish alternative, healthy coping behaviors to manage daily stressors. **Behavioral rehearsal,** or role-playing the practice and application of newly learned skills, is a key element in cognitive-behavioral therapy. The following are the recommended steps for conducting behavioral rehearsal:

- Read the situation or scenario aloud
- Discuss appropriate responses to the situation
- Choose an appropriate response and explain the rationale for the choice
- Model the chosen behavioral response
- Get feedback from the group on the effectiveness of the behavioral response
- Modify the response based on group feedback if necessary
- Read the scenario aloud a second time
- Choose a client to rehearse the behavior
- Ask the group to provide feedback
- Coach the client if necessary
- Rehearse again
- Ask for group feedback again
- Move to the next client and introduce a new situation or scenario (Center for Substance Abuse Treatment, 2005).

12-Step Recovery Programs

Recovery programs based on the 12 Steps of Alcoholics Anonymous (AA) take two basic forms. One is a professionally facilitated therapeutic process (Twelve Step Facilitation Therapy), and the other is in the form of mutual support group programs, like AA and others.

Twelve Step Facilitation (TSF) Therapy is a structured 12–15 session professionally facilitated program for early recovery from substance abuse and dependence. The program is based on the cognitive, behavioral, and spiritual principles of 12-step recovery fellowships such as AA. The TSF counselor assesses the client's substance use, advocates abstinence, provides psychoeducational sessions on 12-step concepts, and facilitates initial and ongoing participation in 12-step recovery support groups. In a large-scale, federally funded research project, TSF therapy clients demonstrated significantly higher rates of substance abstinence than those who participated in cognitive-behavioral therapy (CBT) or motivational enhancement therapy (MET) interventions. In addition, TSF participants had higher rates of involvement in AA group meetings (62%) as compared to those receiving MET (38%) or CBT (25%) (National Registry of Evidence-based Programs and Practices, 2008). TSF can be used by occupational therapists, and an implementation guide can be purchased from the National Institute on Alcohol Abuse and Alcoholism.

Involvement of clients in **mutual support programs** (those programs that do not rely on professional intervention but on the support of group members) is particularly important given the push by managed-care programs to drastically reduce both inpatient and outpatient treatment days. The occupational therapy practitioner encourages and recommends participation in a variety of 12-step programs, such as Alcoholics Anonymous (AA), Cocaine Anonymous, and Narcotics Anonymous. The 12 Steps of AA are listed in Box 20-4.

Research indicates that consistent attendance at 12-step meetings is effective in achieving abstinence for persons with substance abuse disorders (Witbrodt, Mertens, Kaskutas, Bond, Chi, &Weisner, 2011). Miller (1998) stated that spirituality-based programs, such as AA, are more likely to help people remain abstinent when compared to psychological therapy

Box 20-4 The 12 Steps of Alcoholics Anonymous

1. We admitted we were powerless over alcohol—that our lives had become unmanageable.
2. Came to believe that a Power greater than ourselves could restore us to sanity.
3. Made a decision to turn our will and our lives over to the care of God *as we understood Him.*
4. Made a searching and fearless moral inventory of ourselves.
5. Admitted to God, to ourselves, and to another human being the exact nature of our wrongs.
6. Were entirely ready to have God remove all these defects of character.
7. Humbly asked Him to remove our shortcomings.
8. Made a list of all persons we had harmed, and became willing to make amends to them all.
9. Made direct amends to such people wherever possible, except when to do so would injure them or others.
10. Continued to take personal inventory and when we were wrong promptly admitted it.
11. Sought through prayer and meditation to improve our conscious contact with God, *as we understood Him,* praying only for knowledge of His will for us and the power to carry that out.
12. Having had a spiritual awakening as the result of these Steps, we tried to carry this message to alcoholics, and to practice these principles in all our affairs.

Copyright: Alcoholics Anonymous World Services, Inc. (1976). *Alcoholics Anonymous* (3rd Ed.). New York: AA.

devoid of spirituality. In general, AA sees the most pervasive problem of alcoholism as the spiritual decay that results from the distorted perception that the self, rather than a higher power, is at the center of life. (Alcoholics Anonymous World Services, 1976). Committing to abstinence, decreasing preoccupation with the self, and living a life-long program of spirituality are the essential elements of sobriety according to AA (Alcoholics Anonymous World Services, 1970). Achievement of these goals occurs by "working the 12 steps of recovery" and is facilitated by group participation and the support of a sponsor.

Computer technology has made it possible to access self-help resources through e-mail and the Web. The home pages of many of these self-help groups provide information about the organization, about group locations and meeting times, and about ordering literature; some may actually conduct meetings on line. With technology, support for staying sober is immediately available at any time right in the home.

Occupational Therapy in Substance Abuse Programs

Occupational therapists use a client-centered approach to determine the occupational performances that require intervention in order for the client to achieve greater life satisfaction. To identify these occupational performances, the occupational therapist may use an occupational interview or history to highlight for the client the loss of intentionality and the progressive abdication of control over one's life to alcohol and drugs. Reasonable goals are then collaboratively developed to help the client change the deficient occupational performance. For instance, it is important that the client receive help in finding a job and in locating suitable living arrangements. These are two of the critical factors that support the person in recovery. Additionally, the client may need social and leisure counseling and opportunities to attend drug-free social activities.

In addition to helping the client improve occupational performance, the therapist also incorporates into the intervention plan the idea that occupations are opportunities "to progressively reinvent the way in which the self is understood" (Moyers, 1997, p. 211). Therapeutic occupations are used to reinvent the self as abstinent by creating rationales for being sober, developing habits of sobriety, and producing peak experiences when sober. Daily occupations are organized into basic habits such as getting rest, eating balanced meals, keeping the body neat and clean, and following the therapy regimen necessary for maintaining abstinence. Occupations help re-establish intentionality as the individual deliberately selects occupations according to a variety of goals, values, or interests. In fact, occupations may serve as a transition to a valued future goal and thus provide the context for learning and applying new skills needed for personal growth. For instance, occupational therapy intervention might help the client redefine his or her qualifications, select and begin a program of intensive retraining, and eventually obtain a more satisfying and interesting job.

Miller (1998) has noted through a review of 12 different studies that addiction is associated with a lack of meaning and purpose in life. Finding meaning is a spiritual process because the person attempts to discover his or her purpose or reasons for being in the world and clarifies within that scheme the importance of interpersonal relationships, daily events, and goals. Thus, rationales for staying sober are firmly established through meaningful occupations that promote spirituality and one's connectedness to the world.

Underlying performance patterns and performance skills that contribute to impairment in occupational performance are also key recovery factors identified and targeted for intervention. Persons with substance abuse problems often demonstrate dysfunction in habits, routines, and role performance. Cognitive skills, communication and social skills, and emotional regulation skills are other important aspects of functioning that require evaluation and intervention.

To illustrate the influence of performance patterns and performance skills, consider the individual who states that drug and alcohol use negatively affects school performance and interferes with the goal of graduating from college with a degree in accounting. In analyzing the underlying factors or performance components, the client and the occupational therapist determine that managing time, coping with stress and financial worries, developing study habits, and socializing with classmates who are truly supportive of the client's objectives are all important for achieving the goal of obtaining a degree.

The intervention plan outlines strategies to improve skills in time management, coping, academics, and socialization. Coping skills training is important for the client to learn how to cope with frustration when engaging in routine occupations. Coping skills training usually involves teaching relaxation techniques, meditation strategies, alternate coping behaviors, specific control skills (limit setting, planning ahead for potential difficulties), drug refusal skills, and self-monitoring of emotional extremes and negative thinking. However, this training may be ineffective due to the disruption of these skills by the presence of drug-using cues in the environment. Contextual factors, including the physical, social, and cultural environments that facilitate or inhibit recovery, are also identified as parts of the intervention plan.

Environmental modification may involve working with the family to help the person create a supportive atmosphere for change. Typical family behaviors, such as reinforcing drug use through attention and caretaking, protecting the individual from the consequences of substance use, and punishing for infractions related to drug use, have been noted to increase the likelihood of continued substance abuse. However, not only does the family affect the person using substances but also the individual's substance-related behaviors affect family members. Occupational therapy practitioners work with family members to enhance their occupational performance and participation (Moyers, 1991, 1992; Stoffel, 1994). The goals are to help family members learn to cope with their emotional distress and to concentrate on their own motivations for change in performance areas, regardless of whether the individual decides to change his or her substance use.

Finally, occupational therapy practitioners can provide instruction to clients regarding relapse prevention strategies. Many of the risk factors that have been shown to precipitate relapse, for example, negative affect, low self-efficacy, limited coping skills, lack of social support, and poor psychological functioning (Marlatt, Bowen, &Witkiewitz, 2009), are amenable to occupational therapy intervention. The Stages of Change Model (described in Chapter 3) provides a useful framework for developing interventions appropriate for each stage (Table 20-1).

Conclusion

Occupational therapy practitioners working in community settings have tremendous potential to provide an occupation-focused perspective on helping individuals who struggle with substance use disorders by enhancing their occupational performance in environments that support their

Table 20-1	Occupational Therapy Interventions for Substance Abuse Using the Stages of Change Model	
Stage	**Description**	**Appropriate Interventions**
Precontemplation	Little or no awareness of effects of substance use on occupational performance	Increasing awareness of the impact of substance use on occupational performance through self-assessment techniques and motivational interviewing
Contemplation	Some awareness of effects of substance use on occupational performance but no efforts made to address the resulting problems	Decisional balance exercises to explore the positive and negative aspects of substance use and the resulting impact on occupational performance
Preparation	Consideration of potential ways to address the impact of substance use on occupational performance but no implementation of strategies	Exploration of a range of treatment options and community resources to support initiation and maintenance of changes in substance use
Action	Implementation of change strategies to decrease substance use and improve occupational performance	Cognitive-behavioral interventions, participation in 12-step programs, and motivational enhancement therapy
Maintenance	Efforts to maintain improvements in occupational performance and changes in substance use patterns	Community support programs, participation in 12-step programs, and relapse prevention skill development
Relapse	Return to substance use after a period of abstinence and the resulting decline in occupational performance	Revisit motivational strategies and decisional balance exercises to re-engage client in the action stage and identify cues to relapse

CASE STUDIES

CASE STUDY 20•1 Richard

Richard is a single, 30-year-old white male with a 10-year history of cocaine and barbiturate abuse. Richard is currently staying with various "friends" and does not have a primary residence of his own. Richard has been employed off and on for the past 10 years as a heating and air conditioning specialist, and the longest time he has maintained employment was 9 months. Each time he was fired from a job, it was due to being absent or late for work secondary to substance abuse. Richard has a legal history of misdemeanor drug possession and paraphernalia possession, and he has received inpatient treatment for substance abuse three times. He has one daughter who is 9 years old and lives with her mother. Richard is currently not allowed to contact his daughter. Richard has no insurance coverage and no money to pay out-of-pocket expenses for treatment, so he has been referred to state-funded facilities.

Richard has received state-funded medical detoxification treatment at a local facility for the last 14 days, and he has been evaluated for a state-run intensive outpatient program (IOP). Upon evaluation, Richard stated that he would like to return to work in his field and to regain partial custody of his daughter. He currently has no hobbies other than using drugs, and he has isolated himself from all of his friends. The only contacts that he has are people who also use drugs. Richard states that he wants to approach treatment differently this time, and he states that he truly wants to be successful at managing his addictions.

Continued

CASE STUDY 20•1 Richard *cont'd*

CASE STUDY 20•1 Discussion Questions

1. In order for Richard to be successful, what services within the IOP would you recommend?
2. Name five ways in which an occupational therapist could help Richard meet his goals.
3. After Richard completes the IOP, what would be the next step? Find one of these types of facilities in your local area to which Richard could be referred.
4. List five suggestions that an occupational therapist could give Richard to help him manage daily stressors that could trigger him to use substances.
5. Name three interventions that an occupational therapist at the IOP could use to help Richard attain and maintain employment.

---

health and meaningful occupational roles. Occupational therapy intervention includes the following main approaches:

- Facilitating change in occupational performance and participation for the person using substances and for the family members affected by the substance use of others
- Identifying occupations that are satisfying and that contribute to well-being and quality of life
- Removing barriers that interfere with abstinence, such as methods for resolving the financial problems typical for persons with substance use disorders

- Helping the individual make environmental changes that are conducive to abstinence and that compensate for performance impairments
- Developing coping skills that assist the individual in responding to temptations and cravings, and to typical daily hassles and their frustrations with occupational performance.

REFERENCES

Alcoholics Anonymous World Services. (1970). *A member's-eye view of Alcoholics Anonymous.* New York: Author.

Alcoholics Anonymous World Services. (1976). *Alcoholics Anonymous* (3rd ed.). New York: AA.

American Occupational Therapy Association. (2008). Occupational therapy practice framework: Domain and process (2nd ed.). *American Journal of Occupational Therapy, 62,* 625–683.

American Psychiatric Association. (2013). *Diagnostic and statistical manual of mental disorders, fifth edition (DSM V).* Arlington, VA: Author.

Bottlender, M., & Soyka, M. (2005). Efficacy of an intensive outpatient rehabilitation program in alcoholism: Predictors of outcome 6 months after treatment. *European Addiction Research, 11,* 132–137.

Brown, T. G., Seraganian, P., Tremblay, J., & Annis, H. (2001). Process and outcome changes with relapse prevention versus 12-step aftercare programs for substance abusers. *Addiction, 97,* 677–689.

Center for Behavioral Health Statistics and Quality. (2011). The NSSATS-Report: Differences and Similarities Between Urban and Rural Outpatient Substance Abuse Treatment Facilities. Retrieved from http://oas.samhsa.gov

Center for Substance Abuse Treatment. (2005). *Substance abuse relapse prevention for older adults: A group treatment approach.* Rockville, MD: Substance Abuse and Mental Health Services Administration.

Chapleau, A., Seroczynski, A. D., Meyers, S., Lamb, K., & Haynes, S. (2011). Occupational therapy consultation for

Learning Activities

1. Use the Internet to find community resources in your area for patients who have substance abuse problems, specifically local AA or NA meetings. Attend an open AA or NA meeting.
2. Use the Internet to find various types of community-based substance abuse treatment facilities in your area. Call the facilities and ask questions regarding the services that they offer. Find out if there has ever been an occupational therapist employed with the facility.
3. Use the SAMHSA Web site to compile a notebook of informational handouts to offer to clients with substance abuse problems.
4. Identify five occupational therapy assessments that may be appropriate to use with clients who have substance abuse problems.

case managers in community mental health: Exploring strategies to improve job satisfaction and self-efficacy. *Professional Case Management, 16*(2), 71–79.

Christiansen, C., Clark, F., Kielhofner, G., & Rogers, J. (1995). Occupation: A position paper. *American Journal of Occupational Therapy, 49,* 1015–1018.

Everything Addiction. (2011). Importance of Aftercare in Addiction Treatment. Retrieved from http://www.everythingaddiction.com/addiction-treatment/recovery-addiction-treatment/importance-of-aftercare-in-addiction-treatment/

Ewing, J. (1984). Detecting alcoholism: The CAGE questionnaire. *Journal of the American Medical Association, 252,* 1905–1907.

Frydrych, L. M., Greene, B. J., Blondell, R. D., & Purdy, C. H. (2009). Self-help program components and linkage to aftercare following inpatient detoxification. *Journal of Addictive Diseases, 28*(1), 21–27.

Levy, D. T., Mallonee, S., Miller, T. R., Smith, G. S., Spicer, R. S., Romano, E. O., & Fisher, D.A. (2004). Alcohol involvement in burn, submersion, spinal cord and brain injuries. *Medical Science Monitor, 10*(1), 17–24.

Lieberman, D., & Scheer, J. (2002). AOTA's evidence-based literature review project. *American Journal of Occupational Therapy, 56,* 344–349.

Marlatt, G. A., Bowen, S. W., & Witkiewitz, K. (2009). Relapse prevention: Evidence base and future directions. In Peter M. Miller (Ed.), *Evidence-based addiction treatment* (pp. 215–230). Burlington, MA: Elsevier.

Merrick, E. S., Volpe-Vartanian, J., Horgan, C. M., & McCann, B. (2007). Revisiting employee assistance programs and substance use problems in the workplace: Key issues and a research agenda. *Psychiatric Services, 58*(10), 1262–1264.

Mertens, J. R., Weisner, C., Ray, G. T., Fireman, B., & Walsh, K. (2005). Hazardous drinkers and drug users in HOMO primary care: Prevalence, medical conditions and costs. *Alcoholism: Clinical and Experimental Research, 29*(6), 989–998.

Miller, W. R. (1995). Increasing motivation for change. In R. K. Hester & W. R. Miller (Eds.), *Handbook of alcoholism treatment approaches: Effective alternatives* (2nd ed., pp. 88–104). Boston: Allyn and Bacon.

Miller, W. R. (1998). Researching the spiritual dimensions of alcohol and other drug problems. *Addiction, 93,* 979–990.

Miller, W. R., & Munoz, R. F. (1982). *How to control your drinking* (Rev. ed.). Albuquerque, NM: University of New Mexico Press.

Miller, W. R., & Rollnick, S. (2002). *Motivational interviewing: Preparing people for change, 2nd edition.* New York: Guilford Press.

Miller, W. R., & Sanchez, V. C. (1994). Motivating young adults for treatment and lifestyle change. In G. Howard (Ed.), *Issues in alcohol use and misuse by young adults* (pp. 55–82). Notre Dame, IN: University of Notre Dame Press.

Miller, W. R., Zweben, A., DiClemente, C. C., & Rychtarik, R. G. (1992). *Motivational enhancement therapy (MET): A clinical research guide for therapists treating individuals with alcohol abuse and dependence* (DHHS Publication N. ADM 92–1894). Washington, DC: U.S. Government Printing Office.

Moyers, P. A. (1991). Occupational therapy and treatment of the alcoholic's family. *Occupational Therapy in Mental Health, 11,* 45–64.

Moyers, P. A. (1992). Occupational therapy intervention with the alcoholic's family. *American Journal of Occupational Therapy, 46,* 105–111.

Moyers, P. A. (1997). Occupational meanings and spirituality: The quest for sobriety. *American Journal of Occupational Therapy, 51*(3), 207–214.

Moyers, P. A., & Stoffel, V. C. (1999). Alcohol dependence in a client with a work-related injury. *American Journal of Occupational Therapy, 53*(6), 640–645.

National Registry of Evidence-based Programs and Practices. (2008). Twelve step facilitation therapy. Retrieved from http://www.nrepp.samhsa.gov/ViewIntervention.aspx?id=55

O'Day, K. (2009). Effectiveness of treatment techniques for substance abuse in occupational therapy. *Mental Health CATs: Paper 1.* Retrieved from http://commons.pacificu.edu/otmh/1

Reilly, P. M., & Shopshire, M. S. (2002). *Anger management for substance abuse and mental health clients: A cognitive behavioral therapy manual.* Rockville, MD: Center for Substance Abuse Treatment, Substance Abuse and Mental Health Services Administration.

Rollnick, S., & Bell, A. (1991). Brief motivational interviewing for use by the nonspecialist. In W. R. Miller & S. Rollnick (Eds.), *Motivational interviewing: Preparing people to change addictive behavior* (pp. 203–213). New York: Guilford.

Rollnick, S., & Miller, W. R. (1995). What is motivational interviewing? *Behavioural and Cognitive Psychotherapy, 23,* 325–334.

Rumpf, H. J., Hapke, U., Erfurth, A., & John, U. (1998). Screening questionnaires in the detection of hazardous alcohol consumption in the general hospital: Direct or disguised assessment? *Journal of Studies on Alcohol, 59,* 698–703.

Saatcioglu, O., Erim, R., & Cakmak, D. (2006). Role of family in alcohol and substance abuse. *Psychiatry and Clinical Neurosciences, 60*(2), 125–132.

Sadock, B. J., & Sadock, V. A. (2008). *Kaplan & Sadock's concise textbook of clinical psychiatry, 3rd Ed.* Baltimore: Lippincott Williams and Wilkins.

Selzer, M. L. (1971). The Michigan alcoholism screening test: The quest for a new diagnostic instrument. *American Journal of Psychiatry, 127,* 1653–1658.

Stoffel, V. C. (1994). Occupational therapist's roles in treating substance abuse. *Hospital and Community Psychiatry, 45,* 21–22.

Stoffel, V. C., & Moyers, P. A. (2004). An evidence-based and occupational perspective of interventions for persons with substance-use disorders. *American Journal of Occupational Therapy, 58*(5), 570–586.

Substance Abuse and Mental Health Services Administration. (1993). SAMHSA/CSAT Treatment Improvement Protocols: Services in Intensive Outpatient Treatment Programs. Retrieved from http://www.ncbi.nlm.nih.gov/books/NBK25875/

Substance Abuse and Mental Health Services Administration. (1999a). *TIP 34 Brief interventions and brief therapies for substance abuse.* Retrieved from http://www.ncbi.nlm.nih.gov/books/NBK14512/

Substance Abuse and Mental Health Services Administration. (1999b). *TIP 35 Enhancing motivation for change in substance abuse treatment.* Retrieved from http://www.ncbi.nlm.nih.gov/books/NBK14856/

Substance Abuse and Mental Health Services Administration. (2010). *Prevention services: Brief motivational interventions for alcohol and drug use for the elderly.* Retrieved from http://www.samhsa.gov/healthReform/docs/Prevention_Service_Definitions_Brief_Motivational_Interview_Elderly_Reformatted_20101129.pdf

United Behavioral Health. (2011). Substance Use Disorders: Intensive Outpatient Program. *U.S. Behavioral Health Plan, California 2011 Level of Care Guidelines.* Retrieved from https://www.ubhonline.com/html/guidelines/levelOfCareGuidelines/pdf/saIntensiveOutpatient.pdf

U.S. Department of Labor. (2011). Drug-Free Workplace Advisor: Employee Assistance Program. Retrieved from http://www.dol.gov/elaws/asp/drugfree/drugs/assistance/screen89.asp

Weisner, C. J. (1995, June). Distinctive features of the alcohol treatment system. *Frontlines: Linking Alcohol Services Research and Practice,* 1–2.

Wise, E. A. (2010). Evidence-based effectiveness of a private practice intensive outpatient program with dual diagnosis. *Journal of Dual Diagnosis, 6,* 25–45.

Witbrodt, J., Mertens, J., Kaskutas, L. A., Bond, J., Chi, F., & Weisner, C. (2011). Do 12-step meeting attendance trajectories over 9 years predict abstinence? *Journal of Substance Abuse Treatment, 43*(1), 30–43.

Ziedonis, D. M., Smelson, D., Rosenthal, R. N., Batki, S. L., Green, A. I., Henry, R. J., Montoya, I., Parks, J., & Weiss, R. D. (2005). Improving the care of individuals with schizophrenia and substance use disorders: Consensus recommendations. *Journal of Psychiatric Practice, 11*(5), 315–339.

Zweben, A., & Rose, S. J. (1999). Innovations in treating alcohol problems. In D. Biegel and A. Blum (Eds.), *Innovations in practice and service delivery with vulnerable populations* (pp. 197–227). New York: Oxford University Press.

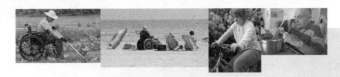

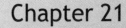

Chapter 21

Forensic Mental Health Practice Within the Community

Roxanne Castaneda, MS, OTR/L, and S. Maggie Reitz, PhD, OTR/L, FAOTA

When in doubt always be human.
—Alfred J. Shulman, M.D.

Learning Objectives

This chapter is designed to enable the reader to:
- Identify and discuss several ways clients in the criminal justice system enter the community mental health system in the United States.
- Describe the reentry process into the community following incarceration or hospitalization.
- Explain and describe the role of occupational therapy within forensic mental health practice.
- Describe the cultural dynamics of criminal justice and forensic mental health contexts and the mental health recovery movement.

Key Terms

Insanity acquitees
Re-Entry After Prison/Jail (RAP)

Specialty courts

Introduction

State mental health agencies attributed an increase in admissions to in-state psychiatric hospitals nationwide in the United States from 2002 to 2005 to the increase of forensic admissions. Although the dynamics of this process are not clearly understood, experts speculate that the influx of individuals with mental health issues into the courtroom is due to the lack of community resources to address their needs (Manderschied, Atay, & Crider, 2009). State behavioral health hospitals, formerly accustomed to only civil admissions, are seeing an influx of forensic clients. For example, in 2010 the population of a 250-bed civil facility in Maryland was 75% forensic clients (P. Langmeade, personal communication, February 2010).

Although the return from incarceration or forensic hospitalization to the community is complex, occupational therapy practice with this population can be very rewarding. However, it is pursued by few. Occupational therapists employed by day and residential programs are rare (A. Thompson, personal communication, March 2008). The presence of forensic and corrections clientele at state institutions seems to increase the challenge of hiring and retaining staff in many areas of mental health practice due to the nature of the crimes and concerns about potential violence. This difficulty in recruitment is even more prevalent in corrections and forensic agencies. An additional factor for limited occupational therapy service provision is the difficulty in obtaining reimbursement.

The focus of this chapter is individuals with mental illness and criminal behavior with forensic involvement. Services for the general prison population are beyond the scope of this chapter. Most of the information in this chapter comes from the primary author's direct experience as a director of community forensics services, as a director of forensic evaluation, and in working with the National Association of State Mental Health Forensic Directors Group. Specific topics covered in this chapter include:

- Entry process to the criminal justice system and/or the forensic mental health system
- Route to community reintegration
- Role of occupational therapy in community re-entry with forensic clients
- Challenges to community intervention
- Cultural dynamics of criminal justice and forensic mental health contexts
- Mental health recovery movement
- Occupational therapy community practice with persons with mental health and criminal justice/forensic involvement

A case study is presented at the end of the chapter.

Entry Process to Criminal Justice System and/or the Forensic Mental Health System: Client, Defendant, or Inmate?

Clients in the criminal justice system can come in contact with the mental health system in several ways in the United States. Forensic clients could include:

- defendants, pre-trial or undergoing evaluation phase inmates, post-conviction phase at jails or prisons
- "**'insanity acquitees'** (those acquitted based on an insanity defense). Insanity acquitees ... typically have mental illness and often also have an additional diagnosis such as mental retardation or substance abuse" (Castaneda, 2010, p. 202).

Those who avail themselves of the insanity defense typically receive evaluation and/or treatment through the formal state mental health forensic system (i.e., maximum security hospital and/or state psychiatric hospital).

Other forensic clients may choose not to disclose mental illness, be asymptomatic, or become symptomatic only after incarceration in a jail or prison. The process of being identified as in need of mental

health services may vary from state to state but is almost always supported by law. Forensic clients are a diverse group of adults in terms of age, gender, and ethnicity. Psychiatric diagnoses vary, and criminal charges range from misdemeanors to serious violent felonies.

In general, defendants/clients who have been arrested and sent to jail could be seen for criminal disposition and possible mental health assessment in three systems: the court system, criminal justice system, and forensic mental health system. Although the court system is technically part of the criminal justice system, for this discussion the courts have been separated to show the path of the defendant/client through the entire complex process. The next step, for all defendants/clients, is to go to court.

Court System

Depending on the nature of the charge, the defendant may go to a district, circuit, or specialty court. Those who are found guilty enter the criminal justice system to serve their sentence in jail, prison, or a correctional mental health facility. Defendants/clients adjudicated through an insanity defense could then be transferred to a court-designated facility (i.e., maximum security mental health hospital, state regional mental health hospital with forensic services) to receive further forensic evaluation and/or treatment to restore competency to stand trial.

Another verdict, "guilty but mentally ill" (GBMI), exists in some states. "Four of the twelve states that adopted the GBMI verdict did so because of the uproar over the Hinckley verdict. The consequence of rendering a GBMI verdict is conviction and a criminal sentence. A defendant will be evaluated by mental health authorities to determine whether psychiatric treatment is warranted under the circumstances. If such treatment is deemed necessary, the offender is hospitalized. If discharged, the offender is sent back to prison to serve the remainder of the sentence" (Collins, Hinkebein, & Schorgl, n.d., ¶ 24).

Specialty Court

Specialty courts were developed to assist defendants who have social or behavioral health issues in addition to their criminal history. "Mental Health and Drug courts have their genesis in the concept of specialty courts and the idea of therapeutic jurisprudence" (Steadman, Davidson, & Brown, 2001, p. 457).

Therapeutic jurisprudence is the study of the law as a potential therapeutic or nontherapeutic agent, with the belief that the integration of the principles of law and care can be used as a social force to enhance quality of life (Wexler, 1999). In 1997, the first Mental Health Court was established in Broward County, Florida, based on the past success of Drug Courts in Dade County, Florida. Mental Health Courts expanded once federal funding was made available upon President Clinton's signing of U.S. Senate Bill S. 1865 (Steadman et al., 2001).

Mental Health Court processes vary by state and jurisdiction, but most:

- Work with persons with mental illness who have entered the criminal justice system whose offenses vary; the offenses are usually misdemeanors but may include serious violent felonies (Callahan, 2011).
- Divert persons with mental illness from the criminal justice system into the community with court-ordered mental health treatment and support (B. Wise, personal communication, December 2009).

Some jurisdictions are investigating the possible benefits of developing other types of specialty courts, such as behavioral health/drug courts (Substance Abuse Mental Health Systems Administration [SAMHSA], 2011a), prostitution court (B. Wise, personal communication, December 2010), and veterans court.

Criminal Justice System

Access to mental health care varies according to how the person enters the criminal justice system and/or the forensic mental health system. If defendants are found guilty in the court system, they may get sentenced to time in jail or prison depending on the nature of the offense. Once incarcerated, if they disclose mental illness or exhibit signs of mental illness, they might be able to access limited psychiatric services. If their illness worsens, they may be transferred from the general population to a correctional mental heath hospital for further assessment and treatment.

Forensic Mental Health System

In states that have the insanity plea, individuals who have been adjudicated as "Not Competent to stand trial" or "Not Criminally Responsible" (NCR) usually receive further evaluation or treatment in a maximum security hospital. This facility provides treatment and rehabilitation to those accused of committing serious violent felonies (e.g., murder, arson, or rape). If the charge is of a lesser nature (e.g., a misdemeanor like vagrancy), the person may be placed at a less-restrictive state behavioral mental health facility for further evaluation and treatment.

It is important to mention that some states have "integrated" criminal justice and forensic mental health services. Facilities within these systems usually provide security and some treatment but are not accredited by The Joint Commission (TJC) or the Centers for Medicare and Medicaid Services (CMS). The priority in these facilities is usually punishment (as per the mandate of the state's penal code) versus active treatment (D. Barton, personal communication, January 2010).

Route to Community Reintegration

Whether released from a maximum security or state psychiatric hospital, jail, prison, or mental health court, an individual will be challenged by multiple legal and psychiatric concerns. There are expectations for adherence to court and conditional release orders, mandated psychiatric appointments, medication compliance, required visits with parole and probation officers, court-appointed legal guardians, scheduled court appearances, and possible ongoing evaluations for risk assessments, psychiatric evaluations, medication reviews, and other stipulated requirements. The path to reintegration varies depending on the original court finding and its disposition. Two routes based on disposition are described below, one for the defendant/inmate and the other for those adjudicated NCR. Those individuals found not competent to stand trial are not discussed in this chapter because they do not have an immediate path to community integration and the process varies significantly by jurisdiction.

Defendant/Inmate

Individuals may be released by the court from a mental health court, jail, prison, or the correctional mental health system into the community. These individuals may have been charged, found guilty, and sentenced for various misdemeanors or serious felonies. They may have completed their sentence or are in the community on parole or probation. Placement or release into the community is complex. States have their own regulations, laws, and procedures that affect this process.

Adjudicated Not Criminally Responsible

In some states, patient-defendants adjudicated as NCR may reside in a maximum security state hospital but no longer need that level of supervision. In some cases, the initial offense might have been so heinous and highly publicized that community agencies are hesitant to accept the individual directly from a maximum security hospital. In these cases, transfer to a state behavioral mental health facility may be warranted. The discharge preparation continues in a less restrictive hospital setting, and placement in the community becomes less stigmatized.

Most states have an entity like an Office of Community Forensic Services/Aftercare that is supported by legislation and the court. The primary purpose of such an organization is to monitor individuals who are on conditional release in the community. Requests for conditional release are usually formulated by the inpatient treatment team, which in some cases includes an occupational therapist, in consultation with the designated forensic psychiatrist or psychologist in the facility, the patient-defendant, and the patient-defendant's legal counsel.

The court is petitioned and conditional release orders are presented to a judge for final approval. Most of these orders are specific to the community living needs of the person (e.g., must reside in a residential setting with 12 hours of supervision) and reflect public safety requirements related to the initial offense. They may include restrictions regarding alcohol and illicit drugs, contact with certain individuals like family members (e.g., children) or alleged victims, and travel across state lines. These orders also may include monitoring for a stipulated amount of time; for example, in Maryland, an initial conditional release is usually monitored for 5 years (B. Wise, personal communication, December 2009).

Role of Occupational Therapy Community Re-entry With Forensic Clients

A variety of knowledge and skills are used by occupational therapists working in community re-entry with forensic clients. A high degree of knowledge of general occupational therapy, mental health and illness, community systems, and the criminal justice system is the minimum required for this role. Occupational therapists receive formal training in the mental health needs of individuals as students but learn about the legal issues their clients are experiencing through "on-the-job training." In an inpatient setting, this usually entails listening to the patient-defendant during evaluation and intervention, reading the patient-defendant's forensic history in his or her chart (if available), or discussing the planned community re-integration with other treatment team members. Occupational therapists working in the community, in a group home, residence, or work setting, may not have any information or knowledge of a client's forensic hospitalization, criminal background, or legal history.

Additional education gained through facility orientation programs, formal continuing education experiences, or a self-directed reading and mentoring program can help occupational therapy practitioners understand "legal concepts and statutes pertaining to insanity acquitees, sex offender registries, parole and probation, conditional release, victim notification, and county and state judicial operation that are important to the life circumstances, treatment, and outcomes of people with mental illness and forensic involvement" (Castaneda, 2010, p. 202).

Programs like **Re-Entry After Prison/Jail (RAP)** can be important resources for community practitioners (Rotter & Massaro, 2008). This program focuses on the effects of "doing time"; cultural competence within penal institutions; cognitive behavioral approaches to assist prisoners transitioning into the community; and ongoing training, research, and intervention approaches for professionals both "behind the walls" and in the community.

With the appropriate knowledge, occupational therapists can assist forensic clients in reentering the community and honoring their freedom of choice and community life as guided by the law.

"Occupational therapy treatment at its best focuses on client inclusion, personal choice, and empowerment" (Castaneda, 2010, p. 203). Smith-Gabai (2007) identifies the occupational therapist's role in assisting clients to develop problem-solving skills and to increase their awareness of their own strengths and barriers to occupational performance. The therapist helps the client to generate strategies and solutions that will foster the client's empowerment and assist the client in achieving his or her stated goals. "However ... the opportunity for true choice is limited by the parameters dictated by the judiciary, and for some the client's concomitant sociopathy" (Castaneda, 2010, p. 203).

Occupational therapists must provide care that is consistent with the *Occupational Therapy Code of Ethics and Ethics Standards 2010* (American Occupational Therapy Association [AOTA], 2010) and avoid breaches of ethical principles such as patient abandonment. An occupational therapy practitioner cannot suddenly stop intervention with an individual (i.e., abandon a patient), regardless of how difficult the circumstances. For example, an occupational therapist working with a client may learn that the client is a pedophile and has history of offending with children the same age as the therapist's children. The occupational therapist must continue to see the client until arrangements for an alternate caregiver (Morris, 2011) are put in place.

Challenges to Community Intervention

When working with defendants/clients in community settings, occupational therapists must be well versed with legal, psychiatric, and public safety issues that are part of the forensic clients' lives at all times. Occupational therapists also must be aware of how these issues may impact their therapeutic use of self, personal safety, and ability to access community supports when needed, such as a mental health court social worker. Many occupational therapists working with forensic clients in the community sole providers. Those who are part of health care agencies may not have access to supervisors who know about legal, psychiatric, public safety, and community issues. It is important for the practitioner to seek out atypical "supervision" by gathering information and mentorship from the legal, psychiatric, and public safety personnel that are a part of the client's "team." Professional judgment and knowledge of the law are important in this area of practice. One must be prepared to answer questions about occupational therapy interventions and be able to maximize community engagement while complying with judicial requirements (Box 21-1).

Public Safety

In addition to the needs and goals of the forensic client, the occupational therapist must consider public safety. The issue of public safety generally refers to protection of person and property from physical or psychological harm from a variety of dangers. Potential dangers to the community include: felony crimes (e.g., arson, assault with a deadly weapon, kidnapping, murder); sex offenses (e.g., pedophilia, rape); intentional transmission of infectious diseases; and acts of terrorism (Castaneda, 2002). It is imperative that the occupational therapist understands probation and parole criteria; state

---

Box 21-1   Compliance With Judicial Requirements

In the state of Maryland, a client on conditional release cannot leave the state without permission from the court. During a bi-weekly meeting with the community occupational therapist, Dutch requests assistance with budgeting. Dutch is planning to purchase hot dog meals for himself and his father at a Washington Nationals baseball game in Washington, DC, in a few weeks. The occupational therapist discusses his conditional release, asking him if he has permission from the judge to cross state lines. Dutch is unaware whether he has permission. Further investigation showed that the case manager, therapist, father, and the director of the residential service of the agency did not know permission was needed for the trip. A call to the community forensic aftercare office by the client's therapist and director of residential services enabled them to request permission to enter another state, for a time limited "sign out" with a parent. The client and his father were reminded of this crucial process. By raising the question, the occupational therapist was able to prevent a situation that could have resulted in the client's revocation of conditional release and subsequent return to a state forensic hospital.

laws regarding victim notification and obligations for reporting antisocial behavior; and therapeutic approaches for individuals with antisocial personality disorder; and knows how to access and appropriately interact with community forensic aftercare entities.

Castaneda (2010) discusses the dilemma occupational therapists face in developing an intervention plan and approach that balances client/defendant choice and public safety. Achieving this balance is more difficult if individual behavior indicates a lack of interest in the promotion of recovery, release, or discharge. Snively and Dressler (2005) identified additional challenges for professionals working with forensic clients, one of which is the need for "developing and maintaining relationships with patients who are impaired in their ability to trust and cooperate with others, find it difficult to express their thoughts and feelings, and are unable to interact in a socially acceptable manner" (p. 544). Antisocial personality and other personality disorders are commonly encountered in the criminal justice system. In the United Kingdom (2009), an estimated "60–80% of male prisoners and 50% of female prisoners have a personality disorder diagnosis compared with 6–15% of the general population" (Sainsbury Centre for Mental Health [SCMH], 2009, p. 3).

Diligent risk assessment and risk management must be a part of daily practice when working in the community with individuals with mental illness and criminal justice histories. Occupational therapists must implement strategies to manage difficult behavior and prevent violence. Understanding the organizational priorities and operation of community agencies is crucial. For example, a common challenge may be the seeming lack of formal, structured rules and rule enforcement for extreme aberrant behavior within a residence, work, or day program. Identifying consequences for breaking those rules is usually viewed as non-normalizing or institutional; thus, the expectation is that it is the clients' responsibility to independently manage their own behavior. Most community organizations will call 9-1-1 and rely on the police to resolve the situation. This plan of action is considered most "normalized," and one any citizen would employ when faced with a possible threat to public safety.

The support and services available in community settings are different from those of more structured institutional treatment settings. In some community agencies, the staff-to-client ratio is significantly lower (e.g., 1 staff to 8 clients for a 12- to 24-hour period) than inpatient client-to-staff ratios (e.g., 2–4 staff for 5 clients for an 8-hour shift). Supports available in inpatient settings, such as PRN medications for anxiety or agitation or additional immediate staff support, are not readily available in the community. If a client experiences a temporary resurgence of symptoms during his or her transition, a practitioner in this setting must be prepared to suggest interventions that do not overly depend on staff or access to limited supports. Examples of appropriate suggestions include strategies such as environmental analysis and adaptations.

Cultural Dynamics of Criminal Justice and Forensic Mental Health Contexts

Barriers, contextual features, or cultural dynamics of multiple systems also may affect transition into the community. The occupational therapist must be aware of difficulties the individual may experience living in an institution, jail, or forensic hospital that may impact his or her ability to make decisions, practice choice, or implement the principles of recovery. Examples of concerns specific to the following three contexts will be explored:

- institutional jail/maximum security hospital
- person
- community agency

Institutional Jail/Maximum Security Hospital

Most penal systems focus on their mandate to implement punishment for crimes first and then provide the needed mental health or substance abuse treatment. Everything is considered contraband. This can impact the individual's performance of areas of occupation (AOTA, 2008), which include activities of daily living (ADLs), instrumental activities of daily living (IADLs), education, work, play, leisure, and social participation. The opportunity to engage in any of these areas of occupation is severely limited for people with mental health issues living in any of these 24/7 types of supervised forensic environments. Regimented schedules, rules, and regulations are part of daily life experiences over which the individual has little or no control. Most, if not all, ADLs and IADLs are completed with close supervision and in groups with no autonomy to exercise individual preferences. The presence of cameras, and in some settings armed guards, changes the dynamics and health benefits of occupational engagement. For example, timing and administration of medications are controlled by staff, and showers are allowed only when scheduled. Eating, a social occupation, is usually an opportunity to select foods which gives one pleasure. This is not the case for individuals restricted to living in these settings. Access to food choice is extremely limited to nonexistent. The only food permitted is prepared by dietary staff and served on a tray, with everyone eating the same food. In addition, this occupation is heavily observed and regulated due to the need to count utensils before and after each meal. While many leisure activities are provided in forensic hospital settings, they do not routinely occur in penal settings. Living in these environments impedes decision making, and the desire to be independent can be lost. There are limited to no opportunities to develop personal or professional contacts outside of the facility. For example, in maximum security prisons, learning how to use public transportation has been considered escape planning. This limits experiences and opportunities to practice community readiness.

Person

Individual patients, defendants, inmates, or clients may experience fear of the "unknown" and may be reluctant to leave their familiar contexts. For example, after 30 years of institutional care, an individual scheduled for release may still be experiencing active symptoms (e.g., being delusional, "hearing voices") and may dread the loss of support and acceptance from staff who in some ways have grown to be his or her "family." The individual has had no practice in being independent with IADLs, and minimal knowledge or use of current technology (e.g., an ATM) due to limited or no community exposure.

This can increase fear and reluctance to engage in release planning. This situation can be more problematic with people who have had an increased length of isolation from society.

Once released, the dual stigma of mental illness and a criminal history with resultant gaps in work history can add to the challenge of finding employment and successful community reentry. Upon release, most of these individuals are faced with pervasive court and legal issues, requiring long-term monitoring. The lack of finances due to limited access to gainful employment while in the hospital or incarcerated and no recent work history make finding gainful employment a challenge. In addition, laws often restrict the types of jobs or employment setting a person who has committed a serious felony can access (e.g., child care, health care, teacher).

Community Agency Context

There are unique challenges faced by clients when they re-enter the community and need to meet the expectations of the agency. These expectations may include being completely independent in ADLs and the ability to structure their own leisure time. Waiting lists for housing are prevalent, so there is limited to no choice in selecting their own roommates; living with strangers or staff-assigned roommates becomes inevitable. The need to pay for rent, food, transportation, and medication for the first time can be a challenge. Agency staff are not as well versed with the legal requirements that a client must follow to stay in the community; some may not be as tolerant of "behavioral" adjustment or symptom increase during the first few months at residence. This may trigger a re-arrest or hospitalization.

Mental Health Recovery Movement

Occupational therapy, with its client-centered perspective, fits well with the principles of the recovery movement. "Recovery is a unique journey for each individual, and each person in recovery must choose the range of services and supports ranging from clinical treatment to peer services...Like other aspects of health care and unless adjudicated by courts of law, people have the right to choose and determine what services and treatments best meet their needs and preferences" (SAMSHA 2011b, p. 49). Pouncy and Lukens (2009) examine the inherent contradictions between the recovery movement and care of the forensic client:

- "The mental health recovery movement promotes patient self-determination and opposes coercive psychiatric treatment" (p. 93).
- "Forensic psychiatrists routinely argue that persons with mental illness who have committed crimes are not full moral agents" (p. 93).
- "The recovery movement has not explored how its principles can extend from civil matters to criminal law" (p. 94).
- Limits to "moral agency in persons with severe mental illness creates an ethical disconnect between forensic psychiatry, medical ethics, and recovery principles" (p. 94).

It is important to recognize the possible conflicts when attempting to integrate and implement the principles of recovery in community practice. It might be difficult to encourage self-determination and empowerment without taking into consideration judicial mandates that dictate the person's community participation. For example, individuals who committed a felony and wished to resume college, for a career in teaching, health care, or the legal profession, may not be able to work in these areas after graduation because of their past forensic history and legal constraints. Many clients who leave the institution, jail, or prison wish to live near friends and family but may not be able to due to restraining orders, victim notification, or conditional release restrictions. Once again, this limits the application of some principles of recovery.

Occupational Therapy Community Practice With Persons With Mental Health and Criminal Justice/ Forensic Involvement

Examples of applications to practice with the forensic population in the United States are limited. However, groundbreaking work has been done by the Duquesne University's Occupational Therapy Department (Eggers, Muñoz, Sciulli, & Crist, 2006). As early as 2003, this group developed several community outreach projects that included a partnership with local industry, the county jail, and homeless shelter, providing necessary occupational therapy transition services to those released (Brachtesende, 2003).

In addition, a Level II fieldwork program for occupational therapy students was established within a jail to assist inmates in learning about and practicing life skills (Provident & Joyce-Gaguzis, 2005). The program's efforts resulted in the hiring of full-time occupational therapists in several community settings. Although these projects did not focus solely on inmates with mental illness, these efforts identified and included services for those who might need this support.

Occupational Therapy Community Consultation-Liaison Service

Community providers and the literature support the development of a community consultation/liaison service. Providing familiar, transitional therapeutic relationships to individuals moving out of the hospital, consultation with and training of community staff will help to bridge the gap between the inpatient stay and life in the community. A consultation liaison service helps the person transfer skills learned in the inpatient hospital setting and adapt skills to live successfully in the community.

In June of 2008 the Director of Rehabilitation Services (an occupational therapist), Social Work and Psychology, of a 350-bed, state-operated behavioral /mental health inpatient hospital in Maryland decided to re-examine the difficulties involved in patients' transition to the community. The majority of patients at this state facility are admitted through the forensic process and were on or pending conditional release.

The social work department requested feedback on several clients during extended stay (i.e., a 6-month period) discharges, in four separate and distinct community placements.

The following client behaviors and needs were observed by community providers:

- Lack of mobility/transportation skills
- Lack of budgeting skills, safety skills, medication management skills

- Lack of awareness of how to use entitlement funds to pay for services
- Refusal to go to a physician
- Urinary incontinence
- Difficulty with boundary issues for male clients with female staff
- Need for medication education
- Need for substance abuse education; community life provoked lapse into old lifestyle
- Financial irresponsibility and subsequent relapse

In addition, a community provider's general observation about clients from the hospital was that "Many clients are not ready for the lack of structure, lack of 24 hr. staffing, they don't know what to do with unstructured time, how to cook, how to keep rooms clean, personal hygiene, how to get along with roommates, how to handle a bank account." Another provider commented on how helpful it was when the client's hospital social worker visited several times to ease the transition into the program.

Based on these findings, a new consultation liaison service was developed by an occupational therapist. Clients were referred by their current treatment team and were seen if a provider:

- had been identified and the client had a targeted discharge date;
- was considering accepting a client for placement but had questions or concerns;
- requested consultation to adapt/modify activities or expectations for successful community living for a client on a trial visit;
- was willing to work with a client returned from an unsuccessful stay in the community;
- observed a client, after successful community placement, having difficulty with daily living activities and coping skills, and in danger of relapse.

Once the occupational therapy consultant receives a referral, it is important to collect intake information, including the client's concerns and perceived needs in IADLs (e.g., health management and maintenance, safety, and emergency maintenance). In addition, clients should be asked to identify possible circles of support (e.g., family, friends, staff) and provide details about the perceived quality of the relationships and the client's expectations. The occupational therapist uses one-on-one interviews, focus groups, and site visits to collect this information for the initial intake. Additional occupational therapy assessments are completed as indicated.

Once the initial intake data is collected, the occupational therapy consultant works with the client, community provider, and hospital to suggest strategies to address concerns raised by all parties in regard to successful community placement. Participation in the consultation/liaison service is strictly voluntary. Clients and agency visits vary from one time a week or month to once every 2–3 months as needed. The end goal is to prevent reinstitutionalization (e.g., return to jail or hospital) and facilitate community integration.

Consultative visits may include, but are not limited to, examining a client's daily routines in detail (i.e., by 15-minute increments), analyzing what occupations are causing the client difficulty. A potential intervention is to compare the client's routine to staff routines to identify conflicts and to determine what might be done differently by the client or staff. For example, a frequent source of conflict is the method used to wake a client. The client, the occupational therapist, and a staff member analyzed the situation and jointly developed a successful adaption (e.g., use of multiple alarm clocks).

In order to facilitate successful community living, it is helpful for the occupational therapist to analyze the interaction of the clients' routines and habits and the contextual features of their new home. Asking the following types of questions can be helpful in suggesting possible adaptations. Is the individual more successful with one staff member versus another? If so, what can the client teach the staff member about his or her learning style? What can staff teach each other about how to bring out the best in the client? How does the individual cope with staffing changes within the home?

Another consultative strategy to maximize the potential for successful community living is to help the client and staff develop an alternate schedule for the client when he or she is not well or is more symptomatic. A "Plan B" is helpful in alleviating feelings of helplessness among the individual and staff. It involves the analysis of the occupation and a recommendation as to what part of the occupation can be done without exacerbating symptoms or adding stress to the individual or staff. It requires a partnership between the client and the staff to obtain the appropriate supports and achieve successful occupational engagement.

Conclusion

In order to work ethically, safely, and effectively with individuals with mental health issues and criminal justice involvement in the community, the occupational therapy practitioner must be well versed in multiple systems. Understanding the legal, mental health forensic, community corrections system, public safety, ethics, risk management, psychiatric, and occupational therapy principles specifically around difficult contexts (e.g., forensic issues/violence) is imperative. One must be knowledgeable of the possible challenges that the releasing institution, the community agency, and the individual himself presents to the process of transition to life in the community. With this knowledge, occupational therapy practitioners can facilitate clients' reclaiming lives outside of an institution.

In her 2006 Eleanor Clark Slagle Lecture, Hasselkus discusses the impact of occupational deprivation in prison and how individuals miss some of the seemingly "mundane" aspects of everyday life. In closing she states: "I believe that the ordinary rhythm of daily living is the deep primordial nourishment of our existence. It is the 'truth'—the primary reality for each one of us. After all, everyday occupation is present in our lives at *all* times and in *all* places.... As occupational therapists—in this profession that we love—we have the potential to be an exception to the generalized *in*visibility of everyday occupation in people's lives....*With our clients,* such a heightened awareness will enable us to enter the rich and singular spaces of their everyday lives, maximizing our abilities to work together effectively toward the maintenance and renewal of meaningful day-to-day living ... May it be so." (Hasselkus, 2006, p. 638).

May this be so with all clients, including those with forensic and mental health issues.

CASE STUDIES

CASE STUDY 21•1 Aretha

Aretha is on conditional release after being hospitalized in a maximum security hospital for 15 years and then transferred to a regional state psychiatric hospital for 10 years following a double homicide (i.e., murder of both her parents). It was hard to find a community placement because of the nature of her offense and difficulty convincing the judiciary that she was psychiatrically stable and thus less likely to be dangerous. After several successful trial visits, Aretha was accepted to a community placement. The agency and Aretha voluntarily agreed to visits from the occupational therapy consultant.

Several meetings were held with an agency case manager, Aretha, and the occupational therapist. The client discussed her anxiety about having lived in a hospital for "half her life" and worried about how to structure her time after attending the day program. Meetings focused around her goal of adjusting to roommates, completing house chores, getting to know the community, and managing with limited money.

Together, Aretha and the occupational therapist reviewed her conditional release requirements, developed simple goals, selected a bi-weekly time to meet, and discussed progress and next steps. Aretha had many artistic hobbies (e.g., painting and playing the piano). Suggestions were made as to where she could go in town to participate in like occupations. She was able to walk to and attend events provided by a free arts council. A suggestion was made to visit with the local peer-run support center. Further discussion revealed Aretha's hesitation in meeting peers and possibly discussing her past. The therapist commended her for "venturing out" and reassured her that there was no need to rush into what she felt was an "uncomfortable" place or situation.

Occupational therapy consultation revolved around providing the therapeutic relationship and transitional bridge between her hospitalization and the community. The client communicated her accomplishments, goals, and concerns to community residential staff. The client thanked the occupational therapist for meeting with her and stated she looked forward to their bi-weekly meetings.

CASE STUDY 21•1 Discussion Questions

1. Would you feel comfortable working with Aretha? Why or why not?
2. What can you do to prepare yourself to work with this type of client?
3. What free activities are available in your community that Aretha might enjoy? Make a list of these activities in rank order from least demanding to most challenging, based on your knowledge of Aretha and activity analysis. What legal or public safety factors would need to be considered prior to engagement in the activities?

Learning Activities

1. Review the theories discussed in Chapter 3. Then select a model and describe how you would use it to support your bi-weekly meetings.
2. Investigate whether your state has a drug or mental health specialty court and the level of occupational therapy involvement within the forensic mental health system.

REFERENCES

American Occupational Therapy Association. (2008). Occupational therapy practice framework: Domain and process (2nd ed.). *American Journal of Occupational Therapy, 62,* 625–683.

American Occupational Therapy Association. (2010). Occupational therapy code of ethics and ethics standards (2010.) [Supplemental material]. *American Journal of Occupational Therapy, 64*(6), S17–S26.

Brachtesende, A. (2003, May 19). Community partnerships: Creating possibilities. *OT Practice, 8,* 1–3.

Callahan, L. (2011, August). *The role of co-occurring disorders in outcomes in mental health Courts* [Webinar presented at SAMHSA by Policy R Associates].

Castaneda, R. (2002, April). *Choice and public safety: A rehabilitation professional's role in seeking to resolve the apparent conflict.* Paper presented at the World Federation of Occupational Therapists Conference, Stockholm, Sweden.

Castaneda, R. (2010). Therapeutic relationships in difficult contexts: Involuntary commitment, forensic settings, and violence. In M. K. Scheinholtz (Ed.), *Occupational therapy in mental health: Considerations for advanced practice* (pp. 200–214). Bethesda, MD: AOTA Press.

Collins, K., Hinkebein, G., & Schorgl, S. (n.d.). The John Hinckley Trial & its effect on the insanity defense. In D. Linder. (2002), *Famous American trials: The John Hinkley Trial, 1982.* Retrieved from http://www.law.umkc.edu/faculty/projects/ftrials/hinckley/hinckleyinsanity.htm

Eggers, M., Muñoz, J., Sciulli, J., & Crist, P. (2006). The Community Reintegration Project: occupational therapy at work in a county jail. *Occupational Therapy in Health Care, 20*(1), 17–37.

Hasselkus, B. R. (2006). 2006 Eleanor Clarke Slagle Lecture—The world of everyday occupation: Real people, real lives. *American Journal of Occupational Therapy, 60*(6), 627–640.

Manderscheid, R. A., Atay, J. E., & Crider, R. A. (2009). Changing trends in state psychiatric hospital use from 2002 to 2005. *Psychiatric Services, 60*(1), 29–34.

Morris, J. F. (2011). Patient abandonment. In D. Y. Slater (Ed.), *Reference guide to the Occupational Therapy Code of Ethics and Ethics Standards.* Bethesda, MD: American Occupational Therapy Association.

Pouncy, C. L., & Lukens, J. M. (2009). Madness versus badness: The ethical tension between the recovery movement and forensic psychiatry. *Theoretical Medicine and Bioethics, 31*(1), 93–105.

Provident, I., & Joyce-Gaguzis, K. (2005). Brief report. Creating an occupational therapy level II fieldwork experience in a county jail setting. *American Journal of Occupational Therapy, 59*(1), 101–106.

Rotter, M., & Massaro, J. (2008). *Re-entry after prison/jail: A therapeutic curriculum for people with mental illness and histories of incarceration.* Unpublished treatment manual.

Sainsbury Centre for Mental Health. (2009). Personality disorder: A briefing for people working in the criminal justice system. London, UK: Author. Retrieved from http://www.centreformentalhealth.org.uk/

Smith-Gabai, H. (2007). Perspectives: Client empowerment. *OT Practice, 12*(13), 23–25.

Snively, F., & Dressler, J. (2005). Occupational therapy in the criminal justice system. In E. Cara & A. MacRae (Eds.), *Psychosocial occupational therapy: A clinical practice* (2nd ed., pp. 567–590). Australia: Thomson Delmar Learning.

Steadman, H. J., Davidson, S., & Brown, C. (2001). Mental health courts: Their promise and unanswered questions. *Psychiatric Services, 52*(4), 457–458.

Substance Abuse Mental Health Systems Administration. (2011a). *FY 2011 Grant Request for Application (RFA) Grants to Develop and Expand Behavioral Health Treatment Court Collaboratives.* Rockville, MD: Author.

Substance Abuse Mental Health Systems Administration. (2011b). *Leading change: A plan for SAMHSA's Roles and Actions 2011–2014.* Rockville, MD: Author.

Wexler, D. B. (1999, October 29). *Therapeutic jurisprudence: An overview.* Retrieved from http://www.law.arizona.edu/depts/upr-intj/

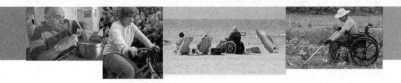

Rehabilitation and Participation

Chapter 22

Accessibility and Community Integration

Janie B. Scott, MA, OT/L, FAOTA

Until the great mass of the people shall be filled with the sense of responsibility for each other's welfare, social justice can never be attained.

—Helen Keller

Learning Objectives

This chapter is designed to enable the reader to:

- Define the terms associated with accessibility and community integration.
- Discuss legislation that supports accessibility and community integration.
- Identify issues that impact home and community accessibility.
- Describe occupational therapy strategies to promote accessibility in the community.
- Discuss transportation options for community mobility.

Key Terms

Accessibility
Accommodation
Advocacy
Architectural barriers

Community integration
Community mobility
Reasonable accommodation
Stakeholders

Introduction

Successful community living and occupational participation depends on the interaction of individuals with their environments as they respond to activity demands using performance skills and patterns (American Occupational Therapy Association [AOTA], 2008). Individuals with disabilities or chronic illnesses, those who are returning home following a traumatic event, and those who are aging in place may have difficulties effectively managing activity demands in community environments.

According to data from the U.S. Census Bureau (2010), 36 million people in the United States have at least one physical disability; this represents 12% of the civilian, non-institutionalized population. Five percent of children age 5–17 years, 10% of adults age 18–64 years, and 37% of adults 65 years and older have a disability. Twenty-one percent of the population age 16 and older with a disability live below the poverty level, as compared to 11% of the non-disabled population of the same age (Disabled World, 2011). According to the *Chartbook on Mental Health and Disability* (Jans, Stoddard, & Kraus, 2004), 3.5% of the adult U.S. civilian non-institutionalized population is estimated to have a mental health disability (6.7 million people). This represents a significant number of community-dwelling individuals who are already integrated or who seek assistance in identifying ways to gain accessibility and participation in community life.

Chronic disease management and improved access to preventive health care services have enabled greater numbers of individuals to continue living independently in the community. The numbers of individuals with chronic illnesses and disabilities is expected to increase in the coming years with the aging of the baby boomer generation. These facts make it imperative for the occupational therapy profession to expand its community-based service delivery focusing on accessibility, community mobility, and community integration.

This chapter contains a brief review of legislation related to accessibility and community integration for persons with disabilities. Accessibility issues in the home and community are explored. This includes access to public and private transportation as well as ways that occupational therapy practitioners can work with individuals and agencies to promote community mobility. Community integration for persons following an injury, illness, or exposure to war is discussed, including ways that occupational therapy practitioners can assist in making this transition safe and successful.

Accessibility Issues

Accessibility is the "degree to which an environment (i.e., site, facility, workplace, service or program) can be approached, entered, operated and/or used safely and with dignity by a person with limitations" (Banks, 2001, p. 120). Public laws and state regulations have increased accessibility to buildings, services, and opportunities by removing barriers (e.g., Americans with Disabilities Act [ADA] of 1990, Architectural Barriers Act of 1968). The Telecommunications Act of 1996 requires manufacturers of telecommunications products and services to ensure that equipment and services are accessible to, and usable by, persons with disabilities. The occupational therapy practitioner can help identify appropriate devices for individual use and public accessibility. Accessibility to businesses, social opportunities, transportation, and other instrumental activities of daily living (IADLs) promotes community participation for work, play, and leisure in a variety of contexts (Fig. 22.1).

Although great strides have been made in the past two decades, persons with disabilities still encounter significant barriers to full participation in society,

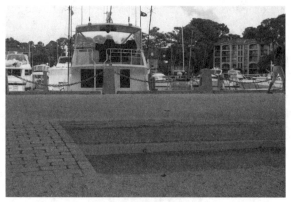

Fig. 22•1 Making the Harbor Accessible: A Ramp That Blends in With the Surroundings. *(Photo by Janie B. Scott, August 20, 2011)*

including architectural, attitudinal, technological, and economic barriers. **Architectural barriers,** "physical structures that present obstacles for individuals who have mobility, visual, or sensory limitations" (Banks, 2001, p. 121), are the most easily changed. Home and community accessibility are critical if the goal of full inclusion is to be achieved.

Home Accessibility

Individuals with disabilities or conditions that impair their performance skills may have greater difficulty getting around inside the home and performing activities of daily living (ADLs). Home modifications (e.g., ramps, widened doorways, lowered counter tops, no step entrances) increase accessibility and ultimately promote independence and quality of life. The majority of home modifications are paid for privately; however, there are some programs that can assist homeowners in making these adaptations. In some states, Medicaid programs offer waivers (funding) for home modifications to eligible individuals. Habitat for Humanity, Rebuilding Together, and other similar organizations offer assistance to individuals who need home modifications. These programs welcome occupational therapists as volunteers and occasionally as paid staff.

The Architectural Barriers Act, Fair Housing Act, and the Americans with Disabilities Act address accessibility in living environments. Public housing is required by law "to allow persons with disabilities to make reasonable modifications. A reasonable modification is a structural modification that is made to allow persons with disabilities the full enjoyment of the housing and related facilities" (U.S. Department of Housing and Urban Development, 2006, para 8). The resident is typically responsible for paying for the modifications; however, loan or grant programs may be available to make the accommodations possible. Owners of public, residential properties may benefit from subsidies to fund the renovations. Information about these programs is available through local Housing and Urban Development (HUD) offices. Additionally, the Veterans Administration provides home modification funding for eligible veterans. Finally, landlords may also be able to take advantage of special loan programs offered by the federal government (Useful Community Development, 2011).

Home modification can also incorporate adaptations to enhance occupational performance for persons with visual or hearing impairments. The technologies that are available for the home include aids for the blind, computer access, environmental controls, speech generating devices, and cognitive prosthetic devices (U.S. Department of Veteran Affairs, 2009). In addition, modifications to the environment can support the sensory needs of residents. Reducing glare, increasing color contrasts, and improving task lighting promotes safety and comfort within the home. Electronic cognitive devices help people with memory, organization, and orientation challenges to compensate for their limitations. These devices can support daily living and participation in work, play, and leisure for people with a wide variety of mental and physical conditions.

The Massachusetts Institute of Technology (MIT) and similar research centers are researching technologies that promote health and safety within the home by using computer technologies to monitor health and alert the consumer or health care provider about the need to update care plans. Many technologies exist that monitor the activities of individuals in the home without on-site supervision. For example, there are devices that track whether a person has taken his or her medications, opened the refrigerator within a specified period of time, gotten out of bed, or performed other activities that are important to health and safety. Refer to Chapter 24 for discussion of the types of accommodations that can be made to promote community living as well as a discussion of the role of occupational therapy in evaluation and training in the use and maintenance of these technologies.

Community Accessibility

State and federal legislation establishes rules for individuals, businesses, and governments that protect the rights of individuals within the community, often addressing issues of accessibility. Businesses, health care systems, and other organizations often implement access to community-based services without the imposition of regulations. Health care programs that offer telehealth services are one example. Telehealth services facilitate the monitoring of a person's health and alert health care providers and caregivers when interventions may be warranted. These programs are particularly helpful when the consumer lives in a remote area with poor access to health care services. Sometimes access is limited due to a lack of transportation, or the needed health care provider does not serve a particular geographic area. Participating pharmacies may ensure delivery of medications to consumers who do not have transportation and for their customers' convenience. Some pharmacies offer mail order service, and others provide home delivery and will set up weekly, biweekly, or monthly medication boxes.

Community accessibility also includes an individual's physical access to community services. This is achieved by removing architectural barriers. For example, ramps are built to provide alternate access to buildings, curb cuts are installed, restrooms are enlarged/adapted, and sign language or language interpreter services are made available.

There are many factors that make community integration possible. Access to education, work, social and leisure opportunities, and health and wellness services is critical for individuals with new, acquired, or lifelong disabilities. The occupational therapist uses evidence-based assessments and interventions to serve clients and can intervene directly or through consultation with the individual, his or her representative, businesses, and agencies.

Occupational therapy students, practitioners, and others can be involved in evaluating the accessibility of their communities. There are many assessment tools available to examine accessibility and barriers in homes and neighborhoods. The Center on Health Promotion Research for People with Disabilities (n.d.) at the University of Chicago provides training materials, checklists, and advocacy activities on its Web site. Occupational therapy students and practitioners can use these materials to evaluate the accessibility of their communities and advocate to businesses and government for public accommodations to meet the needs of persons with disabilities.

Community Mobility

Community mobility is identified in the *Occupational Therapy Practice Framework: Domain and*

Process, 2nd Edition (American Occupational Therapy Association [AOTA], 2008) as an instrumental activity of daily living. **Community mobility** involves "moving around in the community using public or private transportation such as driving, walking, bicycling, or accessing and riding in buses, taxicabs or other transportation systems" (AOTA, 2008, p. 631). Some transportation services are operated by paid employees, and others are run by volunteers at no cost to the individual. In order to access community services, individuals with disabilities and some seniors need to rely on community transportation systems for their mobility. Individuals who are recovering from a traumatic injury or other condition that impairs their mobility, or individuals adapting to functional changes, may need to use alternate means of transportation. Some communities offer or help coordinate ride-sharing programs. For example, someone who is recovering from a traumatic injury may enter into an agreement with one or more individuals that his or her car may be used in exchange for the non-disabled individual's driving services. Traditional ride-sharing programs have focused on carpooling as an environmental or energy conservation strategy.

Personal Transportation

Personal transportation factors are related to an individual's ability to drive, vehicle modification and maintenance, older driver safety, driver education for special groups, and the fit of the vehicle for the individual. Acute injury or chronic illnesses may interfere with the individual's role as driver. Individuals who are newly disabled may need occupational therapy services to develop safe driver skills or to compensate for the change in roles. Driving is an IADL and for many people in the United States is closely associated with their personal identity and roles. Driving cessation impacts an individual's community engagement, occupational participation, and often, self-image (Vrkljan & Polgar, 2007). The occupational therapy practitioner can explore the impact these role changes have on the individual and significant others and suggest transportation options that are available within the community appropriate for the individual's physical, psychosocial, and financial needs. The emphasis of this collaboration is on maximizing the individual's occupational participation. Ignoring these needs may lead to social deprivation, isolation, adverse health outcomes, and decreased access to health care.

Occupational therapy helps people adjust to changed roles and develop alternate transportation options. Qualified veterans can receive adaptive equipment for their cars or vans through the Veterans Administration. Individuals with disabilities with appropriate documentation may apply to the Motor Vehicle Administration (MVA) for temporary or permanent license plates or hang tags to allow them to park in specially designated parking spaces. Disabled drivers may have their vehicles modified, for example, by installing hand controls, or the driver may learn to use strategies to compensate for his or her disability. Occupational therapy practitioners can become certified as driving rehabilitation specialists through AOTA or ADED (Association for Driver Rehabilitation Specialists). Chapter 11 discusses driving and community mobility in more detail.

Public Transportation

Many people with disabilities rely on public transportation to travel where and when they desire in order to participate in school, work, leisure, and health-related activities such as grocery shopping and doctor appointments. The inability to access transportation can impact social opportunities, employment status, and ultimately quality of life. Regulations exist that govern transportation by automobiles, trains, air travel, ships and boats, and other forms of mass transit. The Americans with Disability Act Amendments Act of 2008 (ADAAA) provides specific rules regarding public transportation, paratransit, and other publicly run services. Information about the ADAAA can be found at http://ada.gov. Occupational therapy practitioners who wish to assist their clients with reintegration into the community and utilization of public transportation services should search for local or county departments of disability, transportation, aging, or human resources. Locating on-demand, fixed-route, and escorted services will assist clients to utilize accessible transportation services to enhance their community participation. Occupational therapy practitioners can teach young and old clients how to read maps, use transportation, enter and exit vehicles, and use public conveyances.

Transportation Safety

There are many areas of transportation safety, including the proper use of car seats, safety seat belts, and bicycle helmets. These safety features are regulated by individual states and their jurisdictions. Avoiding further injury or disability is important for everyone, especially persons with disabilities. Occupational therapists have been involved in injury prevention activities focused on child safety seats, access and egress to public transportation, and educating transportation providers with strategies to keep passengers safe. The Air Carrier Access Act prohibits discrimination against individuals with disabilities in air travel. However, if the airline determines that someone is unsafe to travel and can document these facts, it may refuse to transport the individual. In some situations, an airline can require a safety assistant for the disabled traveler (U.S. Department of Transportation, 2005).

Community Integration

Community integration refers to being "happily situated, productively occupied, and effectively supported in the community" (McColl, Davies, Carlson, Johnston, & Minnes, 2001). "Reintegration" refers to returning to the community following an absence due to illness, injury, or traumatic event. The concepts of community integration and reintegration are applicable to individuals of all ages. According to McColl et al. (2001), community integration is a function of four factors: assimilation, social support, occupation, and independent living (Box 22-1).

Often, reasonable accommodations are needed to facilitate the individual's integration into the community and participation in community-based services and activities. Reasonable accommodations, as defined by the ADA, relate to modifications or adjustments to the job application process, work environment, or the ability of an employee with a disability to receive benefits that are available to other employees (U.S. Equal Employment Opportunity Commission, 2002).

The Olmstead Act and Home and Community-Based Waiver programs were created to help individuals transition into the community and/or avoid

Box 22-1	Components of Community Integration

Assimilation

Conformity: fitting in with other people, knowing the rules
Orientation: knowing one's way around the community, being familiar with one's surroundings
Acceptance: being comfortable in the community, feeling understood and acknowledged

Social Support

Close relationships: feeling connected and in close proximity to family and friends, engaged in relationships that are important, reciprocal, mutual, and intimate
Diffuse relationships: interacting with others in the community, neighbors, service providers, co-workers, etc.

Occupation

Leisure: participating in social and recreational activities with others in the community
Productivity: making a contribution, having a sense of purpose, engaging in education, work exploration, employment, and volunteer activities

Independent Living

Personal independence: experiencing autonomy and self-determination, having some control over one's life and choices
Satisfaction with living arrangement: being able to come and go as one pleases, freedom from supervision, living independent of one's family of origin

Data from: McColl, M. A., Davies, D., Carlson, P., Johnston, J., & Minnes, P. (2001). The Community Integration Measure: Development and preliminary validation. *Archives of Physical Medicine and Rehabilitation, 82,* 429–434.

institutionalization. Occupational therapy practitioners have the opportunity to facilitate community integration through rehabilitation, habilitation, and specialized programs in both community settings and institutions. The occupational therapy emphasis is on identifying appropriate contexts for daily living, work, leisure, and social participation. The occupational therapy evaluation determines the client's occupational history, goals, and current level of function in order to maximize the client's potential for successful community integration.

Occupational re-engagement may occur within the school, home, community center, or workplace. Family members often need assistance in how to best support the individual's functional independence and autonomy. The occupational therapy process of evaluation and intervention facilitates the re-entry of the individual and creates the opportunity to support and educate the family and caregivers. Additionally, the occupational therapist can assess the individual in the home and work/school environments to determine the types of supports or environmental modifications that are required and facilitate the acquisition of needed goods and services.

The occupational therapy practitioner works with schools and places of employment to sensitize teachers,

students, employees, and employers about the needs of the individual who is attempting to resume community life. These activities are best undertaken with the participation of the individual in order to promote his or her autonomy and privacy. Collaboration with community stakeholders raises awareness that in turn facilitates successful transitions. The occupational therapy practitioner can advocate for the client's integration into the community by proposing altered work/school schedules or alternate work plans, for example, telecommuting.

Community Integration Post-Injury or Illness

Children, youth, veterans, and adults of all ages may need assistance returning to the community after an injury or prolonged illness. Whether the individual is recovering from a brain injury, spinal cord injury, stroke, relapse from a persistent mental illness or substance use disorder, amputation, or other disabling condition, preparations likely have to be made within the family and community. When children are transitioning from the hospital or rehabilitation setting to home, they may need continued occupational therapy services through outpatient clinics or home-based school, or in the classroom. Occupational therapy interventions incorporate the child's rehabilitation goals, academic priorities, and social adjustment.

The home, school, or work environment may need to be adapted to better suit the individual's mobility and occupational needs. This may take the form of increasing physical or sensory access to the environment through the use of assistive technologies. The occupational therapy practitioner can identify accommodations that meet the individual's and family's needs. Occupational therapy interventions may focus on enhancing the performance of ADLs or IADLs and concurrently teaching family members energy conservation techniques and strategies for stress management, and helping them identify community-based resources that support occupational performance. The opportunity also exists to educate teachers, employers, and others regarding the needs of the individual and potentially advocate when gaps in services are discovered.

Leisure and Recreation

Occupational therapy practice has stressed the importance of balancing work, rest, and play. Engagement in play and leisure typically promotes a sense of fun or enjoyment regardless of whether the activity is planned or spontaneous. Individuals with disabilities are often excluded from recreational activities and consequently do not have the opportunity to develop leisure interests and social connectedness. Occupational therapy practitioners can help individuals and families identify appropriate play and leisure opportunities to promote independence and social participation.

There are also national and state-specific leisure and recreation programs accessible to people with disabilities. These programs may focus on a specific sport (e.g., surfing) or disability (e.g., amputation) and can give the participant a feeling of connectedness to a community while pursuing leisure interests, restoring self-confidence, and developing skills needed for occupational performance in a broader range of activities.

Occupational therapists may develop, lead, or consult for programs that offer leisure activities to community-dwelling individuals with disabilities, and work with schools and community groups to develop and promote playground safety. Occupational therapy practitioners may also serve as consultants on the construction of buildings and stadiums for accessibility as well as recommend the range of adaptive recreational equipment appropriate for community centers, public recreation programs, and other programs where participation of individuals with disabilities should be promoted.

Occupational therapists collaborate with individuals and families to determine social environments and opportunities that are a "good fit." The determination of fit may be based on whether social and recreational activities are in inclusive settings or those specifically for people with disabilities. Collaboration with the individual, family, or community programs may provide greater exposure to play and leisure that may ultimately improve health and quality of life, and decrease adverse health outcomes among older adults and individuals with disabilities.

Work

The unemployment and under-employment of individuals with disabilities have been recognized for decades. According to the U.S. Bureau of Labor Statistics (2011), while 69.7% of working-age adults without a disability were employed in 2010, only 28.6% of adults with a disability were working. In addition, the median earnings of the population age 16 and older with a disability was $18, 865 in 2009, as compared to the median earnings of $28, 983 for their non-disabled peers (Disabled World, 2011). Occupational therapists can assess job readiness skills, identify employment opportunities in the community, determine whether the workplace is accessible, and recommend environmental modifications and adaptations for the employee. The occupational therapy practitioner is in the unique position to identify and address workplace biases, develop in-service educational programs to increase awareness, and create more job opportunities for older adults and individuals with disabilities. Some persons with disabilities will require accommodations to participate fully in work settings.

Accommodation is an adjustment to an environment, program, or service that enables individuals with disabilities to engage in occupations in similar ways as those without disabilities. "A **reasonable accommodation** is any modification or adjustment to a job or the work environment that will enable a qualified applicant or employee with a disability to participate in the application process or to perform essential job functions. Reasonable accommodation also includes adjustments to assure that a qualified individual with a disability has rights and privileges in employment equal to those of employees without disabilities" (U.S. Department of Justice [USDOJ], 2002, ¶12).

In the case of injured workers, the worker and the employer are stakeholders in the outcome of occupational therapy services. Occupational therapists can provide rehabilitation interventions that emphasize occupational performance, encourage clients' self-advocacy efforts, and identify environmental modifications that would facilitate a return to work.

Wounded Warrior Project

With advancements in protective gear and medical management of battlefield injuries, an unprecedented number of service personnel are returning home seriously wounded or disabled. The most common conditions seen in returning warriors are traumatic brain injury (TBI), amputations, and post-traumatic stress disorder (PTSD). Approximately 42,000 service members have returned home injured as a result of combat operations in Afghanistan and Iraq from 2001 to 2011 (Wounded Warrior Project, 2011).

The Wounded Warrior Project (WWP) was founded in 2003 for the purpose of raising awareness of the needs of injured service members, providing programs and services to meet those needs, and facilitating the transition and reintegration of injured and disabled service members into their communities and into civilian life (WWP, 2011).

Services provided by the WWP include rehabilitation, peer support, mental health counseling, adapted sports and recreational activities, technology training, employment assistance, advocacy, and education of service personnel and their families. All services are free to persons with service-related illnesses, wounds, injuries, and disabilities incurred after the September 11, 2001, terrorist attacks on U.S. soil.

The WWP Web site provides visitors with many examples of successful programs for recreation and socialization for injured military personnel in communities around the United States. This Web site (www.woundedwarriorproject.org) posts stories of wounded service persons and the importance they place on becoming reintegrated into their communities and engaging in meaningful activities.

Advocacy

Advocacy is the process of educating others to promote opinions or views that influence policies, attitudes, or the creation/modification of legislation and regulations. This educational process may help to remove attitudinal barriers that exist against individuals with accessibility challenges and those returning to the community with disabilities or special needs through enhanced awareness and sensitivity. It can also involve teaching self-advocacy skills that empower persons with disabilities to act or to represent themselves on issues. The occupational therapist can teach self-advocacy strategies in classrooms, clinics, homes, and elsewhere to individuals of varying needs and abilities.

In order to advocate for accessibility and community integration, it is important for the occupational therapy practitioner to identify who the stakeholders are and promote community-based services that will be most advantageous to clients. **Stakeholders** have an interest in particular businesses or causes, or have a self-interest based on personal need. Stakeholders may be individuals, family members, business owners, employers, advocates, or government entities or officials. When stakeholders want to initiate services, or change existing services or regulations, they become advocates within their organization, in their community, or with legislators.

Conclusion

As stakeholders and advocates, occupational therapy practitioners can use disability data to identify their potential client base and where services may be needed. This data offers a perspective on who is disabled, the impact of the disabilities (e.g., on ADLs or IADLs), the geographic distribution of the population, and employment status of individuals. The occupational therapy practitioner can use data to determine where gaps in services are and how to facilitate accessibility and community integration programs for people with disabilities and special needs. Occupational therapy practitioners also need to understand the population for whom special laws and opportunities were established.

Disability data also informs community planners and health care providers regarding how to provide services that meet the needs of individuals who may require specialized services (e.g., health care, education, support). When demographics and trends are understood, services can be developed or modified that meet the current and future needs of society.

Occupational therapy plays an important role in assisting individuals with disabilities, recovering from traumas, and/or living with chronic conditions to acquire access and achieve community integration. Accessibility and community integration may be mandated legislatively or required because these concepts reflect the core values of communities. Individuals and groups who are stakeholders for this population serve as advocates to increase public awareness, create living and work opportunities, and facilitate transitions from more restricted to less restricted living environments. Accessibility assessments, the development of implementation strategies to remove barriers in built environments, and programs and services will enable a greater number of individuals to live with maximum independence in communities around the United States. Consumer choice and government policies help guide the development and availability of services, including reduction in environmental and programmatic barriers, and improvement in living environments, employment, transportation, and leisure and recreation. Occupational therapists work with individuals, families, agencies, and communities to support independent living and facilitate positive change.

CASE STUDIES

CASE STUDY 22•1 Veretta

Veretta was 19 years old and away at college when she contracted meningitis. She was hospitalized for several weeks and was to be transferred to a nursing home in her community until she could tolerate a full rehabilitation program. Veretta and her family realized that about 10% of people with meningitis do not survive (National Association of School Nurses, n.d.), and they felt fortunate even though Veretta faced a long road in rehabilitation and potentially a life with physical challenges. At the time of transfer, Veretta's cognition, executive functions, and fine and gross motor coordination were impaired.

When Veretta completed rehabilitation, she was discharged to her parents' home. She made this move with the hopes that this would be a temporary situation and that she eventually would be able to return to college even though she might need physical and academic support. Veretta would continue to need outpatient rehabilitation services to continue to strengthen her balance, motor planning, and organizational skills.

CASE STUDY 22•1 Discussion Questions

1. Contact a local college or university and discover the eligibility requirements for student disability services. Would Veretta qualify for services?
2. Based on your assumptions of Veretta's functioning, what occupational therapy services may be beneficial to help her integrate back into the community?
3. What services might a Center for Independent Living (see U.S. Department of Education, 2010) provide that could help Veretta reach her goals?

CASE STUDY 22•2 Paul

Paul is a 61-year-old who was diagnosed with multiple sclerosis when he was in his early 40s. He has managed his symptoms (i.e., fatigue, depression, muscle weakness, and muscle spasms) with medication and exercise. His balance has become significantly impaired and his endurance, upper extremity coordination, and ability to walk are also impaired. He now uses a scooter when traveling outside of his home. Paul's wife has been doing the majority of driving, and he wants to get his own wheels back as he values his independence. Paul owns his own optometric business and recognizes that he will need to have accommodations at home and at work to meet his current and future needs.

CASE STUDY 22•2 Discussion Questions

1. If Paul will need his scooter for all of his mobility needs, what environmental barriers might exist at home and at work that require removal?
2. Visit the Job Accommodation Network (www.jan.org) Web site. Identify the type of assistance that Paul and others with disabilities can use to modify their work sites to meet their physical and cognitive needs. List at least three adaptations that may be useful to Paul as his needs increase.
3. Paul wants to be able to drive again. He wants to locate a driver rehabilitation specialist who can assess his driving ability and what car/van modifications may be appropriate to meet his current and growing needs. Locate the national resources that may help Paul find the occupational therapist with the skill set that would be helpful. Also, visit the local Division of Rehabilitation Services or Center for Independent Living (see U.S. Department of Education, 2010) to learn what additional services and supports are available and their eligibility requirements.

Learning Activities

1. Visit the National Center on Workforce and Disability Web site. Explore which of the Transportation Resources are available in your community and the eligibility requirements for those services.
2. Individuals with disabilities continue to be institutionalized when they would prefer to live in the community. Consider Dave B., who was injured at the age of 13 in a crash while riding his ATV. He was admitted to a nursing home following rehabilitation because his family doubted their ability to care for him at home. Identify the legislation that supports transition from institution to community. Also identify the state agencies that Dave's parents would work with to help make this transition possible.
3. Select one of the following laws: Rehabilitation Act, Developmental Disabilities Act, Assistive Technology Act, or Older Americans Act and:
   a. Determine which agency in your state is responsible for the administration and implementation of the law.
   b. Investigate whether occupational therapy services are delivered through the state or local level. Identify where occupational therapy is available and the services that are available to the community. (If occupational therapy is not a recognized provider, suggest a minimum of three ways that occupational therapy should be involved and where to direct advocacy efforts.)

Acknowledgments: Special thanks to Melissa Kellner, graduate assistant, Department of Occupational Therapy and Occupational Science at Towson University, for her assistance in updating some of the legislative information that appears in this chapter.

REFERENCES

American Occupational Therapy Association. (2008). *Occupational therapy practice framework: Domain and process* (2nd ed.). Bethesda, MD: AOTA Press.

Banks, F. M. (2001). Accessibility issues. In M. E. Scaffa, *Occupational therapy in community-based practice settings.* Philadelphia: F.A. Davis.

Center on Health Promotion Research for People with Disabilities. (n.d.). *Health Empowerment Zone: The Health Empowerment Zone Study Manual.* University of Illinois at Chicago. Retrieved from http://uic-chp. org/Articles/HEZ/HEZ_Manual_Final_forWebsite.pdf

Disabled World. (2011). Latest U.S. disability statistics and facts. Retrieved from http://disabled-world.com/ disability/statistics/census-figures.php

Jans, L., Stoddard, S., & Kraus, L. (2004). Chartbook on mental health and disability in the United States: An info use report. Washington, DC: U.S. Department of Education, National Institute on Disability and Rehabilitation Research. Retrieved from http://infouse.com/ disabilitydata/mentalhealth/index.php

McColl, M. A., Davies, D., Carlson, P., Johnston, J., & Minnes, P. (2001). The Community Integration Measure: Development and preliminary validation. *Archives of Physical Medicine and Rehabilitation, 82,* 429–434.

National Association of School Nurses. (n.d.). *Voices of Meningitis.* Retrieved from http://voicesofmeningitis.com

Useful-community-development.org (2011). Government Housing Assistance Overview Program. Retrieved from: http://useful-community-development.org/government-housing-assistance.html

U.S. Bureau of Labor Statistics. (2011). Employment status of the civilian noninstitutionalized population by disability status and age, 2009 and 2010 annual averages. Retrieved from http://bls.gov/news.release/disabl.a.htm

U.S. Census Bureau. (2010). *Selected social characteristics in the United States.* Retrieved from http://factfinder2. census.gov/faces/tableservices/jsf/pages/productview.xhtml ?pid=ACS_10_1YR_DP02&prodType=table

U.S. Department of Education. (2010). *Centers for independent living.* Retrieved from http://www2.ed.gov/ programs/cil/index.html

U.S. Department of Housing and Urban Development, Home & Communities. (2006). *Disability Rights in Housing.* Retrieved from http://hud.gov/offices/fheo/ disabilities/inhousing.cfm

U.S. Department of Justice. (2002.) *Americans with Disabilities Act: Questions and answers.* Retrieved from http://ada.gov/q%26aeng02.htm

U.S. Department of Transportation. (2005). *What Airline Employees, Airline Contractors, and Air Travelers with Disabilities Need to Know About Access to Air Travel for Persons with Disabilities.* Retrieved from http:// airconsumer.dot.gov/SA_Disability.htm

U.S. Department of Veterans Affairs, Patient Care Services. (October 27, 2009). Prosthetic and Sensory Aids Support Veterans. Retrieved from http://www1.va.gov/women.vet/ docs/ProstheticanSensoryAids.pps

U.S. Equal Employment Opportunity Commission. (2002). *Enforcement guidance: Reasonable accommodation and undue hardship under the Americans with disabilities act.* Retrieved from http://eeoc.gov/policy/docs/accommodation.html

Vrkljan, B. H., & Polgar, J. M. (2007). Linking occupational participation and occupational identity: An exploratory study of the transition from driving to driving cessation in older adulthood. *Journal of Occupational Science, 14* (1), 30–39.

Wounded Warriors Project. (2011). To honor and empower wounded warriors. Retrieved from http://woundedwarriorproject.org/mission.aspx

Chapter 23

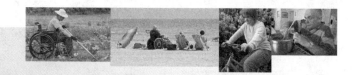

Independent Living Centers

Courtney S. Sasse, MA EdL, MS, OTR/L

Independent living is not doing things by yourself, it is being in control of how things are done.

—Judy Heumann in *Just Like Everyone Else* (World Institute on Disability, 1995, p. 8)

Learning Objectives

This chapter is designed to enable the reader to:
- List and describe the events and factors leading to the advent of the independent living movement.
- Describe the independent living philosophy.
- Identify key advocates and their associated roles in influencing the independent living movement.
- Compare and contrast the independent living movement with other civil rights movements.
- List and describe the four core services of independent living programs.
- Demonstrate an understanding of the role of occupational therapy in independent living centers.

Key Terms

Consumer control
Consumerism
Deinstitutionalization
Demedicalization
Disability rights movement
Independent Living Center (ILC)

Independent living movement
Individualized Written Independent Living Plan (IWILP)
National Council on Independent Living (NCIL)
Statewide Independent Living Council (SILC)
Vocational rehabilitation model
World Institute on Disability (WID)

Introduction

The **disability rights movement** asserts that persons with disabilities have the same rights as their nondisabled peers and opposes discrimination in housing, education, employment, and public accommodations. The independent living movement is part of the broader movement for disability rights. The **independent living movement** is based on the premise that all persons with disability, regardless of the severity, should have the right to live in settings and communities of their choice (University of California Berkeley, 2010).

There are many similarities between the independent living movement and the disability rights movement. Both movements have as the primary goal independence in thoughts, choices, decisions, and actions for the individual with disabilities (Center for Independent Living, SMILES, n.d.a.). The history, philosophy, key leaders, and advocates of the independent living movement are described in this chapter. In addition, the core service principles of independent living programs and the role of occupational therapy are discussed.

History and Philosophy of the Independent Living Movement

History

Beginning as early as the 1900s, people with disabilities ranging from mental illness to physical disabilities were institutionalized and dehumanized. State-run institutions were home to criminals, people with disabilities, abandoned children, and others shunned by society. The process of **deinstitutionalization,** or the release of persons from institutions with the expectation of alternative placements and care within community-based settings, began in the mid-1960s. This was an initial attempt to return individuals to their family, home, or community of origin (McDonald & Oxford, 1995).

The process of giving institutionalized persons their freedom (deinstitutionalization) was one of the first recognized social movements. Deinstitutionalization, spurred by the social model of practice, is rooted in the philosophy of normalization, founded by Canadian sociologist Wolf Wolfensburger. In order to normalize behaviors, Wolfensburger believed that individuals with disabilities needed exposure and immersion in living environments that mimicked "normal." Deinstitutionalization was believed to support the return of people to a more normalized place. Although the philosophical principle was sound, many of those who left state-run institutions found themselves with a lack of alternative homes and placements due to insufficient funding and inadequate political resolve. Initially intended for good purpose, deinstitutionalization at times contributed to the ongoing problem of a lack of suitable housing and care options for those with disabilities. Many young people were wrongly placed in nursing home settings because of this lack of appropriate alternatives (McDonald & Oxford, 1995).

Simultaneously with the deinstitutionalization movement, the Civil Rights Act of 1964, which prohibits discrimination on the basis of race, religion, ethnicity, national origin, and creed, was enacted. Other legislative acts that have influenced the independent living movement are outlined in Box 23-1. Many leaders of the independent living movement recall the Civil Rights Act of 1964 as

Box 23-1 Key Legislative Acts That Influenced the Independent Living Movement	
• Civil Rights Act of 1964	• Established to prohibit discrimination on the basis of race, religion, ethnicity, national origin, and creed. Later, gender was added as a protected class.
• Rehabilitation Act of 1973	• Specific protection under Title V, Sections 501, 503, and 504, prohibits discrimination in federal programs and services and all other programs or services receiving federal funding.
• 1975 Education of All Handicapped Children Act, Public Law 94-142 (currently recognized as the Individuals with Disabilities Education Act (IDEA))	• Requires free and appropriate public education in the least restrictive environment possible for children with disabilities.
• 1975 Developmental Disabilities Bill of Rights Act	• Establishes Protection and Advocacy (P&A) services for individuals with disabilities.
• 1978 Amendments to the Rehabilitation Act	• Provides for consumer-controlled independent living centers (ILCs).
• 1983 Amendments to the Rehabilitation Act	• Provides for the Client Assistance Program (CAP), an advocacy program for consumers of rehabilitation and independent living services.
• 1990 Americans with Disabilities Act	• Provides comprehensive civil rights protection for people with disabilities. This legislative act was modeled after the Civil Rights Act of 1964 and Section 504 of Title V of the Rehabilitation Act and its regulations.

being the model and the impetus that sparked a realization in people with disabilities that they too had a unique culture. They believed they needed to be a protected class, and that they should be afforded the same privileges that all U.S. citizens enjoy. With this realization a further push toward self-advocacy came during the era of "self-help" in the 1970s. During this time, the capacity to help oneself merged with the idea of peer support, and people with disabilities, particularly groups of people with similar types of disabilities, realized strength could be found in numbers (McDonald & Oxford, 1995).

Philosophy

The independent living philosophy emphasizes the rights of persons with disabilities to decide how to live, work, and participate in community life, and can be summarized by the principles outlined in Box 23-2. Three of these, demedicalization, consumerism, and consumer control, will be discussed here in more detail.

Demedicalization, a movement and philosophy characterized by a more holistic approach to health care, evolved slowly and progressively from 1960 through 1980 but then intensified when people began to realize that they had the potential to change their own health and influence their own destiny. The demedicalization movement was a departure from the medical profession's authoritative reign over health decision making and created the demand for a more holistic approach to health care with accessibility to a variety of health care providers. Health care provision no longer comprised medical doctors exclusively; instead, people chose to utilize multidisciplinary teams of professionals who practiced in the community.

A paradigm shift was ushered in, from a medical model of care to a more community-based, individually self-empowered era dominated by the social model of care that is still growing and evolving today (McDonald & Oxford, 1995).

Consumerism, an idea and a movement that was popularized by its vocal advocate, Ralph Nader, focused on societal and consumer demands for product quality, reliability, and fair pricing. Arguably the most critical and foundational element of the independent living movement is the same as that demanded in consumerism, that the user of the product or service has the right to control the choices and decisions that are personally relevant, convenient, necessary, and preferable to him or her.

An extension of consumerism is **consumer control,** which means placing power with the consumer or empowering the individual (McDonald & Oxford, 1995; National Council on Independent Living, n.d.a.; Workforce Investment Act, 1978). In the late 1970s, Gerber DeJong developed the independent living theory as a further extension of the principle of consumer control. In this paradigm shift, the consumer is seen as the expert on his or her life choices; hence, the often-heard expression from the independent living movement, "Nothing about us without us." Although society had long assumed the role of attempting to "fix" people with disabilities, the independent living paradigm helped introduce the idea that no medicine, program, or rehabilitation could "fix" a human being. Because disability is a part of the human experience, it is not an indication of something being broken. Therefore, it is the societal barriers to independence and societal attitudes toward people with disabilities that require "fixing" (Jenkins, 2011; McDonald & Oxford, 1995).

Leaders and Advocates of the Independent Living Movement

Ed Roberts is often called the father of the independent living movement for his role in promoting self-advocacy and empowerment (Box 23-3). He created the first fully funded **independent living center** (ILC) in Berkeley, California. An ILC is a private, non-profit, community-based, grassroots

Box 23-2 Principles of Independent Living
A   Advocacy
B   Barrier removal
C   Civil rights, consumerism, and a cross-disability approach
D   Deinstitutionalization and demedicalization
E   Empowerment of the individual through consumer control, peer role models, and self-help
F   Fix society, not the individual with the disability

Box 23-3 **Ed Roberts is considered the father of the Independent Living Movement. The following is a letter written by Mr. Roberts.**

Forty years ago I contracted polio. At an early age I had been taught not to stare at people with disabilities. Now I was one of "those" people. I had been a healthy, athletic teenager. Suddenly I became a patient. But I was not, as people thought, a helpless cripple.

In my early 20s I enrolled at the University of California. The university set up housing for me in the hospital on campus.

There were other people like me at Berkeley. We began to discuss what we could accomplish if the school provided services for us. We would be able to live outside of the hospital. We would be able to get into restaurants and other public buildings. We would be able to live a life similar to other students. We convinced the university to provide some services, and we began to do these things.

We soon found other people like us throughout the area. The services we had initiated could help people besides students. Shortly thereafter we sought and received funds to begin a community organization, the Center for Independent Living. We provided information about services for people with disabilities, we had wheelchair repair assistance, we referred attendants to people, and we provided an atmosphere for people with disabilities to support each other. We helped make it possible for people with significant disabilities to live independent lives in our community.

Today I travel around the country and the world speaking about the rights of people with disabilities. Independent Living is now an international movement. Wherever I go, I hear similar concerns and needs; people with disabilities simply want to be included in the activities of their communities.

That's what "Independent Living" means—that every one of us (and not just people with disabilities) has the right and capacity to participate in all of society's activities.

From: World Institute on Disability (1995). *Just like everyone else: The changing image of disability.* Oakland, CA: Author.

advocacy organization run by and for people with disabilities. ILCs provide a wide range of services and resources that enhance or support inclusion of people with disabilities in all aspects of community living (Workforce Investment Act, 1978).

In the early 1930s, there was a powerful American leader who lifted U.S. citizens from the oppression of the Great Depression and paved the way for people with disabilities who would follow. President Franklin Delano Roosevelt contracted poliomyelitis as an adult. Fear that being disabled would defeat his efforts toward leadership because of the attitudes of society created his perceived need to hide his disability (Center for Independent Living, SMILES, n.d.b.). Nevertheless, President Roosevelt is well recognized as one of the most powerful, popular, and productive presidents in history despite his disability. He later was revered as one who quietly opened the door to the reality that disability does not define, but rather ability makes people powerfully shine. Additionally, disabilities activists share foundations with leagues of people who organized in the 1940s and 1950s toward political change for people who were blind or deaf. In many ways these diagnosis-specific or disability-specific groups modeled how powerful a "culture" can be when advocating toward positive participation in the community (McDonald & Oxford, 1995).

As Ed Roberts pushed for rights for people with disabilities on the West Coast of the United States, a teacher named Judy Heumann on the East Coast brought the battle to the New York City Board of Education. Heumann wanted to teach school, but when she applied for her teaching credentials she had to be carried up two flights of steps in multiple inaccessible buildings in order to take a written exam, an oral exam, and submit to a physical exam. After passing the written and oral exams and learning she had failed the physical exam because of her inability to walk, she decided to take action. She sued the Board of Education, won, and was hired to teach (National Council on Independent Living [NCIL], n.d.b.).

In 1983, the World Institute on Disability was founded by Ed Roberts, Judy Heumann, and another leading disabilities rights activist, Joan Leon. The **World Institute on Disability (WID)** is a non-profit public policy, research, and training institute that advocates for independence and quality of life for all people with disabilities, regardless of their age. In the same year, Max Starkloff, Charlie Carr, and Marca Bristo founded the National Council on Independent Living. The **National Council on Independent Living (NCIL)** remains one of the only national membership organizations that advances independent living, quality of life, and choice for people with disabilities through consumer-controlled advocacy (NCIL, 2010).

Although the Americans with Disabilities Act (ADA) was not passed until 1990, the original Rehabilitation Act of 1973 had provided the legislative foundation for the ADA. Four primary people, and countless others, were responsible for developing and fighting for the passage of the ADA. Justin Dart is often referred to as the "spiritual leader" of the independent living movement. Liz Savage and Pat Wright were called the maternal arms of the ADA, and together they worked tirelessly for the passage of the ADA. Lex Frieden, a former chairperson of the National Council on Disabilities, is considered the father of the ADA. He was instrumental in conceiving and drafting the original ADA legislation and introducing the philosophies and ideas of the independent living movement to the U.S. Congress for the first time (McDonald & Oxford, 1995).

It is not possible to create a fully inclusive list of the advocates who made the independent living movement possible. However, the unified voices of many led to more meaningful participation in the community for individuals with disabilities through the development of independent living programs.

Independent Living Programs: Meaningful Participation in the Community

The most prominent effect of the increasing push and advocacy toward independent living and the social paradigm, as well as the recognized emergence of the critical importance of community participation, was the development within the community of independent living programs through ILCs. In October of 2000, an evaluative study on the role and performance outcomes of ILCs was conducted. The narrow focus of the

study was the centers' capacity for being a resource to empower individuals with disabilities. The evaluation served three critical purposes: to provide evidence for the consistency of ILCs in reporting outcomes to the Rehabilitation Services Administration's Government Performance and Results Act reporting requirements, to assist ILCs in identification of best practice in service and advocacy, and to inform advocates and legislators about programs made possible through ILCs.

Data for the outcomes-based study were obtained from three sources. A mail-out survey of all ILCs that receive Medicare Part C federal funding was completed. Current and former consumers, totaling 569 individuals, were selected using a random sample of 104 centers as well as an additional random sample selected at the center level to identify consumers who would be interviewed. Finally, the Rehabilitation Services Administration 704 report was used to select and describe the centers and the characteristics of the centers' consumers (U.S. Department of Education, Office of Special Education and Rehabilitative Services, 2004). One finding from the evaluation of ILCs was related to Statewide Independent Living Councils.

Independent living centers typically receive public and private grant funding, but they can also receive federal and state funding as a result of the Workforce Investment Act. In order to be eligible for federal and state funding, each state is required to establish a **Statewide Independent Living Council (SILC)**. The SILC is a state agency designed to

- receive, account for, disburse, and coordinate benefits between federal and state sources,
- document plans recorded and received by the state commissioner for the purposes of matching objectives and outcomes to expenditures, and
- facilitate communication between local ILCs and state and federal government agencies (Rehabilitation Services Administration, 2010; Workforce Investment Act, 1978).

The survey results indicated that even though 89% of the center directors believed that they had minimal to adequate representation at the state level through their SILC, many ILC directors indicated that their SILC was not measuring up to its intended purpose of representation or its responsibility for meeting the requirements of the Rehabilitation Act

Chapter 23 | Independent Living Centers   337

Amendments (U.S. Department of Education Office of Special Education and Rehabilitative Services, 2004). The implication of this finding is what has driven many ILCs to seek more grassroots, local community support in funding as well as in providing a powerful source of legislative strength and a voice to state and national advocacy platforms. Other key findings from the *Final Evaluation Report on the Centers for Independent Living (CIL) Programs* are listed in Table 23-1.

The Four Core Services of Independent Living Programs and Centers

The independent living movement envisioned a future of equality for people with disabilities. The foundation of the independent living philosophy is for services and choices for people with disabilities within a community to be made "by" the people rather than "for" or "about" the people. The concept of consumer control helped support advocacy activists in creating ILCs, which led to the development of best practices for implementing community programs that would provide occupational opportunities for all people within the community.

The four core services that ILCs provide for people with disabilities are:

1. individual and systems advocacy,
2. information and referral,
3. peer support, and
4. independent living skills training (National Council on Independent Living).

Through the first core service, ILC staff advocate on behalf of individuals and for systems change to

Table 23-1	Key Findings From the Final Evaluation Report on the Centers for Independent Living (CIL) Programs
Key Findings	**Key Findings and Community Practice Implications:**
One	Independent Living Centers provide a variety of services while incorporating advocacy within the community by practicing consumer empowerment and control, peer support, and systems change across a variety of disabilities.
Two	Minority groups with disabilities are being served in Independent Living Centers in approximately the same ratio that they are present in the U.S. population.
Three	Items on the evaluation related to accessibility were scored higher on average than the other surveyed items.
Four	Independent Living Centers primarily serve a population who have household incomes of less than $20,000 per year (are considered poor), are typically unemployed or underemployed, and are unmarried. These three risk factors (being unemployed, unmarried, and poor) are correlated with a loss of independence. The typical consumers at Independent Living Centers cannot afford many services to support their independence.
Five	Clients with cognitive disabilities received fewer employment support services than other consumer populations. Additionally, Hispanic clients were less likely to receive adaptive technology or assistance and adaptive equipment than other populations who required similar adaptations.
Six	Significant levels of community change were reported for many centers in the areas of transportation, housing, deinstitutionalization, education, employment, and civil rights. Center directors reported high consumer participation in the majority of the advocacy actions at the local level.
Seven	Consumers indicated significant benefits and concrete changes in their lives as a result of the services provided by Independent Living Centers.

Data from: U.S. Department of Education Office of Special Education and Rehabilitative Services (February 9, 2004). Final Evaluation Report on the Centers for Independent Living (CIL) Program. Rehabilitation Services Administration, Washington, DC. Retrieved from http://ed.gov/policy/speced/leg/eval-studies.html

ensure the civil and human rights of persons with disabilities. ILC leadership can be a local source for providing disability awareness training and advocacy toward enhanced accessibility and community mobility. ILC staff can assist individuals and families with transitions between acute rehabilitation facilities and home, or transitions from skilled nursing facilities to independent living in the community. Advocacy can result in legislation, or alternatively, ILCs can become the watchdog that ensures that ADA legislation is implemented effectively (NCIL, n.d.b.).

The second core service involves providing disability-specific information, referrals, and access to specific services. The goal is to provide the information people need to initiate and maintain independent living in the community. In order to encourage participation and provide equitable community experiences, a primary responsibility of ILC staff is to educate both consumers and the communities in which they live.

The third core service, peer support, is based on the premise that peers with disabilities can be as effective as professionals in providing information and support. Centers for independent living often solicit peer support from within the community to ensure the integrity of consumer control within independent living programs. In this way, people who have needs for independent living services participate in programmatic decisions. Peer support and participation within the boundaries of their unique culture effectively empower people with disabilities to direct their lives, further securing and promoting independence (National Council on Independent Living).

ILCs often design programs that utilize peer support to provide education on skill sets necessary to navigate independence within a community setting. Independent living skills training is the fourth core service. From an occupational therapy perspective, participation is often thought of as active engagement in occupation. However, independent participation within the larger community for people with disabilities is not successful without the seamless integration of desires, choices, decisions, and actions being met. Through sharing of life stories and life histories, and support of person-to-person and person-to-environment interactions, ILC staff can teach coping strategies

and help individuals with disabilities rebuild their identity, improve vocational skills, and adapt to new situations (NCIL, Wiley, 2003). The principles of independent living are continuously improving and emerging, but the four core services of ILCs consistently remain the foundation that supports independence for people with disabilities within the community.

The Role of Occupational Therapy in Independent Living Centers

The principles underlying the independent living movement parallel the philosophy and goals of occupational therapy. Meaningful engagement in occupation requires choice, access, and freedom to engage in activities that are personally relevant. Occupational therapy practitioners work to provide accessibility in order to promote a greater degree of independence among adults with disabilities. Supporting maximum participation in work and leisure, more particularly, maximum participation in community activities for all regardless of ability, enhances quality of life and can contribute to an improved sense of community cohesion (American Occupational Therapy Association [AOTA], 2011; Santoyo, 2011).

Exclusion based on physical disability is no longer the only consideration in accessibility. A wide variety of populations with restricted capabilities are denied access to participation in the community. With over half of the baby boomer generation already diagnosed with a chronic medical condition, commonly high blood pressure, arthritis, high cholesterol, diabetes, obesity, and trauma or disease-related amputations, the reality of accessibility becomes even more critical for all community members (McUsic, 2011). Occupational therapists have a skill set that includes the ability to analyze and identify the barriers to accessibility, which then become barriers to participation.

The independent living movement was founded on the premise of consumer control. Accessibility has historically been designed with the presumption that people with disabilities will be attempting to meet the norms of able-bodied people. Furthermore, the typical accessibility designs for physical adaptations assume that people with any disability, regardless of the nature of the disability, require the same adaptations to enhance accessibility and participation. Now we know this assumption is incorrect. Kielhofner (2002) was among the first to recognize the influence of the environment on performance capacity. Perhaps the most critical role for occupational therapy in the future will be contributions to accessibility design that align the multiple aspects of living with disabilities to the multiple dimensions of occupational engagement, performance capacity, environmental demands, and occupational performance (Jenkins, 2011).

Preventative Occupational Therapy Services

While there are a variety of levels of prevention of disease and disability, independent living programs typically focus on tertiary prevention. The focus of occupational intervention for people with disabilities in tertiary prevention is to minimize further dysfunction while simultaneously improving accessibility to meaningful occupations for this population within the community in a cost-effective way (Hay et al., 2002; Scaffa, Desmond, & Brownson, 2001). Research by Hay et al. (2002) based on the Well-Elderly Study evaluated the cost-effectiveness of a 9-month preventive occupational therapy program for independent living older adults. The study found that the quality of life improvements in health, participation, and function attributable to occupational therapy preventive interventions were significant. Cost-effectiveness of the services was demonstrated by a trend toward decreasing post-intervention health care costs of participants and insurers.

The goals of independent living skills training and preventive occupational therapy overlap in many ways. Both interventions focus on adequate maintenance of affordable health care and the provision of information regarding resources and options available to assist with independent living in the community. It is the goal of occupational therapy to help participants determine goals that are meaningful and purposeful. Independent living programs provide an environment where daily schedules, routines, environments, and interactions are the same for people with disabilities as they are for

their non-disabled peers (AOTA, 1993; NCIL, n.d.c.). Research indicates that the two strongest predictors of return to independent living at discharge from acute care or rehabilitation, or following sub-acute hospitalization, are physical functioning and cognitive status in older disabled adults. Furthermore, research supports the notion that cognition is of equal value in determining fitness to live alone as physical condition (Lysack, Neufeld, Mast, MacNeill, & Lichtenberg, 2003). Preventative occupational therapy interventions should reinforce the importance of community resources when supporting independent living in the community.

Health Promotion Services

One of the underlying philosophies of independent living is that people with different disabilities, when linked together through common experiences and goals, are empowered. Not only is the empowerment a stimulus for advocacy and working collectively toward positive change but also as consumer control is practiced, health promotion is an inherent result. Health promotion, or the combination of approaches and interventions that support positive health outcomes, has traditionally consisted of programs that support individuals setting health-oriented goals. However, new programs like "Living Well with a Disability" incorporate a more innovative approach to independent living and health promotion by following two goals. Participants first establish goal pursuits and then encourage health behavior changes as objectives that focus heavily on the consumer's quality-of-life goals. Hope and positive outcomes are developed through problem solving, through the use of attribution retraining, and by teaching positive self-talk strategies (Ravesloot et al., 2007). Because programs such as this promote consumer control and incorporate independent living philosophies, people with disabilities experience positive improvements in health ranging from fewer limitations from secondary conditions and fewer unhealthy days to fewer trips to seek medical intervention.

Nevertheless, positive physical changes are not the only significant outcomes that affect independent living. Psychosocial and mental health improvements have also been documented through use of health promotion practices (Clark et al., 2001).

Through the independent living movement, health promotion can also mean promoting a culture and a community where independent living is a way of life. Occupational therapy can support independent living in the community by ensuring that people with disabilities have the same choices with regard to housing, education, entertainment, transportation, and employment (World Institute on Disability, 1995). The role of an occupational therapy practitioner within the independent living context will consistently be to make adaptations to the environment that promote independence, participation, and health. Assessment, case management, vocational rehabilitation specialist, driving assessment or driving rehabilitation specialist, consultant, coordinator, or director of independent living programs or centers are all potential roles that can be fulfilled by occupational therapists.

Services for Special Populations

Independent living programs often target specific populations in order to more thoroughly inform practice and concentrate services necessary for greater advocacy and independence of people with similar disabilities. These cohorts also often have similar experiences and needs. Independent living programs for children and youth, the elderly, and adults with acquired brain injury or spinal cord injury exist as a source of support for these populations.

Regardless of the population served, ILC staff members assess the needs and desires of the consumer, and collaboratively determine a plan that includes goals toward independent living in the community and access to opportunities. An **individualized written independent living plan (IWILP)** is a plan that documents the rights and responsibilities of the consumer and the agents of the ILC, as well as a time-bound set of consumer and ILC goals and objectives for progress toward independence of the individual with disability (Bowen, 2001).

Services for Youth

When a geographical area has a greater demand for ILCs or programs, specialty centers are sometimes created. For example, legislation regarding independent living was developed in New York in the mid-1980s as a response to a class action lawsuit filed by former wards of the state, teenagers who had "aged out"

of the foster care system and were turned out to live on the streets with few resources. The lawsuit claimed that New York City's child welfare system failed to prepare youth for independent living, leaving them uniquely "disabled" (Georgiades, 2005). From this legislation came the inception of subsidized independent living programs. Programs like this allow teens 16 years of age or older to live in an approved setting (which cannot be institutional), and by meeting requirements related to education, work, and vocational training, the teens are eligible for a monetary stipend (Georgiades, 2005).

When youth leave the foster care system, research indicates that they are at an increased risk for low levels of achievement in many domains, which often presages their involvement with the criminal justice system and a dependency on public assistance. Youth with disabilities or complex medical needs who leave the foster care system are at an even greater disadvantage, particularly if cognitive disabilities are involved (Georgiades, 2005; Montgomery, Donkoh, & Underhill, 2006). For ILCs that serve special populations such as children and youth, the service-delivery model that often applies is the vocational rehabilitation model. In the **vocational rehabilitation model,** participants are often required to commit to vocational training and form vocational goals in order to participate in the programming (Bowen, 2001).

Services for Older Adults

At the opposite end of the age continuum are older adults, particularly those who have a long-term disability, who will increasingly demand independent living services. People who are aging with a disability require specialized programming through ILCs to support their desire to age productively within the communities where they live.

This cohort includes people who have experienced a traumatic accident, those with degenerative diseases, and those who have survived poliomyelitis and are now making adaptations in their lives to adjust to post-polio syndrome (Wiley, 2003). Adaptation of the environment is a critical consideration for proponents of the independent living paradigm, as disability is considered to be a human condition. Independence and quality of life are not thought to be about changing human beings but instead about changing the environment to meet people's needs.

Independent living centers provide programs that support enabling people with chronic impairments to achieve a cadre of skills that produce achievements of personally meaningful goals in an individual's environment (Yerxa, 1998).

Meaningful occupation is widely recognized as being related to well-being. Because of the advances in medicine, technology, and quality of care, individuals with long-term disabilities, regardless of the origin of the disability, have an increased life expectancy. ILCs and the programs that they offer supply a unique set of services that meet the individual at any stage following the onset or progression of a disability. Older adults and those with more severe cognitive impairments are likely to need increasing community support and community programming through ILCs for a more significant length of time.

Just as consumer control helped shaped the independent living movement, people with disabilities who are aging should help shape the programs and services offered in ILCs and independent living programs. In order for equality to be reached in opportunities and community activities, the life stories of these consumers must be not only heard and considered but also truly embedded in advocacy efforts. Occupational performance is affected by participation in meaningful activities. Performance is not possible unless active participation and engagement occurs. Independence can be supported most successfully when a person's anticipated needs and benefits are achieved through management of a disability (Wiley, 2003). Many occupational therapy interventions, such as energy conservation, joint protection, and physical and environmental modifications, promote the same goals for people with disabilities that the independent living movement demands, those of independence and participation.

Services for Persons With Brain and Spinal Cord Injuries

Although some special populations who use independent living services are defined by age, such as children, youth, and the elderly with chronic health conditions or disabilities, several special populations for whom independent living services are critically necessary are defined by particular diagnoses. Every year it is estimated that more than 2 million people survive an incident that produces traumatic brain injury (TBI) or spinal cord injury (SCI) and then face a lifetime of making adaptations to purposeful occupations (Trombly, Radomski, Trexel, & Burnett-Smith, 2002). Occupational therapy recognizes the positive relationship between participation in goal-specific occupational therapy and improvement in self-identified goals in adults with TBI or SCI.

When people with disabilities are considered truly integrated into a community and products and services are consumer-controlled, self-identified goals are inherent in the process. Research supports that the perception of performance, satisfaction with performance, and attainment of community-related skills are significantly improved and sustained by individuals with TBI or SCI following occupational therapy intervention (Powell, Temkin, Machamer, & Dikmen, 2007; Trombly, Radomski, Trexel, & Burnett-Smith, 2002). Ultimately, it is both the goal and the challenge for occupational therapists to encourage independence through support while mindfully considering that best practice requires that the client self-identifies meaningful goals and maintains consumer control. In many respects this is also the balance that is necessary for ILCs, that of facilitative support.

Although client-centered practice is considered fundamental in occupational therapy, research outcomes and measures often fail to compare the outcomes of an individual against either his or her self-identified goals or the functional performance of those with similar disabilities and circumstances. Furthermore, reductions in length of stay in acute care and rehabilitation services has meant a necessary focus on activities of daily living (ADLs) during this time, and instrumental activities of daily living (IADLs), which are of critical importance for independent living in the community, have received less attention (Powell, Temkin, Machamer, & Dikmen, 2007).

The Future of Independent Living Centers

The traditional service delivery model of ILCs has included providing site-based resources and support in a consumer-controlled context. Today's technology and the Internet have made advances, advocacy, information, and adaptation possible without the need for a physical space. Consumer access to resources on the Internet promotes independence that is immediate and timely for people with disabilities. The core principles and services of independent living—advocacy, information and referrals, peer support, and independent living skills training—are now widely available and accessible to individuals with disabilities. In the presence of so many avenues of support and possibility, the Internet is perhaps the most influential tool of empowerment for advancement of the philosophy of equal opportunity and equal engagement that is held in such high regard for independent living consumers and advocates. Fulfilling community participation for consumers of independent living requires equal access to employment opportunities, assistance with daily living activities, housing options, and meaningful occupational engagement with social participation that includes effective interpersonal relationships with others (Ritchie & Blanck, 2003).

Sources of financial support and budgets of ILCs vary widely and are typically determined by the level of state funding used to supplement funds received from Title VII of the Rehabilitation Act of 1973, as amended in 1998. Therefore, it is fairly common for an ILC to have a modest budget and serve multiple cities across several counties. The Internet has also made services and resources more widely available through ILCs and accessible across the miles (Ritchie & Blanck, 2003). Since accessibility and availability of technology and Internet use can be hindered by financial constraints, many grant-based funding opportunities exist for supporting IL programs that integrate technology into communities with restricted access (Rehabilitation Services Administration, 2010).

Other than financial constraints, the most common barrier to effective use of technology to support independent living is the lack of knowledge, training, and/or practice opportunities for consumers. Since the Internet is arguably one of the most effective consumer voices for choice, the ability of the consumer to use a computer has become an independent living skill (Ritchie & Blanck, 2003). Occupational therapists whose specialty is adaptive technology can play an important role in consulting with the teams in ILCs and with independent living consumers regarding the implementation and integration of computer technology for personal use. Accessibility continues to be enhanced by the emergence of more advanced universal design features. As universal design is integrated into society, ILCs will continue to advocate for fair and equitable use of technology toward the goal of independence and community participation for people with disabilities, just as they have advocated for the enactment of independent living practices historically.

Conclusion

Effectively participating in meaningful occupations for people with a chronic illness or disability has historically been filled with challenge and discrimination (Persson & Rydén, 2006). The independent living movement can be credited with removing barriers that changed community life for people with disabilities. Today, though much work remains to be done in the form of advocacy, the focus is now on what can be accomplished rather than what cannot be accomplished.

In many ways, people with disabilities and minority populations became the teachers and the rest of society became the students, learning from those involved in the civil rights movement, the Americans with disabilities movement, and the independent living movement. These populations find new ways to participate in their community and in meaningful occupation, often demonstrating self-reliance and self-advocacy that is admirable (Yerxa, 1993). Persons with disabilities have taught society that coping with disability is as individual as people are and that with community support, they have used resiliency and hope to become a culture of "I CAN."

People with disabilities find meaning in occupation when they can live as independently as possible. Occupational therapy practitioners are trained to support adaptations, promote occupational balance, and help people develop and maintain independent living skills and manage their environments. Occupational therapy practitioners are therefore valuable assets to ILCs and the independent living movement.

CASE STUDIES

CASE STUDY 23•1 Marianne

Marianne is a 37-year-old female diagnosed with early onset multiple sclerosis (MS). She lives with her husband and two children in a two-story home. She has had a very difficult time coping since the onset of her initial symptoms and dealing emotionally with the news of her diagnosis. Many of her friends are not sure what her needs are and do not visit with her as frequently as they used to. Marianne feels lonely and isolated. She can still perform most of her ADLs and IADLs with little assistance when she is not experiencing exacerbations of the disease. Nevertheless, she and her husband realize that her functional decline could happen quickly, so they would like to begin to make some preparations to their home and their lifestyle.

During a recent visit with her occupational therapist at an outpatient rehabilitation center, Marianne discussed the emotional burden and worry that her diagnosis had brought on. Marianne's husband, who also was present during the visit, openly discussed the worry and concern he had about Marianne being able to continue to care for herself and the children with the progression of her disease. Marianne tearfully acknowledged that she had stopped driving the children to their extracurricular activities because one of her earliest symptoms was blurred vision and at times even double vision. She also mentioned that one of the most difficult tasks she faces involves helping her children understand what is happening to her.

Marianne had worked for much of her adult life as a paralegal assistant. She also delivered a variety of legal documents around town when needed, as a temporary courier for the same law firm that employed her for paralegal functions. She feared not only that her progressive eyesight problems would soon prevent her from driving safely but also that her ability to see the legal documents on her computer screen would become so impaired that she would no longer be able to perform her work tasks.

Marianne's occupational therapist recommended that Marianne and her husband contact the ILC in their town. The occupational therapist suggested that the ILC might be a source of information on resources available in the community for assisting with changes that needed to be made as her MS progressed. Marianne decided after several weeks of contemplation to contact the ILC. An independent living specialist made an appointment for the following day to meet Marianne and her husband.

The initial meeting felt somewhat awkward to Marianne because, as she later told her IL case manager, at first she wasn't ready to acknowledge that her condition was disabling. The sincerity, friendship, trust, and rapport that she soon built with her case manager changed those initial feelings. The services that followed for Marianne and her family included referrals to support groups for her and her husband. Meeting other families who were dealing with MS was a comfort as well as an opportunity to socialize with others, alleviating the feelings of social isolation she had experienced.

Marianne also began attending computer classes at the ILC, where she learned a variety of programs that would allow her to do her paralegal work from home and maintain her job. Marianne became a skilled user of community transportation, which enhanced her feelings of independence and eased her husband's caregiver burden. Finally, and perhaps most importantly, one of the friends that she made at the support group told her about a counselor who specialized in grief counseling. Marianne began weekly visits with the counselor to help alleviate the depression and grief that she felt over her loss of independence. Her counselor also helped guide her and her husband through the process of counseling their children through the progression of her disease. Marianne was grateful for the regained sense of independence she felt that began with the support she received through her occupational therapist and the ILC.

Continued

CASE STUDY 23•1 Marianne   *cont'd*

CASE STUDY 23•1 Discussion Questions

1. Based on the information provided in the case study, what are some additional recommendations that Marianne's occupational therapist could have provided?
2. Other than the services that Marianne took advantage of as suggested by her IL case manager, research two other services, referrals, or recommendations that the IL manager could have suggested.
3. Discuss how the four core services of ILCs are demonstrated in the case study.
4. Define "health promotion" as related to occupational therapy and independent living programs. Discuss how Marianne's IL case manager has supported health promotion.
5. What are three ways that Marianne's community and family will benefit from the services provided for her at the ILC?

Learning Activities

1. Instead of saying ..., say ....
   Supporting independence for people with disabilities within the community is everyone's responsibility. Discuss the appropriate way to communicate with and about people with disabilities.
   - Instead of saying *the disabled,* say....
   - Instead of saying *autistic,* say ....
   - Instead of saying *blind,* say ....
   - Instead of saying *brain damaged,* say ....
   - Instead of saying *normal,* say ....
   - Instead of saying *confined to a wheelchair,* say ....
   - Instead of saying *crippled,* say....
   - Instead of saying *insane or crazy,* say ....
   - Instead of saying *AIDS victim,* say ....

   Data from: United Cerebral Palsy Associations, Incorporated (UCPA Public Service Announcement, n.d.). The ten commandments of communicating with people with disabilities. Retrieved from http://smilescil.org/resources/non-discriminatory-lingo

2. Occupational Therapy in Independent Living Centers
   Research has identified a variety of issues for which people with disabilities continue to need advocacy and intervention. For each of the following areas, suggest a potential program or service that could be offered at an ILC. Describe potential roles for OT within each service or program. The areas are:
   - health care,
   - employment,
   - technology,
   - long-term care, and
   - civil rights enforcement.

REFERENCES

American Occupational Therapy Association. (1993). Statement: The role of occupational therapy in the independent living movement. *American Journal of Occupational Therapy, 47,* 1079–1080.

American Occupational Therapy Association Fact Sheet. (2011). *Occupational therapy's role in adult cognitive disorders.* Bethesda, MD: American Occupational Therapy Association.

Bowen, R. E. (2001). Independent living programs. In M. E. Scaffa (Ed.), *Occupational therapy in community-based practice settings* (pp. 173–187). Philadelphia: F.A. Davis

Center for Independent Living, SMILES. (n.d.a.). Independent living philosophy. Retrieved from http://smilescil.org/about/independent-living-philosophy

Center for Independent Living, SMILES. (n.d.b.). Independent living advocate. Retrieved from http://smilescil.org/about/independent-living-philosophy/advocates-in-the-independent-living-movement

Clark, F., Azen, S. P., Carlson, M., Mandel, D., LaBree, L., Hay, J., Lipson, L. (2001). Embedding health-promoting changes into the daily lives of independent-living older adults: Long-term follow-up of occupational therapy intervention. *Journal of Gerontology: Psychological Sciences, 56b*(1), 60–63.

Georgiades, S., (2005). A multi-outcome evaluation of an independent living program. *Child and Adolescent Social Work Journal, 22*(5-6), 417–439. doi: 10.1007s10560-005-0020-v

Hay, J., LaBree, L., Luo, R., Clark, F., Carlson, M., Mandel, D., Azen, S. P. (2002). Cost-effectiveness of preventative occupational therapy for independent living older adults. *Journal of American Geriatrics Society, 50*(8), 1381–1388.

Jenkins, G. R. (2011). The challenges of characterizing people with disabilities in the built environment. *OT Practice 16*(9), Article Code CEA0511, CE-1–CE-6.

Kielhofner, G. (2002). *A model of human occupation: Theory and application* (3rd ed.). Baltimore: Lippincott Williams & Wilkins.

Lysack, C. L., Neufeld, S., Mast, B. T., MacNeill, S. E., & Lichtenberg, P. A. (2003). After rehabilitation: An 18-month follow-up of elderly inner-city women. *American Journal of Occupational Therapy, 57,* 298–306.

McDonald, G., & Oxford, M. (1995). Standards and more: Beyond compliance. *IL NET Training Manual.* Retrieved from http://ilru.org/html/projects/ilnet/ilnet_manuals.htm

McUsic, T. (2011). The big boom: The country's largest generation will need adaptive help to reach goals in golden years. *Today in OT, 4*(2), 13–14.

Montgomery, P., Donkoh, C., & Underhill, K. (2006). Independent living programs for young people leaving the care system: The state of the evidence. *Children and Youth Services Review, 28,* 1435–1448. doi: 10.1016/j.childyouth.2006.03.002

National Council on Independent Living. (n.d.a.). Consumer control. Retrieved from http://ncil.org/about/Consumer-Control.html

National Council on Independent Living. (n.d.b.).The disability rights and independent living movements. Retrieved from http://ncil.org/about/WhatIsIndependentLiving.html

National Council on Independent Living. (n.d.c.). Centers for independent living. Retrieved from http://ncil.org/about/CentersforIndependentLiving.html

National Council on Independent Living. (2010). Annual report. Retrieved from http://ncil.org/annualreport

Persson, L. O., & Ryden, A. (2006). Themes of effective coping in physical disability: an interview study of 26 persons who have learnt to live with their disability. *Scandinavian Journal of Caring Sciences, 20,* 355–363.

Powell, J. M., Temkin, N. R., Machamer, J. E., & Dikmen, S. S. (2007). Gaining insight into patients' perspectives on participation in home management activities after traumatic brain injury. *American Journal of Occupational Therapy, 61,* 269–279.

Ravesloot, C. H., Seekins, T., Cahill, T., Lindgren, S., Nary, D. E., & White, G. (2007). Health promotion for people with disabilities: development and evaluation of Living Well with a Disability program. *Health Education Research, 22*(4), 522–531. doi: 10.1093/her/cyl114

Rehabilitation Services Administration. (2010). Center for independent living discretionary/competitive grants. Retrieved from http://www2ed.gov/print/programs/cil/index.html

Ritchie, H., & Blanck, P. (2003). The promise of the Internet for disability: A study of on-line services and web site accessibility at centers for independent living. *Behavioral Sciences and the Law,* 5–26. doi: 10:1002/bsl.520

Santoyo, M. M. (2011). ADA made accessible: 20 years after the watershed law was enacted, a new tool kit helps assess compliance. *Today in OT, 4*(2), 22–23.

Scaffa, M. E., Desmond, S., & Brownson, C. A. (2001). Public health, community health, and occupational therapy. In M. E. Scaffa (Ed.), *Occupational therapy in community-based practice settings* (pp. 35–50). Philadelphia: F.A. Davis.

Trombly, C. A., Radomski, M. V., Trexel, C., & Burnett-Smith, S. E. (2002). Occupational therapy and achievement of self-identified goals by adults with acquired brain injury: Phase II. *American Journal of Occupational Therapy, 56,* 489–498.

United Cerebral Palsy Associations, Incorporated (UCPA Public Service Announcement, n.d.). The ten commandments of communicating with people with disabilities. Retrieved from http://smilescil.org/resources/non-discriminatory-lingo

University of California, Berkeley. (2010). The disability rights and independent living movement: Introduction. Retrieved from http://bancroft.berkeley.edu/collections/drilm/introduction.html

U.S. Department of Education Office of Special Education and Rehabilitative Services (February 9, 2004). Final evaluation report on the centers for independent living (CIL) program. Rehabilitation Services Administration, Washington, DC. Retrieved from http://ed.gov/policy/speced/leg/eval-studies.html

Wiley, E. A. (2003). Aging with a long-term disability: Voices unheard. *Physical & Occupational Therapy in Geriatrics, 21*(3), 33–47.

Workforce Investment Act. (1978). Title VII of the Rehabilitation Act of 1973 (29 U.S.C. 796 et seq.). Independent living services and centers for independent living. Chapters 1 and 2 of the Rehabilitation Act of 1973, as amended.

World Institute on Disability (1995). *Just like everyone else: The changing image of disability.* Oakland, CA: Author.

Yerxa, E. J. (1993). Occupational science: A new source of power for participants in occupational therapy. *Occupational Science: Australia, 1*(1), 3–9.

Yerxa, E. J. (1998). Health and the human spirit for occupation. *American Journal of Occupational Therapy, 52,* 412–418.

Chapter 24

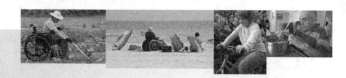

Technology and Environmental Interventions in Community-Based Practice

Rebecca I. Estes, PhD, OTR/L, Paula Lowrey, MOT, OTR/L, and Mary Frances Baxter, PhD, OT, FAOTA

It's mind-boggling when you think of the things that they're coming up with. What higher-level quads like me couldn't do before, we can do now. What a big incentive to keep going. There are so many advantages...I mean, I'm glad I broke my neck in this century!

—Sherer (1996, p. 15)

Learning Objectives

This chapter is designed to enable the reader to:

- Understand the breadth and depth of occupational therapy practice in technology and environmental interventions.
- Describe the key concepts and scope of technology and environmental interventions.
- Identify the principles of universal design.
- Describe some common home modifications recommended by occupational therapy practitioners.
- Discuss the multiple roles and level of training for occupational therapists providing community-based technology and environmental interventions.

Key Terms

Advanced level TEI service
Assistive technology devices
Assistive technology services
Augmentative or alternative communication system
Electronic aid to daily living (EADL)
Entry level of TEI service
Home modification

Home modification process
Home modification product
Input devices
Output devices
Universal design
Wheeled mobility

Introduction

The term technology and environmental intervention (TEI) was coined to embody the vast array of interventions occupational therapists may employ with individuals with disabilities to facilitate full engagement in occupations in accessible environments (American Occupational Therapy Association [AOTA], 2009).

This practice area encompasses technology, including assistive technology services and device prescription, at both the entry and advanced level as well as electronic, information, rehabilitation, and educational technologies.

The Assistive Technology Act of 2004 (Public Law [P.L.] 108-364) defines **assistive technology devices** and **assistive technology services,** respectively, as: "any item, piece of equipment or product systems, whether acquired commercially off the shelf, modified, or customized, that is used to increase, maintain, or improve functional capabilities of individuals with disabilities" (p. 4); "any service that directly assists an individual with a disability in the selection, acquisition, or use of an assistive technology device" (pp. 4–5).

Given these definitions, entry-level occupational therapists who provide low-tech devices such as reachers and sock aids, as well as advanced practice therapists who provide powered wheeled mobility equipment, computer adaptations, and augmentative communications devices, are all providing assistive technology devices and services. Assistive technology devices include appliances or installed equipment (e.g., hospital beds); assistive tools that are used to access inaccessible items or devices (e.g., sip-and-puff wheelchair control); prostheses; and items that assist, augment, or compensate for existing function (e.g., cognitive aids for memory recall).

The AOTA (2009) suggests that occupational therapists may employ TEI interventions at an **entry level of TEI service** by providing the delivery and coordination of technologies basic to occupational performance, acting as an advocate for the client, and acting as a gatekeeper for multiple technology specialist referrals and communication. Therapists who provide more **advanced level TEI services** are involved with the integration of multiple technological devices and deliver more complicated, involved arrangements of technology and environmental modifications.

Whereas entry-level TEI provision is within the skill level of all occupational therapists, the provision of advanced level services requires additional training. Historically, occupational therapists have incorporated current technologies within interventions. Today, although computers and information technologies are commonplace, they are not commonly used in intervention. Combining assistive technology with environmental interventions demonstrates the roles occupational therapists have in accessibility and modification of the different contexts in which clients perform their occupations.

This chapter will focus on the roles of the occupational therapist in both emerging and established community-based TEI practice. The

breadth of service provision, as identified by the AOTA's Centennial Vision, will be discussed as it relates to community-based TEI practice settings, rather than the depth or details of the multitude of service provision areas available.

Technology and Environmental Intervention Outcomes

The occupational therapist may approach technology and environmental interventions using any of the current occupation-based theoretical models used in professional practice, such as the Model of Human Occupation, Occupational Adaptation, Ecology of Human Performance, or the Person-Environment-Occupational-Performance Model (Cole & Tufano, 2008). These models take a holistic approach and consider all aspects of client needs within the multiple contexts and environments in which their occupations are performed. Models discussed specifically as they apply to assistive technology interventions may also guide the therapist providing TEI, such as the Matching Persons and Technology Model, the Human Activity Assistive Technology Model, and the Canadian Model of Occupational Performance (Cook, Polgar, & Hussey, 2008).

The evaluation of TEI outcomes requires the application of appropriate assessments and establishment of the appropriate team for the tasks. In TEI, the team includes not only the therapist and consumer (client, family, caregivers, and significant others) but may also include a variety of specialists, such as assistive technology practitioners, educators, rehabilitation engineers and machinists, vendors, product distributors and manufacturers, architects, contractors and builders, and funders. The team members, whether assembled or brought in as consultants, will depend on the type, extent, and complexity of the TEI being provided. The assessments chosen must be compatible with the types of outcomes being considered. While no single evaluation tool is universally applicable or universally accepted, general guidelines are established and a variety of tools are available for TEI outcomes assessment.

Evaluation of TEI outcomes by the occupational therapist begins with documentation of the client's baseline performance, which may be with no technology device or environmental intervention, or it may be while using a current but outmoded or outgrown technology device or environmental intervention. Traditional occupational therapy assessments may be used to obtain information on performance skills such as speed, accuracy, reliability, and fatigue and endurance. Traditional evaluations may also be used to assess the impact of environmental features on performance. Evaluations may be used to determine the primary physical environments, what is done in each environment, how transitions between environments occur, whether each environment is accessible, and the interface and accessibility of furniture and other items in the environment. Once baseline performance is assessed, a client's seating and positioning needs should be reviewed, if needed, related to the identified occupations and environments. Complex seating and positioning may require specialized assessment and intervention by advanced level therapists.

TEI-focused outcomes assessments are also available to supplement the more traditional occupational therapy evaluations. Commercially available TEI evaluations may focus on matching technology with the person (Assistive Technology Device Predisposition Assessment; Scherer, 1998), matching the environmental needs with the person (Lifespace Access Profile; Williams, Stemach, Wolfe, & Stanger, 1994), or evaluating the user experience and preference of specific devices (QUEST; Demers, Weiss-Lambrou, & Ska, 2000). Due to the high cost of high-tech devices and some home modifications, it is common practice to provide trials, if at all possible, of the top three preferred options before actually proceeding with the most preferred option. Assessment and reassessment must occur with each trial in order to obtain information on the best option for intervention with the consumer.

Universal Design

Environmental modification, an aspect of TEI practice, encompasses the provision of home modifications, assessment of public areas for accessibility, and application of universal design principles. The term **universal design** was coined by Ron Mace, a faculty member at North Carolina State University, home to the Center for Universal Design (CUD). Universal design is defined as "the design of products and environments to be usable by all people, to the greatest extent possible, without the need for adaptation or specialized design" (CUD, 1998, p. 2). Universal design principles (Table 24-1) were established in 1997 by architects, product designers, engineers, and environmental design researchers so products and environments would meet the needs of potential users with a wide variety of characteristics (CUD, 1998). These principles suggest that items designed for universal access should have equitable use, with identical means of access for all users; accommodate a wide range of users and avoid segregation of users; be simple and intuitive to use to allow access by individuals of varying cognitive level; convey information without requiring ideal conditions for function; tolerate user error whether motor or cognition based; require a low level of physical effort to use; and be accessible as relates to both the size of the item and the space for approach and use of the item.

Many universal design items are developed using anthropomorphic measurement standards in order to create items aimed at a generic standard. The problem with these standards is that they do not fit the mainstream individual seeking universal design items because most standards are based on the 18- to 25-year-old male in the military (Panero & Zelnik, 1979).

Occupational therapists acting in the role of practitioner, consultant, or entrepreneur and practicing across all community-based settings and centennial vision areas will find that universal design principles may be applicable and may be incorporated into interventions. Universal design principles apply to site planning and landscaping as well as to internal building floor plans for a variety of contexts, including home, work, school, or leisure. Client dwellings may benefit from overall site planning and landscaping for new or existing buildings, for example, installing maintenance-free exterior and trim; assuring that walkways are wide and level, with little or no slope; planting low maintenance trees, shrubs, and plants; and providing accessible yard and garden areas.

Entrances ideally would be wide enough for wheelchair entry to the main floor at ground level

Table 24-1	Universal Design Principles and Explanations (Center for Universal Design, 1998)
Principle	**Explanations**
Equitable Use	All users should be able to use the device in a similar or equivalent manner. It should be useful and appealing to people with diverse abilities. No users should be segregated or stigmatized, and any user should have privacy, security, and safety during use.
Flexibility in Use	The design should provide a variety of methods of use in order to accommodate a wide range of individual preferences, pace, and accuracy and precision abilities, including right- or left-handed use.
Simple and Intuitive Use	The design should be easy to understand and be consistent with user expectations. Complexity should be minimized, information should be arranged according to importance, and prompting should be available during and after the task. The device should accommodate a wide range of literacy and language skills regardless of the user's experience, knowledge, or concentration skills.
Perceptible Information	The design should effectively provide information to the user, regardless of environment or the user's sensory abilities. Information should be provided in multiple modes (pictorial, verbal, tactile) for important information and be compatible with alternative access modes of individuals with sensory disabilities.
Tolerance for Error	The design should have fail-safe features and minimizes problems and negative outcomes of accidental or unintended actions. Input should be organized so those most used are also the most accessible. Any hazardous components should be eliminated, isolated, or shielded.
Low Physical Effort	The device should be designed for use with the body in neutral positions and avoid repetitive actions. It should be accessed efficiently and comfortably and with a minimum of fatigue.
Size and Space for Approach and Use	The design should allow for use by a seated or standing user, with adequate line of sight; have adequate size and surrounding space for easy approach, use of assistive devices, or personal assistance; accommodate a variety of levels of reach, differing hand grips, and sizes, and allow use regardless of user's body size, posture, or mobility.

with no thresholds, steps, or ramps and would have door locks and lever-style door handles that are easy to operate, peepholes at various heights or sidelights, and good lighting both inside and outside the entrance. Ideally, the entrance would have a roof, canopy, or awning for protection and provide ample landing space both outside and inside the entry door. These are only a few examples of an extensive list of potentially beneficial applications of universal design in the home, school, or work settings. Therapists practicing in this area need awareness of the many options available to assist clients.

The following section briefly describes several areas of TEI practice, including wheeled mobility, communication technology, and computer access, and ends with a discussion of home modifications and electronic aids to daily living.

Wheeled Mobility

Community integration and access would be difficult if not impossible without mobility. Limitations in mobility may be the result of a variety of disabilities and may manifest to varying degrees. Children born with neuromotor conditions or who acquire movement impairments early in life may never ambulate and may rely on wheeled mobility throughout life. Adults with traumatic, degenerative, or acquired neuromotor conditions may lose the ability to ambulate in part or whole and may require wheeled mobility for some or all of their mobility needs. The inability to move effectively in the environment may limit the options for participating in school activities or gainful employment. Mobility limitations affect productive aging, mental health, and overall general health by restricting social participation. In rehabilitation, there is often emphasis on safe mobility, which should include wheeled mobility.

Wheeled mobility is commonly divided into two categories, manual wheelchairs and powered wheelchairs. These categories can be further divided into independent and dependent wheeled mobility. The outcomes of independent mobility include energy efficiency and functional and safe mobility in the environments in which one participates. Independent mobility results in many secondary benefits, such as increased participation in community activities, better access to health care, enhanced self-esteem, and an increased quality of life. Independent mobility can be achieved through the use of manual wheelchairs, power wheelchairs or scooters, or a combination of any of these and other mobility aids such as walkers and canes.

However, independent mobility is not possible for everyone. A child with severe spastic athetoid cerebral palsy, a person with physical limitations and impaired vision, and an elderly person who is very frail are examples of people for whom independent mobility may be difficult to achieve. When independence is not possible, manual wheelchairs, operated by someone other than the client, strollers, and travel chairs become the options of choice.

There are many custom features for seating, positioning, control, and other options available in both manual and powered mobility. When the custom features are combined with user input to meet the users' unique needs, an effective, efficient, and comfortable mobility system can be created for the user. Fundamental wheelchair features include: the seat and back configuration (i.e., height, depth, and seat/back angle), whether the chair construction is rigid or is a folding wheelchair, the type and position of the wheels, and the type and configuration of the casters, if any. Each of these features contributes to the stability or mobility of the wheelchair and therefore the smoothness of the ride and effective and efficient use of the wheelchair. For mobility, further consideration may be given to new technology, such as push rim-activated wheels, power assist features on manual chairs, and the many driving mechanisms of powered wheelchairs. Other features of the wheelchair may not impact the

efficiency and effectiveness of use but may be critical to the client's independence and safety (Giesbrecht, Ripat, Quanbury, & Cooper, 2009). Features such as seat belts or harness supports are important for safety, and tilt or recline capability is important for comfort, transport, or medical reasons. Other features include a variety of armrests and foot and leg supports. These provide comfort, function, or a combination of both.

Arthanat, Nochajski, Lenker, Bauer, and Wu (2009) identify the factors that impact success in wheelchair use. These are: the user's perception of the effect of the wheelchair on participation in activities in contexts; the user's perception of the ease of use, safety, and comfort; the effective use of the wheelchair as measured by the abilities and skills of the user as he or she interacts with the wheelchair; and the influence of environmental or contextual factors that interrelate with mobility. Kreutz and Taylor (2002) indicate independence in community propulsion will depend on factors such as the ability to:

- propel on a variety of indoor and outdoor surfaces and ability to ascend and descend a 1:12 ramp
- manage environmental features such as curb cuts, ramps, and doors
- transfer to and from the wheelchair
- load and unload wheelchair from a vehicle
- manage or communicate information related to wheelchair maintenance and repair, including knowledge of and access to a supplier and funding sources.

Pedersen and Taylor (2004) provide a detailed description of the role of the occupational therapist in wheeled mobility and seating. With input from the user and other team members, the process of wheelchair prescription involves matching the person's abilities with the features of the wheelchair. A knowledgeable wheelchair vendor or supplier is important to this process and an important team member.

A fundamental outcome of wheeled mobility is increased level of function. Cost-effectiveness of the wheeled mobility may also be used as a measurable outcome. Issues such as decreased need for attendant care, decreased occurrence of medical complications such as decubiti, and reduced length of stay in rehabilitation or long-term care facilities are justifiable outcomes of wheeled mobility. Additionally, wheeled mobility can increase access to public transportation and thereby potential work opportunities, and provide a means to engage in or perform activities that would not be possible otherwise, such as attending school for a young child, participating in religious activities and groups for an elderly person, or caring for family members (Mortenson, Miller, & Auger, 2008).

Communication Technology

Communication is a vital function for participation in daily activities, especially when the daily activities intersect with community contexts. From simple daily greetings and pleasantries to ordering a meal at a restaurant to calling 911 in an emergency situation, communication takes many forms. In ddition to verbal interactions, communication also encompasses a wide range of non-verbal forms, including facial expressions, gestures, e-mail, text messaging and tweeting, and computer use.

When communication is difficult or ineffective because of impairment, independence and participation in daily activities may be compromised. The communication disability that results from impairment may be temporary or permanent, and developmental or acquired. Many impairments affect communication, for example, children with cerebral palsy and adults who have had a cerebrovascular accident or cancer of the throat or larynx. The person's diagnosis, symptoms, and age will uniquely influence the communication impairment as well as his or her communication needs and interventions.

Augmentative and alternative communication (AAC) intervention is a practice area with a focus on increasing independence and participation, increasing quality of life, increasing safety, improving personal relationships, and providing access to the environment and communities in which one interacts. AAC intervention often provides a combination of devices and strategies that increases communication for the recipient, often referred to as a communication system. An **augmentative or alternative communication system** is defined as a system that uses an integrated group of components such as symbols, aids, strategies, and techniques to enhance an individual's communication (American Speech-Language-Hearing Association, 1989).

The features of AAC include the output, feedback, input method, symbol type or set and size, language storage and retrieval method, flexibility of use, portability, durability, cost (including warranty), manufacturer support, and ability to integrate with other devices. Because of advances in technology, these features change rapidly (Table 24-2). Regardless, it is important to understand the concept related to each feature and how that feature may impact the individual's ability to use the device successfully.

Communication usually falls under the purview of speech language pathologists (SLPs), and many reimbursement systems will pay for a communication system only when an SLP has performed the evaluation. The role of the occupational therapist (OT) in the evaluation for and intervention in augmentative and alternative communication may include evaluation of physical positioning, both of the individual and the AAC device, and method of device access. Proper positioning of both the client's body and the device will optimize access and usability. The OT also plays an integral role in analyzing the activities and contexts in which the device, strategies, or systems may be used.

It is important to consider that not all persons will be independent communicators in all situations. People with complex communication needs may not have all their needs met with any one device. As mentioned earlier, a system of devices and techniques will increase the likelihood of participation in community settings, yet there may still be communication barriers. One strategy for overcoming communication barriers is the use of communication assistants. A communication assistant might be used to ensure accurate or detailed communication with a third party via face-to-face interactions, over the telephone, or through written communication. Examples of when a communication assistant might be used are when a college student needs to complete a written application, or when a person makes an appointment for medical care or communicates medical needs to a provider. Through the assistance of a communication partner or assistant, access to and interaction in community activities may be successful (Collier, McGhie-Richmond, & Self, 2010).

Table 24-2	Descriptions of Features to Consider in AAC Device Selection	
Function	**Purpose**	**Feature Options**
Output	Helps the user interact with communication partners.	Auditory: digitized or synthesized Visual display: static vs. dynamic display, written output
Feedback	As the user interacts with the device, what type of feedback do they receive?	Auditory: beep, click, tones Visual: lights, written display Tactile: key movement, touch of keys
Input method	Often motoric. How does the user interact with the device; what method is used to access messages?	Direct selection: use of the fingers, hands, mouthstick to access the device Scanning: used with switch access; there are multiple ways to scan and many different switches available.
Symbol type or set and size	What symbols are used in the display; what symbols does the user understand?	Symbols: Photographs, black-and-white line drawings, colored line drawings, or symbol language systems such as Blissymbol or Minspeak. Size matters especially for visual impairments.
Language storage and retrieval method	Messages and words can be stored in combinations for efficient retrieval so each letter of an utterance does not have to be accessed.	Multiple levels of display as in a dynamic display; encoding through color, letters, or icons Prediction: letter, word, or phrase
Flexibility of use	Meeting the client's needs	Accommodates a variety of access methods. Output can be modified for user needs, e.g., print display can be enlarged. Can generate new phrases if needed.
Portability	How easy is it to carry or transport?	Weight for carrying. Method for mounting on wheelchair or walker.
Durability	Will it withstand dropping, rough use, or weather extremes?	Waterproof and cushioned covers
Cost	Overall costs for use	Is it covered by insurance? Is there a warranty available in case of accident or breakage?
Manufacturer support	Overall support from the manufacturer	Is there a local product representative? How available is the manufacturer? Does it have a toll-free number, e-mail access, and available assistance?
Integration with other devices	Can the device be used with other systems?	Environmental controls, power wheelchairs, computer access

Computer Access

In today's society, computers are integral to everyday life. Computers or computer-based devices are used across the life span, by children and youth through older adults, and across occupations and contexts, from schools and universities to private homes, work, and industry. For most individuals, computer access is simple, but for those with age-related deterioration or a disability, adaptations or alternative access may be necessary. Thus, the role of the OT in this TEI practice area may be as a regional education technology specialist, as a consultant, or as a rehabilitation practitioner providing services in evaluation of computer access and computer use at school, in the home, or at a work site. Whatever the setting and age of the client, the evaluation of computer access is a process that includes assessment of the consumer's abilities and limitations, analysis of contextual and environmental factors, and matching the client's abilities and interests to appropriate computer access options.

Universal Design in Computer Use

As in other areas, there is a trend toward increased incorporation of universal design principles in the development of new computer hardware, software, and peripherals. Numerous options abound in computer peripherals with universal design characteristics such as detachable keyboards, monitors that tilt, compact disks, external memory sticks, large hard drives, power switches and strips at convenient locations, touch screens, and many others. Software options with built-in universal design characteristics include word processing software that allows changes in the size and/or color of the text, as well as speech-to-text and text-to-speech options.

Numerous universal design accessibility options are now built into most computer operating systems and are available for any user population in any context. The Windows accessibilities options are discussed below; however, similar options are available for other popular computer operating systems. Windows accessibility options may be accessed through the accessibility wizard, control panel, properties, Internet Explorer options, and a variety of other locations. A caution is offered to practitioners with limited experience: the Windows accessibility wizard may seem easy and simple to use; however, while it provides alternatives for individuals with hearing, vision, or physical limitations, they are "canned" alternatives and do not allow for the application of the great diversity of options that may make the computer optimally accessible to each unique client.

The ability to alter the display and readability of the content displayed on the computer screen is available. These controls allow for alteration of font size and style and icon size as well as manipulation of the font and background colors. These options may be useful for individuals with decreased vision, those with poor figure ground discrimination, or those who need alteration to facilitate cognitive organization. A screen magnifier may be built in, allowing for magnification of specific areas the consumer has difficulty

viewing. Voice narration may also be a built-in feature, providing auditory output of content on the screen and benefitting those with visual or cognitive limitations. A few of the keyboard and mouse operations that may be adjusted include:

- keyboard layout or use of an onscreen keyboard,
- speed of response and sensitivity,
- cursor size and shape,
- alternative controls for mouse use and mouse buttons,
- visual or auditory feedback for actions performed, and
- shortcuts that allow information to be automatically filled in on Web addresses, routine forms, and user name and password fields.

Additionally, numerous options are available to make navigating the Web and use of the Web browser more streamlined and accessible.

Adaptations for Computer Access

Alternative computer access may be considered in the two broad areas of input and output devices. **Input devices** provide ways to enter information into the computer, for example through typing on a computer keyboard, manipulating the mouse, or voicing commands. **Output devices** provide ways to obtain information from the computer; common examples are visually from the monitor or in written format from the printer. Alternative computer access is an area in need of ongoing research to address, in part, the safe use of alternative input or output devices, the issue of device abandonment, and concerns about unique health issues related to computer overuse by disabled users (Burton, Nieuwenhuijsen, & Epstein, 2008).

Adaptations for inputting data to the computer may be found in the form of software to increase typing speed and efficiency, such as abbreviation expansion software or word prediction software. Software is also available to access the keyboard from the screen level through on-screen keyboard programs that may be used through touch screens, scanning, or hands-free access devices. Hardware devices that alter the method of keyboard input include expanded keyboards, mini keyboards, and touch screens. Devices are also available that alter the method of mouse access through infrared control, switch control for scanning, sip-and-puff options, and many others. Universal design options are also plentiful, such as ergonomic mouse options, trackballs, joysticks, and graphic pads. The type of alternative input device must be chosen to meet the unique needs of individuals with disabilities. Clients with spinal cord injuries may benefit from low-cost alternative computer input devices such as mouthsticks, sticky keys, mouth-controlled joysticks, trackballs, onscreen keyboards, mouse emulators, or speech recognition software (McKinley, Tewksbury, Sitter, Reed, & Floyd, 2004). Individuals with complex or multiple motor performance impairments will need more complex alternative computer access solutions to meet their unique needs (Capilouto, Higginbotham, McClenaghan, Williams, & Dickerson, 2005; Man & Wong, 2007).

Adaptations for obtaining output from the computer include options such as a larger monitors for clients with difficulty seeing items on the screen as well as software programs to change text size and text and background contrast. Various refreshable braille display screen reader options are available for individuals who are blind to provide real-time access of information on the computer screen; hard copies may be provided using a braille printer/embosser. Software programs may be installed that read each character, word, or sentence as it is typed or that read all typed text or graphics on the screen and transform those images into voice output for clients with visual, cognitive, or learning disabilities who would benefit from auditory presentation.

Home Modifications and Electronic Aids to Daily Living

Home modification, defined in the most straightforward way, is making changes or adaptations to a home to increase safety, accessibility, independence, security, or comfort (Sanford, 2004). These changes may be needed for immediate access or may be the result of planning for needs that might arise in the future; either way, modifying a home is customizing based on an individual's needs to increase independence (Sebring-Cale, 2008). Home modifications may take a variety of forms, such as replacing or

adding fixtures, appliances, or features in a home; changing or adding to the structure; or automating environmental controls (Jones & Sanford, 2002). The modification may be as simple as an alternate doorknob, a grab bar in the shower, or a ramp to provide access to the house. It may be as complex as rebuilding an entire bathroom to meet a client's accessibility and functional needs. Home modification interventions may be instrumental in providing safe, accessible housing environments across the life span and across disabling conditions, including those with physical or mental health conditions. There is a growing need to increase awareness within our communities of the potential for home modifications to allow individuals to remain in their homes.

The OT may simply recommend a home modification product to minimize environmental demands on the client and/or his or her caregivers. However, a more holistic approach, using a home modification process, may be needed to meet the complex situational and contextual needs for promoting performance of occupations as independently and safely as possible. A **home modification product** is defined as any alteration, adjustment, or addition to the layout or structure of the home to improve the client's functional capability. A **home modification process** is a combination of activities and delivery of services that contributes to change, adjustment, or addition to the home environment and includes assessing needs, identifying solutions, implementing solutions, training in use of solutions, and evaluating outcomes.

Many OTs are involved in fundamental home modifications, such as replacing or adding fixtures, appliances, or features in a home. Therapists frequently evaluate client homes before discharge and make recommendations to increase safety, function, mobility, and access to increase the client's ability to participate in activities in his or her home and community. This level of home modifications includes low-tech adaptive equipment for the home, such as a tub transfer bench, grab bars, raised seating, brighter lighting, and many other recommendations.

Home modifications may require changing or adding to the structure, such as when considering bathroom accessibility for an individual in a wheelchair (Sebring-Cale, 2008). The first priority in bathrooms designed for people who use wheelchairs is adequate space for access and maneuvering. Wheelchairs need a minimum of a 32-inch door width for a straight-in approach. If the doorway is located in a typical hallway and requires turning a wheelchair, a 36-inch door width is needed. A home modification project for a person in a wheelchair may include projects such as installation of a swing-away door hinge that will increase the width by a few inches, installation of a pocket door, or remodeling to widen the doorway. Additionally, the bathroom door should swing outward rather than inward, and should be fitted with a lever-type handle, not a knob, for easier accessibility. For wheelchair accessibility, the shower stall should have no threshold to impede entrance and exit and should include a handheld nozzle that may be accessed from a seated position. Sink access may be attained by removal of vanity cabinets to provide knee space underneath or installation of a pedestal-style or a wall-mounted sink. Additional features that may be needed include faucets with single lever controls, an anti-scald temperature control, grab bars beside the tub and toilet, a bidet, a telephone, an emergency notification system, and lower light switches.

A supportive home environment is important for successful aging-in-place, and home modifications can enhance the home as a place of personal and social meaning in addition to improving safety and comfort for the disabled or older person (Tanner, Tilse, & de Jonge, 2008). With the aging of the "baby boomers," productive aging and aging-in-place are growing concerns, and baby boomers are a key population that may benefit from modifications to the physical environment. Home modifications can accommodate individuals across the life span and address the needs of most health conditions, whether physical, cognitive, or psychosocial.

Electronic Aids to Daily Living

Making a home accessible may involve installation of an automated environmental control or **electronic aid to daily living (EADL),** previously referred to as environmental control units. EADLs range from simple to complex technology options that provide a way to access and control items in the environment. These may turn on appliances, lights, and small electronic devices; control thermostats or

window treatments; or open doors. EADLs may be configured to control one device or a variety of devices. An EADL sends a signal to the device through infrared rays, ultrasound waves, radio frequency waves, or alternating current house wiring. The first three utilize remote control transmitters; the fourth sends out its signals over the home's electrical wires. The EADL provision requires the consideration of a variety of options including the number and types of devices to be controlled, type of transmission, access methods, setting changes, type of user feedback provided (i.e., auditory, visual, or tactile), sequencing required to operate, training requirements, flexibility, reliability, maintenance, and price (Rakoski, 2006). Another consideration is the ability of the EADL to integrate with other technologies such as computers, augmentative communication devices, and powered wheelchair controls. The occupational therapist will need to provide training in the use of the EADL and other modifications after they have been installed.

Outcomes of improved functional performance after home modifications may be assessed through traditional occupational therapy evaluations such as the Canadian Occupational Performance Measure or the Functional Performance Record. Evaluations designed especially for home modifications range from detailed measurements to simple checklists. The Comprehensive Assessment and Solution Process for Aging Residents (CASPAR) is a home modification assessment tool designed for use by a health care professional to collect information on client goals, problems, and abilities (MM&I Construction & Design, 2007). HomeFit is available through AARP and is a checklist of questions to help clients make a decision on whether their home is suitable or if modifications need to be made. LifeEase is a company that sells a variety of computer-generated assessments that look at environmental barriers and functional performance. Regardless of which evaluation tool is used, the evaluation should be performed in the home, preferably with the client present to contribute to the evaluation of environmental requirements and concerns, and for cultural sensitivity.

Funding for Home Modification

Home modifications can be expensive, and funding is difficult to obtain. Most modifications are paid for using personal savings, but there are some alternatives, such as home mortgage loans or even reverse mortgages if the client is 62 or older (Fagan, 2007). Medicare and Medicaid generally require substantiation of medical necessity for any funding; therefore, they do not pay for most low-tech adaptive equipment, much less home modifications. Home modifications are found in the majority of these waivers, but coverage applies only to the limited number of persons enrolled. Individuals with disabilities who have served in the armed forces may be eligible for limited funding through the Veterans Administration (VA), and some veterans may qualify for a VA home loan that can be used to simultaneously purchase and modify a home. The U.S. Department of Housing and Urban Development awards Community Block Development Grants (CBDGs) to eligible city and county housing and community development departments to revitalize neighborhoods and improve community facilities and services. Communities develop their own funding priorities, and many choose to provide home modification programs with part of their CBDG funds. The U.S. Department of Agriculture has created the Rural Development Home Repair Loan and Grant Programs to provide assistance to individuals who live in areas with a population fewer than 10,000. Finally, there are a few foundations and national organizations, such as Easter Seals, that may provide a limited amount of home modification funding for specific conditions and disabilities. In some cases, automobile insurance policies, workers' compensation programs, accident insurance plans, or other insurance programs will pay for home modifications, especially if the need for home modifications arose as the result of an accident or injury.

Advanced Training in Home Modification

There are expanding opportunities available for occupational therapists to work with contractors as they build accessible housing. In this situation, the role of the occupational therapy practitioner is as a consultant to contractors, builders, architects, remodelers, interior designers, or lawyers that specialize in elder law, and community programs. Frequently, occupational therapists are a part of a team of experts that work together to meet with and ascertain the needs of the client. The National Association of Home Builders (NAHB) offers training to become a Certified Aging in Place Specialist (CAPS). This series of three courses teaches the strategies and techniques for marketing, designing, and building aesthetically enriching barrier-free living environments, and addresses the communication and technical needs of the older adult population. The training is available to occupational therapists, and AOTA collaborates with NAHB to assure that occupational therapy is fully integrated into the training. CAPS training and certification is valuable as it increases the occupational therapists' knowledge base and improves consultation skills with a variety of home modification organizations and entities.

In addition, AOTA offers an Environmental Modification Specialty Certification, available to all occupational therapy practitioners, that covers implementing environmental modifications in senior housing, assisted living, long-term-care facilities, and private homes. The Home Modification Network, within the AOTA Home and Community Special Interest Section, was formed in 2004 and is an excellent resource for accurate information and networking.

Conclusion

The role of OTs in the community-based TEI practice area is multi-faceted. Practitioners may function as consultants, entrepreneurs, educators, trainers, advocates, or direct service providers. OTs have expertise and training in recommending and applying TEI that may increase and promote independence, quality of life, health, and safety in the environment as well as prevent further decline or injury. TEI may be provided, at either the entry or advanced level, by a licensed occupational therapist with or without additional specialty certification. OTs incorporate the physical, sensory, psychological, cognitive, and social aspects of disabilities, illness, and aging as they analyze occupational performance, assess needs, identify solutions, and evaluate outcomes of TEI. OTs incorporate TEI on a daily basis in both traditional practice areas and emerging practice areas; this expertise in TEI is a valuable contribution to clients in their communities.

CASE STUDIES

CASE STUDY 24•1 RP

RP is a 56-year-old female who was diagnosed with Amyotrophic Lateral Sclerosis (ALS) 8 years ago. She is currently in a manual wheelchair that has tilt in space and recline functions, elevating leg rests, and a head rest. She has limited mobility in her right thumb, and in neck flexion, extension, and rotation. She has no other controllable movement. She speaks in a whisper and is able to control her eye gaze. Her mobility is currently accomplished by her husband and caretaker pushing her wheelchair. She is experiencing ongoing, slow deterioration in function as a result of ALS and is declining from stage 3 to stage 4. She is referred to occupational therapy for evaluation of her technology needs. She indicates that she used to work on the computer, using e-mail to interact with friends as well as Web sites for shopping and support group partici-pation. She is no longer able to access the computer. Her husband reports difficulty in understanding her and is concerned about leaving her alone in another room because he cannot hear her call for help.

CASE STUDY 24•1 Discussion Questions

1. What are the evaluation issues the occupational therapist needs to consider, and what would be the best process to address them?
2. There are at least two major assistive technology needs imbedded in the scenario. What needs are you able to identify? How would you prioritize the needs?
3. What specific recommendations and justification would you determine for your AT choices priori-tized in #2 above? Resources may include the Internet, texts, journal articles, equipment catalogs, and other professionals.
4. What considerations need to be included to address RP's continuing functional decline as a result of ALS?
5. What are the expected outcomes of the TEI for this scenario?

Learning Activities

1. Access the Internet and go to: http://lifease.com/ PracticalGuideToUniversalHomeDesign.pdf and download a free copy of "A Practical Guide to Universal Home Design," produced by East Metro Seniors Agenda for Independent Living, Saint Paul, Minnesota with support from the Minnesota Department of Human Services. Review the guide and use the checklist to determine the accessibility of your home or apartment for a wheelchair-bound person, an elderly person using a walker, or a person with low vision.
2. Access the Internet and go to: http://microsoft. com/enable Go to the sections on *training* and guides *by disability*. In the *Training* option select Step-by-Step. Complete the training for the Windows version you have. Experiment with some of the options on your own computer (be sure to write down what changes you make so you can undo them later).

3. Access the Internet and go to: http://aarp.org Search for HomeFit and download the check-list. Use the checklist to evaluate your home environment for an aging person with debili-tating arthritis. What recommendations would you make after reviewing the results?
4. Access the Internet and go to: http://abilityhub. com . Click on the link on the left under Computer Access for blind and visually impaired. Explore the options listed there and learn the difference between screen reader, screen magnifier, and text reader. Which options would best suit an individual with low vision as compared to a person who is blind?
5. Wheelchair resources.
   Access the Internet and go to: http:// wheelchairnet.org. Click on the first-time user link to learn about the resources and information available through this Web site. What areas would you suggest for a client who is new to using a wheelchair?

REFERENCES

American Occupational Therapy Association (AOTA). (2009). Specialized knowledge and skills in technology and environmental interventions for occupational therapy. *American Journal of Occupational Therapy, 63*(6), 1–13.

American Speech-Language-Hearing Association (ASHA). (1989). Competencies for speech language pathologists providing services in augmentative communication. *ASHA: A Journal of the American Speech-Language-Hearing Association, 31,* 107–110.

Arthanat, S., Nochajski, S. M., Lenker, J. A., Bauer, S. B., & Wu, Y. W. B. (2009). Measuring usability of assistive technology from a multicontextual perspective: The case of power wheelchairs. *American Journal of Occupational Therapy, 63,* 751–764.

Burton, M., Nieuwenhuijsen, E. R., & Epstein, M. J. (2008). Computer-related assistive technology: Satisfaction and experiences among users with disabilities. *Assistive Technology, 20,* 99–106.

Capilouto, G. J., Higginbotham, D. J., McClenaghan, B., Williams, H. G., & Dickerson, J. (2005). Performance investigation of a head-operated device and expanded membrane cursor keys in a target acquisition task. *Technology and Disability, 17,* 173–183.

Center for Universal Design. (1998). *The universal design file: Designing for people of all ages and abilities.* Raleigh, NC: Author.

Cole, M. B., & Tufano R. (2008). *Applied theories in occupational therapy.* Thorofare, NJ: SLACK Inc.

Collier, B., McGhie-Richmond, D., & Self, H. (2010). Exploring communication assistants as an option for increasing communication access to communities for people who use augmentative communication. *Augmentative and Alternative Communication, 26*(1), 48–59.

Cook, A. M., Polgar, J. M., & Hussey, S. M. (2008). *Assistive technologies: Principles and practice.* St. Louis, MO: Mosby Elsevier.

Demers, L., Weiss-Lambrou, R., & Ska, B. (2000). Item analysis of the Quebec User Evaluation of Satisfaction with Assistive Technology (QUEST). *Assistive Technology, 12*(2), 96– 105.

Fagan, L. A. (2007, September). Funding sources for home modifications. *Home and Community Health Special Interest Section Quarterly, 14*(3), 1–3.

Giesbrecht, E. M., Ripat, J. D., Quanbury, A. O., & Cooper, J. E. (2009). Participation in community-based activities of daily living: Comparison of a pushrim-activated, power-assisted wheelchair and a power wheelchair. *Disability and Rehabilitation: Assistive Technology, 4*(3), 198–207.

Jones, M. L., & Sanford, J. (2002). Home environments, automation, and environmental controls. In D. A. Olson & F. DeRuyter (Eds.), *Clincian's guide to assistive technology* (pp. 405–424). St Louis, MO: Mosby.

Kreutz, D., & Taylor, S. J. (2002). Wheelchair mobility. In D. A. Olson & F. DeRuyter (Eds.), *Clincian's guide to assistive technology* (pp. 311–330). St Louis, MO: Mosby.

Man, D. W. K., & Wong, M-S. L. (2007). Evaluation of computer-access solutions for students with quadriplegic athetoid cerebral palsy. *American Journal of Occupational Therapy, 61*(3), 355–364.

McKinley W., Tewksbury, M. A., Sitter, P., Reed, J., & Floyd, S. (2004). Assistive technology and computer adaptations for individuals with spinal cord injury. *NeuroRehabilitation, 19,* 141–146.

MM&I Construction and Design, Inc. (2007). CASPAR: Comprehensive assessment and solution process for aging residents. Nashville, TN: Author. Retrieved from http://design101.tv/uploads/CASPAR-worksheet1.pdf

Mortenson, W. B., Miller, W. C., & Auger, C. (2008). Issues for the selection of wheelchair- specific activity and participation outcome measures: A review. *Archives of Physical Medicine and Rehabilitation, 89,* 1177–1186.

Panero J., & Zelnik, M. (1979). *Human dimension and interior space.* New York: Whitney Library of Design.

Pedersen, J. P., & Taylor, S. J. (2004). Wheeled-mobility seating: The occupational therapist's role. *OT Practice, 9*(18), 11–14.

Public Law 108-364. (2004). Retrieved from http://ataporg.org/atap/atact_law.pdf

Rakoski, D. (2006, October). *Assessment for and exploration of current electronic aids to daily living.* Presentation at the 30th Annual Occupational Therapy Association of California Conference in Costa Mesa, California.

Sanford, J. A. (2004, May). *Definition of home modifications.* Presentation at the American Occupational Therapy Association Annual Conference & Expo, Minneapolis, MN.

Scherer, M. J. (1998). *Matching persons to technology.* Webster, NY: Institute for Matching Persons to Technology.

Sebring-Cale, N. J. (2008). Accessibility issues with long-term disabilities. *Neurological Research, 30,* 437–440.

Sherer, M. J. (1996). *Living in the state of stuck.* Cambridge, MA: Brookline Books.

Tanner, B., Tilse, C., & de Jonge, D. (2008). Restoring and sustaining home: The impact of home modifications on the meaning of home for older people. *Journal of Housing for the Elderly, 22*(3), 195–215.

Williams, W. B., Stemach, B., Wolfe, S., & Stanger, C. (1994). *Lifespace access profile upper extension: Assistive technology assessment and planning for individuals with physical disabilities.* Sebastopol, CA: Lifespace Access.

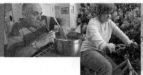
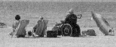
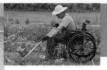

Health Promotion and Wellness

Chapter 25

Occupational Therapy in Faith-Based Organizations

Lynn M. Swedberg, MS, OT, and Shirley A. Blanchard, PhD, ABDA, OTR/L, FAOTA

I hosted a booth on "Occupational Therapy in the Church" at the American Occupational Therapy Association Conference in St. Louis. The booth was swamped the entire time. Practitioners said, "This is what I've been looking for. I've wanted to integrate my faith and my practice."

—R. Mourey, personal communication, September 4, 2009

Learning Objectives

This chapter is designed to enable the reader to:

• Discuss the rationale and roles for occupational therapy involvement in faith-based organizations.
• Identify background requirements, training needs, cautions, and resources for practitioners interested in developing health programs in faith-based settings.
• Describe the seven functions of a faith-community health minister.
• Compare and contrast the roles of faith-community practitioner with those of home health practitioner and faith-community nurse.

Key Terms

Denomination
Disability ministry
Faith-based intervention
Faith-based organization
Faith-placed
Health minister

Health ministry
Missions
Parachurch
Parish (or faith-community) nurse
Stewardship

Introduction

Amid the noise of politically based health care reform, a quiet health-care revolution is taking place in faith communities around the United States and many other nations. The revolution comes from the realization that medical model interventions are not the whole answer to achieving health. Faith-based organizations are showing leadership in implementing health promotion strategies that affect their members and reaching out to underserved populations in their communities. While nursing is leading this movement, occupational therapists also are playing a role.

The purpose of this chapter is to describe occupational therapy in community-based, faith-based organizations. **Faith-based organizations** include churches, synagogues, and mosques, but also outreach programs sponsored by religious groups. These may include cultural community centers, religious camping programs, and social service agencies that target specific populations such as people who are homeless or recent immigrants.

With few exceptions (Shamberg & Kidd, 2010; Smith, 2003a, 2003b; Swedberg, 2001; Voltz, 2005), there is little published by occupational therapy practitioners working in faith-based settings, so interviews were a primary source of information for this chapter. Other material comes from the literature of the nursing, health promotion, health ministry, and disability ministry fields and from the authors' experience.

Historical Background

Faith Community as a Resource

As occupational therapy moves into the community, faith communities are natural partners for addressing health disparities and promoting optimal health and participation. The U.S. government has recognized the potential benefit of partnerships between faith-based and health care organizations and has developed resources (e.g., National Center for Cultural Competence, 2001) to facilitate interaction. The Healthy People 2010 initiative included churches among recommended organizations that should be cooperating to improve health outcomes (Public Health Foundation, 2002, pp. 71–72). Eleven U.S. federal agencies have Centers for Faith-Based and Neighborhood Partnerships, with a goal of coordinating agency services with local faith-based organizations and with other agencies and the White House (Dubois, 2009).

In the United States, there are an estimated 345,000 faith communities (Peterson, Atwood, & Yates, 2002). Despite membership declines in mainline Protestant denominations, 80% self-identify as belonging to a faith tradition (Kosmin & Keysar, 2009). Of these, 76% claim the Christian faith; 4% relate to other religious traditions, including Judaism, Islam, Buddhism, and other less well-known religions (Kosmin & Keysar, 2009); these numbers are growing with the influx of immigrants from non-European countries (Pew Forum on Religion and Public Life, 2008). Recent surveys indicate that 39% of residents in the United States attend religious services once a week, 15% once or twice a month, and another 18% attend at least several times a year (Pew Forum).

Some congregations are organized independently of other bodies, but most are part of a larger religious umbrella organization or **denomination.** This means there are networks and communication systems in place to reach large numbers of people and to disseminate information about new initiatives and ideas.

Faith Communities and Health

Faith communities have provided health care and noted the connections between physical and spiritual well-being for centuries. In the United States, many hospitals were founded by religious organizations and staffed by nuns and deaconesses. When medicine became more science-driven and the body was reduced to a series of organs and systems, the effects of spirituality were dismissed as irrelevant, and the medical community and the church went separate ways (Olson, 2000).

In the late 1970s, Granger Westberg, a hospital chaplain, attempted to integrate spirituality and health. He established health care clinics, operated in partnership with hospitals, in a number of congregations (Westberg, 1999). He believed that nurses were best equipped to speak the languages of the faith community and of medicine, and could serve as interpreters between both worlds. As medical practice and insurance issues became more complex, the clinics closed, but the movement of parish nursing (now called faith-community nursing/health ministry) endured and is expanding on a worldwide basis.

Spirituality and Health

There is growing interest in the relationship between spiritual health and well-being. Spirituality and health research investigates assumptions such as whether religious behaviors including attending church and praying have a positive impact on health (Mueller, Plevak, & Rummans, 2001). Research suggests that spirituality aids in the development of coping skills, which may result in longevity. Mueller and colleagues used a meta-analysis to examine health outcomes following intervention for major disease states, including cardiovascular disease and mental illness, when religion or spirituality was included. Both systolic and diastolic blood pressure levels were lower among patients with who attended church once a week; frequent attendees who engaged in private religious activities such as prayer were 40% less likely to have diastolic hypertension. Religiously involved persons also were more likely to be compliant with pharmacological interventions for blood pressure.

Persons diagnosed with depression and treated with a combination of cognitive behavioral therapy (CBT) and spiritual pastoral care had less post-treatment depression than with CBT alone. Religious involvement was associated with less anxiety and substance abuse, and there was an inverse relationship between suicidal ideation and attendance at religious services (Mueller et al., 2001).

Health-related quality of life diminishes when spiritual and religious involvement is compromised. Mueller and colleagues (2001) found that persons involved in faith communities were more likely to practice health-enhancing lifestyles including consuming a healthier diet and decreased participation in risky behaviors such as smoking and substance use. Religiously active persons were more likely to participate in health prevention screenings and comply with recommended treatment. Prayer, worship,

and meditation are associated with positive emotional responses that calm the autonomic nervous system. This calming effect may reduce release of the stress hormones norepinephrine and cortisol, thus decreasing anxiety, blood pressure, and heart rate.

Occupational Therapy and Spirituality

The founders of occupational therapy recognized a spiritual component as vital to restoring health, function, and well-being (Stevenson, 2003). Reed (2006) summarized the values and beliefs of the profession during the formative years, listing principles derived from the literature of that time, including:

- "The primary goal of occupational therapy is to return the person to active life and for the person to function in normal society as a whole person in body and soul.
- Occupational therapy is the making of a man (individual) stronger physically, mentally, and spiritually than he was before.
- Sick minds, bodies, and souls can be healed through occupation." (pp. 24–25)

The American Occupational Therapy Association (AOTA) includes spirituality as a client factor within the *Occupational Therapy Practice Framework* (AOTA, 2008). Values, beliefs, and spirituality explain why individuals select and engage in various occupations. The occupation of attending worship services is important to the development of relationships, connectedness, meaning, beliefs, and well-being (Faull & Hills, 2006; Meyer, 1977; Reilly, 1962). Spirituality often implies resilience and coping. It is a fundamental need to perceive life experiences as manageable, comprehensible, and meaningful (Faull & Hills, 2006).

Because illness interrupts spiritual and religious routines, occupational therapy practitioners need to understand how spirituality may positively affect health during an acute episode, during the recuperation period, or when living with disability or chronic conditions. Occupational therapy practitioners who practice in the medical model may perceive that they do not have the knowledge to address the spiritual needs of the client (Belcham, 2004; Egan & Swedersky, 2003). Occupational therapists use the occupational profile to connect client narratives to past and present life experiences and health. Similar to obtaining an occupational profile, Puchalski and Romer (2000) suggest the need for a spiritual history using the Faith, Importance, Community, and Address (FICA) assessment:

- "**F**aith: Do you consider yourself spiritual? Do you have a religious faith?
- **I**mportance: How important are your religious beliefs and spirituality, and how might they influence decisions related to your health?
- **C**ommunity: Are you part of a religious or spiritual or other community? If so, how does this community support you?
- **A**ddress: How might I address your spiritual needs?" (Puchalski & Romer, 2000, p. 131)

This tool allows the practitioner to discern the spiritual need of the client and whether or not the client is open to faith-based intervention.

Need for Occupational Therapy Involvement in Faith-Based Organizations

Occupational therapy literature increasingly addresses wellness ("a state of mental and physical balance and fitness" [AOTA, 2008, p. 676]) and health promotion interventions. The AOTA has issued statements on the role of occupational therapy in health promotion and disease prevention (Scaffa, Van Slyke, & Brownson, 2008) and in the management of obesity (Reingold & Jordan, 2013), among others. Yet the potential impact of occupational therapy skills and the profession's unique perspective are largely unrecognized in the larger arenas of health ministry and health promotion.

Health disparities point to another direction that occupational therapy involvement may take (Bass-Haugen, 2009). Persons with disabilities have decreased access to health and wellness services (Smeltzer, 2007). Underserved and marginalized populations, including Native Americans, homeless persons with mental illness, persons with disabilities, and ethnic communities, often have unmet health-related needs. Due to inequitable distribution of health care resources as well as historic distrust,

many underserved groups have difficulty accessing traditional health care providers (Black & Wells, 2007). Faith-based outreach programs within neighborhoods and communities may be a first point of contact.

A major area of need is the lack of accessibility and inclusion in many faith communities. Persons with disabilities, who could benefit from the support and fellowship they might find, are underrepresented in nearly every congregation (Carter, 2007, p. 6). Physical inaccessibility of buildings is a primary barrier, yet many people with disabilities report that attitudinal and programmatic barriers have a stronger impact on participation. Most able-bodied persons fail to realize that a ramp alone does not guarantee that persons with disabilities will feel welcome and included in the activities of the community (National Organization on Disability, 1992). Yet having a ramp or level entrance is a necessary starting place. Faith communities have been slow to make physical accommodations, due in part to the fact that denominations lobbied for and won exemption from the landmark Americans with Disabilities Act (Pridmore, 2006). Opponents cited concerns about potential expenses and separation of church and state. Only congregations employing more than 15 persons are currently required to comply with the standards for workers.

Leaders in the profession have urged practitioners to become involved in enhancing community participation and inclusion (Grady, 1995; Hansen & Hinojosa, 2009; Neufeld, 2004). Yet Carter's comprehensive book, *Including People with Disabilities in Faith Communities: A Guide for Service Providers, Families, and Congregations* (2007), has no mention of occupational therapy as a potential resource for addressing the concerns identified.

Health Ministry

Health ministry describes an overall process of health-related activities carried out in or through the faith community in order to promote health and wholeness (Chase-Ziolek, 2005; Wylie & Solari-Twadell, 1999). Health ministry is carried out by professionals, acting on a volunteer or paid basis, with the assistance of lay volunteers. The most common health ministry worker is the **parish**

(or faith-community) nurse, who assumes a staff role in the parish, addressing health needs. Non-nurses are called **health ministers.**

One aim of health ministry is to help persons in faith communities take the necessary steps to avoid preventable illnesses and conditions by utilizing spiritual and faith-community resources. Ministries of health benefit all, clergy and laypersons alike. In fact, clergy exceed the general population in the percentage who are overweight and obese: 76% of clergy are obese or overweight, compared with 61% of adults in general (Maykus, 2006). Clergy responsibilities that sometimes require being on call 24 hours a day lead to neglect of self-care (Rediger, 2000).

Health promotion interventions in faith-based settings can be viewed on a continuum. Programs held in churches and other faith-based settings as an outreach to members or the community but planned or carried out by outside leadership, and not including faith-related content, are considered **faith-placed** (Steinman & Bambakidis, 2008). These efforts may target the faith community but are not tailored, or specifically designed (Walker, Pullen, Boeckner, Hageman, Hertzog, Oberdorfer, & Ruthledge, 2009), to meet the values, needs, and culture of the participants. An example of a faith-placed program is offering classroom space to groups such as the Red Cross for CPR and first aid courses.

A **faith-based intervention** for health promotion incorporates faith-related content and is a program of the sponsoring group (Steinman & Bambakidis, 2008). While outside persons may provide leadership, the need for the program is established from within and there is joint planning. An example of this would be university–faith community partnerships where the educational component is developed or taught by faculty or students but the faith community adds the religious and cultural content.

In faith-based initiatives, persons are encouraged to practice good **stewardship** as caretakers of the gift of their bodies (Peterson, Atwood, & Yates, 2002; Rediger, 2000) because they need health in order to carry out the ongoing ministries to which they are called. Living out their faith is the motivator, not losing weight or exercising for the sake of health. This understanding of health is similar to the definition of health in the Ottawa Charter of the World Health Organization (WHO, 1986): health is "a resource for living" and not as an end in itself. Holistic health in this sense is not absence of disease but rather well-being in all spheres of life, including the physical, the emotional, and the spiritual realms.

Functions and Roles of the Faith-Community Practitioner as Health Minister

The functions of health ministers, including occupational therapists, fall primarily into one or more of seven areas of practice: health education, health counseling, health advocacy, referral advising, volunteer coordination, development of support groups, and integration of faith and health (Brudenell, 2003; Holstrom, 1999; Patterson, 2003), which are described in Box 25-1.

Box 25-1 **Roles of the Health Minister**

- **Health Educator:** implements health fairs, health screenings, and back-to-school backpack safety events; creates newsletter articles and bulletin board displays on health topics; recruits speakers or teaches classes; expands the faith-community library to include books on caregiving and living with chronic illness.
- **Health Counselor:** supports individuals in modifying occupations to make needed lifestyle changes; helps interpret medical findings and recommendations, assisting the individual to formulate questions to ask his or her provider; accompanies individuals through the maze of health care services; provides home safety assessments for persons who do not otherwise qualify; monitors follow-through and home programs.
- **Health Advocate:** empowers clients to become self-advocates; helps the congregation identify physical, communication, and programmatic barriers to full participation, along with recommendations for overcoming these in order to achieve accessibility.
- **Referral Advisor:** researches community resources and collaborates with other agencies; refers clients to service providers and follows up to ensure that the client's needs were met; helps families develop criteria for making placement decisions.

Continued

Box 25-1 Roles of the Health Minister—cont'd

- **Volunteer Coordinator:** develops job descriptions for volunteer placement, then recruits, trains, assigns, and supervises volunteers who carry out programs such as caregiving teams and respite services; provides ongoing support, periodic evaluation, and recognition for services rendered; works with a health committee/cabinet of laypersons and health professionals, which shares in oversight and development of programs.
- **Developer of Support Groups:** identifies needs and sets up or runs support groups for caregivers, recently widowed persons, people with a specific chronic illness or disability, siblings of children with disabilities, or those wanting to band together for weight loss support; helps group members access their beliefs and spirituality to facilitate coping or making needed changes.
- **Integrator of Faith and Health:** educates the congregation regarding the role of healing and health in their particular faith tradition through articles, workshops, sermons, and other means of communication; provides visitation in homes and health care facilities and offers listening, supportive presence, touch, and prayer (Tuck, Pullen, & Wallace, 2001); assists persons to find meaning and hope in illness, disability, or loss; helps members explore personal values around end-of-life decisions; educates the congregation on ethical issues from a faith perspective; helps plan and implement healing services.

Faith-community nursing does not involve direct hands-on care (Cassidy, 2002; Patterson, 2003), nor should faith-community occupational therapy. The roles and tasks are to supplement available resources and fill in the gaps. The seven functions of health ministry are the same whether being carried out by a nurse or an occupational therapy practitioner, but specific implementation reflects the professional's background, experience, and scope of practice. For instance, either professional may take blood pressure readings. The nurse provides more specific medical teaching while the occupational therapy focus is on occupations of shopping and meal preparation, and those that increase physical activity and decrease stress. Both document their interventions in order to provide continuity and assess outcomes (Johnson, Ludwig-Beymer, & Micek, 1999).

Faith-community occupational therapy differs from home health therapy in that the therapist does not provide treatment, is not focused on remediation of deficits, and does not need a physician's referral. Many interventions are on a group basis. Faith-community occupational therapy incorporates the client's beliefs and spirituality as an important component of any intervention. See Tables 25-1 and 25-2 for further examples of how health promotion initiatives can be adapted by practitioners in faith-based settings.

Table 25-1 Examples of Faith-Based or Easily Adaptable Interventions

Program Area	Description	Faith-Based Component
Children and Youth		
*Camp Noah for Disaster Survivors (Zotti, Graham, Whitt, Anad, & Replogle, 2006)	Structured curriculum for school age children followed "disaster cycle of recovery" (p. 401) using skits, crafts, fun activities	Study materials/ activities are based on Noah's ark story; includes spiritual coping strategies
*Project Transformation (Campbell, Rhynders, Riley, Merryman, Scaffa, 2010) for at-risk children	After-school academic and enrichment programs with games, meal, play time, presentations; served as Level I fieldwork site	Faith-based setting, activities included scripture lessons; trained young adult interns; outreach to community
*Jump Kids Jump (Yamkovenko, 2009)	Fun, progressive exercise programs for obesity prevention and bone health	Easily adapted to faith-based programs and groups

Table 25-1 Examples of Faith-Based or Easily Adaptable Interventions—cont'd		
Program Area	**Description**	**Faith-Based Component**
*Healthy Homes Assessments (U.S. Dept. of Health and Human Services, 2009)	Assessed homes for safety and accessibility, but also for toxins and allergens that may affect child development	Can be carried out through faith communities and organizations, using pool of volunteers for modifications
Productive Aging *Exercise for Fall Risk Reduction (Arnold, Sran, & Harrison, 2009; Voltz, 2005)	Evidence for effectiveness of exercise in reducing fall risk in community-dwelling older adults.	Faith-community exercise and walking groups offer support, accountability, and motivation for change.
*Energy Conservation Workshop for Well Elderly (Bunyog & Griffin, 2007)	Instruction in work simplification for ADLs/IADLs, including use of adaptive equipment	Participants were recruited from churches; program easily adaptable to faith-based setting
*Designing a Life of Wellness for Community Elders (Matuska, Giles-Heinz, Flinn, Neighbor, & Bass-Haugen, 2003)	Six months of weekly classes based on Lifestyle Redesign concepts with focus on increasing communication and participation	Easily adaptable to faith-based setting, with benefit of additional spiritual and community resources
Work and Industry *Ergonomic Consultation (Fecko, Errico, & Jabobs, 2004; Noack, 2005)	Analysis of job requirements and design of specific interventions	Addresses specific needs of clergy, office staff, youth worker, custodian
*Clergy Wellness (Rediger, 2000)	Lifestyle modification for clergy on disability leave or at risk for burnout	Includes spiritual fitness along with mental and physical fitness
*Job Development for Persons with Developmental Disabilities (Carter, 2007)	Analysis of volunteer tasks that can be shadowed and learned for skills development; job referral and placement	Taps volunteer base and spirit of faith-based organization, addresses occupational deprivation
Mental Health *Caregiver Training and Support Groups (Brachtesende, 2004; Dooley & Hinojosa, 2004)	Education on balance of daily occupations, strategies for promoting occupational involvement for care recipient	Support group includes devotionals, sharing, prayer support for members
*Community Practice with Persons who are Homeless (Herzberg & Petrenchik, 2010; Hotchkiss & Fisher, 2004)	Identified needs of shelter residents and developed empowering interventions, addressed mental health needs, high in this population	Many shelters and day programs are faith-based and welcome interventions that address spirituality
Rehabilitation and Participation *Accessibility Consultation (Shamberg, 1993; Shamberg & Kidd, 2010; Swedberg, 2001)	Analyzed faith-community building and programs, adapted ADA concepts to enable full participation of all members	Requires knowledge of religious occupations and of aspects of building that serve religious functions
*Emergency Preparedness for Persons with Disabilities (Scaffa, Gerardi, Herzberg, & McColl, 2006)	Addressed specialized needs and developed individualized plans that address support personnel, DME and service animals	Mobilizes faith communities to develop safety net; offer spiritual support to persons displaced by disaster

Continued

Table 25-1   Examples of Faith-Based or Easily Adaptable Interventions—cont'd

Program Area	Description	Faith-Based Component
*Skill Development for Immigrants and Refugees (Gupta & Sullivan, 2008)	Assessed skills, role changes, IADL needs; developed training for mentors to facilitate participation in society	Faith communities will offer space and volunteers; need to assess cultural and religious worldview of immigrants
Health Promotion and Wellness		
*Self-Management Programs for Persons with Chronic Conditions (Neufeld & Kneippman, 2003)	Focus is on training, exercise for specific needs of persons with multiple sclerosis, Parkinson's, etc.; included group process, workbook	Easily adapted to a faith-based program, empowers individuals and caregivers to stay positive, find support.
*Faithfully Fit Forever (White, Drechsel, & Johnson, 2006)	Educated trainers/group leaders in faith-based exercise program for body, mind, and spirit	Leaders come from faith communities; program incorporates inspirational readings and spiritual support.
*Faith-Based Health Training Program (Kotecki, 2002)	Educated lay health ministers in health promotion based on *Healthy People 2010;* included updates for graduates	Participants offer prayer, faith-based resources; pastors are involved and speak at graduation
*Health Ministry Fair (Wilson, 2000)	Identified priorities, invited resources, ensured accessibility of venue and materials, evaluated program effectiveness	Both secular and faith-based services and products are included in booths and activities

Table 25-2   Examples of Occupational Therapy Faith-Based Interventions

Topic	Faith-Based Organization	Occupational Therapy Roles	Contact
Health Ministry	Greater Pleasant Branch Missionary Baptist Church; Primary affiliation: University of Central Arkansas	Educator, program developer, community-based participatory research partner, health ministry coordinator, speaker—local and national levels	Letha Mosley, PhD, OT, Conway, AR
Disability Ministry	Twin Oaks Presbyterian Church, Special Needs Ministry	Disability ministry coordinator, program developer, speaker—local church and community levels	Robin Mourey, OT, St. Louis, MO
Parachurch Disability Ministry	Joni and Friends	Disability ministry coordinator, program developer, consultant, writer, speaker, short-term missionary—local, regional, and national/international levels	Care Tuk, OT, MEd, Elk, WA; and Kim Schartow, OT, Bay Area, CA
Missionary Work	JianHua Foundation (Hong Kong–based Christian non-governmental organization)	Long-term missionary, program developer, consultant— local level (international)	Ann Churchwell, OT, RN, Tianjin, China

Table 25-2 Examples of Occupational Therapy Faith-Based Interventions—cont'd

Topic	Faith-Based Organization	Occupational Therapy Roles	Contact
Consultation to Faith-Based Organization	UMCOR Health, United Methodist Church	Consultant, advocate, writer, researcher—local and national/denominational levels	Jennifer Yound, OTD, St. Louis, MO, and New York
Advocacy with Jewish Faith Communities	Samuel Merritt University; Jewish Family and Children's Services of the East Bay	Program developer, board member of community agency, community-based researcher, advocate, educator, grant writer—local and regional levels	Marcia Goodman-Lavey, OT, JD, Walnut Creek, CA
Initiatives of an Occupational Therapy Educator	Presbyterian Outreach; Creighton University; International Child Care (Dominican Republic)	Program developer, community-based researcher, university, educator, grant writer, writer, board member of community agency—local, regional, international levels	Joy Voltz Doll, OTD, Omaha, NE
Ordained Ministry		Health educator, health counselor, advocate, referral advisor, program developer—local level—in addition to primary role as deacon/pastor	Charmaine Kathmann, New Orleans, LA; Suzanne Trump, Allentown, PA; and Donna Twardowski, Sarasota, FL
Initiatives of an Occupational Therapy Assistant	Cadence International—Port of Call Hospitality House	Program developer, community-based health ministry coordinator, long-term missionary within the United States—local level	Sunny Anderson, OTA; BS (nutrition), Bremerton, WA

Disability Ministry

A natural fit for occupational therapy practitioners is **disability ministry,** a form of ministry that focuses on expanding opportunities for full participation of persons with disabilities. Inclusion ministry would be a better term for this combination of advocacy and practical suggestions that enables faith communities to embrace all persons and families as essential participants (Saliers, 1998). Inclusion focuses on helping persons carry out their lives in community locations they select, participating in all feasible aspects of activities they choose. National disability ministries include **parachurch** organizations, which are faith-based groups that operate independently of a specific denomination.

Missions and Outreach

Another model of ministry is that of mission work, which may incorporate health ministry, disability ministry, and/or other roles. To be in **mission** means to be sent out from the parent religious organization, either to an underserved area in one's own country or to another country. Mission trips are usually short-term ventures involving a group that partners with a local hosting organization over a several-week period to accomplish a specific objective. Examples include medical clinics for underserved groups or raising the walls for a building and providing activities for the children of a community. Orloff (2007) shared her pediatric occupational therapy experience with and learned from professionals and families during a team outreach to

Moldova through Jewish Healthcare International. Service-learning trips offered by some occupational therapy educational programs fall into this category if they incorporate a faith-based component. Other initiatives take place in urban areas of the United States, such as the Door of Hope program for homeless persons (Stokes & Nolan, 2006).

Another example of a short-term mission trip that includes occupational therapists is wheelchair distribution outreach. Team members travel to developing countries to fit persons who could otherwise not afford a wheelchair with donated, refurbished wheelchairs. While wheelchairs may not be appropriate for persons in some environments (Zollars & Ruppelt, 1999), for many Eastern Europeans and others who live in cities with paved surfaces, a restored wheelchair facilitates community access and participation. Both short- and long-term programs need to ensure that the intervention benefits the indigenous people as well as the trip participants (DeCamp, 2007). Ethical considerations include local participation in planning the outreach, training team members about cultural issues they will face, consideration for long-term sustainability, and having evaluation built into the process (DeCamp, 2007; U.S. Standards of Excellence in Short-Term Mission, 2009).

Long-term mission work involves assignment of individuals for a period of a year or more. While the missionaries themselves experience a religious calling to the work, the faith-based component of their work is often subtle and introduced only after they are specifically asked what motivates them to leave a comfortable life at home and reach out to others.

Other Community-Based Occupational Therapy Roles in Faith-Based Organizations

Consultation

The *Occupational Therapy Practice Framework* (AOTA, 2008) includes consultation as a valid occupational therapy intervention. A therapist providing consultation services to a faith-based organization will equip the organization with skills to improve services and programming in arenas defined by the organization. A consultant may come from outside the organization and offer a fresh, objective view (Epstein & Jaffe, 2003). The practitioner who

belongs to the organization functions as an internal consultant with the advantage of understanding more of the context and performance patterns underlying the current status. The request for consultation may originate from the organization, but astute therapists who note areas in need of improvement may also initiate the process. Consultation is provided on a contractual, time-limited basis, for a specific project. At the end of the time or project, renegotiation for an additional period may be possible.

Occupational therapy education equips therapists with basic skills for task analysis, problem solving, and group process, which are useful in consulting. A practitioner needs to gain advanced skills and experience, and to develop an extensive toolkit of resources pertaining to the area of consultation, prior to offering consultation services (Epstein & Jaffe, 2003; Scott, 2009).

A practitioner provides person-level (case) consultation (AOTA, 2008) when developing individualized plans for inclusion of children or adults who need adaptive supports in faith-community programs. Examples of organization-level consultation are helping a congregation or camp complete an accessibility audit and prioritize recommendations for action, or working with the education department to adapt the overall curriculum for children with differing learning abilities. At both levels the therapist helps the organization understand the need to modify activity demands, contexts, and environments for successful participation. Population-level consultation might involve working with an entire denomination to change policies and implement procedures, or developing awareness and training materials to be used throughout the system (Herzog, 2006).

Board Member and Advocate

Practitioners who engage in community-based practice find they are more effective if they work in conjunction with other individuals and groups (Stokes & Nolan, 2006). Serving as a board member for a local, state, or national faith-based organization is one way of influencing the community. Occupational therapy practitioners have skills that make them valued board members (Daly, 2008). Most start with serving on a local level and then gradually progress to state or national levels. Like consultants, board members must understand organizational behavior and the change process (Braveman, 2006).

Advocacy means speaking or acting on behalf of another person or group to help them achieve services, status, or support that has been denied. Advocacy is not limited to lobbying legislators and other politicians (Patterson, 2007) but rather is applied to systems wherever power and resources are unequally distributed and marginalized persons are excluded. Practitioners working with such populations teach self-advocacy and community-building skills (Hammel, Charlton, Jones, Kramer, & Wilson, 2009). Causes that occupational therapy advocates embrace may include health care access for the uninsured (Voltz, 2006) or improved services for mentally ill homeless persons.

The first author has applied her occupational therapy skills and interest in accessibility by serving as a chairperson of a state-level denominational committee on disability concerns. She is now chair of a national task force on disability ministries that is charged with advocating for and increasing inclusion of persons with disabilities throughout the denomination.

Communications

One reason so little is known about occupational therapy practitioners' involvement in faith-based organizations is that few have written about their programs. There are no books about faith-based occupational therapy and few articles written about evidence-based interventions or practice models in faith communities. Several scholar-writers have published on spirituality and occupational therapy, but the articles are focused on theory, applications for occupational therapy education, or practice in medical model settings (Donica, 2008; Egan & Swedersky, 2003; Unruh, Versnel, & Kerr, 2004). The profession will lack credibility until there is more published evidence of effective faith-based occupational therapy interventions. The *Journal of Religion, Disability and Health* is the premier interdisciplinary journal addressing concerns of disability ministry.

Speaking opportunities abound for approaching health and disability ministry from an occupational therapy perspective. The first author presented workshops at state and AOTA conferences on using the skills of occupational therapy to facilitate full participation in faith communities and on the role of the faith-community occupational therapist (Swedberg & Tuk, 2001; Swedberg, 2004). Parish nursing and health education association meetings and symposia on local, state, and national levels provide receptive audiences. Presenting to groups outside occupational therapy develops partnerships and expands awareness of the skills occupational therapists offer as team players in faith communities and faith-based organizations. Practitioners who are drawn to faith-based work often realize the need for credentials recognized within their religion. Many denominations offer lay speaking training, and practitioners who earn this certification can lead worship in their own and other congregations, preaching sermons that illustrate scriptural principles of wholeness and inclusion and draw on their occupational therapy perspective and experience.

Ordained Ministry

A minority of occupational therapists involved in faith communities become ordained as ministers. Three pastors interviewed for this chapter sensed a calling to the ministry earlier in life, but when ordination for women was not an option they discovered occupational therapy as a means to be in service to others. After traditional occupational therapy careers in direct services and academic settings, they chose to pursue formal seminary training and ordination.

Recommended Training and Experience

Before taking formal training in a faith-community nursing/health ministry program, significant self-examination is called for. A new practitioner or one who lacks experience in community practice could start as a volunteer in an existing program. Another entry point is participation in a structured mission experience. The therapist must have a sense of calling to this service and a desire to grow spiritually. Experience in home and community health, in case management, or in settings where the therapist must operate independently is an advantage for health ministry. A holistic orientation is crucial, and the therapist should supplement traditional occupational therapy education with information about health promotion, community organizing, religion, and the particular denomination or faith community.

Formal training is provided through faith-community (parish) nursing programs, many of which—but not all—are open to including other professionals who have the appropriate background and experience. The International Parish Nurse Resource Center sets the standards for program curriculum so the content is similar even though the venue and time frame for the course varies (McDermott, Solari-Twadell, & Matheus, 1999; Patterson, 2003).

Within occupational therapy the question of roles needs clarification. The likely outcome of a dialogue would be that occupational therapy assistants and occupational therapists alike may become faith-community practitioners if each group restricts their activity to tasks and roles within their respective scope of practice for which they have training and experience.

Ethical Considerations

A practitioner working or volunteering in a faith-based organization will encounter circumstances that require ethical analysis and decision making. The *Occupational Therapy Code of Ethics and Ethics Standards (2010)* (AOTA, 2010) provides guidance regarding principles that help the therapist determine the best course to take. Principle 3, Autonomy and Confidentiality, provides guidance and is upheld when the practitioner empowers parishioners to learn skills for making their own decisions and assesses the values of each individual, avoiding assumptions based on religious affiliation.

Occupational therapy practitioners should be familiar with standard health care ethical approaches that emphasize rights and rules and treat persons as autonomous agents. While these principles are effective in addressing typical dilemmas in medical model settings, they have less to offer those in community practice (Racher, 2007). The Ethic of Care, which comes from the nursing feminist ethics perspective (Vollbrecht, 2002), is more readily applied to community-based faith-community settings. This theory emphasizes relationships and community, assuming that persons operate out of a natural sense of caring rather than in response to principles. Concepts

germane to this frame of reference are "inclusion, diversity, participation, empowerment, social justice, advocacy, and interdependence" (p. 65), which form an effective foundation for practice in the community. The Public Health Leadership Society developed a Code of Ethics (2002) that further elaborates on the application of ethics in community practice.

A growing number of occupational therapy publications address the need for the profession to address social justice and/or occupational injustice issues (Arnold & Rybski, 2010; Kronenberg & Pollard, 2006; Wilcock & Townsend, 2009), including the *Occupational Therapy Code of Ethics and Ethics Standards (2010)* (AOTA, 2010). Many faith-based organizations reach out to underserved groups within their communities, offering partnering practitioners a chance to bring about social change and increased participation in occupational opportunities.

Self-Care

Self-care is vital to successful health ministry. Prochnau, Liu, and Boman (2003) discuss coping strategies for hospice therapists, including finding appropriate means to ventilate and practicing self-nurturance, which would benefit therapists in faith-based settings. Attention to one's spiritual life allows continued reserves to serve others. Authenticity is required; the practitioner must model any behaviors that he or she expects others to follow. Beyond that, if the practitioner is not leading a balanced life, burnout and the tendency to try to carry out the program alone are probable consequences. Each practitioner needs to seek out support from others doing similar work; this may be possible through a local organizations. A community health ministry or disability ministry group also enables sharing of program ideas and resource information, and may offer retreats and continuing education.

Future Directions

The nursing profession has standards of practice for faith-community nursing. As more occupational therapy practitioners work in this area, they can contribute to setting standards for faith-based occupational therapy practice. Standards should be developed collaboratively, in a similar manner to the nursing standards that were jointly written by representatives from the American Nursing Association and the Health Ministry Association. A preliminary step would be a position paper or white paper developed through the AOTA.

Before standards of practice are created, more informal and formal networking is needed among practitioners working in faith-based settings. Options for communication include establishing a listserv or online group through AOTA or another organization, affinity group meetings at national or regional conferences of both occupational therapy and health ministry, and use of social networking sites.

Occupational therapists working in faith-based settings can contribute to the expansion of this specialty by offering fieldwork placements through occupational therapy schools that emphasize emerging practice areas and community-based fieldwork. Educators can collaborate with community practitioners and students to carry out needed research on the effectiveness of faith-based health and inclusion initiatives.

While currently nearly all occupational therapy faith-based involvement is in Judeo-Christian organizations, future growth will be in diverse settings. Occupational therapy is less developed in predominately Muslim countries and will succeed only if faith-based factors are incorporated. Asian occupational therapists have realized that the Western focus on independence and autonomy has limited relevance in their cultures where the family and society are more prominent than the individual. Developed initially for Asian clients, the Kawa (river) model of rehabilitation (Iwama, 2005) may prove a better conceptual fit for persons from Native American cultures as well as for immigrants in North America. As therapists become attuned to considering the cultural context and spiritual domain, and as they look for trends in society that point to opportunities and concerns that occupational therapists can address, there is no limit to the types of services that can be developed in faith-based settings.

Conclusion

By partnering with faith-based organizations, occupational therapy can contribute to the development of a new health care system that fosters well-being and participation rather than merely addressing disease. Dehaven, Hunter, Wilder, Walton, and Berry (2004) completed a comprehensive literature review of health programs in faith-based organizations and concluded that for programs that assessed outcomes, results were overwhelmingly positive. Outcomes included improved cholesterol and blood pressure levels, decreased weight, and increased screening for potential breast cancer.

Clearly, health promotion will play an increasingly important role in reducing the current costly health care focus on extensive diagnostic workups and high-tech and pharmaceutical interventions. If occupational therapists are to fully embrace their claim to holistic practice, they need to address the spiritual domain along with the physical, social, emotional, cognitive, and environmental influences. All practitioners can become more comfortable with addressing spiritual and religious occupational performance. Practitioners from health care settings can routinely ensure that clients can fully participate in their faith communities. Practitioners within faith communities can use their skills as agents of change so that congregations become places where all are welcome and healthy behaviors are upheld.

CASE STUDIES

CASE STUDY 25•1 Elaine

Elaine is a woman in her mid-70s who has always been active in her church and community, with music as her passion. After receiving a degree in voice and communications, she married Scott, an Air Force officer, and raised two children. Both children are grown, have their own families, and live at a distance. When Elaine had a major stroke with deficits including left-sided paralysis that required using a wheelchair, left visual field loss and neglect, and voice and swallowing impairment, she felt a loss of self-identity. "Where is Elaine?" was a common question. She had looked out for her husband, so he was

Continued

overwhelmed when confronted with the myriad decisions and tasks involved with the onset of a disability. The son and daughter visited as often as possible, but there was a gap in support. When the occupational therapist who had been their small group leader at the church offered to accompany Scott and Elaine through the rehabilitation process, they graciously accepted. Several months later, Elaine was overheard to tell someone that while her church didn't have a parish nurse, it had a parish occupational therapist. Some of the functions carried out by the occupational therapist included the following:

Health Counselor: Throughout the active therapy phase, the faith-community occupational therapist helped interpret interventions provided by the facility therapists and reinforced what was taught. The occupational therapist assisted Scott with the home evaluation form and supplemented information provided by the inpatient program regarding accommodations needed to allow Elaine to return home from the rehabilitation facility. When the dietitian provided education on following a modified diet, Scott and Elaine needed support to learn to read labels, select appropriate foods, and find new favorites to replace items no longer allowed.

Health Advocate: The faith-community occupational therapist supplemented the social work interventions by assisting the couple to fill out forms needed for long-term care insurance. When issues arose regarding care and follow-through in the rehabilitation center and later the skilled nursing facility, the occupational therapist provided advocacy.

Referral Advisor: The occupational therapist helped the family sort through the options available for rehabilitation after Elaine's short hospital stay, as the brief visit by social services was not sufficient for an informed decision. When Elaine was not strong enough to return home at discharge from the rehabilitation center, the occupational therapist assisted the family in planning for continuing care.

Volunteer Coordinator: After Elaine came home with her husband and part-time caregivers, the occupational therapist helped the family determine how and when church volunteers could assist without giving direct care. The primary task selected was providing respite—staying with Elaine so that Scott could continue his involvement in musical groups.

Integrator of Faith and Health: Elaine was able to verbalize that her angst was more spiritual than physical, so the occupational therapist's interventions focused on supporting Elaine's continued involvement in valued spiritual occupations. Elaine appreciated being informed of prayer concerns from each Sunday service, happy to pray for others when she could do little else. Later, when Elaine was able to attend church, the occupational therapist modified the bulletin and hymns by printing them in a large font with narrow columns and a red anchor line on the left. Though she never recovered from her paralysis, Elaine reclaimed her faith and discovered a new sense of self through the spiritual journey she faced in her tenacious style.

CASE STUDY 25•1 Discussion Questions

1. After discharge from the skilled nursing facility, Elaine intentionally opted to use the home health agency where the faith-community therapist was the sole occupational therapist. Describe potential conflicts of interest and boundary issues that would need to be very clear for such an arrangement to work.
2. What are additional spiritual occupations and interventions that Elaine may find meaningful?
3. What criteria does the practitioner use to decide when to assist the caregiver and when to empower him or her to carry out the necessary task independently with support? Task examples in this case were the completion of long-term-care insurance paperwork and the home assessment form.

Learning Activities

1. Locate a faith-community nurse (parish nurse) in your community and arrange to interview him or her to discuss roles and functions. Identify which roles could be carried out by a faith-community occupational therapist. If no one is available, search nationally and interview a faith-community nurse by telephone.

2. Select an accessibility audit from the resources and carry out an assessment of a house of worship or a faith-based organization. Interview a person with a disability who uses the building to get his or her input. Make preliminary recommendations based on your findings and the Americans with Disabilities Act (ADA) regulations.

3. Interview a client about how participation in a faith community affects that person's health and well-being, and about any current limitations to participation.

4. Design a faith-based occupational therapy intervention that could be conducted during a health fair in a faith community.

REFERENCES

American Occupational Therapy Association. (2008). Occupational therapy practice framework: Domain and process (2nd ed.). *American Journal of Occupational Therapy, 62*(6), 625–683.

American Occupational Therapy Association (2010). *Occupational therapy code of ethics and ethics standards.* Retrieved from http://aota.org/Practitioners/Ethics/Docs/Standards/38527.aspx

Arnold, C. M., Sran, M. M., & Harrison, E. L. (2009). Exercise for fall risk reduction in community-dwelling older adults: A systematic review. *Physiotherapy Canada, 60*(4), 358–372.

Arnold, M. J., & Rybski, D. (2010). Occupational justice. In M. E. Scaffa, S. M. Reitz, & M. A. Pizzi, *Occupational therapy in the promotion of health and wellness* (pp. 135–156). Philadelphia: F.A. Davis.

Bass-Haugen, J. D. (2009). Health disparities: Examination of evidence relevant for occupational therapy. *American Journal of Occupational Therapy, 63*(1), 24–34.

Belcham, C. (2004). Spirituality in occupational therapy: Theory in practice? *British Journal of Occupational Therapy, 67*(1), 39–46.

Black, R. M., & Wells, S. A. (2007). *Culture & occupation: A model of empowerment in occupational therapy.* Bethesda, MD: AOTA Press.

Brachtesende, A. (2004). Helping caregivers cope. *OT Practice, 9*(6), 13–17.

Braveman, B. (2006). *Leading and managing occupational therapy services: An evidence-based approach.* Philadelphia: F.A. Davis.

Brudenell, I. (2003). Parish nursing: Nurturing body, mind, spirit, and community. *Public Health Nursing, 20*(2), 85–94.

Bunyog, V. M., & Griffin, C. (2007). Educating the well elderly on work simplification and energy conservation techniques. *OT Practice, 12*(6), 11–12.

Campbell, R. M., Rhynders, P. A., Riley, M., Merryman, M. B., & Scaffa, M. E. (2010). Educating practitioners for health promotion practice. In M. E. Scaffa, S. M. Reitz, & M. A. Pizzi, *Occupational therapy in the promotion of health and wellness* (pp. 512–527). Philadelphia: F.A. Davis.

Carter, E. W. (2007). *Including people with disabilities in faith communities: A guide for service providers, families, & congregations.* Baltimore: Paul H. Brookes.

Cassidy, K. (2002). Partners in healing: Home care, hospice, and parish nurses. *Home Healthcare Nurse, 20*(3), 179–183.

Chase-Ziolek, M. (2005). *Health, healing, and wholeness.* Cleveland, OH: Pilgrim Press.

Churchwell, A. (2007). JHF classroom recognized as model classroom by central government. Retrieved from https://jhfchina.org/cms/index.php?id=22&L=&tx_ttnews[backPid]=71&tx_ttnews[tt_news]=47&print=1&no_cache=1

Daly, C. (2008). Expanding the role of OT to board rooms. *OT Practice, 13*(21), 23–24.

DeCamp, M. (2007). Scrutinizing global short-term medical outreach. *Hastings Center Report, 37*(6), 21–23.

DeHaven, M. J., Hunter, I. B., Wilder, L., Walton, J. W., & Berry, J. (2004). Health programs in faith-based organizations: Are they effective? *American Journal of Public Health, 94*(6), 1030–1036.

Donica, D. K. (2008). Spirituality and occupational therapy: The application of the psychospiritual integration frame of reference. *Physical and Occupational Therapy in Geriatrics, 27*(2), 107–121.

Dooley, N. R., & Hinojosa, J. (2004). Improving the quality of life for persons with Alzheimer's disease and their family caregivers: Brief occupational therapy intervention. *American Journal of Occupational Therapy, 58*(5), 561–569.

Dubois, J. (2009). *Inside the federal centers for faith-based and neighborhood partnerships.* Retrieved from http://whitehouse.gov/blog/2009/11/17/inside-federal-centers-faith-based-and-neighborhood-partnerships

Egan, M., & Swedersky, J. (2003). Spirituality as experienced by occupational therapists in practice. *American Journal of Occupational Therapy, 57*(5), 525–533.

Epstein, C. F., & Jaffe, E. G. (2003). Consultation: Collaborative interventions for change. In G. L. McCormack, E. G. Jaffe, & Goodman-Lavey, M. (Eds.), *The occupational therapy manager* (4th ed., pp. 259–286). Bethesda, MD: AOTA Press.

Faull, K., & Hills, M. D. (2006). The role of the spiritual dimension of the self as the prime determinant of health. *Disability and Rehabilitation, 28*(11), 729–740.

Fecko, A., Errico, P., & Jacobs, K. (2004). Everyday ergonomics for therapists. *OT Practice, 9*(15), 16–18.

Grady, A. P. (1995). Building inclusive community: A challenge for occupational therapy. *American Journal of Occupational Therapy, 49*(4), 300–310.

Gupta, J., & Sullivan, C. (2008). Enabling immigrants to overcome participation challenges. *OT Practice, 13*(5), 25–32.

Hammel, J., Charlton, J., Jones, R., Kramer, J. M., & Wilson, T. (2009). From disability rights to empowered consciousness. In E. B. Crepeau, E. S. Cohn, & B. A. B. Schell (Eds.), *Willard & Spackman's occupational therapy* (11th ed., pp. 868–887). Philadelphia: Wolters Kluwer/Lippincott Williams & Wilkins.

Hansen, R. H., & Hinojosa, J. (2009). Occupational therapy's commitment to nondiscrimination and inclusion. Retrieved from http://aota.org/Practitioners/Official/Position/39198.aspx

Herzberg, G., & Petrenchik, T. M. (2010). Health promotion for individuals and families who are homeless. In M. E. Scaffa, S. M. Reitz, & M. A. Pizzi, (Eds.), *Occupational therapy in the promotion of health and wellness* (pp. 434–453). Philadelphia: F.A. Davis.

Herzog, A. A. (2006). Disability advocacy in American mainline Protestantism. In A. Herzog (Ed.), *Disability advocacy among religious organizations: Histories and reflections* (pp. 75–92). Binghamton, NY: Haworth Press.

Holstrom, S. (1999). Perspectives on a suburban parish nursing practice. In P. A. Solari-Twadell & M. A. McDermott (Eds.), *Parish nursing: Promoting whole person health within faith communities* (pp. 67–74). Thousand Oaks, CA: Sage.

Hotchkiss, A., & Fisher, G. S. (2004). Community practice for the homeless: OT education at the Mercy Center for Women. *OT Practice, 9*(8), 17–21.

Iwama, M. K. (2005). The Kawa (river) model: Nature, life flow, and the power of culturally relevant occupational therapy. In F. Kronenberg, S. S. Algado, & N. Pollard, (Eds.), *Occupational therapy without borders: Learning from the spirit of survivors* (pp. 213–227). New York, NY: Elsevier, Churchill Livingston.

Johnson, B., Ludwig-Beymer, P., & Micek, W. T. (1999). Documenting the practice. In P. A. Solari-Twadell & M. A. McDermott (Eds.), *Parish nursing: Promoting whole person health within faith communities* (pp. 233–245). Thousand Oaks, CA: Sage.

Kosmin, B. A., & Keysar, A. (2009). American religious identification survey (ARIS 2008). Retrieved from http://americanreligionsurvey-aris.org/reports/ARIS_Report_2008.pdf

Kotecki, C. N. (2002). Developing a health promotion program for faith-based communities. *Holistic Nursing Practice, 16*(3), 61–69.

Kronenberg, F., & Pollard, N. (2006). Political dimensions of occupation and the roles of occupational therapy. *American Journal of Occupational Therapy, 60*(6), 617–625.

Matuska, K., Giles-Heinz, A., Flinn, N., Neighbor, M., Bass-Haugen, J. (2003). Outcomes of a pilot occupational therapy wellness program for older adults. *American Journal of Occupational Therapy, 57*(2), 220–224.

Maykus, J. (2006). Condition: Critical: Exploring the causes of poor clergy health. Retrieved from http://152.3.90.197/programs/spe/articles/200601/critical.html?printable=true

McDermott, M. A., Solari-Twadell, P. A., & Matheus, R. (1999). Educational preparation. In P. A. Solari-Twadell & M. A. McDermott (Eds.), *Parish nursing: Promoting whole person health within faith communities* (pp. 269–276). Thousand Oaks, CA: Sage.

Meyer, A. (1977). The philosophy of occupational therapy. *American Journal of Occupational Therapy, 31*, 639–642. (Original work published 1922.)

Mueller, P. S., Plevak, D. J., & Rummans, T. A. (2001). Religious involvement, spirituality, and medicine: Implications for clinical practice. *Mayo Clinical Proceedings, 76*, 1225–1235.

National Center for Cultural Competence. (2001). *Sharing a legacy of caring: Partnerships between health care and faith-based organizations.* Retrieved from http://11.georgetown.edu/research/gucchd/nccc/documents/faith.pdf

National Organization on Disability. (1992). *That all may worship.* Washington, DC: Author.

Neufeld, P. S. (2004). Enabling participation through community and population approaches. *OT Practice, 9*(14), CE-1–8.

Neufeld, P., & Kneippmann, K. (2003). Wellness and self-management programs for persons with chronic disabling conditions. *OT Practice, 8*(13), 17–21.

Noack, J. (2005). Development of an employer-based injury-prevention program for office workers using ergonomic principles. *OT Practice, 10*(7), CE-1–8.

Olson, J. K. (2000). Health, healing, wholeness, and health promotion. In M. B. Clark & J. K. Olson (Eds.), *Nursing within a faith community: Promoting health in times of transition* (pp. 31–41). Thousand Oaks, CA: Sage.

Orloff, S. N. S. (2007). Miracles in Moldova. *OT Practice, 12*(16), 40.

Patterson, D. L. (2003). *The essential parish nurse.* Cleveland, OH: The Pilgrim Press.

Patterson, D. L. (2007). Eight advocacy roles for parish nurses. *Journal of Christian Nursing, 24*(1), 33–35.

Peterson, J., Atwood, J. R., & Yates, B. (2002). Key elements for church-based health promotion programs: Outcome-based literature review. *Public Health Nursing, 19*(6), 401–411.

Pew Forum on Religion & Public Life. (2008). *US religious landscape survey.* Retrieved from http://religions.pewforum.org/pdf/report-religious-landscape-study-full.pdf

Pridmore, E. (2006). The Christian Reformed Church as a model for the inclusion of people with disabilities. In A. Herzog (Ed.), *Disability advocacy among religious organizations: Histories and reflections* (pp. 93–107). Binghamton, NY: Haworth Press.

Prochnau, C., Liu, L., & Boman, J. (2003). Personal-professional connections in palliative care occupational therapy. *American Journal of Occupational Therapy, 57*(2), 196–204.

Public Health Foundation. (2002). *Healthy people 2010 toolkit*. Retrieved from http://healthypeople.gov/state/toolkit/ToolkitAll2002.pdf

Public Health Leadership Society. (2002). *Principles of the ethical practice of public health*. Retrieved from http://phls.org/CMSuploads/PHLSposter-68526.pdf

Puchalski, C., & Romer, A. L. (2000). Taking a spiritual history allows clinicians to understand patients more fully. *Journal of Palliative Medicine, 3*, 129–137.

Racher, F. E. (2007). The evolution of ethics for community practice. *Journal of Community Health Nursing, 24*(1), 65–76.

Rediger, G. L. (2000). *Fit to be a pastor: A call to physical, mental, and spiritual fitness*. Louisville, KY: Westminster John Knox Press.

Reed, K. L. (2006). Occupational therapy values and beliefs— The formative years: 1904–1929. *OT Practice, 11*(7), 21–25.

Reingold, F. S., & Jordan, K. (2013). *Obesity and occupational therapy*. Retrieved from http://www.aota.org/practitioners/official/position/41262.aspx

Reilly, M. (1962). Occupational therapy-A historical perspective: The modernization of occupational therapy. *American Journal of Occupational Therapy, 25*, 243–246.

Saliers, D. E. (1998). Toward a spirituality of inclusiveness. In N. L. Eiesland & D. E. Saliers, *Human disability and the service of God: Reassessing religious practice* (pp. 19–31). Nashville, TN: Abingdon Press.

Scaffa, M. E., Gerardi, S., Herzberg, G., & McColl, M. A. (2006). The role of occupational therapy in disaster preparedness, response, and recovery. *American Journal of Occupational Therapy, 60*(6), 642–649.

Scaffa, M. E., Van Slyke, N., & Brownson, C. A. (2008). *Occupational therapy in the promotion of health and the prevention of disease and disability*. Retrieved from http://aota.org/Practitioners/Official/Concept/39464.aspx

Scott, J. B. (2009). Consultation. In E. B. Crepeau, E. S. Cohn, & B. A. B. Schell (Eds.), *Willard & Spackman's occupational therapy* (11th ed., pp. 965–972). Philadelphia: Wolters Kluwer/Lippincott Williams & Wilkins.

Shamberg, S. (1993). The accessibility consultant: A new role for occupational therapists under the Americans with Disabilities Act. *Occupational Therapy Practice, 4*(4), 14–23.

Shamberg, S., & Kidd, A. (2010). Making places of worship more accessible. *OT Practice, 15*(18), 18–20.

Smeltzer, S. C. (2007). Improving the health and wellness of persons with disabilities: A call to action too important for nursing to ignore. *Nursing Outlook, 55*(4), 189–195.

Smith, C. (2003a). The case for faith-based services [Electronic version]. *Advance for Occupational Therapy Practitioners, 19*(9), 7.

Smith, C. (2003b). The case for faith-based services: Part 2. [Electronic version]. *Advance for Occupational Therapy Practitioners, 19*(22), 8.

Steinman, K. J., & Bambakidis, A. (2008). Faith-health collaboration in the United States: Results from a nationally representative study. *American Journal of Health Promotion, 22*(4), 256–263.

Stevenson, C. S. (2003). The Christian heritage of occupational therapy [Electronic version]. *The Newsletter of International Occupational Therapists for Christ, 7*(1). Retrieved from http://otforchrist.org/newsletter_2003_spring.htm

Stokes, G., & Nolen, A. (2006), Community partnerships: Perspectives, pitfalls, principles, and players. *OT Practice, 11*(13), CE-1–8.

Swedberg, L. (2001). Facilitating accessibility and participation in faith communities. *OT Practice, 6*(9), CE-1–8.

Swedberg, L. (2004, April). *Parish occupational therapist: An emerging role in community-based practice*. Paper presented at the meeting of the American Occupational Therapy Association Conference and Exposition, Minneapolis, MN.

Swedberg, L., & Tuk, C. (2001, April). *Beyond ADA: Tools for facilitating accessibility and inclusion in faith communities*. Paper presented at the meeting of the American Occupational Therapy Association Conference and Exposition, Seattle, WA.

Tuck, I., Pullen, L., & Wallace, D. (2001). A comparative study of the spiritual perspectives and interventions of mental health and parish nurses. *Issues in Mental Health Nursing, 22*(6), 593–605.

U.S. Department of Health and Human Services. (2009). The Surgeon General's call to action to promote healthy homes. Retrieved from http://surgeongeneral.gov/topics/healthyhomes/calltoactiontopromotehealthyhomes.pdf

U.S. Standards of Excellence in Short-Term Mission. (2009). *The 7 standards*. Retrieved from http://soe.org/explore/the-7-standards/

Unruh, A. M., Versnel, J., & Kerr, N. (2004). Spirituality in the context of occupation: A theory to practice application. In M. Molineux (Ed.), *Occupation for occupational therapists* (pp. 33–45). Oxford: Blackwell.

Vollbrecht, R. M. (2002). *Nursing ethics: Communities in dialogue*. Upper Saddle River, NJ: Prentice Hall.

Voltz, J. D. (2005). Health ministry: A role for occupational therapy. *Advance for Occupational Therapy Practitioners, 21*(5), 40–41.

Voltz, J. D. (2006). The uninsured: A call for advocacy. *Advance for Occupational Therapy Practitioners, 22*(15), 20–22.

Walker, S. N., Pullen, C. H., Boeckner, L., Hageman, P. A., Hertzog, M., Oberdorfer, M. K., & Rutledge, M. J. (2009). Clinical trial of tailored activity and eating newsletters with older rural women. *Nursing Research, 58*(2), 74–85.

Westberg, G. (1999). A personal historical perspective of whole person health and the congregation. In P. A. Solari-Twadell & M. A. McDermott (Eds.), *Parish nursing: Promoting whole person health within faith communities* (pp. 35–41). Thousand Oaks, CA: Sage.

White, J. A., Drechsel, J., & Johnson, J. (2006). Faithfully fit forever: A holistic exercise and wellness program for faith communities. *Journal of Holistic Nursing, 24*(2), 127–131.

Wilcock, A. A., & Townsend, E. A. (2009). Occupational justice. In E. B. Crepeau, E. S. Cohn, & B. A. B. Schell (Eds.), *Willard & Spackman's occupational therapy*

(11th ed., pp. 192–199). Philadelphia, PA: Wolters Kluwer/Lippincott Williams & Wilkins.

Wilson, L. C. (2000). Implementation and evaluation of church-based health fairs. *Journal of Community Health Nursing, 17*(1), 39–48.

World Health Organization (WHO). (1986). Ottawa Charter for Health Promotion. Retrieved from http://who.int/hpr/ NPH/docs/ottawa-charter-hp.pdf

Wylie, L. J., & Solari-Twadell, P. A. (1999). Health and the congregation. In P. A. Solari-Twadell & M. A. McDermott (Eds.), *Parish nursing: Promoting whole person health*

within faith communities (pp. 25–33). Thousand Oaks, CA: Sage.

Yamkovenko, S. (2009). The power of a jump rope: An evidence-based movement. *OT Practice, 14*(14), 17–19.

Zollars, J. A., & Ruppelt, P. (1999). Appropriate assistive technology. In R. L. Leavitt (Ed.), *Cross-cultural Rehabilitation* (pp. 125–136). Philadelphia: W. B. Saunders.

Zotti, M. E., Graham, J., Whitt, A. L., Anad, S., & Replogle, W. H. (2006). Evaluation of a multistate faith-based program for children affected by natural disaster. *Public Health Nursing, 23*(5), 400–409.

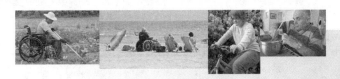

Chapter 26

Lifestyle Redesign Programs

Camille Dieterle, OTD, OTR/L

Live a balanced life—learn some and think some and draw and paint and sing and dance and play and work every day some.

—Robert Fulghum (2004)

Learning Objectives

This chapter is designed to enable the reader to:

- Understand the need for Lifestyle Redesign intervention.
- Identify the key components that make up "lifestyle."
- Describe the history and development of Lifestyle Redesign.
- Describe different types of Lifestyle Redesign programs and how Lifestyle Redesign interventions can be applied to various populations and settings.
- Identify reimbursement and education/marketing issues relevant to Lifestyle Redesign programming.

Key Terms

Accountability structure
Didactic presentation
Direct experience
Lifestyle
Lifestyle Redesign
Obesogenic

Occupational self-analysis
Occupational storytelling and story making
Peer exchange
Personal exploration
Wellness

Introduction

According to the Centers for Disease Control and Prevention (CDC), chronic diseases such as heart disease, diabetes, and cancer are the leading causes of death and disability in the United States (CDC, 2010). Among its residents in 2005, 7 out of 10 deaths could be attributed to such chronic diseases (Kung, Hoyert, Xu, & Murphy, 2008), with almost one half of adults living with at least one chronic condition (CDC, 2007). Heart disease, cancer, and stroke account for more than 50% of deaths per year (Kung et al., 2008), and of the top 30 causes of self-reported disability in adults, the following chronic conditions were ranked among the top 15: arthritis, spine and back pain, heart disease, lung and respiratory problems, mental health

and emotional issues, diabetes, stroke, cancer, hypertension, and kidney problems (CDC, 2009). Additionally, the number of U.S. adults age 65 and older is projected to double by 2030, and experts are expecting to see an increase in the incidence of disability from chronic conditions (CDC, 2009). Although the statistics within the United States alone are staggering, such health concerns appear internationally. The World Health Organization (WHO) reports that chronic diseases, such as heart disease, stroke, cancer, chronic respiratory diseases, and diabetes, are the most common cause of mortality in the world and represent 60% of all deaths (WHO, 2012).

The need for prevention and self-management of chronic conditions is paramount, and both the CDC and WHO, among others, are calling for more health professionals to address these conditions with more vigor. According to the CDC, "Greater numbers of trained professionals will be needed to expand the reach of effective community-based programs to mitigate the effects of disability. Modifiable lifestyle characteristics (e.g., physical inactivity, obesity, and tobacco use) are major contributors to the most common causes of disability, and sometimes stem from a primary disabling condition" (2009, Editorial Note, ¶ 4).

Occupational therapists, with their emphasis on the impact of activity on health, are among the key health professionals to provide preventive interventions and management of chronic conditions. As a community-based occupational therapy approach and set of techniques and tools specifically developed to address chronic conditions, Lifestyle Redesign intervention can both prevent chronic conditions and help to better manage them after onset. Through clinical trial research, Lifestyle Redesign was demonstrated to be an effective preventive technique in community-based settings. It enhances health, improves quality of life, and reduces health care costs (Clark, Azen, Zemka, Jackson, Carlson, Mandel,...Lipson, 1997; Mandel, Jackson, Zemke, Nelson, & Clark, 1999). Occupational therapists can use Lifestyle Redesign as an approach for widening the scope of occupational therapy practice to include facilitating self-management of chronic conditions on a broader scale.

Presently, the University of Southern California (USC) Occupational Therapy Faculty Practice (OTFP) provides occupational therapy interventions for the prevention and management of chronic conditions. The OTFP is an outpatient clinic situated on the campus of USC, where occupational therapists utilize the Lifestyle Redesign approach to address chronic conditions.

Lifestyle Redesign Defined

Lifestyle Redesign is defined by Clark as "the process of developing and enacting a customized routine of health promoting and meaningful daily activities" (Mandel et al., 1999, Introduction page). The term **lifestyle** includes several occupational factors, such as activities of daily living (ADLs), instrumental activities of daily living (IADLs), habits, and routines, as well as other factors, such as health status, environmental press, attitude, and mood.

Lifestyle also refers to daily choices, great and small, and includes the tangible and intangible aspects of a person's occupational repertoire, such as nutritional choices, cultural preferences, physical activity patterns, and sources of pleasure and motivation. The various components of lifestyle are listed in Box 26-1. Lifestyle is created by what an individual places his or her attention on throughout daily and weekly occupations and routines. Lifestyle Redesign is the intentional process of analyzing occupations and lifestyle choices, and then making changes based on articulated personal priorities, values, and health-related goals. Lifestyle Redesign places the client as an empowered director over his own life, his health, and what he does. It helps clients to become their own health advocate and to see how what they do affects their health and life satisfaction.

Often during the process of Lifestyle Redesign a need to make considerable changes in lifestyle arises, such as a change in living environment, employment, relationship status, or a significant meaningful occupation. Throughout this process of transformation, Lifestyle Redesign *always* targets the minutia of

---

Box 26-1   Lifestyle Components

- Attitude and Mood
- Daily Habits and Routines
- Eating Routines and Nutrition
- Health Status
- Meaningful Activities
- Pacing and Energy Conservation
- Personal Motivation and Habit Change
- Physical Activity Patterns
- Pleasure, Play, and Leisure
- Relaxation and Sleep
- Roles and their impact on daily routines
- Social Relationships, Demands, Support, and Community
- Spirituality
- Stressors and Stress Management
- Time Management

Additional client factors related to lifestyle:

- Abuse
- Increased risk factors for chronic condition(s) and/or disability
- Occupational deprivation
- Occupational role overload
- Poverty
- Presence of chronic condition(s) and/or disability

life, such as daily water or caffeine consumption, specific nutritional choices, taking the stairs to increase physical activity, taking deep breaths to relax while stuck in traffic, listening to a portable music device while engaged in an activity, or keeping a gratitude journal. Occupational therapists have an in-depth knowledge of the importance of detail and how it can completely change occupation or motivate one to stop an undesirable habit or begin to cherish a new one. It is these kinds of finely calibrated changes that can have powerful radiating effects on many aspects of lifestyle and lead to total lifestyle redesign.

The Lifestyle Redesign approach aims to facilitate gradual lifestyle changes over a prolonged period, which has a profound and extensive effect on occupation, health outcomes, and quality of life. The goal is to help clients determine lifestyle changes that *they want to make* and would like to maintain indefinitely since Lifestyle Redesign is an ongoing lifelong process. As the client undergoes the process of Lifestyle Redesign, he or she acquires the tools, including attitudes, beliefs, strategies, and actions, that will eventually allow the client to continue this process for the rest of his or her life.

The wellness construct is an important part of Lifestyle Redesign. The American Occupational Therapy Association (AOTA) defines **wellness** as "more than a lack of disease symptoms. It is a state of mental and physical balance and fitness" (AOTA, 2008, p. 676). Each client can develop his or her own sense of what wellness means for him or her, taking into account individual factors, preferences, and situations. Occupational therapists can work with clients to analyze the activities, environments, and people that either energize and restore or drain and deplete. Then the client and therapist work to decrease any barriers to enacting a customized routine of health promoting activities while utilizing supports. This analytic process

becomes a practice or tool that the client can use perpetually.

Development of Lifestyle Redesign

In *Lifestyle Redesign: Implementing the Well Elderly Program*, Mandel and colleagues summarize four core ideas from the occupational therapy profession that shaped the development of Lifestyle Redesign:

- Occupation is life itself.
- Occupation can create new visions of possible lives.
- Occupation has a curative effect on physical and mental health and on a sense of life order and routine.
- Occupation has a place in preventive care. (pp. 12–13)

Additionally, occupational science greatly influences Lifestyle Redesign (Carlson, Clark, & Young, 1998). Mandel et al. and Jackson, Carlson, Mandel, Zemke, and Clark describe four occupational science concepts that shape Lifestyle Redesign as:

- the "dynamic and generative quality of occupations," which have the power to create transformation,
- the meaning evoked from occupation including life narratives,
- dynamic systems theory, and
- the "view of the human as occupational being" (pp. 14–17) (1998).

Other theoretical and philosophical influences on Lifestyle Redesign are listed in Box 26-2.

Box 26-2 Theoretical and Philosophical Influences in the Creation of Lifestyle Redesign

- Grounded theory for qualitative research (Polkinghorne, 1988)
- Grounded theory for occupational narrative analysis (Clark, 1993; Clark, Ennevor, & Richardson, 1996)
- Narrative Analysis and Reasoning (Mattingly, 1991)
- Problematiques and Technologies of the Self (Foucault, 1984)
- Human Condition—Heidegger (Calhoun & Solomon, 1984)
- Hermenuetics (Chessick, 1990)
- Stages of Change (Prochaska & Norcross, 2001)
- Motivational Interviewing—used more recently in treatment and in the Pressure Ulcer Prevention Study (PUPS) after the original development of Lifestyle Redesign (Miller & Rollnick, 2002)

With its many theoretical and philosophical influences, the Lifestyle Redesign approach was created to be the intervention for the University of Southern California (USC) Well Elderly Study, a randomized clinical trial that was conducted with community-dwelling seniors living in Los Angeles, California, from 1994–1997. The primary objective of the study was to determine if occupational therapy was effective for preventing declines in function and well-being in a healthy aging population. Funded by the National Institute of Health and the American Occupational Therapy Foundation, the study had 361 men and women participants over the age of 60 (with a mean age of 74.4) who were African American, Asian, Caucasian, and Hispanic. The participants were randomly assigned to one of three groups: occupational therapy, social activities led by a non-professional, and no treatment. Treatment lasted 9 months, and groups of 8–10 participants met once per week for 2 hours and once per month individually with their occupational therapist.

Results demonstrated that the participants who received occupational therapy experienced greater gains or fewer declines in physical health, physical functioning, social functioning, vitality, mental health, and life satisfaction with *p* values < .05 (Clark et al., 1997). Not only were the results maintained after the 6-month follow-up period but additional findings also demonstrated that the Lifestyle Redesign intervention was cost-effective (Clark, Azen, Carlson, Mandel, LaBree, Hay,...Lipson, 2001) (Hay, LaBree, Luo, Clark, Carlson, Mandel,...Azen, 2002).

Several steps were taken to develop the Lifestyle Redesign intervention implemented in the study. The following summarizes this process as described by Mandel et al. in their Well Elderly manual. The needs assessment phase included conducting focus groups, interviewing key informants, administering surveys, community profiling, and literature reviews. Formal studies to identify what the intervention would target included two qualitative pilot studies and a literature review (Mandel et al., 1999).

The first was a qualitative study that identified seven categories of adaptation used by community dwelling elders *living with disabilities.* Jackson found that the adaptations they made to promote their success in living in the community were: "personal themes of meaning as motifs for occupations, risk and challenge in occupations, activity patterns and temporal rhythms, control, identity through occupations, maintaining continuity, and promoting social change" (Jackson, 1996, p. 345).

The second qualitative study examined the adaptive strategies that were being utilized by successful community-dwelling elderly persons *not living with disabilities.* Researchers interviewed 29 community-dwelling well older people and found that the following 11 life domains were most threatening to the participants: activities of daily living (ADL), adaptation to a multicultural environment, use of free time, grave illness and death, spirituality, health maintenance, mobility maintenance, personal finances, personal safety, psychological well-being and happiness, and relationships with others (Clark, Carlson, Zemka, Frank, Patterson, Ennevor, ...Lipson, 1996). This study was especially significant because it identified certain areas that occupational therapy had not traditionally addressed at the time with elders. These needs were specific to this particular group of elders and their environment, an urban multicultural high-rise apartment building. This pilot study was important because it highlighted the need for occupational therapists to perform extensive needs assessments for the specific populations they work with to tailor interventions. Thorough needs assessments allow occupational therapists to identify significant factors affecting a unique population that may be different from those associated with the general population.

Another step was the development by Clark of **occupational self-analysis** in a course taught for several years at USC. The students were challenged to analyze their own occupational patterns and then make changes according to what they thought would make their lives more satisfying, productive, and meaningful. Specifically, they looked at how their childhood occupations shaped their current occupational choices, how their daily occupations and choices affect their health and well-being, and how their everyday routines were promoting or inhibiting the achievement of personal goals. Interveners in the Well Elderly study utilized this process throughout the sessions.

Key Components of the Lifestyle Redesign Intervention Created for the USC Well Elderly Study

The following summarizes the work of Mandel et al. and Jackson et al. in describing the Lifestyle Redesign intervention of the USC Well Elderly Study. As the process of Lifestyle Redesign unfolded, each client developed a personal action plan. The occupational therapist educated the client about how to harness the "power of ordinary occupations" in order to "optimize health and wellbeing" (Jackson, et al., 1998, p. 329). For example, the occupational therapists educated the participants about how occupational engagement contributes to physical health, productivity, creativity, and satisfaction, and, conversely, depression, loneliness, helplessness, and both physical and cognitive fatigue. The participants gained "occupational knowledge and reflective skills" and then could "imagine and enact healthy occupational lives as they age" (1998, p. 329).

Several components were crucial to the success of Lifestyle Redesign. The attitude of the therapist and the environment that she/he created for intervention was paramount. The therapist created an environment where the participant was the expert and where he or she felt safe and inspired to take risks and initiate change. For example, the occupational therapist would prepare a document of the participants' thoughts, feelings, and ideas from a previous session and then distribute them to the participants at the following session to create a notebook. Such physical representations validated their ideas and contributions (Mandel et al., 1999).

Service delivery incorporated four key methods, as outlined by Mandel et al.: didactic presentation, peer exchange, direct experience, and personal exploration (1999). **Didactic presentation** included new information about a topic relevant to the participant(s) as well as about occupation and how it affects each participant. Occupational therapists led the participants through a process of occupational self-analysis in regard to the topic (1999). The therapist facilitated **peer exchange,** where each participant had the opportunity to tell stories from his or her own life and how his or her experiences relate to the topic at hand. Time was provided for group problem solving, and group members were encouraged to offer solutions to each other. The Lifestyle Redesign intervention also provided **direct experience** through an activity or outing. Some examples from the Well Elderly study include: creating resource booklets with transportation information, inexpensive things to do in the community, the range of motion (ROM) dance, planning, shopping for and preparing a meal together, and creating and displaying personal history time lines. Direct experience, both inside and outside of sessions, provided participants with the opportunity to increase their self-efficacy and sense of control, and to better self-regulate (1999).

Personal exploration and application happened throughout each of these processes and consisted of specific time for reflection on the content of each session. This reflection could take shape in a writing exercise, discussion, or another format. These activities allowed the participants to see how far they have come and increased their awareness of the graduated nature of the Lifestyle Redesign process (1999). The process of intervention is described in Box 26-3.

Box 26-3 Mandel et al.'s Outline of the Lifestyle Redesign® Intervention Process

1. Acquiring knowledge of the factors related to occupation that promote health and happiness
2. Performing a personal inventory and reflecting on one's fears and occupational choices, interests, life goals, and so forth (occupational self-analysis)
3. Overcoming one's fears by taking incremental risks in the real world of activity in small steps over time
4. Weaving together the outcomes of prior steps to develop a health-promoting daily routine

Data from: Carlson, Clark & Young, 1998; Mandel et al., 1999, p. 29.

Four keys ideas that participants learned that contributed to the success of the intervention were:

"**1.** Experience in occupation creates radiating, not linear change.

2. Occupational self-analysis is possible," and through this process participants are encouraged to identify barriers to desired changes and the small next steps to get them there.

"**3.** When people understand the elements of occupation, they have the tool kit to redesign their lives." Selection of occupations becomes more intentional, and participants are guided through the process of recognizing and experiencing meaning in their selected occupations.

"**4.** Occupation is the impetus that propels people forward." (Mandel et al., 1999, pp. 30–31).

Both the therapist and the participant engage in **occupational storytelling and story making** to create the future lifestyle they will begin to enact. Through this approach, participants are able to see that their life, or story, is still moving forward and they are experiencing transformation (pp. 30–31).

Lifestyle Redesign interventions can be conducted in both group and individual formats, and often participants utilize both formats to maximize their experience. The benefits from group and individual formats share similarities and differences, yet when done concurrently can enhance one another (Carlson, Franchiang, Zemke, & Clark, 1996). Groups and individuals meet with their occupational therapist one time per week for an extended period of time, usually 12–16 weeks or longer. In the group sessions, the same participants meet together for the duration and become sources of support for one another. This format intentionally allows for a feeling of both familiarity and novelty simultaneously. Meetings occur at the same location and time weekly; however, the occupational therapist presents a different topic each week, providing spontaneity and variation. Activities and outings also sprinkle the process with more variety as well as the continual social shifting as participants get to know one another better (Mandel et al., 1999).

Lifestyle Redesign Programs and Applications Since the USC Well Elderly Study

All of the Lifestyle Redesign programs created since the USC Well Elderly Study contain the same key components outlined previously. Differences include the content of the didactic material, which is based on each population's needs, and variations in format (e.g., individual, group, or a combination of both), frequency, duration, and location. The occupational therapist may see clients in an outpatient occupational therapy clinic, physician clinics, university offices and conference rooms, or clients' homes. A list of Lifestyle Redesign programs offered by the OTFP is provided in Box 26-4.

Box 26-4 Lifestyle Redesign Programs Developed at the USC Occupational Therapy Faculty Practice

- *Weight Management, including bariatric surgery*—Development and enactment of a customized routine of health promoting and meaningful activities designed to result in weight loss and improved life satisfaction.
- *Type II Diabetes*—Integration of health promoting and meaningful activities into one's daily routine to prevent or management diabetes, improve life satisfaction, and increase quality of life.
- *Chronic Pain Management*—Development and enactment of a customized routine of health promoting and meaningful activities designed to decrease debilitating habits; reduce pain levels; increase ability to cope with pain; and utilize strategies including energy conservation, pacing, adaptive equipment, and time management.
- *Chronic Headaches*—Identification of triggers and other lifestyle factors associated with headaches and incorporation of strategies to prevent headaches throughout routines.
- *College Student*—Development and optimization of routines to improve overall well-being and academic performance through increasing time management, stress management, organization, lifestyle balance, motivation, and focus.

| **Box 26-4** | **Lifestyle Redesign Programs Developed at the USC Occupational Therapy Faculty Practice—cont'd** |

- *Movement Disorders / Parkinson's Disease / Multiple Sclerosis*—Integration of healthy routines and habits that focus on engagement in occupation, stress management, ergonomics, energy conservation, pacing techniques, healthy eating, relaxation, and fall safety.
- *Mental Health*—Integration of health promoting and meaningful activities into one's daily routine to improve mental wellness, stress management, lifestyle balance, time management, organization, and life satisfaction.
- *Breast Cancer*—Integration of healthy habits to support remission and life re-integration, increase functional and meaningful activity, and prevent chronic conditions through eating routines, physical activity, stress management, and more.
- *Smoking Cessation and Relapse Prevention*—Development of health promoting daily habits and routines to replace smoking and manage triggers, including eating routines, physical activity, and stress management.
- *Truck Drivers*—A 7-week pilot program which utilized a combination of group and individual sessions in response to the health risks associated with the trucking industry including weight and stress management, and incorporation of physical activity while on the road.
- *Green Lifestyle Redesign*—Integration of environmentally sustainable activities into daily habits and routines to strengthen stewardship of the environment and improve physical and mental health and well-being.

Lifestyle Redesign Weight Management Program

In 2007–2008, a third of adults in the United States were categorized as obese (body mass index (BMI) >30) and another third as overweight (BMI of 25–29.9) (Flegal, Carroll, Ogden, & Curtin, 2010). The Lifestyle Redesign Weight Management Program was created to address the growing need to address overweight, obesity, and associated co-morbid conditions. By far the largest program at the OTFP, its therapists have seen hundreds of clients since its inception in 2000. Due to the chronic nature of overweight/obesity and common co-morbidities, Lifestyle Redesign is an appropriate method and has yielded positive results. According to a 2006 analysis, after attending eight or more Lifestyle Redesign sessions, participants lost, on average, 4.2% of their original body weight and 7.5% of their original fat mass. The more sessions a client attended, the more weight he or she lost. Clients attend group or individual sessions for 16 consecutive weeks and often continue as needed. Because healthy weight loss (about 1–2 pounds per week) is critical (National Institutes of Health [NIH], 1988), in a 16-week program clients lose a maximum of 32 pounds. As many clients have more weight to lose, they may choose to continue treatment and/or often continue to lose weight on their own following intervention.

The most common co-morbid conditions associated with overweight/obesity include: hypertension, hypercholesterolemia, heart disease, and type 2 diabetes. Other common diagnoses for weight management include: pre-diabetes, glucose intolerance, metabolic syndrome, coronary heart disease (CHD), coronary artery disease (CAD), hypertriglyceridemia, fatty liver, candidates for bariatric surgery, joint pain, sleep apnea, thyroid issues, depression, anxiety, and multiple sclerosis, among others. A co-morbid diagnosis is usually necessary for reimbursement by a third-party payer, since overweight/obesity is not currently considered a reimbursable diagnosis. This requirement is especially challenging for pediatric clients who are overweight or obese but have not yet acquired a co-morbid condition.

Weight management intervention is based on implementing gradual lifestyle changes, which affect weight, co-morbid conditions, overall physical and psychosocial health, self-efficacy, and life satisfaction. Emphasis is placed on goal setting and accountability during each session. First clients learn to analyze their own habits and routines and relate their personal experience to the weekly topic. Topics include eating routines, meal/snack preparation, physical activity, time management, and addressing occupational role overload and deprivation. Throughout the intervention, clients consider how their routines and environments impact their weight management, sleep, relaxation, lifestyle balance, stress management, and emotional eating.

Through occupational self-analysis, clients can begin to enact change. They become savvy consumers regarding food labels, dining out, and fad diets. They address psychosocial and emotional issues related to healthy habit formation and find new healthy pleasures and meaningful activities to replace habits related to overeating. Weight Management Program occupational therapists ensure that clients have the experience and understanding to independently make the best choices for themselves to manage their weight effectively. Clients gain experience in reading food and menu labels, and learn how to reach comfortable satiety while consuming less calories, how to balance blood sugar, and how to choose foods to decrease cholesterol and blood pressure. A registered dietitian provides consultation during the development of the program and approves an eating plan.

Next, the sessions focus on problem solving with the therapist and other participants (if applicable) on how to make the best choices within a client's current occupational repertoires and environments and how to overcome barriers to the changes the client has decided he or she would like to make. The occupational therapist places emphasis on the relationship between stress, occupation, and eating, and helps the client see and transform reactionary eating patterns that contribute to weight gain. Clients establish accountability structures for their short-term action oriented goals each week.

The occupational therapist helps the client to create his or her own **accountability structures** in order to increase the likelihood of achieving short-term goals and to have accountability when occupational therapy intervention is complete. Examples of accountability structures include making an appointment to walk or exercise with a friend or family member; being responsible for walking the dog once or twice per day; or paying for a service in advance, such as a class or massage. It is essential for the client to determine his or her own goals and accountability structures each week with the therapist and other group members (if applicable). Developing relationships with other group members and the occupational therapist, practicing the new habit, and performing the weekly

check-in are each a crucial part of the habit change process (Clark, 2000).

Additionally, the weight management program places particular emphasis on the environments in which the clients are situated in their daily lives. The built environment includes the foods they are exposed to and is a key contributor to weight gain or loss. The built environment also includes sidewalks, transportation, local parks, neighborhood safety, and density of the surrounding area. Occupational therapists in Los Angeles frequently address the built environment because it has become so **"obesogenic,"** defined by the CDC as an environment that "offers access to high-calorie foods but limits opportunities for physical activity" (CDC, n.d., para 1). Many clients find it impossible or inconvenient to walk or bike to their daily activities such as work, markets, restaurants, and other recreational activities. With longer commutes and more sedentary jobs, physical activity embedded into daily routines can become very limited. The therapist works with the client to increase physical activity in home, work, and transportation environments when possible, and advises how to navigate the deluge of calorie-dense food available at every turn (Clark, Saliman Reingold, & Salles-Jordan, 2007).

Bariatric Surgery

Many insurance companies now require lifestyle intervention/modification programs before authorizing bariatric surgery. Because bariatric surgery is only one of the tools clients may use to maintain a healthy weight, it is crucial for clients to learn and incorporate the skills and habits necessary to continue to lose and maintain their desired weight for life after surgery. The surgery is essentially a jumpstart and can enable clients to engage in physical activity more comfortably as well as decrease or eliminate symptoms and co-morbidities associated with type 2 diabetes and obesity. Lifestyle Redesign intervention for bariatric clients emphasizes preparation for engagement in increased meaningful activity that is not associated with food.

Because clients must drastically decrease their caloric intake and food options after surgery, many clients lose some of their cherished meaningful occupations that revolve around mealtimes and pleasure from food. As a result, they must begin to identify other healthy pleasures, reward systems, and emotional outlets to replace eating. Similarly, eating routines change drastically. Prior to surgery, as part of the Lifestyle Redesign program, bariatric clients prepare to change their eating routines to eat more frequently, decrease portion sizes, and incorporate new nutritional needs such as supplements and protein. Clients who undergo bariatric surgery must also increase their physical activity in order to prevent muscle loss. The OTFP has partnered with the bariatric surgeons at USC to provide this service. At the time of this writing, two large insurance companies require clients to complete the Lifestyle Redesign program before surgery.

Lifestyle Redesign for Diabetes

The Lifestyle Redesign for Diabetes program naturally evolved from the weight management program to address the growing population with diabetes. In 2008, 8% of people in the United States, or 24 million, had diabetes (CDC, 2008). This program utilizes similar didactic content but adds information about both preventing and managing diabetes and its associated co-morbid conditions, sustaining healthy eating routines and blood sugar levels, and engaging in physical activity and stress management to help to decrease blood sugar levels and symptoms of diabetes.

Lifestyle Redesign for Chronic Headaches

As was the case with the diabetes program, the Lifestyle Redesign program for clients with headaches and migraines grew out of the pain management program. The prevalence of migraines is 18% of American women and 6% of American men, which is more than 28 million people (Sun-Edelstein & Mauskop, 2009). Inspired by Lifestyle Redesign, a neurologist at USC requested occupational therapy for her patients with headaches, where lifestyle factors play such an important part in pain and pain management. The chronic headache population lends itself well to a group format because of commonly shared traits and demographics. Depending on their needs, many clients with chronic headaches often choose individual or both group and individual sessions simultaneously. The program lasts for 8 weeks, though many clients continue for additional sessions.

Lifestyle Redesign for the College Student

In 2007, the Association for University and College Counseling Center Directors reported that 87% of college counseling centers observed an increase in the number of students who visit their centers and are taking psychotropic medications (Nauert, 2008). College students experience frequent habit and routine changes every year and often every semester. Many students, away from home for the first time, have to learn how to engage in new occupations, create their own occupational routines, and structure their time independently. Lifestyle Redesign helps students acquire skills to successfully meet academic, social, and other developmentally appropriate demands. The program helps students manage time, become more self-motivated, improve focus, problem solve, better organize their activities, decrease procrastination, optimize study/work environments, reduce stress, engage in dating and other social occupations, and promote lifestyle balance. Other topics include leisure, money management, community transportation, effective communication, eating routines/cooking, exercise, substance abuse, psychosocial issues, learning styles, and goal setting. Common diagnoses include difficulty adjusting to college roles, learning disabilities, attention deficit disorder (ADD), attention deficit hyperactive disorder (ADHD), mental health diagnoses, and acute reactions to stress as well as diagnoses related to weight management and chronic pain.

The intervention is usually delivered individually because most students prefer this format. In addition, OTFP affects six to eight open-enrollment occupational therapy groups in conjunction with counseling per semester on topics such as lifestyle balance, time management, stress management, communication/conflict resolution, self-awareness and embracing diversity, and relationship success. In the community setting of a large university campus, intervention can conveniently occur in work, home, and leisure environments, including dorm rooms, eating places, grocery stores, and the student fitness center.

Lifestyle Redesign for Mental Health

Lifestyle Redesign for any population addresses the psychosocial realm of clients and their lifestyle, health status, and situations. This can be an appropriate intervention method for people who have moderate to mild symptoms from psychosocial disease. For more serious and severe mental health issues, a client may not be able to set appropriate goals and follow through with them independently. Intervention emphasizes using lifestyle factors and lifestyle changes as a way to improve self-regulation, mood, attention, concentration, and motivation. For example, maintaining proper blood sugar and getting consistent physical activity can greatly improve concentration and mood, which can lead to greater gains in motivation and productivity. Addressing lifestyle factors also gives clients a sense of control over themselves and their daily lives. This population receives weekly individual sessions, usually over several months.

Lifestyle Redesign Interventions Outside of USC Settings

The name "Lifestyle Redesign" has been registered and trademarked by USC in order to maintain the precision and consistency of its successful clinical trial interventions. In addition to the Well Elderly study, USC is creating other Lifestyle Redesign research trials, such as the Pressure Ulcer Prevention Study (PUPS). Occupational therapy practitioners are encouraged to draw from the Lifestyle Redesign format and methods in their settings; however, they must use a different name.

The following are three examples of interventions in other settings using a Lifestyle Redesign approach. *Employee Wellness* is an 8-week program for employees at USC designed to encourage acquisition of health promoting habits in the workplace by Daley. *Live Your Best Life,* created by Chu, is a stroke prevention program at Rancho Los Amigos Rehabilitation Center in Downey, California, near Los Angeles, that targets women age 35–65 who have had a stroke or transient ischemic attack (TIA) and are interested in learning healthy lifestyle habits to prevent a second stroke. *Lifestyle Matters* is an adapted version of the USC Well Elderly Study in Great Britain (Mountain, Craig, Mozley, & Ball, 2006).

Reimbursement for Lifestyle Redesign

Reimbursement for the weight management program and for the other Lifestyle Redesign programs offered at the OTFP primarily comes from the clients' health insurance. Common occupational therapy codes are used, such as evaluation, therapeutic group, functional therapeutic activity, ADLs, and therapeutic exercise. Even though the diagnoses treated using Lifestyle Redesign may be different than those of more traditional occupational therapy practice, many insurance companies pay for occupational therapy services for these diagnoses.

Self-pay, grants, and special contracts also have demonstrated to be viable methods of reimbursement. Grants also may be secured because there are many specific populations that need weight management interventions and are often prioritized by funding agencies. For the past 8 years, a major insurer of USC employees has contracted with OTFP to create a prevention model for reimbursement. Those covered by this plan do not need a diagnosis or physician prescription to participate and are incentivized to lose weight and maintain their weight loss. The member has a co-payment for each visit for the 16 weeks of services. If he or she loses weight and keeps it off for 3 months, the insurance company reimburses the member for co-pays. Members of this plan may participate in the 16-week program and receive reimbursement up to three times. This arrangement significantly increases access to the Lifestyle Redesign service.

Students who have the USC student health insurance are entitled to 26 visits per academic year for occupational therapy shared with physical therapy and chiropractic services and pay either a small or no co-payment. Often students have not used any of these visits for other services, so they are able to come once per week for almost two full semesters per year. Again, the reimbursement arrangement significantly increases clients' access to Lifestyle Redesign.

Conclusion

Lifestyle Redesign provides occupational therapists with a community-based intervention approach that addresses the critical need for prevention and self-management of chronic conditions. This method draws from the roots of occupational therapy but also looks to the future by widening the scope of practice to include a much broader client base.

Anyone who wants to live a healthier and happier life and to prevent or better manage chronic conditions can benefit from this approach. With both the evidence to support its efficacy with certain populations and a practical format, Lifestyle Redesign programs are situated to directly address each of the goals in the AOTA Centennial Vision to become a more "powerful, widely recognized, science-driven, and evidence-based profession with a globally connected and diverse workforce meeting society's occupational needs" (AOTA, 2006, ¶1). As the needs of society shift, occupational therapy intervention must shift as well. With the sheer numbers of people living with chronic conditions and diseases and predicted to acquire chronic conditions in the coming years, the profession must more fully utilize its unique and effective Lifestyle Redesign approach to increase the role of occupational therapy practice in prevention and health promotion.

CASE STUDIES

CASE STUDY 26•1 Linda

Linda is a 58-year-old female with a diagnosis of obesity and diabetes. After being referred by her physician, Linda started the Lifestyle Redesign program for diabetes. Biomeasures on her first session were: weight: 227.4 pounds, BMI: 37.8, fat mass: 102.8 pounds, and blood pressure: 142/72 (with medication). Her concerns included diabetes and escalating blood sugar, continued weight gain from increased amounts of insulin required to manage her blood sugar, fatigue, and increased stress at work. Linda is a registered nurse and the manager of a large nursing unit in a hospital. Her work demands high energy, constant communication with others, and attention to detail. She attended a Lifestyle Redesign for Diabetes group for 24 sessions. During these sessions, Linda realized that she focused most of her attention throughout her long workday and at home on other people. She is a caregiver in some capacity for most of her time. Additionally, while completing a "balance wheel" activity in which she colored a circular picture of a wheel divided into 24 hours according to how she spends her typical day, Linda realized that she spends very little time engaging in leisure activities. In another session, she learned that her caffeine consumption of six to eight diet sodas per day was excessive and could be contributing to her weight gain.

Linda was guided in prioritizing her own health and well-being, planning ahead for healthy eating, engaging in consistent physical activity, improving self-esteem, managing stress and relaxation techniques, cultivating happiness in daily routines, and substituting new healthy pleasures for caloric rewards. After 24 weeks, Linda lowered and maintained her blood sugar to a level where she was able to stop using insulin completely. She also stopped her weight gain. She lost 2 pounds overall and 5 pounds of fat mass. She developed and maintained consistent exercise for three days per week. She started a routine at the YMCA and had a trainer there who guided her through both cardiovascular and resistance exercises that were appropriate for her and made her feel good. Linda was able to reduce her caffeine consumption by 75%, and she reported that she felt happier at work and less stressed most of the time. When reflecting on her accomplishments, she wrote, "I feel great! I have so much more energy now."

CASE STUDY 26•1 Discussion Questions

1. Identify the lifestyle factors that contribute to Linda's concerns.
2. Identify additional lifestyle factors that Linda discovered were contributing to her presenting concerns through occupational self-analysis.
3. Identify and discuss lifestyle changes that Linda made and how they had radiating effects in other aspects of her lifestyle and health outcomes.
4. What do you think motivated Linda to stay consistent with her lifestyle changes over 24 weeks?

Learning Activities

1. Find articles from popular media (e.g., newspapers, magazines, Web sites, etc.) about a situation, issue, or population that could benefit from Lifestyle Redesign both in the United States and in another country.

2. Create a list of 8–10 interview questions to use as part of a needs assessment for a particular community-based population that you think may have a need for a lifestyle intervention. Craft the questions in order to obtain specific detailed information about this population's threats to health, well-being, and engagement in occupation as well as their current occupational patterns and lifestyle factors.

3. Plan a group activity for a specific population in a community-based setting that engages the participants in the process of occupational self-analysis. Determine the population and setting, and take into consideration the clients' occupational and lifestyle factors.

4. Think of a habit that you would like to start or stop. What are some accountability structures that you could set up to help you to engage in or cease this habit?

REFERENCES

American Occupational Therapy Association. (2006). *Centennial vision* [electronic version]. Retrieved from http://aota.org/News/Centennial/Background/36516.aspx

American Occupational Therapy Association. (2008). Occupational therapy practice framework: Domain and process. *American Journal of Occupational Therapy, 56,* 625–683.

Calhoun, C., & Solomon, R. C. (1984). Martin Heidegger. In C. Calhoun & R. C. Solomon (Eds.), *What is an emotion?: Classic readings in philosophical psychology* (pp. 229–243). New York, NY: Oxford University Press.

Carlson, M., Clark, F., & Young, B. (1998). Practical contributions of occupational science to the art of successful aging: How to sculpt a meaningful life in older adulthood. *Journal of Occupational Science, 5,* 107–118.

Carlson, M., Fanchiang, S., Zemke, R., & Clark, F. (1996). A meta-analysis of the effectiveness of occupational therapy for older persons. *American Journal of Occupational Therapy, 50*(2), 89–98.

Centers for Disease Control and Prevention. (n.d.). *Genomics and health: Genes and obesity.* Retrieved from http://cdc.gov/genomics/resources/diseases/obesity/obesedit.htm

Centers for Disease Control and Prevention. (2007, Nov.). *Obesity among adults in the US* [electronic version]. *NCHS Data Brief.* Retrieved from http://cdc.gov/nchs/data/databriefs

Centers for Disease Control and Prevention. (2008). *Number of people with diabetes increases to 24 million.* Retrieved from http://cdc.gov/media/pressrel/2008/r080624.htm

Centers for Disease Control and Prevention. (2009). *Common Causes of Disability Among Adults—United States 2005* [electronic version]. *MMWR Weekly, 58*(16), 421–426. Retrieved from http://cdc.gov/mmwr/preview/mmwrhtml/mm5816a2.htm

Centers for Disease Control and Prevention. (2010). *Chronic disease prevention and health promotion.* Retrieved from http://cdc.gov/chronicdisease/index.htm

Chessick, R. D. (1990). Hermeneutics for psychotherapists. *American Journal of Psychotherapy, 44*(2), 256–273.

Clark, F. (1993). Occupation embedded in a real life: Interweaving occupational science and occupational therapy. *American Journal of Occupational Therapy, 47*(12), 1067–1078.

Clark, F. A. (2000). The concepts of habits and routine: A preliminary theoretical synthesis. *Occupational Therapy Journal of Research, 20* (supplement I), 123S–137S.

Clark, F., Azen, S. P, Carlson, M., Mandel, D., LaBree, L., Hay, J.,...Lipson, L. (2001). Embedding health-promoting changes into the daily lives of independent-living older adults: Long-term follow-up of occupational therapy intervention. *Journal of Gerontology: Psychological Sciences, 56,* 60–63.

Clark, F., Azen, S. P., Zemke, R., Jackson, J., Carlson, M., Mandel, D.,...Lipson, L. (1997). Occupational therapy for independent-living older adults: A randomized control trial. *JAMA 278*(16), 1321–1326.

Clark, F., Carlson, M., Zemke, R., Frank, G., Patterson, K., Ennevor, L.,... Lipson, L. (1996). Life domains and adaptive strategies of the low income well elderly. *American Journal of Occupational Therapy, 50,* 99–108.

Clark, F. A., Ennevor, L. E., & Richardson, P. (1996). A grounded theory of techniques or occupational storytelling and occupational story making. In R. Zemke & F. Clark (Eds.), *Occupational science: The evolving discipline* (pp. 373–392). Philadelphia, PA: F.A. Davis.

Clark, F., Saliman Reingold, F., & Salles-Jordan, K. (2007). American Occupational Therapy Association Obesity Position Paper. *American Journal of Occupational Therapy, 61*(6), 701–703. doi: 10.5014/ajot.61.6.701

Flegal, K., Carroll, M., Ogden, C., & Curtin, L. (2010). Prevalence and trends in obesity among US adults, 1999–2008. *JAMA, 303*(3), 235–241.

Foucault, M. (1984). On the genealogy of ethics: An overview of work in progress In P. Rabinow (Ed.), *The Foucault reader* (pp. 340–372). New York, NY: Pantheon Books.

Fulghum, R. (2004). *All I really need to know I learned in kindergarten, 15th anniversary edition.* New York, NY: Ballantine Books.

Hay, J., LaBree, L., Luo, R., Clark, F., Carlson, M., Mandel, D.,...Azen, S. P. (2002). Cost-effectiveness of preventative occupational therapy for independent-living older adults. *JAGS, 50,* 1381–1388.

Jackson, J. (1996). Living a meaningful existence in old age. In R. Zemke & F. Clark (Eds.), *Occupational science: The evolving discipline* (pp. 339–361). Philadelphia, PA: F.A. Davis.

Jackson, J., Carlson, M., Mandel, D., Zemke, R., & Clark, F. (1998). Occupation in lifestyle redesign: The well elderly study occupational therapy program. *American Journal of Occupational Therapy, 52*(5), 326–336.

.Kung, H. C., Hoyert, D. L., Xu, J., & Murphy, S. L. (2008). Deaths: Final Data for 2005. *National Vital Statistics Report, 56*(10). Retrieved from http://cdc.gov/nchs/data/nvsr/nvsr56/nvsr56_10.pdf

Mandel, D. R., Jackson, J. M., Zemke, R., Nelson, L., & Clark, F. A. (1999). Lifestyle redesign°: Implementing the well elderly program. Bethesda, MD: American Occupational Therapy Association.

Mattingly, C. (1991). *Healing dramas and clinical plots: The narrative structure of experience.* Cambridge, UK: Cambridge University Press.

Miller, W. R., & Rollnick, S. (2002). *Motivational Interviewing: Preparing People to Change.* New York, NY: Guilford Press.

Mountain, G., Craig, C., Mozley, C., & Ball, L. (2006). *Lifestyle matters: An occupational approach towards health and wellbeing in later life.* Sheffield, England: Sheffield Hallam University.

National Institutes of Health. (1998). *Clinical guidelines on the identification, evaluation, and obesity in adults: The evidence report.* Retrieved from http://nhlbi.nih.gov/guidelines/obesity/ob_gdlns.htm

Nauert, R. (2008). *Medication management for college students.* Retrieved from http://psychcentral.com/news/2008/08/25/medication-management-for-college students/2816.html

Prochaska, J. O., & Norcross, J. C. (2001). Stages of change. *Psychotherapy, 38*(4), 443–448.

Polkinghorne, D. (1988). *Narrative knowing and the human sciences.* Alban, NY: State University of New York Press.

Sun-Edelstein, C., & Maskop, A. (2009). Foods and supplements in the management of migraine headaches [electronic version]. *Clinical Journal of Pain, 25,* 446–452. Retrieved from http://clinicalpain.com.

World Health Organization. (2012). *Chronic diseases and health promotion.* Retrieved from http://who.int/chp/en/

Chapter 27

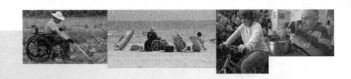

Occupational Therapy in Primary Health Care Settings

S. Blaise Chromiak, MD; Marjorie E. Scaffa, PhD, OTR/L, FAOTA; and Shannon Norris, OTR/L

Primary health care is essential health care based on practical, scientifically sound and socially acceptable methods and technology made universally accessible to individuals and families in the community through their full participation and at a cost that the community and country can afford to maintain at every stage of their development in the spirit of self-reliance and self-determination.

—World Health Organization [WHO], 1978, section VI

Learning Objectives

This chapter is designed to enable the reader to:

- Describe primary health care, including the types of providers, settings, and populations served.
- Identify the objectives of *Healthy People 2020* that apply to primary health care.
- Discuss potential roles for occupational therapy in primary care settings.
- Discuss the most commonly addressed prevention and health promotion issues in primary health care practice.
- Describe the impact of health literacy on individual health and strategies for addressing the problem of health illiteracy.
- Discuss the evidence-based components of chronic disease self-management programs.

Key Terms

Brief office intervention
Chronic disease self-management
Health literacy
Health risk appraisals (HRAs)

Medical home
Primary care physician
Primary health care
Teachable moments

Introduction

Over the past century or so, public health measures have spurred major gains in health, mostly by controlling infectious diseases. In recent decades, advances in preventive medicine have significantly reduced or delayed the morbidity and mortality associated with cardiovascular disease, hypertension, stroke, diabetes, and some types of cancer (Ganiats & King, 2003). This has been aided by improved medications and technological breakthroughs.

However, the stress of today's complex lifestyles is resulting in new epidemics of illness that seriously endanger the health of individuals and families in the United States. Deleterious societal influences and living conditions are accelerating the prevalence of risk factors for illness and impeding opportunities for promoting health.

The incidence of obesity, poor nutrition, sedentary lifestyle, and diabetes is increasing and has negative implications for the cardiovascular system and other body structures. As a result, today's youth will likely experience increased morbidity and earlier mortality when compared to their parents (Olshansky, Passaro, Hershow, et. al, 2005). In addition, other contributors to the epidemic of poor health include behaviorally influenced diseases and rising numbers of those with mental health conditions, including depression and post-traumatic stress disorders. These physical and mental illnesses may present acutely, but their risk of morbidity may become chronic and persist throughout the life span.

Although the challenges of modern life may be a barrier to achieving sustained positive changes in health and quality of life, primary care physicians are ideally situated to address many types of medical problems and disabilities, whether physical or mental and emotional. The focus of this chapter is on the most common lifestyle-related health problems treated in the primary health care setting and the potential roles for occupational therapists as service extenders for individuals throughout the life span in these settings **(Box 27-1)**.

Primary Health Care Services

The American Academy of Family Physicians (AAFP) defines **primary health care** as "care provided by physicians specifically trained for and skilled in comprehensive first contact and continuing care for persons with any undiagnosed sign, symptom, or health concern (the "undifferentiated" patient) not limited by problem origin (biological, behavioral, or social), organ system, or diagnosis. Primary care includes health promotion, disease prevention, health maintenance, counseling, patient education, diagnosis and treatment of acute and chronic

---

Box 27-1   Selected Occupational Therapy Contributions to Health Promotion in Primary Care Settings throughout the Life Span

Children

- Childhood developmental assessments, including infant reflexes
- Evaluation of and intervention for learning disabilities
- Identification of sensory integration deficits
- Assessment and intervention for infant and child feeding problems
- Safety and injury prevention education for parents, including the appropriate use of car safety seats, playground safety, stranger safety, etc.
- Suggestions for "child-proofing" the home
- Providing parents with toilet training strategies
- Facilitating parent-child attachment, bonding, and communication
- Parental education regarding developmental toys and facilitating age-appropriate play
- Identification of child neglect and abuse
- Guiding families in their search for and evaluation of appropriate child-care services
- Assisting families in identifying governmental and community resources
- Childhood mental health screenings
- Preschool readiness screening
- Educating parents regarding strategies for preventing childhood obesity
- Providing handwriting assessment and intervention for school-aged children
- Assisting parents with problem-behavior management

Adolescents

- Mental health screenings
- Sexuality education
- Prevention and intervention for tobacco, alcohol, and other drug use
- Identification of and intervention for eating disorders
- Encouraging the development of healthy habits
- Facilitating adaptive coping and use of healthy stress management strategies
- Educating parents about signs of suicide and suicide prevention strategies

Continued

Box 27-1   Selected Occupational Therapy Contributions to Health Promotion in Primary Care Settings throughout the Life Span—cont'd

- Educating teens about injury prevention, including high-risk behaviors, sports injuries, etc.
- Development of conflict resolution skills and anger management
- Coping with peer pressure
- Promoting health literacy

Adults

- Work injury prevention, assessment, and treatment
- Chronic pain management
- Parenting training and support
- Ergonomics, body mechanics
- Facilitating adaptive coping and managing psychosocial stress
- Smoking cessation
- Prevention of and intervention for back pain
- Weight loss and healthy meal planning
- Mental health screening
- Promoting health literacy
- Identification of and intervention for alcohol and other drug abuse
- Identification of family violence
- Grief and bereavement support
- Identification of resources for elder care, evaluating assistive living and long-term care options
- Managing caregiver stress and preventing burnout
- Incorporating physical activity into the daily routine
- Reducing or managing disability associated with chronic conditions
- Promoting chronic disease self-management

Elderly

- Medication management
- Energy conservation
- Joint protection
- Fall prevention
- Driving evaluations and identifying alternative transportation
- Low vision adaptations
- Retirement preparation and adjustment
- Adaptive equipment
- Dementia management
- Work simplification strategies
- Identification of elder neglect and abuse
- Mental health screening
- Identification of and intervention for alcohol and other drug abuse
- Grief and bereavement support
- Reducing or managing disability associated with chronic conditions
- Weight management
- Incorporating physical activity into the daily routine
- Managing health care visits and insurance issues
- Home assessment and modification to increase safety and functional independence
- Incontinence management
- Assisting elders in identifying governmental and community resources
- Facilitating adaptive coping and managing psychosocial stress
- Facilitating "aging-in-place"
- Promoting health literacy
- Chronic disease self-management

illnesses in a variety of health care settings (e.g., office, inpatient, critical care, long-term care, home care, day care, etc.). Primary care is performed and managed by a personal physician often collaborating with other health professionals, and utilizing consultation or referral as appropriate" (AAFP, 2011, para 3–4).

Primary health care is continuous, comprehensive care designed to maximize health and prevent disease that is provided near where people live, work, and play (Edelman & Mandle, 2002). The term **primary care physician** "is used to describe all physicians whose practice includes the provision of medical care for well individuals and who act as 'gatekeepers' to specialist services" (Goel & McIsaac, 2000, p. 230). The physicians who today provide the bulk of primary health care are family and general practitioners, medical internists, and pediatricians. In addition, there are obstetrician-gynecologists for women's primary health care and psychiatrists for primary mental health services. Physician extenders, such as nurse practitioners and physician assistants, are also involved in the delivery of primary care services.

There are many types of primary care settings. Usually the physical setting is an office or hospital, but primary care physicians and physician extenders may provide services in the home and for assisted living, rehabilitation, long-term, and hospice care. Patient populations include all age groups: infants, children, adolescents, pregnant women, adults, and the elderly.

The long-term relationships that primary care physicians develop and share with those in their care make the primary physician the entry point in accessing the health care system. This makes the primary physician's office the patient's medical home. The primary care **medical home** "is accountable for meeting the large majority of each patient's physical and mental health care needs, including prevention and wellness, acute care, and chronic care. Providing comprehensive care requires a team of care providers. This team might include physicians, advanced practice nurses, physician assistants, nurses, pharmacists, nutritionists, social workers, educators, and care coordinators. Although some medical home practices may bring together large and diverse teams of care providers to meet the needs of their patients, many others, including smaller practices, will build virtual teams linking

themselves and their patients to providers and services in their communities" (Agency for Healthcare Research and Quality, 2011, para 3).

Health Promotion in Primary Care Settings

Health promotion is an important component of helping patients reach their health goals. The purpose of health promotion is "to enable people to gain greater control over the determinants of their own health" (World Health Organization [WHO], 1986, p. iii). According to the U.S. Preventive Services Task Force [USPSTF], modifying personal health behaviors is the most promising approach for health promotion within current medical practice (USPSTF, 2007). Health promotion and disease prevention activities in primary care settings are guided by *Healthy People 2020,* the national health agenda in the United States (USDHHS, 2011). Many objectives in *HP 2020* refer to primary care, a selection of which appears in Table 27-1.

Primary care physicians' offices are ideal settings for disease prevention and health promotion. Physicians are generally viewed as authoritative and credible sources of information and advice on health and illness. A significant number of studies have demonstrated that physician advice is a strong determinant of compliance with preventive practices, such as mammograms. In addition, brief office interventions have demonstrated effectiveness for smoking cessation, reducing alcohol consumption, and other health-related behaviors. **Teachable moments,** when direct links can be made between symptoms, behavior, and outcome, occur routinely during office visits. For example, an office visit for angina is a teachable moment to address smoking cessation, nutrition, and weight loss with a patient. However, due to time constraints, physicians may not be able to utilize these opportunities effectively.

Occupational therapists providing services in primary care settings need to recognize that health promotion and prevention interventions do not immediately resolve health problems, and that individuals will progress in their own incremental and idiosyncratic ways. Appropriate theoretical perspectives for health promotion practice in these settings are the PRECEDE-PROCEED Model

Table 27-1	Healthy People 2020 Objectives Related to Health Promotion in Primary Care
Area	**Objective**
AHS-3	Increase the proportion of persons with a usual primary care provider
AHS-5	(Developmental) Increase the proportion of persons who receive appropriate evidence-based clinical preventive services
AOCBC-7	Increase the proportion of adults with doctor-diagnosed arthritis who receive health care provider counseling
C-18	Increase the proportion of adults who were counseled about cancer screening consistent with current guidelines
D- 16	Increase prevention behaviors in persons at high risk for diabetes with pre-diabetes
HC/HIT-1	(Developmental) Improve the health literacy of the population
HC/HIT-4	(Developmental) Increase the proportion of patients whose doctor recommends personalized health information resources to help them manage their health
MHMD-5	Increase the proportion of primary care facilities that provide mental health treatment on-site or by paid referral
MHMD-11	Increase depression screening by primary care providers
MICH-12	Increase abstinence from alcohol, cigarettes, and illicit drugs among pregnant women
MICH-30	Increase the proportion of children, including those with special health care needs, who have access to a medical home
NWA-5	Increase the proportion of primary care physicians who regularly measure body mass index of their patients
NWS-6	Increase the proportion of physician office visits that include counseling or education related to nutrition or weight
OA-7	Increase the proportion of health care workforce with geriatric certification
PA-11	Increase the proportion of physician office visits that include counseling or education related to physical activity
RD-6	Increase the proportion of persons with current asthma who receive formal patient education
SA-10	Increase the number of Level I and Level II trauma centers and primary care settings that implement evidence-based alcohol screening and brief intervention
TU-9	Increase tobacco screening in health care settings
TU-10	Increase tobacco cessation counseling in health care settings

Data from: USDHHS (2011). *Healthy people 2020.* Retrieved from http://healthypeople.gov/2020/about/default.aspx

(Green & Kreuter, 2004) and the Transtheoretical (or Stages of Change) Model (TTM) by Prochaska, DiClemente, and Norcross (1992) described in Chapter 3.

Assessing the person's health promotion needs includes identifying his or her readiness to change and the predisposing, reinforcing, and enabling factors that impact the targeted health behavior. The

TTM can be utilized to identify the individual's readiness to change. The health program strategies used should correspond with the stage of readiness, whether precontemplation, contemplation, preparation, action, or maintenance. Acquiring the skills, habits, and lifestyle behaviors that promote health provides individuals with a sense of self-efficacy regarding their health, that may lead to better and longer lasting results, and can be generalized to other health issues.

Applying the stages of change to prevention and health promotion involves:

- bringing the risky behavior(s) to the person's attention,
- helping the person to determine the need to change these risky behaviors,
- facilitating the decision to change and selecting strategies for change,
- maintaining the new healthy behaviors, and
- reinstituting the healthy behaviors when lapsing into old habit patterns and behaviors (Moyers & Stoffel, 2001, p. 329).

The health promotion process in primary care consists of assessing the person's health promotion needs; providing appropriate, culturally sensitive health education; collaboratively setting realistic health goals; facilitating the person's acquisition and development of skills needed to implement health behaviors; assisting individuals and their families to integrate health behavior change into their daily lives; facilitating access and use of community resources; and follow-up monitoring and evaluating the outcomes (Goel & McIsaac, 2000). This approach is consistent with occupational therapy's emphasis on client-centered care. Occupational therapists can offer a wide variety of prevention, health promotion, evaluation, and intervention services in primary care settings.

Some of the most common areas for lifestyle intervention in today's primary care medical practice include weight loss, tobacco use and smoking cessation, low back pain, domestic violence, and mental health problems, including alcohol abuse (Zapka, 2000). Several of these health problems and the role of occupational therapy in the primary care setting are discussed in the next section.

Weight Loss

Obesity has been a well-recognized concern even before the *Surgeon General's Call to Action on Obesity* (U.S. Public Health Service [USPHS], 2001) stated that reducing obesity was a national priority. As many as 300,000 deaths per year are related to obesity caused by unhealthy diet and insufficient physical exercise, although this number is probably an underestimate (Ganiats &

King, 2003). Most of these deaths are attributed to complications of obesity, such as heart disease, stroke, and diabetes.

The American Heart Association (AHA) guidelines for the prevention of cardiovascular disease recommend a target body mass index (BMI) between 18.5 and 24.9 regardless of age (Pearson, Blair, Daniels, et al., 2002). Of the approximately 65% of all adults who are above normal weight, 30% are overweight (BMI 25–29.9), 30% are obese (BMI 30–39.9), and 5% are extremely obese (BMI 40 and over) (Purnell, 2005). Several studies have indicated that abdominal obesity, regardless of overall weight, is a significant predictor of metabolic disturbances and disease risk. Even persons with a BMI in the normal range can be at higher risk if they have a large waist circumference. Therefore, waist circumference measurements are recommended as part of a routine physical examination (Dobbelsteyn, Joffres, Mac Lean, & Flowerdew, 2001). A waist circumference of more than 36–40 inches in men and more than 32–35 inches in women is highly correlated with obesity-related conditions, such as hypertension, sleep apnea, diabetes, and heart disease (Dobbelsteyn et al., 2001; Mosley, Jedlicka, LeQuieu, & Taylor, 2008).

The medical approach to weight management combines healthy nutrition, appropriate physical activity, behavior modification, psychotherapy, hypnosis, and stress reduction techniques, along with fat-binding medications to block fat absorption and anti-depressants to decrease cravings for food. Diet support groups, such as Weight Watchers, self-help, and 12-step groups (Overeaters Anonymous), may also be useful. Stimulant-based weight-loss medications may have severe risks or unpleasant side effects; thus, there is no safe, effective weight-loss drug for the general population.

Role of Occupational Therapy

Mosley, Jedlicka, LeQuieu, and Taylor (2008) provide a succinct overview of the role of occupational therapy in prevention and intervention for obesity in children and adults. They address the importance of occupation weight reduction and the prevention of obesity. In addition, they describe adaptations and modifications that can be made to facilitate bariatric clients' abilities to perform and participate in daily life activities. Occupational therapists can assess an individual's overall pattern of daily activity and make recommendations for occupational participation in instrumental activities of daily living (IADLs), work, and leisure that increase the level of physical activity in which the person engages and thereby enable a person to maintain or lose weight more easily.

Moderate intensity physical activity, such as a brisk walk for 30 minutes daily, is the level recommended by the American Heart Association (AHA) for raising the heart rate from 40% at baseline to 60% of its maximal capacity. Regular exercise, sports, yard work, and job activities may confer the benefits as well (Pearson et al., 2002). For the less active, even 10 minutes of daily walking improves stamina.

Occupational therapists can provide guidance to patients regarding incorporating physical activity into their daily routines. Integrating a variety of occupations into one's routine can provide needed physical activity, for example, washing and waxing a car, housework, gardening, pushing a stroller, raking leaves, and climbing stairs. Occupational therapists can introduce and encourage active leisure pursuits such as bicycling, volleyball, dancing, and swimming. Providing interventions that are developmentally appropriate and addressing safety issues are important considerations (Reitz, 2010).

Tobacco Use and Smoking Cessation

Cigarette smoking has gradually declined over the years, but nearly one in five adults and one in four high school students still smoke (Centers for Disease Control and Prevention, 2011a). The National Cancer Institute (NCI, 2003) concluded the following: tobacco smoking is the leading cause of lung cancer, secondhand smoke is a risk factor for lung cancer, and smoking cessation reduces the likelihood of death from primary lung cancer. Cigarette smoking is a risk factor for several other cancers as well, including mouth, pharynx, larynx, esophagus, pancreas, kidney, bladder, and uterine cervix (American Cancer Society [ACS], 2002). Smoking is also a significant contributor to heart disease, arterial vascular disease, stroke, and chronic obstructive lung disease (USDHHS, 2011).

Most smokers attempting to quit need a combination of pharmacotherapy and behavior modification, which includes supporting their decision to quit, helping them develop practical problem-solving skills and a support system, utilizing meditation and breathing techniques, teaching stress management, encouraging exercise, and prescribing appropriate medications (USPHS, 2000). Medications include first-line agents like nicotine, in forms such as gum, lozenge, skin patch, nasal spray, or oral inhaler. Prescription medications used as adjuncts include those with anti-craving effects, such as the antidepressant bupropion hydrochloride (Wellbutrin, Zyban) and vareniclidine (Chantix), a partial nicotine agonist. Some contraindications to pharmacotherapy include unstable medical conditions, drug interactions (i.e., seizure disorder and use of buproprion), medication side effects, pregnancy, and breastfeeding (Ganiats & King, 2003).

Relapse prevention involves the continuation of stress management and behavioral modification techniques and support from health care providers, including encouragement to remain abstinent, positive reminders of the benefits of smoking cessation, and congratulations on continuing successes. Encouragement and re-motivation for slips may help the return to a tobacco-free lifestyle, along with examining the triggers to smoking that can be changed to avoid further relapse. More intensive treatment may be necessary for those with persisting symptoms of depressed mood, anxiety, insomnia, weight gain, and difficulty maintaining motivation, and for those with withdrawal symptoms or medication side effects (Ganiats & King, 2003).

Role of Occupational Therapy

The smoking cessation program sponsored by the Department of Occupational Science and Occupational Therapy at the University of Southern California (2011) assists smokers to:

- Identify and manage physical, emotional, and social triggers
- Modify work and home environments to decrease cues to smoking
- Address psychosocial and emotional issues related to smoking
- Prevent and control chronic conditions that are the result of smoking
- Discover healthy pleasures and non-tobacco rewards
- Learn and practice stress management and relaxation techniques

- Incorporate exercise and physical activity into their weekly routines
- Develop healthy eating habits
- Increase their energy and improve overall health
- Achieve occupational balance in work, rest, and play

This occupation-based smoking cessation program uses the theoretical premises and evidence-based practices of Lifestyle Redesign that are discussed more fully in Chapter 26.

Low Back Pain

Low back pain (LBP) is the most common musculoskeletal complaint seen in primary care medical practice and is a major source of activity limitation and disability. LBP is experienced by one in five adults each year and affects 60%–80% of adults at some time in their lives. It is often persistent or recurrent and is a significant cost to individuals, businesses, and society. It is the fifth most common reason to seek health care. LBP can be due to a single event resulting in acute injury or to a cumulative process of stress and strain (Gaunt, Herring, & O'Connor, 2008; Rosenwax, Semmens, & Holman, 2001).

The longer a person is out of work due to chronic pain, the more disabling the condition becomes and the less likely the person is to recover and return to work. A work absence of 1–3 months puts the worker at a 10%–40% risk of remaining unemployed at 1 year. Returning to work after a 1- to 2-year absence is highly unlikely even with further treatment (Waddell & Burton, 2001). Therefore, the primary goal of intervention is to return the worker to the job as soon as possible. Strong epidemiological evidence indicates that most workers with LBP can continue working or return to work within a few days or weeks of injury. There is no need for a person with LBP to wait for complete resolution of pain prior to returning to work, as this does not increase risk of reinjury and actually reduces recurrences and missed workdays during the next year. Due to the recurrent and persistent nature of LBP, a complete cure is an unrealistic expectation regardless of work status. Job reassessment, modified work, and employer support increase the likelihood of successful job reentry (Waddell & Burton, 2001).

Role of Occupational Therapy

According to Karjalainen, Malmiraara, van Tulder, Roine, Jauhiainen, Hurri, & Koes, (2003, p. 4), "prolonged low back pain can lead to a combination of physical, psychological, occupational and social impairment." Therefore, a biopsychosocial approach, including psychological, behavioral, and educational interventions, is likely to produce the best results. Rosenwax, Semmens, and Holman (2001) provide examples of how occupational therapists can adapt and apply clinical guidelines for LBP from evidence-based reviews to occupational therapy practice. For example, strong evidence exists that bed rest is counterproductive in the management of LBP. Occupational therapists can assess clients' functional limitations and lifestyles and modify activities to achieve a tolerable comfort level (not necessarily pain-free) that enables a person to maintain participation in a variety of occupations.

For persons with subacute LBP, grading of activities as the client progresses can enable a return to work more quickly with less disability. In addition, there is moderate evidence to support workplace intervention involving the worker, medical team, and employer to facilitate a prompt return to work. Occupational therapists can make recommendations for workstation design and modification of work tasks, provide instruction on appropriate body mechanics in job performance, and address psychosocial risk factors in the work environment (Rosenwax, Semmens, & Holman, 2001). For more information on ergonomics and prevention of work-related injury, see Chapter 16.

Family and Intimate Partner Violence

Intimate partner violence is an abusive pattern of behavior one uses to gain power and control over an intimate partner whether married, living together, or dating. Abuse comes in many forms, including verbal, emotional, psychological, physical, sexual, religious, and economic. Domestic violence can happen to anyone regardless of race, ethnicity, age, gender, sexual orientation, religion, socioeconomic status, or educational level. Typically, domestic violence continues for a long period of time and escalates in frequency and severity (Nelson, Nygren, McInerney, & Klein, 2004). Victims and abusers are from all age and social groups, and women are much more (seven to 14 times) likely to be seriously injured by their partners than men are. One-third of women are abused in their lifetime (USPSTF, 2004).

Each year at the hands of intimate partners, women experience 4.8 million physical assaults and rapes, and men experience 2.9 million physical assaults. These result in more than 2,300 deaths overall (Centers for Disease Control and Prevention, 2011b). Psychological and emotional abuse is much higher in numbers and frequency but is much more difficult to identify and track than physical and sexual abuse is. Fifty percent of men who abuse their female partners also abuse their children. For victims, awareness of the abuse of their children is another way they may be abused. Child abuse also pertains to the trauma endured by children who witness abuse and violence (Nelson et al., 2004).

Long-term effects on victims are many and include: denial, self neglect, self injury, depression, anxiety and panic disorders, alcohol and drug abuse and other addictions, chronic pain syndromes, sleep and eating disorders, sexual dysfunction, aggression toward themselves and others, and suicide attempts (USPSTF, 2004). Many of these symptoms are also found in people with post-traumatic stress disorder (PTSD) (American Psychiatric Association [APA], 2000). Children who witness abuse also develop many of the same symptoms.

Physicians and health professionals suspect abuse when there are: repeated or unusual injuries, persisting or worsening depression or other problems noted above, unexplained physical and psychological symptoms (e.g., fear of the abuser or of being at home alone with the abuser), and absences from school or work (USPSTF, 2004). Abusers are not likely to seek or obtain help unless mandated by their employer or the courts, so victims must usually initiate intervention. It is paramount that health professionals identify the abuse and encourage and support victims in getting help.

Role of Occupational Therapy

Survivors of intimate partner violence often experience difficulty with IADLs, including money management, community mobility, home management, and parenting. In addition, they may struggle with concentration, problem solving, decision making, and coping skills. Women who have been abused also face obstacles obtaining and maintaining employment.

Occupational therapy services for this population "may include working on the development of a realistic budget; facilitating the use of effective decision-making skills regarding employment opportunities; learning parenting skills and calming techniques to use with their children; encouraging and supporting efforts to attain further education; learning assertiveness skills; and teaching stress management and relaxation techniques to improve sleep patterns" (American Occupational Therapy Association [AOTA], 2011, p. 6).

Occupational therapy practitioners may also work with children who have witnessed domestic violence. These interventions may include the facilitation of age-appropriate developmental skills, social skills training, improving attention and concentration for school tasks, stress management, and coping strategies. In addition, occupational therapy practitioners have a professional and ethical responsibility to facilitate the health and ensure the safety of victims of domestic violence. This may involve reporting to local and state authorities and assisting survivors to find temporary shelter, housing, work, and educational opportunities (AOTA, 2011).

Mental Health

According to the World Health Organization UK Collaborating Centre (WHO, 2004), at least 25% of the patients who visit primary care physicians have significant mental health problems. Mental health problems in primary health care settings are frequently manifested by physical symptoms such as chronic pain, insomnia, gastrointestinal disturbance, headaches, and difficulty breathing, among others. The most common mental health problems encountered in primary care are depression, anxiety, substance abuse, eating disorders, and PTSD (WHO, 2004).

Excessive alcohol use is a concern because it is associated with a high rate of injuries and deaths, as well as liver disease, ischemic heart disease, cardiomyopathy, and hemorrhagic stroke (Jaen, 2003). The primary care office is an important setting for screening and brief interventions aimed at reducing alcohol use (Jaen, 2003). When screening reveals at-risk drinking, the four-item CAGE questionnaire is very reliable in diagnosing problem drinking (NIAAA, 2003). See Chapter 20 for more information about this assessment and potential occupational therapy interventions for substance abuse disorders.

Mental health problems, particularly major depressive disorder, impose a significant burden on society in terms of lost work productivity, increased use of health services, and increased morbidity and mortality from chronic illnesses, and as a leading cause of disability. In addition, mental disorders have adverse effects on adherence to medical regimens and health habits, including poor diet, increased alcohol consumption and smoking, and sedentary lifestyle (National Institute of Mental Health, 2010). Therefore, it is of critical importance to screen primary care patients for mental health problems.

Role of Occupational Therapy

Although the United Kingdom has a much different health-care system than the United States has, there is much to be learned from occupational therapists in the UK regarding providing mental health services in primary care venues. Several models have been used, including:

1. providing services in primary care offices,
2. direct referrals from physicians to a service provided at a community site, and
3. a collaboration between a mental health service and primary care physicians (Creek, Beynon, Cook, & Tulloch, 2002).

In the first model, two occupational therapists working on an inpatient psychiatric unit of a hospital decided to pilot mental health services in a local general practice. They discussed the role of occupational therapy in mental health with the physicians and provided them with a written description of the services that could be provided and referral criteria. The potential benefits to the physician included: "reduced time seeing patients with social and emotional problems, reduced prescriptions for anxiolytics and antidepressants, and status in offering an extra service to patients" (Creek et al., 2002, p. 457). The physicians agreed and the occupational therapists began providing evaluations and individual and group interventions. The patients (aged 21–76) presented with a variety of problems, including:

anxiety, stress, obsessions, tranquilizer dependence, depression, post-natal depression, bereavement, marital disharmony, loneliness, child abuse, and lack of self-confidence. Some of the positive aspects of the service were:

- People needed fewer visits than in a hospital-based program because they were identified at an earlier stage, and
- Patients were more likely to accept the services provided in the primary care setting because the stigma of going to a mental health setting was eliminated (Creek et al., 2002).

The second model involved occupational therapists working for a home health–like agency that marketed their mental health services to physicians. They provided individual and group interventions in homes, physician offices, and other community settings. Several group interventions were run on a regular basis, including groups addressing anger management, anxiety management, and assertiveness skills. The types of client problems seen were similar to the first model, but there were some additional psychosocial issues, including women going through menopause, chronic fatigue syndrome, myocardial infarction (for stress management and lifestyle changes), PTSD, and employment/unemployment issues. A biopsychosocial approach was used, with access to psychiatrists and primary care physicians readily available. Referring physicians noted that patients were requesting referral to the occupational therapy services because a friend, family member, or neighbor recommended it (Creek et al., 2002).

The third model utilized the services of a multidisciplinary Community Mental Health Team (CMHT) that provided services to eight primary care practices. The CMHT comprised an occupational therapist, psychiatric nurse, and social worker. A pilot project was set up at one of the practice sites. The goals of the project were to: increase access to mental health services, offer services within the familiar surroundings of a primary care office, provide timely and effective brief interventions, and develop stronger relationships with primary care providers. During the 6 months of the pilot program, referrals increased dramatically and a waiting list had to be developed. Patients expressed a need for evening hours due to work and school schedules, and stated that attending mental health services provided in the primary care setting was convenient and less stressful than traveling to another location (Creek et al., 2002).

These models individually, or the development of a hybrid model, could be useful to occupational therapists in the United States as a starting point for establishing mental health services in primary care settings. The benefits of this type of program are impressive, including identifying clients with psychosocial problems earlier before the problem becomes severe and chronic, reducing the need for psychotropic medication prescriptions, and increasing quality of life.

Integrating Health Promotion Practices Into Routine Primary Care

Specific populations and the health promotion services they could benefit from were just described. In this next section three evidence-based, health promotion approaches that can be used by occupational therapists will be introduced: brief office interventions, health literacy interventions, and chronic disease self-management.

Brief Office Interventions

Brief office interventions are short, targeted interactions between patients and health care professionals for the purpose of changing health behaviors. They are practical and cost-effective and can be implemented by a variety of health care professionals, including occupational therapists (Moyers & Stoffel, 2001). The Counseling and Behavioral Interventions Work Group of the U.S. Preventative Services Task Force (USPSTF) evaluated the features of six models of behavior change and recommended an adaptation for brief office interventions in primary care settings. The model, briefly described in Table 27-2, is based on 5As: Assess, Advise, Agree, Assist, and Arrange (Jaen, 2003).

Medication adherence is a significant concern in primary care practice that can be addressed by occupational therapists through brief office interventions. Barriers to medication compliance, which are magnified with advancing age and increased medical and psychiatric problems, include multiple drugs, multiple doses per day, problematic side effects or interactions, and lack of family/social support. Effective motivational strategies to improve medication adherence include daily reminder charts, use of daily pill holders, packaging medications in combination, training in self-determination, social/family

Table 27-2	Brief Office Intervention Model: The 5 As
Step	**Description**
1. Assess	• Target a risky behavior identified by patient complaint, and/or medical and social history
2. Advise	• Emphasize the importance of discontinuing the risky behavior, the improvements that can be gained in health status, and the willingness of the health care provider to assist the patient in making the needed changes • Clear, simple, and personalized advice provided in a warm, empathic, non-judgmental way
3. Agree	• Collaboratively design and agree upon a course of action to change the target risk behavior • Assess the patient's readiness to change and design interventions accordingly
4. Assist	• Provide specific behavioral interventions • Encourage and facilitate follow-up counseling and health education sessions • Assess the effectiveness of physician-provided medications in assisting behavior change
5. Arrange	• Reinforce positive changes • Revise intervention plans if necessary • Provide ongoing follow-up and support by telephone, electronic communication, or office visits

Data from: Jaen, C. R. (2003). Integrating Health Behavior Counseling into Routine Primary Care. *AAFP CME Bulletin, (2)*7, pp. 1–5. Leawood, KS: AAFP.

support, phone calls from nurses, and phone-linked computer counseling (Domino, 2005).

Health Literacy Interventions

Health literacy refers to "the degree to which individuals have the capacity to obtain, process, and understand basic health information and services needed to make appropriate health decisions" (USDHHS, 2000, pp. 11–20). Osborne (2005) believes health literacy goes beyond the individual and it is the mutual responsibility of the health care provider to communicate information in ways that can be understood and applied. The national emphasis on health literacy is based, in part, on research that demonstrates relationships among health literacy, health disparities, and health outcomes. According to the National Center for Education Statistics, "adults with low literacy levels are more likely than those with high literacy levels to be poor and to have health conditions which limit their activities" (National Network of Libraries of Medicine, 2006, p. 3). Low health literacy is also linked to higher hospitalization rates, more frequent use of emergency room services, less compliance with health recommendations, and more frequent errors with medication management. Studies on health literacy and health outcomes have elucidated the connections between low health literacy and cancer incidence, mortality and quality of life (Merriman, Ades, & Seffrin, 2002), glycemic control and rates of retinopathy in persons with type 2 diabetes (Schillinger, Grumbach, Piette, Wang, et al., 2002), and other health conditions (Williams, Baker, Parker, & Nurss, 1998; Williams, Baker, Honig, Lee, & Nowlan, 1998).

Primary health care settings provide an excellent opportunity for occupational therapists to promote health literacy, thereby enhancing health outcomes. Health literacy services may include:

- Informal assessment of health literacy,
- Creation and provision of culturally relevant, "plain language" health communications for persons with limited health literacy,
- Health information sessions on a variety of topics,
- Training office staff in effective communication with patients,
- Health counseling,
- Facilitating in-person and online self-help and support groups,
- Educating patients on how to prepare for and participate in health care interactions with providers,
- Assisting patients with medication management, and
- Teaching patients to assess the relevance, quality, and credibility of health information, particularly on the Internet.

Chronic Disease Self-Management

In the elderly population over 70 years of age, approximately 80% have at least one of the following chronic diseases or conditions: arthritis, cancer, diabetes mellitus, heart disease, hypertension, respiratory disease, and cerebrovascular accident (CVA) (Chodosh, Morton, Mojica, Maglione, Suttorp, Hilton, Rhodes, & Shekelle, 2005). In addition, chronic diseases are often accompanied by depression and other mental health problems. As a result of rising health care costs, patient self-management of chronic disease is being increasingly emphasized. There are varying definitions in the literature, but essentially **chronic disease self-management** involves individuals and families actively participating in the health care process, self-monitoring symptoms or physiological processes, making informed decisions about their health, and managing the impact of the disease on their daily lives. Chronic disease self-management programs are designed to enable individuals to prevent, control, and manage complications of their conditions, including the mental health sequelae (Chodosh et al., 2005).

Several recent reviews have been published regarding the nature and efficacy of chronic disease self-management programs with mixed results. Program elements vary, but generally they feature:

- tailoring the program and messages to specific individual needs and circumstances,
- grouping interventions in order to facilitate peer support,
- giving frequent feedback to the patient regarding his or her progress in meeting his or her self-management goals,
- addressing psychosocial concerns, and
- involving the health care provider in program delivery (Chodosh et al., 2005).

It is important to note that the Lifestyle Redesign program includes all of these elements, and incorporates occupational therapy principles and practices.

Stanford University's School of Medicine (2006) has developed a model chronic disease self-management program (CDSMP). The program is provided in a workshop format for a total of 15 hours over several sessions and is facilitated by two trained leaders, one a health care professional and the other a person with a chronic disease. The content of the program was derived from information provided by focus groups of people with chronic disease. The topics covered include:

- techniques to deal with problems such as frustration, fatigue, pain, and isolation,
- appropriate exercise for maintaining and improving strength, flexibility, and endurance,
- appropriate use of medications,
- communicating effectively with family, friends, and health professionals,
- nutrition and meal planning, and
- evaluating new treatments and making informed treatment decisions (Stanford University, 2006, para. 2)

More than 1,000 people participated in a randomized controlled evaluation of the program. Participants were followed for up to 3 years. Those who participated in the program, as compared to those who did not, demonstrated significant improvements in a number of areas, as described in Box 27-2. Many of the improvements noted persisted for as long as 3 years. The study showed that for every dollar spent on the self-management program, 10 dollars were saved in health care costs (Stanford University, 2006). Replication of the study in 21 community primary care sites with 489 patients yielded similar results (Lorig, Sobel, Ritter, Laurent, & Hobbs, 2001).

Occupational therapists have knowledge of chronic diseases and their effects on daily life functioning, which enables them to develop chronic disease self-management programs in primary care settings, train persons with chronic diseases to instruct and lead groups, and evaluate the outcomes. The research available supports the efficacy of generic chronic disease self-management programs and their cost-effectiveness. This is a service that

---

Box 27-2   Stanford University's Chronic Disease Self-Management Program

Participants in Stanford University's Chronic Disease Self-Management Program (2006) demonstrated improvements in the following.

Health status:
- Disability
- Social/role limitations
- Energy/fatigue
- Health distress
- Self-reported general health

Health care utilization:
- Fewer hospitalizations
- Fewer days in the hospital
- Fewer outpatient visits

Self-management behaviors:
- Exercise
- Cognitive symptom management
- Communication with physician

Data from: Stanford University (2006). *Chronic disease self-management program.* Retrieved from http://patienteducation.stanford.edu/programs/cdsmp.html

---

occupational therapists could market to primary care providers.

Developing Health Promotion Programs for Primary Care

The nature of primary care is such that practitioners follow a panel of patients intermittently over an extended period, providing health promotion, prevention, and treatment services at times of need. This is much different than typical occupational therapy services, which are often provided continuously and intensely over a short period. However, patients may need fewer visits for intervention because they are seen at an earlier stage of the health problem. Therefore, occupational therapists working in primary care settings must be flexible, adaptive, and readily available when the physician refers a patient with a particular need. Allowing the patient to leave the office and attempting to schedule a follow-up appointment for occupational therapy is likely to be unsuccessful.

A comprehensive health promotion program in a primary care setting would include:

- Health risk appraisals, including mental health screenings,
- Patient health education and counseling,
- Caregiver education and training,
- Phone call follow-up,
- Home visits, and
- Brief office interventions.

Health risk appraisals (HRAs) are assessments that profile an individual's risk factors and estimate the probabilities of manifesting certain diseases. HRAs ask the participant a number of questions related to health behaviors and thereby raise awareness about the impact of lifestyle on health. In addition, some HRAs provide suggestions for improving one's health status. These assessments are a useful tool for initiating dialogue about lifestyle concerns and may motivate the individual to action. Educating patients regarding their health status is the next logical step. Information tailored to the individual's needs can enable and empower the individual to assume more responsibility for his or her health.

Caregivers are also in need of health education and counseling regarding the needs of the care recipient and their own health needs as caregivers. Providing support, information about community resources, and training to prevent caregiver injury can reduce caregiver burden and improve caregiver well-being. Follow-up phone calls to patients and caregivers can reinforce plans made during a health promotion visit, encourage compliance with medical recommendations, and identify barriers to health behavior change. Home visits to assess safety, support systems, psychosocial issues, and home modification can also be helpful. Home visits are particularly beneficial for those who have a difficult time getting to health care facilities and who might otherwise need to move to a long-term care facility (Devereaux & Walker, 1995). Brief office interventions, as described earlier, should be used routinely to address tobacco use, alcohol abuse, mental health, physical fitness, obesity, risky sexual behavior, and other health behaviors.

Developing a health promotion program for a primary care setting is much like developing other community-based health initiatives, with a few additional considerations. The basic steps are outlined in Figure 27.1.

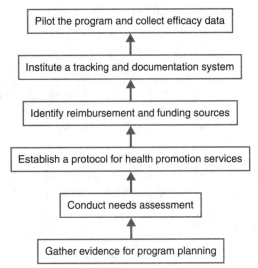

Fig. 27•1 Developing a Health Promotion Program for Primary Care Settings.

The first step is to be well informed and gather evidence for program planning. As is true in all areas of practice, preventive interventions should be based on the best research evidence available. Evidence on appropriate assessment strategies, early detection procedures, and effectiveness of known interventions is essential.

The second step is to conduct a needs assessment of the primary care physician's patient panel. This can be done in a variety of ways using surveys, focus groups, epidemiological data, and chart reviews (Scaffa, 2001). The choice of targets for health promotion interventions should be based on current morbidity and mortality profiles of the community in which the primary care practice is situated (Zapka, 2000). Health promotion approaches are complex and must be flexible, adaptable, and tailored to the individual or group to be effective.

The third step is to establish a protocol that outlines how patients will be evaluated, potential interventions that may be used, and community resources that are available as support services. The protocol should include clear referral criteria and describe the services the occupational therapist can provide. Administering the Canadian Occupational Performance Measure (COPM) provides an excellent opportunity for the occupational therapist to gain an understanding of the patient's needs, desires, and priorities as a basis for individualized health promotion planning (Law, Baptiste, Carswell, McColl, Polatajko, & Pollock, 2005). Health behavior contracts that specify the number of sessions, goals, and strategies may enhance patient motivation and commitment to long-term change.

The fourth step is to identify reimbursement and funding sources for the program. In addition to private health insurance, Medicare, Medicaid, and other reimbursement mechanisms for billable services, sources of revenue may include grants, fee-for-service, and foundation funding. Next is establishing a tracking and documentation system. Tracking may involve creating flow sheets, checklists, and other strategies for monitoring the provision of screenings and other health promotion services. Documentation style and content are often dictated by the funding source.

Finally, the health promotion program is ready to be piloted and evaluated. Quarterly process assessments of services provided, patient satisfaction, and outcome measures are needed to document the efficacy and cost-effectiveness of the program. Data is collected and used to modify and enhance program components. Although program evaluation is the last step in this sequence, it must be systematically planned throughout the earlier stages of program development.

Working With Primary Care Physicians

Primary care physicians are generally unaccustomed to working directly with occupational therapists. Therefore, physicians may need to be informed regarding the potential benefits of offering occupational therapy services to their patients. In addition, the benefits to the physicians themselves should be stressed, for example, increased physician efficiency, enhanced patient adherence to treatment recommendations, and improved outcomes. It is important to assess primary care physicians' knowledge and attitudes toward occupational therapy in order to market services effectively.

An unpublished pilot study conducted by one of the authors was designed to examine physicians' referral patterns regarding occupational therapy and the possible effects that experience and specialty area may have on referral rates. Questionnaires were distributed to rehabilitation and medical facilities along the Mississippi and Alabama Gulf Coast. The survey collected demographic information, reasons for referral, and knowledge of occupational therapy.

The results of this pilot study indicated that physicians with 17 years or more of practice experience were more likely to refer for occupational therapy services than their less experienced counterparts. Physicians practicing in specialty areas referred at a rate 10% higher than the primary care physicians did. Among all physicians, the services most referred for included: range of motion (74%), gross motor skills (71%), fine motor skills (71%), mobility (68%), home assessment (68%), environmental modification (68%), grooming (65%), dressing (62%), and bathing (62%). Other services referred for demonstrate a need for expansion of occupational therapy services into settings other than rehabilitation and offer support for the notion of occupational therapy services in primary care. For example, a significant percentage of physicians referred to occupational therapy for the following services: safety issues (50%), meal preparation (44%), work/job performance (44%), lifestyle modifications (38%), assessment of supports (32%), and emergency response (21%).

Clearly, if occupational therapy is to have a role in primary care, educating physicians about occupational therapy practitioners' contributions to health promotion and prevention, as well as their evaluation and intervention skills, is paramount.

Marketing Occupational Therapy Services to Physicians in Primary Care

Attitudes, personal beliefs, and lifestyle habits of physicians have a major impact on the likelihood of implementing prevention and health promotion strategies in their practices. Primary care physicians tend to be more prevention- and health promotion–focused than physicians in other specialties. In addition, reimbursement issues and energy, time, and resource constraints also limit physicians' participation in patient-centered health promotion (Goel & McIsaac, 2000). Employing or collaborating with other professionals, such as occupational therapists, who have the expertise and time to address lifestyle modifications and health literacy can enhance the health outcomes in primary care settings. The physician can then focus on treating illness and preventing disease, identifying patients in need of specific prevention and health promotion interventions, and referring these individuals to an occupational therapist for follow-up services.

The benefits to primary care physicians of utilizing occupational therapists (as an employee or a contractor) to provide health promotion and prevention services in their practice settings potentially include:

- availability of high-quality prevention and health promotion services on-site, thus increasing the physician's time to focus on medical interventions,
- better patient health outcomes as a result of comprehensive health promotion services,
- less need for medications and better compliance with self-management regimens,
- identification of patients who have mental health needs not readily recognizable in a short medical office visit, including alcohol and drug abuse problems, domestic violence, depression, anxiety, bereavement, etc.,
- detection of performance deficits that may impact the safe participation in everyday activities, and
- prevention of secondary complications of medical conditions.

In addition, it has been noted that providing occupational therapy and other services in-house can enhance a physician's earnings. Out of 11 factors that are associated with high-earning family physicians (those earning $160,000 or more as compared with those earning $100,000 or less), provision of adjunctive services ranks fourth (Carter, 2005).

The benefits to patients include more time with staff, immediate access to occupational therapy services without the need to leave the physician's office, opportunities to learn to manage their own health problems, and improved quality of life.

Funding Occupational Therapy Services in Primary Care

Funding for health promotion services can come from a number of sources. There are office visit and procedural codes for time spent in health counseling that can be billed to insurance, for either individual or group sessions.

Occupational therapy evaluation and treatment is a billable service under Medicare and many private health insurance plans. Many preventive interventions, such as energy conservation, work simplification, and safety awareness, are already being reimbursed through these mechanisms. However, before developing a health promotion program, it is essential that occupational therapists are cognizant of, and adhere to, state licensure laws that define the scope of occupational therapy practice.

Other revenue sources may be foundation grants, fees-for-service, health maintenance organizations (HMOs), workers' compensation, and other government programs. Physicians can also use billing codes for health counseling. In addition, many people may be able and willing to pay for occupational therapy services, as is evidenced by the amount spent for complementary and alternative medical care, which typically is not reimbursed by insurance (National Center for Complementary and Alternative Medicine, 2006).

Conclusion

Health promotion and the medical model can be effectively blended in primary care office practice. Physicians and other primary health providers are in a position to identify their patients' risky behaviors and health practices, determine patients' willingness to change, and encourage changes for better health. Brief visits in the office are a good way to carry out these interventions. More extensive health counseling also could ideally be provided in the office setting. Occupational therapists may be able to establish a niche on the primary health care team by assisting primary care physicians with the provision of health education, prevention, health promotion, and intervention services in the physician office environment and elsewhere.

Integrating occupational therapy and health promotion services into primary care practice is an opportunity and challenge worth pursuing. According to Devereaux and Walker (1995), "occupational therapy can be a major force in the delivery of primary health care" (p. 393). Occupational therapy's focus on physical, cognitive, emotional, social, and spiritual well-being provides a useful, and increasingly necessary, adjunct to primary care medical services.

CASE STUDIES

CASE STUDY 27•1 Doris

Doris is a recently widowed 68-year-old African American woman with diabetes who presents to her family physician with complaints of fatigue, poor concentration, insomnia, and binge eating. She has gained 20 pounds in the 6 months since the death of her husband. The physician, a member of a multidisciplinary practice, diagnoses depression, prescribes an antidepressant medication, and refers the patient to an occupational therapist who works in the office. The occupational therapist conducts an interview, administers several assessments including the COPM, and develops an occupational profile. Prior to her retirement, Doris worked as a middle school teacher. Doris lives alone and has two grown children and six grandchildren who live approximately two hours from her home. She enjoys movies, reading, gardening, and walking her dog. In the past, Doris was very active in her church, but over the past two years while caring for her ill husband, her participation diminished significantly. She has a limited income, but her home mortgage is paid off and she has good health insurance coverage as a benefit of her teacher's retirement plan.

In collaboration with Doris, the occupational therapist develops an intervention plan that includes the following:

- chronic disease self-management and health literacy to address the client's diabetes
- Lifestyle Redesign for weight management to increase the client's level of physical activity and to improve the quality of her sleep, and
- mental health services to facilitate the grief process and re-establish life goals.

CASE STUDY 27•1 Discussion Questions

1. What types of occupational therapy services could be provided to Doris in the primary care physician's office? How would the occupational therapy services be unique and different from services provided by other health care professionals in this setting?
2. What intervention strategies would you use to improve Doris's health literacy and chronic disease self-management? To help Doris achieve her weight loss goals?
3. What intervention strategies would you use to facilitate the grief process and improve her mental health?
4. How would the provision of occupational therapy services in this case benefit the primary care physician?

Learning Activities

1. Write a brief article for *OT Practice* or *Advance for Occupational Therapists* describing how the 5As model of health behavior change could be applied to weight management in a primary care setting.
2. Interview a primary care physician to assess the potential services an occupational therapist could provide to patients in the practice.
3. Conduct a needs assessment and write a brief proposal for occupational therapy services in a primary care setting in your community.

REFERENCES

Agency for Healthcare Research and Quality. (2011). AHRQ's definition of the medical home. Retrieved from http://pcmh.ahrq.gov/portal/server.pt/community/pcmh__home/1483/what_is_pcmh_

American Academy of Family Physicians. (2011). Primary care. Retrieved from http://aafp.org/online/en/home/policy/policies/p/primarycare.html

American Cancer Society (ACS). (2002). *Cancer Prevention and Early Detection*. Atlanta: ACS.

American Occupational Therapy Association. (2011). *Occupational therapy services for individuals who have experienced domestic violence*. Retrieved from http://aota.org/Practitioners/PracticeAreas/Aging/Official-Docs/41261.aspx?FT=.pdf

American Psychiatric Association (APA). (2000). *Diagnostic and statistical manual of mental disorders, text revision (DSM IV-TR)*. Washington, DC: APA.

Carter, J. (2005). What makes a high-earning family physician? *Family Practice Management, 12*(7), 16–23.

Centers for Disease Control and Prevention (CDC). (2011a). CDC reports vital information about smoking. Retrieved from http://cdc.gov/features/vitalsigns/adultsmoking/

Centers for Disease Control and Prevention (CDC). (2011b). *Understanding intimate partner violence: 2011*. Retrieved from http://cdc.gov/violenceprevention/pdf/IPV_factsheet-a.pdf

Chodosh, J., Morton, S. C., Mojica, W., Maglione, M., Suttorp, M. J., Hilton, L., Rhodes, S., & Shekelle, P. (2005). Meta-analysis: Chronic disease self-management programs for older adults. *Annals of Internal Medicine, 143,* 427–438.

Creek, J., Beynon, S., Cook, S., & Tulloch, T. (2002). Occupational therapy in primary care. In J. Creek, *Occupational therapy and mental health*. Edinburgh: Churchill Livingstone.

Devereaux, E. B., & Walker, R. B. (1995). The role of occupational therapy in primary health care. *American Journal of Occupational Therapy, 49*(5), 391–396.

Dobbelsteyn, C. J., Joffres, M. R., MacLean, D. R., & Flowerdew, G. (2001). A comparative evaluation of waist circumference, waist-to-hip ratio and body mass index as indicators of cardiovascular risk factors. *International Journal of Obesity, 25*(5), 652–661.

Domino, F. J. (2005). Improving adherence to treatment for hypertension. *American Family Physician 71*(11), 2089–2090.

Edelman, C. L., & Mandle, C. L. (2002). *Health promotion throughout the lifespan*. St. Louis, MO: Mosby.

Ganiats, T., & King, V. (2003). *Prevention strategies in family practice*. AAFP Video CME Program, Jan. 2003. Leawood, KS: AAFP.

Gaunt, A. M., Herring, S. A., & O'Connor, F. G. (2008). Caring for patients who have acute and subacute low back pain. *CME Bulletin, 7*(2), 1–6.

Goel, V., & McIsaac, W. (2000). Health promotion in clinical practice. In B. D. Poland, L. W. Green, & I. Rootman (Eds.), *Settings for health promotion*. Thousand Oaks, CA: Sage.

Green, L., & Kreuter, M. (2004). Health program planning: An educational and ecological approach (4th ed.). New York: McGraw-Hill.

Jaen, C. R. (2003). Integrating Health Behavior Counseling into Routine Primary Care. *AAFP CME Bulletin, (2)*7, pp. 1–5. Leawood, KS: AAFP.

Karjalainen, K., Malmivaara, A., van Tulder, M., Roine, R., Jauhiainen, M., Hurri, H., & Koes, B. (2003). Multidisciplinary biopsychosocial rehabilitation for subacute low-back pain among working age adults. *Cochrane Database of Systematic Reviews*, Issue 2. Art. No.: CD002193. doi: 10.1002/14651858.CD002193

Law, M., Baptiste, S., Carswell, A., McColl, M. A., Polatajko, H., & Pollock, N. (2005). *Canadian Occupational Performance Measure*. Ottawa, CA: Canadian Association of Occupational Therapists.

Lorig, K. R., Sobel, D. S., Ritter, P. L., Laurent, D., & Hobbs, M. (2001). Effect of a self-management program on patients with chronic diseases. Effective Clinical Practice (online). Retrieved from www.acponline.org/journals/ecp/novdec01/lorig.htm

Merriman, B., Ades, T., & Seffrin, J. R. (2002). Health literacy in the information age: Communicating cancer information to patients and families. *CA: A Cancer Journal for Physicians, 52,* 130–133.

Mosley, L. J., Jedlicka, J. S., LeQuieu, E., & Taylor, F. D. (2008). Obesity and occupational therapy practice. *OT Practice, 13*(7), 8–15.

Moyers, P. A., & Stoffel, V. C. (2001). Community-based approaches for substance use disorders. In M. Scaffa (Ed.), *Occupational therapy in community-based practice settings*. Philadelphia: F.A. Davis.

National Cancer Institute. (2003). *Lung cancer PDQ: Prevention*. Web site http://cancer.gov/cancerinfo/pdq/prevention/lung/healthprofessional.

National Center for Complementary and Alternative Medicine. (2006). *News & events, Use of Complementary and Alternative Medicine in the United States*. Retrieved from http://nccam.nih.gov/news/camsurvey_fs1.htm#top

National Institute of Mental Health. (2010). *Statistics*. Retrieved from http://nimh.nih.gov/statistics/index.shtml

National Institute on Alcohol Abuse and Alcoholism. (2003). *Helping patients with alcohol problems: a health practitioner's guide*. Bethesda, MD: National Institutes of Health (NIH). NIH publication 03-3769.

National Network of Libraries of Medicine. (2006). *Health literacy*. Retrieved from http://nnlm.gov/outreach/consumer/hlthlit.html

Nelson, H. D., Nygren, P., McInerney, Y., & Klein, J. (2004). Screening women and elderly adults for family and intimate partner violence: A review of the evidence for the U.S. Preventive Services Task Force. *Annals of Internal Medicine 140*(5), 387–396.

Olshansky, S. J., Passaro, D. J., Hershow, R. C., et al. (2005). A potential decline in life expectancy in the United States in the 21st century. *The New England Journal of Medicine, 352*(11), 1138–1145.

Osborne, H. (2005). *Health literacy from A to Z: Practical ways to communicate your health message*. Boston: Jones and Bartlett.

Pearson, T. A., Blair, S. N., Daniels, S. R., et al. (2002). AHA Guidelines for Primary Prevention of Cardiovascular Disease and Stroke: 2002 update. *Circulation 106,* 388–391.

Prochaska, J. O., DiClemente, C. C., & Norcross, J. C. (1992). In search of how people change. *American Psychologist, 47,* 1102–1114.

Purnell, J. Q. (2005). Obesity. In D. C. Dale & D. D. Federman (Eds.), *WebMD Scientific American Medicine*, Section 3, Chapter X. New York: WebMD.

Reitz, S.M. (2010). Promoting exercise and physical activity. In M. Scaffa, S. M. Reitz, & M. Pizzi, *Occupational therapy in the promotion of health and wellness*, pp. 225–252. Philadelphia: F.A. Davis.

Rosenwax, L. K., Semmens, J. B., & Holman, C. D. (2001). Is occupational therapy in danger of 'ad-hocery'? An application of evidence-based guidelines to the treatment of acute low back pain. *Australian Occupational Therapy Journal, 48,* 181–186.

Scaffa, M. (2001). *Occupational therapy in community-based practice settings.* Philadelphia: F.A. Davis.

Schillinger, D., Grumbach, K., Piette, J., Wang, F., Osmond, D., Daher, C., Palacios, J., Sullivan, G. D., & Bindman, A. (2002). Association of health literacy with diabetes outcomes. *Journal of the American Medical Association, 288*(4), 475–482.

Stanford University. (2006). *Chronic disease self-management program.* Retrieved from http://patienteducation.stanford.edu/programs/cdsmp.html

University of Southern California, Department of Occupational Science and Occupational Therapy. (2011). *smoking cessation and relapse prevention.* Retrieved from http://ot.usc.edu/patient-care/faculty-practice/smoking/

U.S. Department of Health and Human Services. (2000). *Healthy people 2010: Understanding and improving health.* Retrieved from http://healthdisparitiesks.org/download/Hllthy_People_2010_Improving_Health.pdf

U.S. Department of Health and Human Services. (2011). *Healthy people 2020.* Retrieved from http:// healthypeople.gov/2020/about/default.aspx

U.S. Preventive Services Task Force. (2004). Screening for Family and Intimate Partner Violence: Recommendation Statement. *American Family Physician 70*(4), 747–751.

U.S. Preventive Services Task Force. (2007). *The guide to clinical preventive services-2007: Recommendationsof the U.S. Preventive Services Task Force.* Rockville, MD: Agency for Healthcare Research and Quality.

U.S. Public Health Service. (2000). The Tobacco Use and Dependence Clinical Practice Guidelines Panel, staff and consortium representatives: A clinical practice guideline for treating tobacco use and dependence. *Journal of the American Medical Association, 283,* 3244–3254.

U.S. Public Health Service. (2001). *Surgeon general's call to action on obesity.* Washington, DC: Author.

Waddell, G., & Burton, A. K. (2001). Occupational health guidelines for the management of low back pain at work: Evidence review. *Occupational Medicine, 51*(2), 124–135.

Williams, M. V., Baker, D. W., Honig, E. G., Lee, T. M., & Nowlan, A. (1998). Inadequate literacy is a barrier to asthma knowledge and self-care. *Chest, 114,* 1008–1015.

Williams, M. V., Baker, D. W., Parker, R. M., & Nurss, J. R. (1998). Relationship of functional health literacy to patients' knowledge of their chronic disease: A study of patients with hypertension and diabetes. *Archives of Internal Medicine, 158,* 166–172.

World Health Organization. (1978). *Declaration of Alma-Ata.* Retrieved from www.who.int/hpr/NPH/docs/declaration_almaata.pdf

World Health Organization. (1986). Ottawa charter for health promotion. *Health Promotion, 1*(4), iii–v.

World Health Organization, UK Collaborating Centre. (2004). *WHO Guide to mental and neurological health in primary care.* Retrieved from http://mentalneurologicalprimarycare.org

Zapka, J. G. (2000). Commentary: On finding common ground. In B. D. Poland, L. W. Green, & I. Rootman (Eds.), *Settings for health promotion.* Thousand Oaks, CA: Sage.

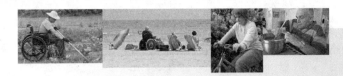

Chapter 28

Health Promotion Initiatives Within Academic Communities

Jenna Yeager, PhD, OTR/L, S. Maggie Reitz, PhD, OTR/L, FAOTA, M. Beth Merryman, PhD, OTR/L, FAOTA, and Sonia Lawson, PhD, OTR/L

The result of the educative process is capacity for further education.

—John Dewey

Learning Objectives

This chapter is designed to enable the reader to:

- Engage in community health promotion activities in partnership with local primary and secondary schools, community colleges, colleges, and universities.
- Develop community-based programs that address knowledge obtainment and skill development to assist in the selection of healthy occupations and lifestyle choices that promote well-being.
- Articulate the benefits of offering health promotion services to an academic community.

Key Terms

Academic community
Flow
Health promotion

Healthy Campus 2010: Making It Happen
Leisure ethic
Well-being

Introduction

As early as the 1930s, in an article in *Occupational Therapy and Rehabilitation,* the forerunner of the *American Journal of Occupational Therapy,* concerns were raised regarding the health and well-being of college students. In this article, Shaffer (1938) criticized colleges for commercializing college sports and abandoning the original goals of such programs, which were to enhance social and health benefits of individual student participants. Shaffer commended Johns Hopkins University's decision to make available "organized play activities to all students instead of concentrating on the development of a special skill in a very limited group" (Shaffer, 1938, p. 102). Discussions continue today regarding the appropriate role of collegiate athletics in campus life (Sperber, 1990, 2000) and access of all students to environments that promote health and well-being (American College Health Association [ACHA], 2002).

The developers of the *Jakarta Declaration on Leading Health Promotion into the 21st Century* document (World Health Organization [WHO], 1997) declare that there is clear evidence that schools and the workplace are ideal locations to provide comprehensive health promotion strategies. **Health Promotion** is defined in the *Jakarta Declaration* as "a process of enabling people to increase control over, and to improve, their health" and is considered an "essential element of health development" (WHO, 1997, p. 1). Academic communities are one of many possible settings where occupational therapy practitioners (i.e., occupational therapists and occupational therapy assistants) can become change agents, preferably within an interdisciplinary team, to meet the challenges of the *Jakarta Declaration.*

Academic occupational therapy departments have ready access to a population in need of health promotion services: the faculty, staff, and students at their home institution and the surrounding community (e.g., Campbell, Rhynders, Riley, Merryman, & Scaffa, 2010). In addition, occupational therapy faculty members have knowledge of human development and the use of occupation as a preventive and a healing tool, expertise in group process, and appreciation for issues such as transition to college life, college athletics, student drinking, and safety that can be used to significantly contribute to the health of academic communities. Occupational therapy and occupational therapy assistant faculty and their respective students can favorably impact the health and well-being of their own and other local academic communities (i.e., primary schools, secondary schools, community colleges, colleges, and universities) in many ways.

For the purposes of this chapter, an **academic community** is defined as the participants in a community that includes faculty, staff, students, and parents who have a shared focus and value of education. **Well-being** is defined as the outcome of a proactive lifestyle, which includes both active engagement in life and reflection on life choices that impact the health, safety, and welfare of self and others. Active engagement is not limited to the pursuit of physically active or challenging occupations, and the state of well-being is not precluded by the occurrence of illness or disability. Access to health information, health services, and the prerequisites to health identified by the Ottawa Charter (WHO, 1986) are, however, required to reach this state.

Four types of health promotion initiatives that can be replicated at any academic campus—with or without an occupational therapy department or major—will be described. Ideas regarding adapting these initiatives to primary and secondary educational settings as well as new avenues to consider for future program development also will be shared. Prior to describing these initiatives, two public health reports will be reviewed that provide support and a context for these and other potential initiatives directed at promoting health and well-being of faculty, staff, and students in academic communities. The initiatives to be discussed include:

- involvement with a university's Healthy Campus Task Force,
- provision of education and training services to faculty, staff, and students to promote an inclusive environment for individuals with mental illness,
- facilitation of a stroke support group, and
- development and provision of college courses.

Policy Support for Occupational Therapy Involvement in Health Promotion in Academic Communities

The U.S. government has used an interdisciplinary approach to develop policies and documents that can assist occupational therapy practitioners in developing or joining health promotion initiatives. One of these documents is *Healthy People 2020* (USDHHS/ODPHP, 2010). Many of the national health objectives identified in this document relate to academic settings along the educational continuum (i.e., primary through post-baccalaureate education). A sampling of objectives from *Healthy People 2020* (USDHHS/ODPHP, 2010) that could be the target of a health promotion initiative in an academic community is provided in Table 28-1.

Healthy Campus 2010: Making It Happen (ACHA, 2002) is a document designed to support colleges and universities as they assess the health status of their campuses in order to make informed decisions regarding priorities and interventions. This document can be instrumental in identifying possible opportunities for occupational therapy students and faculty to contribute to their community's health and well-being. Occupational therapy practitioners can be valuable additions to interdisciplinary task forces or committees seeking to improve the quality of life and well-being for students, staff, and faculty.

Data collected and reported by the ACHA through the National College Health Assessment (NCHA) can also be helpful to both programming and policy decision making. The NCHA collects

Table 28-1	Examples of Healthy People 2020 Objectives for Academic Community Interventions
Objective Number	**Objective**
AH-1	Increase the proportion of adolescents who have had a wellness checkup in the past 12 months
FP-7	Increase the proportion of sexually active persons who received reproductive health services
IID-11	Increase routine vaccination coverage levels for adolescents
IVP-34	Reduce physical fighting among adolescents
IVP-35	Reduce bullying among adolescents
MHMD-2	Reduce suicide attempts by adolescents
MHMD-3	Reduce the proportion of adolescents who engage in disordered eating behaviors in an attempt to control their weight
MICH-4	Reduce the rate of adolescent and young adult deaths
NWS-10	Reduce the proportion of children and adolescents who are considered obese
PA-1	Reduce the proportion of adults who engage in no leisure-time physical activity
PA-3	Increase the proportion of adolescents who meet current Federal physical activity guidelines for aerobic physical activity and for muscle-strengthening activity
PA-13	Increase the proportion of trips made by walking
PA-14	Increase the proportion of trips made by bicycling
SA-14	Reduce the proportion of persons engaging in binge drinking of alcoholic beverages
STD-1	Reduce the proportion of adolescents and young adults with Chlamydia trachomatis infections
STD-10	Reduce the proportion of young adults with genital herpes infection due to herpes simplex type 2
TU-3	Reduce the initiation of tobacco use among children, adolescents, and young adults
TU-15	Increase tobacco-free environments in schools, including all school facilities, property, vehicles, and school events

Adapted from: "Healthy People 2020: Topics and Objectives," by U. S. Department of Health and Human Services (n.d.a.).

data nationally on college and university students' health behaviors and perceptions on a variety of occupations, including alcohol, tobacco, other drug use, sexual intimacy, and physical activity (ACHA, 2004, ¶2).

In addition to data gathered specific to the health topics listed above, data on the perceptions of factors that impact academic success are also collected. With time to degree completion and student graduation becoming important outcome measures for colleges and universities, this data translates general health issues into real-life impacts on student achievement (ACHA, 2004).

Healthy Campus Task Force

The president of a large metropolitan university appointed a Healthy Campus Task Force during his first year in office. This team was charged with developing a comprehensive, long-term, campus-wide health plan (Towson University, 2003). Specifically, the Task Force was charged with completing an environmental scan as the basis for the development of recommendations. These recommendations were to address modifications or additions to current programs as well as strategies to improve the health and health-enhancing behaviors of students, faculty, and staff. The university health center medical director and the chairperson of the Department of Occupational Therapy and Occupational Science (DOTOS) were named task force co-chairs. This shared leadership role helped blend the perspectives of the academic and student affairs divisions, and was further augmented via the appointment of representatives from both divisions. The task force was an interdisciplinary team and included faculty as well as the police chief, safety officer, head of campus recreation, students, and other university officials. The interdisciplinary nature of the task force was one of its strengths and is a key to successful health promotion activities.

The report *Healthy Campuses: Making it Happen* (ACHA, 2002) was the foundation for the work of the task force. Each member received and reviewed a copy of the report prior to conducting the next step, the environmental scan. The task force took approximately 1 year to complete the environmental scan. The scan included documenting current university services, programs, and opportunities for students, staff, and faculty to promote their health and well-being. This process included inviting key university personnel and service providers to meet with the task force and discuss their particular unit or service. Two of these services were offered by faculty members from the DOTOS: (a) ergonomic consultations (Scaffa, Chromiak, Reitz, Blair-Newton, Murphy, & Wallis, 2010) and (b) an awareness program designed to increase others' understanding of people with mental illness (National Empowerment Center, 2010; Merryman & Uhland, 2005). The awareness program will be discussed next in this chapter.

During the fact-finding phase of the task force, the ACHA–National College Health Assessment (ACHA, 2005) survey was administered to a random sample of undergraduate students. The task force reviewed the survey data as well as reference group data from the ACHA-NCHA survey and other survey data available at the university. This data, combined with discussions and results of the year-long fact-finding process, served as the foundation for the development of the task force recommendations. The *Healthy Campus 2010* (ACHA, 2002) document was referenced frequently during the Task Force's deliberations.

Through the provision of services and participation in the *Healthy Campus Task Force*, faculty and students can directly contribute to the health and well-being of the university, and the university community gains an appreciation for the health promotion and healing powers of occupation

Promoting a More Inclusive Environment for Individuals With Psychiatric Disabilities

According to *Healthy People 2020,* mental health conditions are a result of complex interaction between social, emotional, and genetic factors (USDHHS, n.d.b). An overarching goal involves the creation of a social environment that promotes the health of all. Specific objectives address improved access to treatment for persons with mental health disorders. A reduction in stigma toward mental illness by focused education initiatives aimed at knowledge, attitudes, and behavior would support the development of an inclusive environment that promotes the health of all and facilitates treatment access by those who may otherwise avoid it (Mechanic, 2002).

Wilcock (2006) argues that occupational therapists support health beyond the individual level by intervening socially to support community and ecological well-being. According to Sinclair (2004), occupational therapists possess the skills to support community workers and individuals with disabilities to actively participate in valued activities that support occupational performance in environments of choice. In addition the *Occupational Therapy Practice Framework* (AOTA, 2008) and the *International Classification of Functioning, Disability and Health* (WHO, 2001) provide language to describe this advancement in occupational therapy service provision.

The evolution of collaboration between the Office of Disability Support Services (ODSS) and the DOTOS was sparked by an increase in students with serious mental health issues enrolling at the university. The occupational therapy faculty's knowledge of the impact of serious mental illness on healthy role execution, as well as their skills in group facilitation and active advocacy with the local National Alliance on Mental Illness (NAMI) chapter, were valued and needed. This expertise was used to assist the campus as it sought to accommodate a growing number of students with mental health needs. Of particular concern was the need for faculty and staff to develop knowledge and understanding about mental illnesses and their impact on daily life. The goal was to improve knowledge and attitudinal response toward individuals with serious mental illnesses to support a more inclusive campus community.

It is well documented that social stigma negatively impacts the recovery process of individuals with serious mental illnesses (Corrigan & Penn, 1999; Smart, 2009). When asked what they wanted most from providers, people with disabilities revealed that a sense of hopefulness and an understanding of the prejudice and discrimination that they faced were among the top priorities (Marrone, 1997). In an effort to more fully understand the challenges that individuals with mental illnesses face, a consumer advocacy group called the National Empowerment Center offers an educational kit that involves participants experiencing simulated auditory hallucinations (Deegan, 1992). This experience, called *Hearing Voices That Are Distressing,* has been adopted by faculty from the DOTOS and the Towson University ODSS as a key component of an education and training opportunity to make the campus more inclusive for individuals with disabilities that involve hearing voices.

Participants use an individual headset with a cassette tape reflecting content typical of what individuals who hear voices experience. The tapes have been made by people who actually experience auditory hallucinations (i.e., hear voices). While the tape is playing, participants visit four stations and are asked to perform tasks typical of that setting. These stations include a psychiatric day hospital task room, a hospital emergency room, a vocational testing center, and the broader campus.

At the end of the visits to the four stations, participants are asked to discuss the experience. This facilitated discussion includes, when possible, an individual or family member of an individual who is a consumer of mental health services. Having a first-person account during the discussion reinforces the philosophy of inclusion and empowerment by having people speak for themselves. It also supports the work of Kolodzei and Johnson (1996), who found that interpersonal contact between students and people with mental illness was associated with improved attitudes toward persons with mental disorders. The facilitation aspect encourages participants to reflect on their own struggles and use of coping skills during the activity and share observations in a structured group setting that encourages potential applications to daily life.

A mixed methods study was conducted to assess effects of this simulation experience on students' understanding of mental illness (Merryman, 2010). Students completed a pretest including the Mental Illness Disorder Understanding Scale (MIDUS) developed by Tanaka (2003) prior to the exercise and again at the end of the semester. In addition, student qualitative comments during the debriefing and at the end of the semester were systematically collected and analyzed. T-test results were statistically significant on two of three factors. These were that mental illness was treatable and that medications were effective. Student qualitative comments revealed a new awareness of the challenges that hearing voices presents in daily life.

The training has involved a variety of student groups from various disciplines, faculty, counseling center staff, and campus police. Students often comment that it is the most powerful aspect of their mental health course experiences. Staff members have commented on the value of the experience to broaden their understanding of the challenges students face in navigating the campus and fulfilling their student roles (Merryman & Uhland, 2005). According to Baum and Baptiste (2002), occupational therapy practitioners are reframing practice by intervening beyond the individual level to impact communities through attention to the environment and contextual factors that support or impede social participation. An intervention that promotes knowledge and understanding of a marginalized population supports a more inclusive atmosphere for all. In this manner, such an intervention promotes community health and occupational justice (Wilcock, 1998, 2003, 2006; Wilcock & Whiteford, 2003).

Stroke Support Group

Health promotion programs for stroke survivors and their caregivers, such as support groups, are frequently offered through a health care facility or health system. These programs may or may not open their programs to members of the immediate community. Community-based health promotion programs that target individuals who have disabilities, such as stroke, and their families can be offered through academic institutions as well.

Academic campuses that have health-related majors are in an excellent position to offer a community support group for stroke survivors and their caregivers. There are several benefits of this type of program for students, stroke survivors, and caregivers. Students benefit from the opportunities to interact with stroke survivors and caregivers and to develop and deliver presentations on health-related topics, such as yoga for relaxation or driving after a stroke. This enables the students to develop their presentation skills and also benefits the stroke survivor in gaining valuable information to optimize participation in health-promoting activities.

Stroke survivors benefit from an academic institution–based support group as they are able to engage with stroke survivors who have received services from varying rehabilitation facilities; receive unbiased valuable information on community resources in the area that are not associated with a particular health care system; and participate in activities held during the meetings with the extra support of students and faculty who lead the group. Another benefit that stroke survivors receive is current information related to research studies in which the survivor may participate to gain additional physical or speech-related rehabilitation. Many academic institutions have access to this kind of information, perhaps more readily than programs offered in non-academic settings.

Caregivers of stroke survivors, a group that typically is not targeted for support group intervention, benefit from a community-based support group located within an academic institution. Studies have shown that caregivers report fewer negative feelings and believe they gain valuable information and support the more support group sessions they attend (Brereton, Carroll, & Barnston, 2007; Franzen-Dahlin, Larson, Murray, Wredling, & Billing, 2008). For caregivers, support groups can be a primary prevention strategy, helping them cope with emotions by sharing with other caregivers and obtaining information that can help relieve the stress associated with caring for a stroke survivor.

When planning a support group to be offered on an academic campus, faculty, student, and space resources are important considerations. Faculty members in health-related disciplines are ideal candidates to target to serve as leaders of the support group; however, this additional responsibility would need to be evaluated for its impact on the faculty member's workload. In addition, due to the typical semester organization of classes on academic campuses, there may be breaks in the meeting schedule that can impact the continuity of the group and group process. Care should be taken to have some kind of "bridge" activity during semester breaks. Classroom or meeting room space must be allocated for the group meetings, and this space must be fully accessible. With the changing course schedules from semester to semester, finding a permanent meeting space may prove difficult.

The Stroke Survivors Group at Towson University has been in existence for approximately 8 years with 10–20 participants in attendance for each monthly meeting. The group was initially co-led by faculty from nursing and speech language pathology with a faculty member from occupational therapy added in the second year. More recently, the group has been lead by faculty from occupational therapy and speech language pathology.

The Stroke Survivors Group runs during the fall and spring semesters with a break over the summer. Because participants verbalized their desire to continue meetings over the summer, a summer activity-based meeting is planned, with the participants taking the lead for planning this event. This summer event serves as a bridge between the spring and fall semester meetings. A database of participants and their contact information is kept by one of the faculty leaders. Students from the academic disciplines mentioned assist in maintaining the database and sending out information about meeting times, topics, and announcements.

Both participants and students have reported enjoying and benefitting from their experiences attending the group meetings. Because students are required to assist participants as needed, help set up materials for meetings, and reflect on their experiences, they become deeply engaged, and this promotes future professional activities of this type. Participants enjoy engaging with the students and assisting them in their learning. It proves to be a very meaningful activity for the participants, and they take their role as educators very seriously. Many participants are very willing to participate in classroom activities to help train future health professionals.

Overall, academic campuses provide an excellent environment to offer community-based support groups for stroke survivors and for individuals with other types of disabilities. It provides a wonderful learning opportunity for all involved: faculty, students, stroke survivors, and their caregivers.

General Education/Core Curriculum Courses

Occupational therapy faculty and graduate students possess the expertise to develop and provide undergraduate courses that focus on prevention and health promotion using an occupation-based approach. Learning activities from one of three courses offered by an academic occupational therapy department will be described. The course was approved as meeting the university's General Education Requirements, which were "designed to help students gain the essential intellectual skills and knowledge that will be important throughout life" (Towson University, 2010, p. 4).

Offering college courses to address students' health, quality of life, and academic success is consistent with occupational therapy practice as described in the *Occupational Therapy Practice Framework: Domain and Process [Framework]* (American Occupational Therapy Association [AOTA], 2008). Course content is directly related to instrumental activities of daily living (IADL) categories of health management and maintenance, care of others, and child rearing (AOTA, 2008). As noted in the *Framework* (AOTA, 2008), health promotion and other health care service provision must be considered in relation to contextual features, such as health care advances, societal beliefs, cultural factors, and financial constraints. Accordingly, these university courses provide an enhanced awareness of health care contexts and issues in order to enhance students' abilities to make informed decisions regarding health promotion activities, which is a component of health management and health maintenance.

Leisure and Health Course: Overview

This 100-level course targets first- and second-year undergraduate students as they transition to university life, a time when they leave family and old friends and activities and acquire new occupations and habits (Towson, 2011). This course is marketed to students who are not occupational therapy majors. Sometimes students who take the course decide to switch their major to pre-occupational therapy. After a review of the history and philosophy of leisure and leisure studies, the course addresses health promotion via content related to healthy (e.g., moderate physical activity) and unhealthy (e.g., unsafe sexual activity, substance use and abuse) habits of this population, as indicated by national surveillance data. The role of leisure in promoting health and well-being across the life span is discussed and reinforced throughout the course. Examples of course topics include leisure theories, health behaviors, consumerism, and leisure occupations.

Leisure and Health Course: Philosophical and Theoretical Foundation

Teaching methodologies for this course are consistent with the occupational therapy principle of learning through activity engagement (Fidler & Fidler, 1978; Wilcock, 1998). The course is based on the importance and value of a leisure ethic (Kelly, 1982), Csikszentmihayli's construct and theory of flow (Csikszentmihayli, 1990), the Model of Human Occupation (MOHO) developed by Kielhofner and Burke (Kielhofner, 2002; Kielhofner & Burke, 1980; Rosenfeld, 1993), and the Health Belief Model, a health behavior model (Becker, 1974; Rosenstock, Strecher, & Becker, 1994). Constructs from social norms theory (Perkins, 2003) also have been incorporated into the theoretical base of the course.

A primary goal of the course is the facilitation of the development of a healthy leisure ethic and engagement in healthy leisure occupations. The term **leisure ethic** has been described by Kelly as "the process of stressing the quality of life's experience and environment rather than occupational prestige" (1982, p. 10). It is noted that social and internal pressures to pursue power or financial success may result in the abandonment of the value of leisure to enhance quality of life. Accordingly, the course invites students to engage in reflection and discussion regarding the influence of values on lifestyle choice, with an emphasis on the health benefits of an occupationally balanced life (Wilcock, 1998, 2006).

Flow Theory

Csikszentmihayli (1990) articulated an inherent quality of leisure activities, flow, that renders health benefits in various dimensions of wellness. **Flow** is defined as the way in which people "describe their state of mind when consciousness is harmoniously ordered, and they want to pursue whatever they are doing for its own sake" (Csikszentmihayli, 1990, p. 6). Although flow can be reached through engagement in a physical activity, it also can be experienced when playing an instrument, when writing a poem, or through participating in a variety of other skilled leisure or work occupations (Godbey, 1994). This notion is useful in the college classroom as a means of expanding students' awareness of the benefits associated with participation in creative and expressive activities in addition to the more commonly acknowledged health benefits gained through physical activities.

Model of Human Occupation (MOHO)

The *Leisure and Health* course is conceptualized as an avenue to favorably impact the volitional and habituation subsystems described in the MOHO by improving the performance subsystem through enhanced knowledge and skills. It is theorized that a solid foundation for a lifetime of healthy leisure choices, including a balance of physical, social, creative, and reflective occupations, will be established by enhancing the performance subsystem through experiential learning. The rationale behind this assertion is that "volition is reflected in the wide range of thoughts and feelings people have about the things they have done, are doing, or might do" (Kielhofner, 2002, p. 15). Experiential activities and assignments in this course promote student reflection regarding values and interests as well as the resultant choices that impact health and future health through patterns reflected in the habituation subsystem.

Health Belief Model

The Health Belief Model (see Chapter 3 of this text for an introduction to this model) was used to provide the basis for the delivery of health education to maximize adoption or continuation of health screening habits, such as testicular and breast self-examination. These habits were targeted due to the students' average age and recommended age-appropriate health screenings. Age-specific health screenings for later life span periods are also identified.

Peer educators are used to provide course sessions on topics including healthy eating habits, alcohol abuse, and safer sex practices. A novel use of campus resources was illustrated via the involvement of the social action campus theater group to provide theater-based experiential class activities. Student actors perform scenarios pertaining to health issues, such as date rape, eating disorders, and suicide. These scenarios are followed by interactive class discussion exploring perspectives of the various portrayed characters.

Leisure and Health Course: Assignments

Course assignments are designed to engage students in experiential learning. The goal of the assignments is to establish habits consistent with healthy living. Examples of such assignments include the Activity Analysis and Leisure History and Plan.

Fundamental principles of occupational therapy (Fidler & Fidler, 1978; Ludwig, 1993) are evident in the Activity Analysis assignment. Students are required to select two leisure occupations in which to engage for purposes of analysis, one on a favorite familiar activity and one on a new activity. Invoking the notion that positive gains arise from engagement in creative and expressive pursuits as well as physical activities, students are urged to try something new as a means of expanding the repertoire of occupations available for their health and leisure engagement. A structure is provided to assist them in articulating aspects of activity engagement that typically remain tacit. The analysis includes a description of the preparation needed, materials, and costs of the activity. Potential and existing barriers are identified, as well as health benefits and risks of the activity.

Deconstructing their favorite activities provides students with an opportunity to identify the healthy and unhealthy aspects of their own leisure engagement. Furthermore, some students use the assignment as a catalyst to engage in an activity that they "have always wanted to try." For example, students often use the assignment as incentive to "work out" in campus recreational facilities, or attempt a novel activity such as meditation. Students are encouraged to involve friends in these activities, and they often report interest in the assignment among their peers.

In this way, course activities have the potential to make an impact on the health of students beyond those enrolled in the course.

The Leisure History and Plan is a culminating paper, which requires the integration and application of principles learned. In this assignment, students describe their history of leisure and detail a plan for future health-promoting leisure activities. Students engage in a developmental analysis of their occupational engagement since birth, identifying factors that contribute to their current pattern of healthy and unhealthy habits. Integrating constructs gained throughout the course, students devise a plan for leisure that incorporates principles of health promotion and demonstrates an increased awareness of the health risks and health benefits associated with leisure and other occupations.

Leisure and Health Course: Assessment

Student course evaluations have been used through the years to assess and adjust course delivery and content. The course has been offered for more than 30 years, and since that time there has been a long-standing positive trend in qualitative and quantitative student feedback for this course (Reitz, 1994; Reitz & Castaneda, 1995). A total of 699 students took the course from fall 2005 through spring 2010. Student course evaluations were examined for this time period; the mean overall score was 4.52 on a 5-point scale, with 5 being "excellent." Student comments frequently reflect interest in the material and appreciation of experiential and personally relevant activities. A representative comment was made by one student who noted that the course was fun, interesting, and "made a difference in my life." Other comments included, "all the information was relevant," "[I] learned about society and myself at the same time," and "good class to take in college; had a lot of valuable information that could actually be used."

Additionally, students' integration and application of course content to their individual health development is assessed in the culminating assignment, the Leisure History and Plan, described earlier. The engaging nature of class activities and the personal relevance of topics addressed create a context where students actively participate to apply constructs learned to personal lifestyle redesign.

Thus, the course offers a unique opportunity for occupational therapy practitioners to engage in health promotion with college students.

With the exception of the course evaluation process described above, no formal evaluation or long-term follow-up on the impact of this course has been conducted. However, the work of Dermody, Volkins, and Heater (1996) and Hilton, Ackermann, and Smith (2011) may serve as a model for future research into the impact of *Leisure and Health* and other such courses. Dermody et al. investigated the impact of instruction during a course addressing health promotion, prevention, and occupation as a health promotion tool for a group of occupational therapy graduate students. Results indicated that occupation-based health promotion instruction appears to broaden students' perceptions of health promotion and the power of occupation to enhance health and well-being. In addition, the researchers concluded that study participants had achieved perspective transformation, which is a step in behavior change.

Hilton et al. explored the outcomes of a wellness assignment provided to 58 undergraduate occupational science students. The goal of the assignment was to instill healthy habits, while the objective of the study was to determine the barriers and supports for students' success with the assignment. Follow-up data was collected 6 months and 1 year after completion of the course assignment. Continued engagement in healthy habit goals appeared to be sustained, with 86% of the students still working "on at least one goal and almost half still working on two goals a year after completion of the course" (Hilton et al., 2011, p. 70).

Leisure and Health Course: Replicability

This course has been easily adapted for various formats of delivery, suggesting a wider application to other academic communities and community settings. Although originally taught in a traditional semester structure, the course has successfully been offered once a week for a 3-hour time block, as well as in a 7-week format over summer. Therefore, the course serves as a potential model for the development of Leisure and Health Workshops that could be targeted for populations such as teens or elders in community settings.

In addition, it may be taught at a community college as a non-credit life enrichment course or a for-credit health course. Many of the assignments also can be adapted for use in middle and high school courses or programs.

Conclusion

Occupational therapy practitioners can enhance personal health and healing for individuals and groups within academic communities. While occupational therapy practitioners may be most familiar with occupational therapy service delivery in the primary school setting, occupational therapy health promotion interventions also can be delivered at community colleges, colleges, and universities. The populations served in these settings can greatly benefit from occupation-based health education initiatives to influence choices of life habits and activity patterns. These benefits can be achieved through a variety of recommendations and programs, such as pedestrian safety for grade school students, backpack awareness programs (Jacobs et al., 2010), advocating for appropriate size and type of classroom furniture (Wingrat & Exner, 2005a, 2005b), dating etiquette for middle school students, and healthy transitions to university life. Programs can be aimed at healthy individuals and groups or individuals with a specific diagnosis. One such program that focuses on the needs of college students with depression, anxiety, and other similar disorders, *Lifestyle Redesign® for the College Student and the Student Veterans*, is offered through the faculty practice at the Department of Occupational Therapy and Occupational Science, University of Southern California (n.d.).

While access to academic settings may be easier for faculty or future practitioners while in their student roles, it does not need to be the exclusive domain of faculty and students. Practitioners with expertise in population-based or community-based practice have the potential to offer occupation-based health promotion services to academic communities in their local area, whether or not those settings offer occupational therapy degree programs.

Learning Activities

1. Determine, through an investigation of campus resources, the persons on your campus who are responsible for monitoring and facilitating a healthy campus environment. Request a meeting to collect data on an area of health that you are concerned about (e.g., current rates of suicides, accidents/injuries, hate crimes) and information about current programming to reduce those rates. Write a thank-you letter including any suggestions you have for the potential contribution of occupational therapy faculty and students to enhance the academic community through current or additional programs.

2. Review the course catalog at your college or university. Write a course description for a possible new elective course that could be developed and taught by occupational therapy or occupational science faculty.

3. Request an appointment with a member of the campus police to discuss the possible replication of the *Hearing Voices That Are Distressing* program. Before your meeting, develop a one-page fact sheet explaining the program.

Acknowledgment: *The authors would like to thank Stacey Schilling, Shira N. Zapinsky, and Hollie Hatt for their assistance with this manuscript while they were occupational therapy graduate students at Towson University.*

REFERENCES

American College Health Association. (2002). *Healthy campus 2010: Making it happen.* Baltimore: Author.

American College Health Association. (2004). *ACHA-National College Health Assessment.* Retrieved from http://acha.org/projects_programs/assessment.cfm

American College Health Association. (2005). *ACHA: National College Health Assessment.* Retrieved from http://acha.org/projects_programs/ncha_background.cfm

American Occupational Therapy Association. (2008). Occupational therapy practice framework: Domain and process (2nd ed.). *American Journal of Occupational Therapy, 62,* 625–683.

Baum, C., & Baptiste, S. (2002). Reframing occupational therapy practice. In M. Law, C. Baum, & S. Baptiste (Eds.), *Occupation-based practice: Fostering performance and participation* (pp. 3–15). Thorofare, NJ: SLACK.

Becker, M. (Ed.). (1974). *The health belief model and personal health behavior*. Thorofare, NJ: SLACK.

Brereton, L., Carroll, C., & Barnston, S. (2007). Interventions for adult family carers of people who have had a stroke: A systematic review. *Clinical Rehabilitation, 21,* 867–884.

Campbell, R. M., Rynders, P. A., Riley, M., Merryman, M. B., & Scaffa, M. E. (2010). Educating practitioners for health promotion practice. In M. E. Scaffa, S. M. Reitz, & M.A. Pizzi (Eds.), *Occupational therapy in the promotion of health and wellness* (pp. 512–527). Philadelphia: F.A. Davis.

Corrigan, P. W., & Penn, D. L. (1999). Lessons from social psychology on discrediting psychiatric stigma. *American Psychologist, 54*(9), 765–776.

Csikszentmihayli, M. (1990). *Flow: The psychology of optimal performance*. New York: Harper and Row.

Deegan, P. (1992). *Instructor's guide to the training and simulated experience of hearing voices that are distressing*. Lawrence, MA: National Empowerment Center.

Dermody, J. L., Volkens, P. P., & Heater, S. L. (1996). Occupational therapy students' perspectives on occupations as an agent that promotes healthful lifestyles. *American Journal of Occupational Therapy, 50*(10), 835–841.

Fidler, G., & Fidler, J. W. (1978). Doing and becoming: Purposeful action and self-actualization. *American Journal of Occupational Therapy, 32*(5), 305–310.

Franzen-Dahlin, A., Larson, J., Murray, V., Wredling, R., & Billing, E. (2008). A randomized controlled trial evaluating the effect of a support and education programme for spouses of people affected by stroke. *Clinical Rehabilitation, 22,* 722–730.

Godbey, G. (1994). *Leisure in your life: An exploration* (4th ed.). State College, PA: Venture.

Hilton, C. L., Ackermann, A. A., & Smith, D. L. (2011). Healthy habit changes in pre-professional college students: Adherence, supports, and barriers. *OTJR: Occupation, Participation, and Health, 31*(2), 64–72.

Jacobs, K., Sanders, M. J., Dapito, D., Flores, A., Hellman, M., Markowitz, J., Wuest, E.,...Trowbridge, N. (2010, July 26). Backpack awareness across the lifespan. *OT Practice, 15*(13), 15–18.

Kelly, J. (1982). *Leisure*. Englewood Cliffs, NJ: Prentice-Hall.

Kielhofner, G. (2002). Introduction to the model of human occupation. In *Model of human occupation* (3rd ed., pp. 1–9). Baltimore: Lippincott Williams & Wilkins.

Kielhofner, G., & Burke, J. (1980). A model of human occupation: Part 1 conceptual framework and content. *American Journal of Occupational Therapy, 34*(9), 572–581.

Kolodzei, M. E., & Johnson, B. T. (1996). Interpersonal contact and acceptance of persons with psychiatric disorders: A research synthesis. *Journal of Consulting and Clinical Psychology, 64,* 1387–1396.

Lawson, S., Johnson, I., & Lee, L. (2004, November). *Stroke survivors and health professions education: A service learning project*. Poster presented at the Maryland Occupational Therapy Association Annual Conference, Catonsville, MD.

Ludwig, F. M. (1993). Gail Fidler. In R. J. Miller & K. F. Walker (Eds.), *Perspective on theory for the practice of occupational therapy* (pp. 17–40). Gaithersburg, MD: Aspen.

Marrone, J. (1997, May 21). *Job placement for individuals with psychiatric disabilities*. Presented at the Utah State Office of Rehabilitation, 75th Anniversary Conference, Provo, UT.

Mechanic, D. (2002). Removing barriers to care among persons with psychiatric symptoms. *Health Affairs, 21,* 137–147.

Merryman, M. B. (2010). Effects of simulated learning and facilitated debriefing on student understanding of mental illness. *Occupational Therapy in Mental Health, 26,* 18–31.

Merryman, M., & Uhland, R. (2005, April 1). *Virtual voices: A simulated experience of the distressing symptoms of hearing voices*. Paper presented at the Lilly Conference on College and University Teaching: East. Towson, MD.

National Empowerment Center. (2010). *National Empowerment Center store: Hearing voices curriculum*. Retrieved from http://power2u.org/mm5/merchant.mvc?Screen=PROD&Store_Code=NEC&Product_Code=Curricula-HearingVoicesDistressing&Category_Code=hearingvoices

Perkins, H. W. (2003). *The social norms approach to preventing school and college substance abuse: A handbook for educators, counselors, and clinicians*. San Francisco: Jossey-Bass.

Reitz, S. M. (1994, July 10). *Facilitating wellness in the university community*. Paper presented at the CAN-AM 1994 Joint Conference of the Canadian Association of Occupational Therapists and the American Occupational Therapy Association, Boston.

Reitz, S. M., & Castaneda, R. (1995, March 17). *Facilitating a leisure ethic in university students*. Paper presented at the Therapeutic Activities and Leisure Skills 13th Annual Conference, Philadelphia.

Rosenfeld, M. (1993). *Wellness and lifestyle renewal*. Rockville, MD: American Occupational Therapy Association.

Rosenstock, I. M., Strecher, V. J., & Becker, M. H. (1994). The health belief model and HIV risk behavior change. In R. J. DiClemente & J. L. Peterson (Eds.), *Preventing AIDS: Theories and methods for behavioral interventions* (pp. 5–24). New York: Plenum Press.

Scaffa, M. E., Chromiak, S. B., Reitz, S. M., Blair-Newton, A., Murphy, L., & Wallis, C. B. (2010). Unintentional injury and violence prevention. In M. E. Scaffa, S. M. Reitz, & M.A. Pizzi (Eds), *Occupational therapy in the promotion of health and wellness* (pp. 350–375). Philadelphia: F.A. Davis.

Shaffer, G. W. (1938). Recreation as a preventive and therapy for social maladjustments. *Occupational Therapy and Rehabilitation, 17*(2), 97–106.

Sinclair, K. (2004). International perspectives on occupation and participation. *WFOT Bulletin, 50,* 5–8.

Smart, J. (2009). *Disability, society, and the individual* (2nd ed.). Austin, TX: Pro-Ed.

Sperber, M. (1990). *College sports inc.: The athletic department vs. the university*. New York: Henry Holt.

Sperber, M. (2000). *Beer and circus.* New York, NY: Henry Holt.

Tanaka, N. (2003). Development of the mental illness and disorder understanding scale. *International Journal of Japanese Sociology, 12,* 95–107.

Towson University. (2003, December 1). *University senate minutes.* Retrieved from http://new.towson.edu/senate/minutes/2003-12-1.html

Towson University. (2010). *Undergraduate catalog, 2010–2011.* Towson, MD: Author.

Towson University, Department of Occupational Therapy. (2011, Spring). *OCTH 103: Leisure and health* [syllabi]. Towson, MD: Author.

University of Southern California, Department of Occupational Therapy & Occupational Science. (n.d.) *Lifestyle redesign® for the college student and student veterans.* Retrieved from http://ot.usc.edu/patient-care/faculty-practice/lr-for-the-college-student/

U.S. Department of Health and Human Services. (n.d.a). *Healthy People 2020: Topics and objectives.* Retrieved from http://healthypeople.gov/2020/topicsobjectives2020/default.aspx

U.S. Department of Health and Human Services. (n.d.b). *Mental health and mental disorders.* Retrieved from http://healthypeople.gov/2020/TopicsObjectives2020/overview.aspx?topicid=28

U.S. Department of Health and Human Services, Office of Disease Prevention and Health Promotion. (2010). *Healthy People 2020* [ODPHP Publication No. B0132]. [Brochure] Retrieved from http://healthypeople.gov/2020/TopicsObjectives2020/pdfs/HP2020_brochure.pdf

U.S. Department of Health and Human Services, Office of Disease Prevention and Health Promotion. (n.d.b). *Mental health and mental disorders.* Retrieved from http://www.healthypeople.gov/2020/TopicsObjectives2020/overview.aspx?topicid=28

Wilcock, A. A. (1998). Reflections on doing, being and becoming. *Canadian Journal of Occupational Therapy, 65,* 248–256.

Wilcock, A. A. (2003). Occupational therapy practice: Section II population interventions focused on health for all. In E. B. Crepeau, E. S. Cohn, & B. A. Schell (Eds.), *Willard & Spackman's occupational therapy* (10th ed., pp. 30–45). Philadelphia: Lippincott, Williams & Wilkins.

Wilcock, A. A. (2006). *An occupational perspective of health* (2nd ed.). Thorofare, NJ: SLACK.

Wilcock, A., & Whiteford, G. (2003). Occupation, health promotion, and the environment. In L. Letts, P. Rigby, & D. Stewart (Eds.), *Using environments to enable occupational performance* (pp. 55–70). Thorofare, NJ: SLACK.

Wingrat, J. K., & Exner, C. (2005a, May). *Classroom furniture and performance: How furniture size affects task and sitting behaviors.* Poster session presented at the annual conference of the American Occupational Therapy Association, Long Beach, CA.

Wingrat, J. K., & Exner, C. E. (2005b). The impact of school furniture on fourth grade children's on-task and sitting behavior in the classroom: A pilot study. *WORK: A Journal of Assessment, Prevention, and Rehabilitation, 25*(3), 263–272.

World Health Organization. (1986). *Ottawa charter for health promotion.* Retrieved December 4, 2004, from http://who.int/hpr/NPH/docs/ottawa_charter_hp.pdf

World Health Organization. (1997). *Jakarta declaration on leading health promotion into the 21st century.* Retrieved from www.who.int/hpr/NPH/docs/jakarta_declaration_en.pdf

World Health Organization. (2001). *The international classification of functioning, disability, and health.* Geneva, Switzerland: Author.

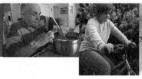
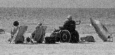
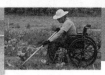

Looking Ahead

Chapter 29

Future Directions in Community-Based Practice

Marjorie E. Scaffa, PhD, OTR/L, FAOTA, Erin Guillory Caraway, MS, OTR, and Shun Takehara, OTR

What we see depends on how we look.
—Capra and Steindl-Rast (1991)
Only people who see the big picture ... are the ones who step out of the frame.
—S. Rushdie (1999, p. 43)

Learning Objectives

This chapter is designed to enable the reader to:
- Discuss the principles of futurist thinking.
- Describe the characteristics of an ecological worldview, applying it to community-based practice.
- Identify strategies that occupational therapy practitioners can use to develop ideas for community-based practice.
- Describe the role of occupational therapy in emerging community-based practice areas.
- Discuss potential curricular and fieldwork options for teaching community-based practice concepts.
- Describe the role of community-based participatory action research in occupational therapy practice and scholarship.

Key Terms

Community-based participatory action research (CBPAR)
Community service learning (CSL)
Ecological worldview
Innovation
Integration
Mixed methods research

Obesity
Occupational justice
Self-assertion
Telehealth
Telerehabilitation
Transition services

Introduction

In ancient Greece and Rome, an oracle was a place where, or a medium by which, deities were consulted for advice or prophecy about the future. The modern futurist movement, which began in the 1960s, was fueled by the desire to understand and shape the future and is guided by three basic principles (Cornish, 1980). The first principle, or conviction, is the unity or interrelatedness of reality. It is the perception that the whole is greater than the sum of its parts, an insistence on the interconnectedness of everything in the universe (Cornish, 1980).

The second principle that directs futurist thinking is the crucial importance of time. The world of the future is shaped by the decisions made today and the determinations made in the past (Cornish, 1980). Futurists believe that almost anything can be accomplished in a period of 20 years.

The third principle on which futurists rely is the importance and power of ideas, particularly ideas about the future. The future is created out of ideas, the tools of thought. Without them, change is not possible. Futurists believe that human achievement is constrained more by conceptual restrictions or limitations in our ideas than by our access to material resources (Cornish, 1980).

Some advocate that the profession should re-create or re-invent itself. However, this is not the only available choice of action. An alternative is to embrace a vision that incorporates the fundamental principles of the profession, with its focus on occupation and one that expands the scope of practice to include populations not typically served in settings not commonly utilized. The profession would not be where it is today if it had not survived the challenges of the past century. Thus, it is not possible or desirable to discard what has been part of the profession's heritage.

Some predictions can be made about the future of occupational therapy based on current trends. The following statements reflect the authors' beliefs regarding the future of occupational therapy and are offered as "food for thought." We anticipate:

- An increased role for occupational therapy in prevention and health promotion
- A significant shift in services from medical institutions to decentralized, coordinated, community-based settings
- An increased focus on the consumer as the driving force in health care
- Changing demographics, including increased cultural diversity of the population, requiring a need for increased cultural competence among practitioners
- Increased numbers of elderly with a full range of health, illness, and disability
- Health care reform that includes increased emphasis on mental health and quality of life
- A developing role for occupational therapy in preventing and addressing social problems such as violence, crime, and alcohol and drug abuse

What occupational therapy needs most to move forward in the 21st century are creative ideas and thoughtful decisions put into action. Only in this way can the profession fulfill its destiny as "health agent" (Finn, 1972), enhance community health, and facilitate "community occupational development" (Bockhoven, 1968).

An Ecological Worldview

To become health agents, occupational therapy practitioners must make a paradigm shift from a holistic perspective to an **ecological worldview.** "An ecological worldview is holistic, but it's more than that. It looks not only at something as a whole, but also how this whole is embedded into larger wholes" (Capra & Steindl-Rast, 1991, p. 69). Ecological awareness recognizes the interrelatedness and interdependence of all phenomena.

The root of the word "ecological" comes from the Greek "oikos," which means house. In a broader context, it refers to "the inhabited world, the house of humanity" (Capra & Steindl-Rast, 1991, p. 70). The house of humanity includes the biological, psychological, and spiritual aspects of life embedded in a physical, social, and cultural reality. The shift to an ecological paradigm reflects not only a change in thinking but also a change in values. Overall, the shift in values is characterized by a shift from self-assertion to integration (Capra & Steindl-Rast, 1991). **Self-assertion** is a living system's tendency toward domination in an effort to preserve and protect itself, while **integration** is the tendency to partner with other systems in order to fulfill the greater good. Table 29-1 provides a synopsis of the changes in values required by the ecological paradigm.

Table 29-1	Change in Paradigm, Change in Values
From a Holistic Perspective With an Emphasis on	**To an Ecological Paradigm With an Emphasis on**
Self-assertion	Integration
Rational thought	Intuitiveness
Analysis	Synthesis
Competition	Cooperation
Expansion	Conservation
Quantity	Quality
Domination	Partnership
Individuality	Community

Self-assertion is not completely lost in the ecological paradigm because it is essential for survival. However, left unchecked, self-assertion can become destructive, evidenced by the variety of community health problems experienced today, such as violence, poverty, racism, homelessness, substance abuse, and destruction of the environment. Self-assertion must be tempered with integration to be useful and healthy. Koestler (1978) speaks of this dichotomy as the *Janus* nature. A living system is an integrated whole that asserts itself to protect its individuality. However, as part of a larger whole, the living system is required to integrate itself into the larger system. According to Capra and Steindl-Rast (1991), "it is important to realize that those are opposite and contradictory tendencies. We need a dynamic balance between them, and that's essential for physical and mental health" (p. 74).

Creating Opportunities in the Community

To develop creative ideas for community-based practice, one must simply be observant, open-minded, and reflective. Opportunities are abundant, but one must know *where* to look and *how* to see potential. Getting to know the community and becoming involved in community affairs are necessary first steps. Volunteering one's time and talents begins the networking process. Communities typically have a variety of groups, organizations, and agencies that need volunteers and may be potential recipients of occupational therapy services.

To be successful in community-based practice settings, practitioners must see themselves providing a wide range of interventions. Direct service to individuals is only a small part of what occupational therapy has to offer. In community-based practice, the client is often not an individual but rather a group, organization, agency, or collective. Potential interventions may include case management, training, consulting, program coordination, policy development, and advocacy. These levels of intervention and their strategies and goals are described in Table 29-2.

Effective community-based interventions share some characteristics in common with effective occupational therapy interventions for individuals. Both are client-centered, involve the recipient of services in the planning and implementation of the intervention, utilize existing environmental resources, and prepare clients to become self-managers and self-advocates. Occupational therapy practitioners can learn much from the professional literature in health education

Table 29-2	Strategies, Goals, and Levels of Occupational Therapy Intervention		
Intervention Type	**Strategy or Process**	**Goals/Outcomes**	**Target/Level**
Direct service	Providing occupational therapy intervention	Improved occupational performance	Individual
Counseling	Helping people learn how to achieve personal goals, resolve problems, make decisions, or change behaviors	Goal attainment, healthy behaviors, empowerment	Individual, interpersonal
Case management	Coordinating care plans	Improved client outcomes, comprehensive, coordinated care	Individual, interpersonal, organizational

Continued

Table 29-2 Strategies, Goals, and Levels of Occupational Therapy Intervention—cont'd

Intervention Type	Strategy or Process	Goals/Outcomes	Target/Level
Education	Providing information and employing the methods, strategies, and tools that facilitate learning	Positive change in knowledge, attitude, or behavior	Individual, interpersonal, organizational, societal/community, governmental/policy
Training	Providing information to enhance a skill or process	Competence in targeted skills, processes, techniques	Individual, interpersonal, organizational
Consulting	Using the knowledge and experience of an "expert" to help a person or organizational leaders make better decisions or deal more effectively with situations	Problem solving in area of concern	Individual, interpersonal, organizational, societal/community, governmental/policy
Program development	Assessing the need for, planning, and evaluating programs and services	Improved services/care for target population	Organizational, societal/community
Program coordination	Managing the resources (e.g., staff, materials, space, finances, etc.) to accomplish the objectives of a program	Effective and efficient use of resources	Organizational, societal/community, governmental/policy
Policy development	Formulating rules, laws, policies, procedures	Laws, rules, policies, and procedures that are favorable to area of concern	Governmental/policy
Advocacy	Using the power of persuasion to alter public opinion and mobilize resources in favor of a policy or issue	Favorable change in policies, regulations, resource allocation	Organizational, societal/community, governmental/policy
Research	Building knowledge through systematic study	Improved practice, evidence-based practice	Organizational, governmental/policy

Data from: Washington University Community Practice Model.

and public health regarding the design and implementation of community health interventions. Basic principles of effective community interventions are listed in Box 29-1.

Innovative Ideas Put Into Action

Occupational therapy practitioners have begun to put some innovative ideas into action. These ideas and

actions expand the scope of practice. Each of these examples, taken from recent literature, is described briefly. Some involve expansion of professional roles, some include populations not typically served, and others describe practice in settings not typically utilized.

Transition Services for Youth With Disabilities

The Individuals With Disabilities Education Act (IDEA) of 2004 requires schools to provide

Box 29-1	Principles of Effective Community Interventions

- Tailor to a specific population within a particular setting.
- Involve the participants in planning, implementation, and evaluation.
- Integrate efforts aimed at changing individuals, social and physical environments, communities, and policies.
- Link participants' concerns about health to broader life concerns and to a vision of a better society.
- Use existing resources within the environment.
- Build on strengths found among participants and their social networks and communities.
- Advocate for the resources and policy changes needed to achieve the desired health objectives.
- Prepare participants to become self-managers and self-advocates.
- Support the diffusion of innovation to a wider population.
- Seek to "institutionalize" successful components and to replicate them in other settings.

Data from: Freudenberg, N., Eng, E., Flay, B., Parcel, G., Rogers, I., and Wallerstein, N., (1995). Strengthening individual and community capacity to prevent disease and promote health: In search of relevant theories and principles. *Health Education Quarterly, 22*(3), 290–306.

individual transition plans (ITPs) for youth with disabilities age 16 to 21. **Transition services** are specifically designed to "facilitate the child's movement from school to post-school activities, including postsecondary education, vocational education, integrated employment (including supported employment), continuing and adult education, adult services, independent living, or community participation" (U.S. Department of Education (USDE), 2006, p. 46762). ITPs are based on the "individual child's needs, taking into account the child's strengths, preferences, and interests; and include:

- Instruction;
- Related services;
- Community experiences;
- The development of employment and other post-school adult living objectives; and
- If appropriate, acquisition of daily living skills and provision of a functional vocational evaluation" (USDE, 2006, p. 46762).

In addition to transition services mandated by IDEA, young adults with disabilities can receive transition-planning services in the community through adult disability services' community-based long-term care services funded by Medicaid Home and Community-Based services (HCBS) waivers (Orentlicher & Dougan, 2011).

Occupational therapy involvement in transition planning for youth can extend beyond the school system to community-based programs. Although transition services for individuals with all types of

disabilities are important, there is a growing need for these services for individuals with autism spectrum disorder. The Southwest Autism Research & Resource Center (SARRC) of Phoenix, Arizona, has made an effort to support people with autism spectrum disorder (ASD) throughout the life span. In its vocational and life skills training program, the Center seeks to advocate for independence in individuals aged 13 and older with ASD. The Center provides opportunities to learn skills required for various jobs and/or independence, including art, job and social skills training, cooking, entrepreneurial skills, landscaping/gardening, and basic life skills. Internships and job coaches are offered for individuals interested in obtaining employment (SARRC, 2012).

Similarly, the Hussman Center for Adults with Autism at Towson University in Maryland, established in 2008, provides mutual learning opportunities for students at the university, professionals in the community, families of people with autism, and transitioning youth/adults aged 18 years and older with autism spectrum disorders. Six to 15 transitioning youth/adults with autism are paired with university students and participate in 4- to 12-week-long programs. Some programs include recreation and fitness classes; introduction to college and peer support; social experience classes; and arts, music, and dance classes. These programs utilize university students in various majors, including occupational therapy, kinesiology, the arts, and family studies to address language, fitness, social, self-advocacy, problem-solving, communication, leadership, and relational skills with individuals with autism (Crabtree, 2011).

As occupational therapists begin to provide transition services for individuals with autism, critical deficits must be targeted to increase independence and occupational participation in transitioning youths/adults. Although deficits associated with autism are on a spectrum from higher to lower functioning, self-determination, self-advocacy, community participation, relationship development, career and employment preparation, and independent living are common areas of concern (Crabtree, 2011). It is important to maintain a client-centered approach, building on the strengths of the individual to foster success and independence during transition into adulthood (Kotler & Koenig, 2012). Finally, when helping a transitioning youth/adult integrate into a particular community/role, it is important to educate the people he or she will encounter about autism, behaviors associated with the disorder, and specific strategies to overcome any associated barriers in order to foster a smooth transition (Baugher & Pyne, 2012).

Obesity Prevention and Intervention

Health management and maintenance is categorized as an instrumental activity of daily living (IADL) and is within the scope of practice for occupational therapists (American Occupational Therapy Association [AOTA], 2008). It incorporates development, management, and maintenance of performance patterns for health and wellness promotion. Interventions focusing on fitness, nutrition, behaviors, and medication routines are appropriate strategies to address health management and maintenance (AOTA, 2008). As a result, there is an increasing awareness in occupational therapy of the need to address community health and wellness, especially regarding the issue of obesity (Clark, Reingold, & Salles-Jordan, 2007). **Obesity** is defined as body mass index greater than or equal to 30 in adults and greater than or equal to the 95th percentile on age- and sex-specific growth charts in children. In 2009–2010, 35.7% of U.S. adults and 16.9% of U.S. children were obese (Odgen, Carroll, Kit, & Flegal, 2012).

Occupational therapists have begun to address this nationwide health concern with the use of primary, secondary, and tertiary prevention approaches with children, adolescents, and adults. Primary prevention involves the implementation of health education and health promotion intervention strategies with healthy people to decrease the incidence of obesity and decrease its prevalence. Secondary prevention involves the early detection and implementation of strategies to prevent or diminish the negative health effects in individuals who are already overweight. Finally, tertiary prevention involves treatment of obesity to prevent disability and to promote engagement in occupation despite the presence of severe obesity (Scaffa, Van Slyke, & Brownson, 2008).

In building a community-based program for health promotion and obesity prevention, occupational therapists consider the *OT Practice Framework* and the functional implications of obesity. Occupational therapists address areas of need relevant to the framework (Clark, Reingold, & Salles-Jordan, 2007). In children's programs some of the areas addressed include arousal, concentration, family education on community resources, safety awareness, nutrition and meal preparation, leisure/play, flexibility, strength, activity level, goal setting, and self-efficacy (Cahill, Daniel, Nelson-Stitt, Brager, Dostal, & Hirter, 2009; Kugel, 2010; Lau, 2011). Similarly, programs geared toward adults focus on establishing and enhancing a client's environment; independence in activities of daily living (ADLs) and IADLs; activity tolerance; range of motion; and performance patterns, habits, and rituals for weight reduction and/or maintenance (Mosley, Jedlika, Lequieu, & Taylor, 2008). These programs may also include education on use of adaptive equipment, stress management, community resources, leisure/physical activity, and compensatory strategies (Mosley, Jedlika, Lequieu, & Taylor, 2008).

In response to the nation's increased incidence of obesity and its limiting effects on occupational performance, occupational therapists can make a difference through prevention and promotion of health within the community. A number of community-based programs have been established to address both childhood and adult obesity, including: *The Healthy Lifestyle Initiative,* by LaGrange Area Department of Special Education and University of Illinois at Chicago (Cahill et al., 2009); *Healthy Choices for Me*, a partnership between Henderson, Nevada, Recreation and Touro

University Nevada OT School (Lau, 2011); and *Madonna ProActive* at Madonna Rehabilitation Hospital in Lincoln, Nebraska (as cited in Mosley et al., 2008). In addition to these sources, the AOTA position paper on obesity can guide practitioners in establishing community-based obesity programs (Clark, Reingold, & Salles-Jordan, 2007).

Driving Across the Life Span

Community mobility involves use of private and/or public transportation to move within one's geographic neighborhood. It includes walking; driving automobiles; and riding bicycles, buses, taxicabs, or other forms of transportation (AOTA, 2008). Driving is an IADL, which contributes to increased independence. Impairments leading to loss of ability to drive can limit a client's occupational performance and participation, especially in locations with limited public transportation options. Driving and community mobility can be addressed through occupational therapy intervention. Both non-specialized occupational therapists and those practicing as driving rehabilitation specialists can and should address this area of occupation to provide needed services for maximization of occupational independence and client well-being (McKenna, 2011).

Many different types of clients can benefit from driving rehabilitation services. Older adults with age-related decline are particularly vulnerable to deficits that may prevent them from driving (McKenna, 2011). Additionally, clients diagnosed with traumatic brain injury, post-traumatic stress disorder (Stern, Prudencio, & Sadler, 2011), vision deficits, amputation, and limited mobility due to cerebral vascular accidents or orthopedic conditions may have decreased safety and independence during driving. Because occupational therapists not only work to restore lost occupations but also create and promote skills for new occupations (AOTA, 2008), young people with disabilities can also benefit from driving rehabilitation programs (Strzelecki, 2011).

Driving programs focus on evaluation and intervention to improve skills related to safe driving for clients, passengers, and other motorists. Some skills important for safe and independent driving include: higher-level cognition, attention, vision, proprioception, muscle power, joint mobility, muscle endurance, muscle tone, motor reflexes, control of voluntary and involuntary movements, cardiovascular functions, and respiratory functions. Specifically, driving programs may focus on:

- independence in car transfers with loading of assistive devices,
- orientation to environment and following directions,
- emotional regulation,
- reaction time,
- bilateral coordination,
- visual perception, processing, and scanning,
- multitasking, attention, decision making, problem solving, and
- recommendation and operation of vehicle modifications (Stern, Prudencio, & Sadler, 2011; Strzelecki, 2011).

Some community-based driving programs are specific to older adults, while others are geared to the needs of young adults or war veterans (McKenna, 2011; Stern, Prudencio, & Sadler, 2011; Strzelecki, 2011). The AOTA has many resources on its Web site to support the development of a driver rehabilitation program. In addition, the Association for Driver Rehab Specialists (ADED) provides certification courses and continuing education to increase competence in driving rehabilitation. Finally, the National Highway Traffic Safety Administration (NHTSA) and state departments of transportation are important resources to increase familiarity with the laws of the road and legal issues regarding adaptive equipment and license restrictions. Driving as an IADL is an enabler of occupational participation and independence and should be addressed in all clients of driving age to ensure safe, effective, and client-centered care.

Aging-in-Place Home Modifications

In the United States in 2009, 12.8% of the population was over age 65, and by 2025 the percentage of older adults is expected to climb to 17.9% (Shrestha & Heisler, 2011). The vast majority of older adults desire to remain in their homes as they age. With aging, natural decline occurs, creating new barriers to living in an environment that was once functional. To address these barriers, occupational therapists work to modify home environments to promote successful aging in place.

Occupational therapists are teaming with building contractors in communities to increase awareness about the role of occupational therapy in home modification and the creation of accessible environments. Through the National Association of Home Builders (NAHB), occupational therapists can be trained as Certified Aging in Place Specialists (CAPS). Additionally, AOTA offers a course for a Specialty Certification in Environmental Modifications (SCEM) (Waite, 2011). Through these courses, therapists can network with contractors, architects, interior designers, and others who advocate for accessible environments for productive aging. Occupational therapists like Lizzette Davis, OTR, CAPS, from San Antonio, Texas; Carolyn Sithong, OTR/L, CAPS, SCEM, from Orlando, Florida; and Marnie Redna, MEd, OTR/L, CAPS from Cincinnati, Ohio, all began home modification businesses by partnering with contractors after recognizing that their recommendations to clients often were not implemented. They noticed that often the modifications were not completed due to lack of professional guidance from occupational therapists to properly implement the recommendations (Waite, 2011).

Considering the functional declines common in the aging population, there are many different recommendations that can be made to increase accessibility of a home and thus enhance occupational participation. The addition of ramps for easy entry, and grab bars to improve safety are commonly recommended modifications. Home lighting and organization of the environment are also important as aging residents' vision and balance decline. In many homes, kitchens and bathrooms are inaccessible due to lack of space to access sinks, stoves, showers, and toilets from a wheelchair or walker. Bathroom tub/shower barriers are often renovated to curbless showers to increase independence in performance of ADLs. Multiple-level houses may require installation of elevators or chairlifts to access upper levels (Fagan & Sabata, 2011; Waite, 2011; Chase & Roche, 2011; Morris, 2009). Although many different recommendations can improve ease of access to home environments and improved independence, it is important to develop a strong network of qualified contractors to support construction and installation of accessible environments (Morris, 2009).

In addition to the AOTA and the NAHB, there are other resources that can facilitate the achievement of aging-in-place goals. Non-profit organizations such as Rebuilding Together, the National Aging in Place Council, and AARP can provide information and potential funding to assist in providing safe home environments promoting occupational performance for productive aging (Waite, 2011; Young, 2011). It appears that this area of practice will continue to grow in the years ahead due to the aging baby boomer generation.

Telerehabilitation

Jana Cason, an early intervention occupational therapy practitioner, uses the emerging telehealth model of practice to provide services to clients who would otherwise not receive occupational therapy. Long distances and hours on the road characterize the jobs of many in-home occupational therapy practitioners (Cason, 2011). Rather than serving more clients, these practitioners exhaust their resources traveling between clients. Despite their efforts, therapists remain unable to provide needed services due to provider shortages or lack of specialized knowledge, creating health disparities in many geographic areas. In an effort to be more cost effective, a new practice model is emerging. **Telehealth** is the use of technology and electronic information to support health care, health administration, or health education delivery across a distance (Health Resources and Services Administration, n.d.). From an occupational therapy perspective, **telerehabilitation** is the use of communication technology to provide clients with evaluative, preventative, diagnostic, and therapeutic services (AOTA, 2010). Telehealth is used to provide health care in underserved areas, homes, hospitals, nursing homes, schools, and workplaces (Cason, 2012). Telerehabilitation has been effective for consultative purposes in situations when therapists can seek advice from expert therapists, or across disciplines for collaborative efforts. Additionally, it has been used successfully to educate caregivers and serve clients with many diagnoses, including traumatic brain injuries, cerebral vascular accidents, multiple sclerosis, cerebral palsy, polytrauma, post-traumatic stress disorder, and chronic diseases (Cason, 2012).

Before using the telehealth model, some concerns/barriers must be considered. Funding of services is limited, so practitioners must be knowledgeable about reimbursement sources and advocate for their clients (U.S. Department of Health and Human Services, n.d.). Research regarding the effective use of assessment and intervention tools is also limited, so care must be taken to ensure services are efficacious (Cason, 2012). Practitioners must be aware of appropriate technology and be competent in its use. This is especially important, as there is an increased risk for a breach in patient privacy due to the use of technology. Care must be taken to ensure the use of protected systems, especially when the Internet is involved (Cason, 2012). Ethical principles must be adhered to just as in any other practice model (AOTA, 2010). Additionally, practitioners are expected to abide by all state licensure laws when performing services across state lines; this may require licensure in more than one state (American Telemedicine Association, 2011). As researchers continue to discover the effective use and benefits of telerehabilitation, opportunities expand for occupational therapists to incorporate advanced communication technology into practice to achieve a globally connected and widely recognized workforce meeting society's occupational needs (AOTA, 2006).

The Influence of Occupational Justice: An International Example

Many of the emerging areas of community-based practice are predicated on the construct of occupational justice. The next section briefly describes the construct and the implications for practice, and provides a case study submitted by an occupational therapist in Japan.

Occupational justice is based on the belief that humans are occupational beings and that participation in occupation is essential for health, well-being, and quality of life. Therefore, all persons should have the right to engage in meaningful occupation; this is their occupational right. Occupational injustice exists when this right is violated or goes unfulfilled (Stadnyk, Townsend, & Wilcock, 2010). When occupational injustice persists, occupational dysfunction is often the result.

Risk factors that cause occupational dysfunction due to occupational injustice include occupational imbalance, deprivation, and alienation (Wilcock, 1998). Occupational imbalance is a lack of balance between self-sustaining, productive, and leisure occupations that fails to meet an individual's physical or psychosocial needs, thereby resulting in decreased health and well-being. Occupational deprivation is the result of external circumstances or limitations that prevent a person from participating in necessary and meaningful occupations. Conditions that lead to occupational deprivation may include poor health, disability, poverty, isolation, and homelessness. Occupational alienation is a lack of satisfaction in one's occupations that leads to experiencing life as purposeless and meaningless. Tasks that are perceived as stressful, meaningless, or boring may result in an experience of occupational alienation.

Occupational therapy practitioners are ethically bound to address occupational injustice wherever it exists, in health care institutions, communities, or social and political policies and practices. A case study at the end of this chapter illustrates the ideas, beliefs, and principles associated with occupational justice as they relate to a Japanese woman, Yuriko, who lives in a nursing home.

Implications for Professional Preparation and Education

As occupational therapy services continue to increase in a diverse array of community-based settings, it is imperative to prepare students for community practice (Fagan, Van Oss, Cabrera, Olivas De La O, & Vance, 2008). In order to respond to changes in practice settings and to fulfill its mission to produce competent practitioners for the future, professional education must develop new curricular and fieldwork models. A primary challenge will be to balance the need to prepare students for traditional biomedical practice with the new demands of community health roles. McColl (1998) identifies the knowledge needed by occupational therapy students and practitioners in order to participate effectively in community programs (Box 29-2).

Box 29-2	What Students and Practitioners Need to Know to Participate Effectively in Community Programs

- What a community is
- How organizations and communities form
- How organizations and communities are governed
- How to identify community resources
- How to identify community needs
- How to facilitate change
- How persons with disabilities live in the community
- How persons develop and pursue occupations in the community
- What supports and barriers to participation in occupation exist in the community

Data from: McColl, M. A. (1998). What do we need to know to practice occupational therapy in the community? *American Journal of Occupational Therapy, 52*(1), 11–18.

In December 2011, the Accreditation Council for Occupational Therapy Education (ACOTE), the organization responsible for accrediting entry-level occupational therapy educational programs, adopted new standards for occupational therapy assistant and occupational therapist (master's and doctoral level) preparation programs to be implemented by July 31, 2013. One entire section of the accreditation standards (the minimum essential requirements for accreditation of educational programs) is devoted to the context of service delivery. This section describes, in some detail, the competencies required for practicing in a variety of environments, with a major emphasis on community and social systems. Community-related competencies also can be found as minor components in other sections of the standards, including:

- Foundational content requirements
- Basic tenets of occupational therapy
- Occupational therapy theoretical perspectives
- Intervention plan formulation and implementation
- Management of occupational therapy services
- Professional ethics, values, and responsibilities
- Fieldwork education.

Box 29-3 provides examples of standards that emphasize community and social systems from the

Box 29-3	ACOTE Standards Related to Community-Based Practice

SECTION B: CONTENT REQUIREMENTS

1.0   Foundational Content Requirements

1.4   Demonstrate knowledge and appreciation of the role of sociocultural, socioeconomic, and diversity factors and lifestyle choices in contemporary society.

1.5   Demonstrate an understanding of the ethical and practical considerations that affect the health and wellness needs of those who are experiencing or are at risk for social injustice, occupational deprivation, and disparity in the receipt of services.

1.6   Demonstrate knowledge of global social issues and prevailing health and welfare needs of populations with or at risk for disabilities and chronic health conditions.

2.0   Basic Tenets of Occupational Therapy

2.5   Explain the role of occupation in the promotion of health and the prevention of disease and disability for the individual, family, and society.

2.9   Express support for the quality of life, well-being, and occupation of the individual, group, or population to promote physical and mental health and prevention of injury and disease considering the context (e.g., cultural, personal, temporal, virtual) and environment.

3.0   Occupational Therapy Theoretical Perspectives

3.5   Apply theoretical constructs to evaluation and intervention with various types of clients in a variety of practice contexts and environments to analyze and effect meaningful occupation outcomes.

5.0   Intervention Plan: Formulation and Implementation

5.4   Design and implement group interventions based on principles of group development and group dynamics across the life span.

5.5   Provide training in self-care, self-management, health management and maintenance, home management, and community and work integration.

5.9   Evaluate and adapt processes or environments (e.g., home, work, school, community) applying ergonomic principles and principles of environmental modification.

Box 29-3 ACOTE Standards Related to Community-Based Practice–cont'd

5.13 Provide recommendations and training in techniques to enhance community mobility, including public transportation, community access, and issues related to driver rehabilitation.

5.17 Develop and promote the use of appropriate home and community programming to support performance in the client's natural environment and participation in all contexts relevant to the client.

5.18 Demonstrate an understanding of health literacy and the ability to educate and train the client, caregiver, family and significant others, and communities to facilitate skills in areas of occupation as well as prevention, health maintenance, health promotion, and safety.

5.21 Effectively communicate and work interprofessionally with those who provide services to individuals, organizations, and/or populations in order to clarify each member's responsibility in executing an intervention plan.

5.26 Understand when and how to use the consultative process with groups, programs, organizations, or communities.

5.27 Describe the role of the occupational therapist in care coordination, case management, and transition services in traditional and emerging practice environments.

5.29 Plan for discharge, in collaboration with the client, by reviewing the needs of client, caregiver, family, and significant others; available resources; and discharge environment. This process includes, but is not limited to, identification of client's current status within the continuum of care; identification of community, human, and fiscal resources; recommendations for environmental adaptations; and home programming to facilitate the client's progression along the continuum toward outcome goals.

5.33 Provide population-based occupational therapy intervention that addresses occupational needs as identified by a community. (Doctoral degree level only)

6.0 Context of Service Delivery

6.1 Evaluate and address the various contexts of health care, education, community, political, and social systems as they relate to the practice of occupational therapy.

6.2 Analyze the current policy issues and the social, economic, political, geographic, and demographic factors that influence the various contexts for practice of occupational therapy.

6.3 Integrate current social, economic, political, geographic, and demographic factors to promote policy development and the provision of occupational therapy services.

6.4 Articulate the role and responsibility of the practitioner to advocate for changes in service delivery policies, to effect changes in the system, and to identify opportunities in emerging practice areas.

6.5 Analyze the trends in models of service delivery, including, but not limited to, medical, educational, community, and social models, and their potential effect on the practice of occupational therapy.

7.0 Management of Occupational Therapy Services

7.1 Describe and discuss the impact of contextual factors on the management and delivery of occupational therapy services.

7.5 Demonstrate the ability to plan, develop, organize, and market the delivery of services to include the determination of programmatic needs and service delivery options and formulation and management of staffing for effective service provision.

7.9 Demonstrate knowledge of and the ability to write program development plans for provision of occupational therapy services to individuals and populations. (Doctoral degree level only)

7.11 Identify and develop strategies to enable occupational therapy to respond to society's changing needs. (Doctoral degree level only)

9.0 Professional Ethics, Values, and Responsibilities

9.12 Describe and discuss strategies to assist the consumer in gaining access to occupational therapy services.

SECTION C: FIELDWORK EDUCATION

1.12 Provide Level II fieldwork in traditional and/or emerging settings, consistent with the curriculum design. In all settings, psychosocial factors influencing engagement in occupation must be understood and integrated for the development of client-centered, meaningful, occupation-based outcomes. The student can complete Level II fieldwork in a minimum of one setting if it is reflective of more than one practice area, or in a maximum of four different settings.

Data from: American Occupational Therapy Association. (2011). Accreditation Council for Occupational Therapy Education (ACOTE) Standards and Interpretative Guide (effective July 31, 2013). Retrieved from http://aota.org/Educate/Accredit/Draft-Standards/50146.aspx?FT=.pdf

Standards for an Accredited Educational Program for the Occupational Therapist (AOTA, 2011).

A number of educational approaches can be developed, implemented, and evaluated for their effectiveness in meeting the demands of emerging practice arenas. The accreditation standards allow the flexibility to create a variety of curricular models that qualify for accreditation. As every community is different, so too may educational programs differ in how they meet the need to produce a new type of occupational therapy practitioner.

Some educational programs are meeting the challenge by infusing community practice content throughout the curriculum, while others are creating new courses that focus entirely on community health concerns. Some programs are using community-based sites in creative ways for level I fieldwork. Other programs place students in community programs for both level I and level II fieldwork. In addition, community service learning has become an attractive educational methodology within occupational therapy programs to address the competencies needed for effective community-based practice. Integrating community service learning opportunities in occupational therapy curricula can facilitate students' understanding and appreciation of social, economic, and environmental factors and their impact on occupational participation, health, and quality of life (Horowitz, 2012).

Community Service Learning

Community service learning (CSL) is defined as "a teaching and learning strategy that integrates meaningful community service with instruction and reflection to enrich the learning experience, teach civic responsibility, and strengthen communities" (National Service Learning Clearinghouse, 2012, para. 1). Through CSL, occupational therapy students not only have the opportunity for practical application of what they have learned in the classroom to a real world problem but also increase the awareness of occupational therapy in the community and provide much-needed services to underserved populations.

CSL has several characteristics that distinguish it from volunteerism. Volunteerism, although a highly valued occupation, is not an educational pedagogy. The purpose of volunteerism is to serve one's neighbors and communities in order to enhance the quality of life for all. Volunteers donate their time, effort, and talents to a need or cause they value out of a sense of social responsibility. In high-quality community service learning programs, students are involved in identifying community needs, planning and implementing a service project, and structured reflection on what was learned through the service experience. CSL is designed to meet a community need while facilitating the development of skills in the learner.

Much research has been conducted on the effects of community service learning. The effects appear to be broad based and enduring, many of which are congruent with occupational therapy's history and philosophical base. Regardless of the discipline, service-based learning appears to:

- Develop open-mindedness
- Increase awareness of one's own values, beliefs, and attitudes (an essential aspect of therapeutic use of self)
- Increase problem-solving ability
- Increase empathy
- Be as effective as traditional instruction in conveying knowledge
- Increase self-efficacy and enhance a belief that a person can make a difference in other people's lives
- Increase social and personal responsibility (an important aspect of ethical behavior)
- Enhance communication skills
- Reinforce the development of professional behaviors (good practice for students early in their academic program)
- Instill a healthy work ethic
- Enable students to assess their strengths and weaknesses (Conrad and Hedin, 1991; Giles and Eyler, 1994; Markus, Howard, & King, 1993; Sankaran, Cinelli, McConatha, & Carson, 1995)

In addition, several potential benefits specific to the discipline of occupational therapy are evident. CSL can increase the students' understanding of the role of occupational therapy in community-based settings, providing an opportunity to integrate theory with practice and networking opportunities with professionals in a variety of disciplines. CSL also allows community-based organizations, which currently may not have occupational therapy services, to experience occupational therapy firsthand, thereby increasing the potential development of new job opportunities for occupational therapy practitioners in community-based programs.

CSL also increases the probability that students might choose a community-based setting for future practice. It has been demonstrated that practitioners who are trained in institutions want to work in institutions (Weissert, Knott, & Steiber, 1993). What students learn in school is most likely how they will practice. Providing students, early in their academic career, with opportunities to experience the potential for community-based practice is one of the goals of this community service-learning approach to level I fieldwork.

The overall goal of a CSL program is to develop students' skills and competencies in the provision of community-based occupational therapy services to agencies and organizations in the local community, which have typically been underserved. An effective program is designed to:

- Respond to actual community needs
- Provide community-based organizations with the opportunity to experience occupational therapy services firsthand
- Increase the potential for the development of new job opportunities in community-based programs
- Increase the probability that students will choose a community-based setting for future practice

According to Horowitz (2012), "service learning provides occupational therapy education with a flexible, relatively low-cost pedagogy that advances the Centennial Vision and provides opportunities to community practice through reflective, active learning experiences" (p. 3).

Implications for Research in Community-Based Practice

Baum and Law (1998) outlined a number of research areas relevant for community practice. Occupational therapy researchers need to:

- Identify the factors that contribute to successful employment, self-sufficiency, and social integration.
- Determine the conditions that enable persons with chronic disabilities to participate fully in

their families, schools, work settings, and community.
- Identify the personal, social, and environmental circumstances that promote acceptance and use of assistive devices.
- Investigate how the interaction of biopsychosocial and environmental factors contribute to the development of functional limitations, disabilities, and impairments.
- Identify the personal, developmental, and environmental attributes that contribute to successful community living.

Traditional approaches to quantitative research may not be the most effective ways of investigating the impact of occupational therapy in community settings or the impact of occupational therapy on community health. Typically, quantitative studies do not capture the unique experiences of community members nor the complex interactions that impact health (Christiansen & Matuska, 2010). As a result, researchers in public and community health have advocated for the use of community-based participatory action approaches and mixed methods research. Kielhofner (2005) eloquently argues that participatory action research may be one strategy for bridging the divide between scholarship and practice in occupational therapy.

Community-based participatory action research (CBPAR) takes place in real-world contexts and is client-centered and collaborative, action-oriented, and designed to solve a community health problem. In CBPAR, participants are involved in a collaborative relationship with the researcher to identify the problem to be addressed, determine the research questions, design the research methods, conduct data collection and analysis, and interpret and apply the results. CBPAR often involves the use of a mixed methods approach combining quantitative and qualitative methods.

Although there are few examples of CBPAR in the occupational therapy literature, Letts (2003) argues that participatory research is an approach that is consistent with the values of the profession and can make significant contributions to the knowledge base in occupational therapy. Taylor, Braveman, and Hammel (2004) describe two case examples of how community-based services, for persons with AIDS and individuals with chronic fatigue syndrome, were developed and evaluated using participatory action research. One CBPAR project, involving occupational therapy faculty and students, was based on the principles of occupational justice and addressed the importance of clean water in the ability of persons in Appalachian Kentucky to carry out the necessary and desired occupations of family and community life (Blakeney & Marshall, 2009). In each of these studies, mixed methods research strategies were employed.

Mixed methods research combines elements of both the quantitative and qualitative research traditions in an attempt to expand our understanding of a phenomenon and confirm findings from a variety of data sources. Using mixed methods helps to neutralize the inherent biases and draw on the respective strengths of each, thereby increasing the validity and usefulness of the information obtained. Researchers intentionally combine the quantitative and qualitative data in order to gain a larger perspective on the phenomenon of interest. Mixed methods studies incorporate both deductive and inductive reasoning. Depending on the research questions, mixing quantitative and qualitative methods may be done sequentially with one method following the other, or concurrently where both methods are used simultaneously. Mixed methods research provides multiple perspectives on a problem, contextualizes the information obtained, and allows the examination of the relationships between processes and outcomes (Office of Behavioral and Social Sciences Research, National Institutes of Health, 2011).

Diffusion of Innovations

Through research, publication, and entry-level and continuing education, innovations are disseminated for implementation into practice. These innovations and changes are diffused and perpetuated in professions through a variety of communication channels.

An **innovation** is an idea, method, practice, or object that is perceived to be new or novel. Some innovations are not really new from an objective historical perspective but are new to the perceiver by virtue of a lapse of time since their initial discovery or introduction (Rogers, 1995).

Innovations often require a significant period of time for diffusion before being adopted by practitioners, academics, and researchers in a discipline. Diffusion refers to "the process by which an innovation is communicated through certain channels over time among the members of a social system" (Rogers, 1995, p. 5). Diffusion of innovation

produces changes, both planned and unplanned, in the structure and function of a social system.

Time is a factor in the diffusion process. Some individuals are early adopters of innovation, while others tend to lag behind. Some innovations are adopted very quickly. Others may take significantly longer periods of time. In a profession, diffusion of innovation requires a "critical mass" of adopters before the innovation becomes the standard.

The occupational therapy profession is at an important crossroads in its history. Do we re-adopt the innovation of community practice and all that it entails and move ahead quickly and deliberately, or do we reinforce the status quo and work within the existing parameters of practice? While some practitioners are losing their jobs in the managed-care arena, other opportunities are becoming available in community settings. These emerging practice areas are very much in harmony with the founders' visions of the profession. Will we respond quickly and enthusiastically to these challenges? Fidler (2000) clearly supports change and suggests moving "beyond the therapy model." She advocates that practitioners become "occupationalists," who have the capability to practice and conduct research in a variety of areas, including but not limited to (Fidler, p. 101):

- services and programs of wellness, of prevention, of learning enhancement, and lifestyle counseling;
- community planning and design;
- organizational, agency, and institutional design and operations; and
- treatment, restorative interventions, and rehabilitation.

Conclusion

"We envision that occupational therapy is a powerful, widely recognized, science-driven, and evidence-based profession with a globally connected and diverse workforce meeting society's occupational needs." (AOTA, 2006)

To paraphrase Barker (1992) in *Future Edge: Discovering the New Paradigms of Success*, the three keys to the successful achievement of the AOTA Centennial Vision are excellence, innovation, and anticipation. Excellence refers to the ability to do whatever it is one does with the utmost quality, in a cost-effective manner, while seeking continuous improvement.

Innovation is the ability to initiate or introduce something new and different, and in unison with excellence is a powerful combination. Anticipation is the ability to be in the right place at the right time with an excellent, innovative product or service. Anticipation allows one to predict or foresee future needs, trends, and priorities. If, in some small way, one can anticipate the future, then there is no need to fear it. The future can be embraced as an opportunity for growth and revitalization.

The ideas presented in this chapter serve as a catalyst to stimulate further dialogue and the dissemination of community practice models in these emerging practice areas. Successful entry into community practice will require occupational therapy practitioners to expand their:

- Conceptualization of the usefulness of occupation
- Perspective on the role of occupational therapy
- View of the profession
- Identification of potential opportunities
- Capabilities as program planners, consultants, advocates, and grant writers

The only real barriers are the limits of one's creativity. Occupation is fundamental to human life. It improves physical and mental health, contributes to a sense of well-being, enhances life satisfaction, and provides meaning to everyday existence. Opportunities for professionals with expertise in occupational performance are evident in all spheres of human endeavor. One need only look with fresh eyes and an open mind.

"Do not follow where the path leads, rather go where there is no path and leave a trail" (Author unknown).

CASE STUDIES

CASE STUDY 29•1 YURIKO

Occupational Justice: An International Case Study
Yuriko is an 85-year-old female who resides in a nursing home in Japan. Twenty years ago, she sustained a cerebrovascular accident (CVA), with right hemiplegia and flaccidity of the right upper and lower extremities. She does not exhibit any cognitive or perceptual deficits. She has right knee pain due to osteoarthritis. She is ADL independent but uses a wheelchair for mobility due to fear of falling.

Yuriko's typical daily pattern was as follows:

- She gets out of bed at 6 a.m. and eats breakfast at 7:30 a.m.
- During the day, she often sleeps in bed or watches some TV in her room.
- At 4 p.m., she watches a TV program with samurai dramas and sumo wrestling in the multipurpose hall.
- At 6 p.m. Yuriko eats supper and then goes to bed.

Yuriko shares a room with three other residents, and has little living space and only a curtain for privacy. She participates in functional rehabilitation that includes stair-climbing exercises and outdoor gardening with a care-worker and other clients once a week. She does not have any opportunities to go out into the community. Her daughter has been able to visit Yuriko only once in three months.

Occupational Therapy Evaluation
Yuriko was evaluated using the occupational justice checklist designed for older adults. The checklist consists of 10 items. For instance, one item reads: "sitting alone in nursing homes or other confined settings with nothing to do except to watch others in the same situation or television programs that they did not choose."

The checklist results suggested that Yuriko was experiencing occupational injustice in the following areas:

1. Occupational imbalance: She had few occupations in the facility except for self-care, and reported boredom in her free time.
2. Occupational deprivation: She had few opportunities for new role acquisition.
3. Occupational alienation: She did only the activities that had been offered in the facility.

Continued

She reported that every day was monotonous because she did not have meaningful occupation. The occupational therapist at the facility developed an intervention blending Occupational Science, Person-Occupation-Environment Model, and the Model of Human Occupation.

Occupational Therapy Goals

The first step was for the occupational therapist to understand Yuriko's occupational history narrative in order to improve her motivation and adjustment to the environment. Yuriko and her occupational therapist collaborated in the identification of meaningful occupations and valued roles, and in the determination of her occupational goals.

Yuriko said, "I was gardening and found value in growing vegetables," before the CVA. "I want to do anything that I am able to do, but what opportunities do I have in the facility?" For Yuriko, her internal expectancies of maximal independence and choice in roles and activities conflicted with the rules and routines of the facility. In choosing to follow the nursing home's rules and routines, she increasingly experienced occupational imbalance, occupational deprivation, and occupational alienation.

Occupational Therapy Intervention

The occupational therapist learned that Yuriko had been a farmer prior to her CVA, so she took Yuriko to the campus of a local university where Yuriko was given the opportunity to teach agriculture to the students. She lectured the students on how to plant a potato crop and sometimes went out to the field to observe. Although she only taught the students the skills and did not manage the crops herself, she enjoyed the challenge of teaching farming skills, which gave her a sense of accomplishment and satisfaction and provided an experience of flow. Yuriko's occupational role as a farmer was expanded to include the role of teacher, and this was very meaningful to her.

Afterwards, the students sent Yuriko photographs of the crop growth and their work in the fields. They wrote about how Yuriko taught them to plant and farm, and they invited her to the campus festival. By this time, the students had already become practicing occupational therapists. In addition to learning how to farm, the students also learned some important occupational therapy principles. The occupational therapist from the nursing home explained the meaning that growing crops had for Yuriko and how motivation is improved when a client is able to enact a chosen role. The students also learned clinical reasoning skills and the meaning of improvised occupational therapy.

Yuriko said that after her stroke she did not know if she would ever be able to work to raise farm products like this again. So she wrote a heartfelt letter of thanks to the students using her non-dominant hand. In the letter, she shared her feelings and thanked them for the photographs they sent and the memories. She said "when I met you one year ago, I was embarrassed and uncertain of what needed to be done. However, I can enjoy the results of the planting thanks to you this year. The potatoes and green soybeans appear to be growing well. I think that this is because 21 students' minds united into one. This experience has become one of the happiest memories of my life, and I am thankful to you every day. I hope to live long, and look forward to the time when we meet again." She also encouraged them to work hard when they graduated from the university and become independent. Then she invited them to the summer festival at the nursing home.

Conclusion

According to Wilcock (1998), occupation is a synthesis of being, doing, and becoming and occupational participation enhances health and well-being. The case of Yuriko is instructive in three ways. First, through being, doing, and becoming, Yuriko emerged as a new occupational being. Prior to occupational therapy intervention, "being" for Yuriko was egocentric and anxiety-producing, with a very limited perspective of the future; "doing" was the once-a-week recreational activity of gardening. As a result of minimal occupational participation, "becoming" was occupational dysfunction, occupational injustice, loss of role, and decreased motivation. After occupational therapy intervention, using an occupational narrative approach, "being" for Yuriko became consideration of the students' needs, a calm and soft manner, and a future perspective; "doing" became a meaningful occupation (teaching) based on her previous role as a farmer. As a result, "becoming" developed into occupational function, occupational justice, role acquisition, and improvement of motivation.

Secondly, Yuriko's activity participation in the nursing home might be considered an unstable occupation. Occupational therapy intervention can transform unstable occupation into occupation with energies. As a result, vitalized unstable occupation becomes "true" occupation and can have the health-enhancing power of occupation. Finally, occupation gives color to the client's daily life and changes the facility environment in which the client lives. As this process is repeated for others, the positive outcomes spread and produce a wonderful, healthier community and region.

CASE STUDY 29•1 Discussion Questions

1. What aspects of occupational justice are illustrated in this case study?
2. How might culture impact Yuriko's daily routine? How might Yuriko's culture have impacted the practice of occupational therapy in this case study?
3. What strengths does Yuriko demonstrate? How might these strengths be incorporated into future therapy sessions?
4. Why were Yuriko's interactions with the occupational therapy students significant for her and for the students?
5. What strategies could be employed in the nursing home to facilitate occupational participation and enhance occupational justice?

Learning Activities

1. Identify a need in your community and describe how occupational therapy could address that need. Develop a program idea to address the need and outline the basic occupational therapy program components.
2. Discuss how your occupational therapy educational program meets the accreditation standards related to community-based practice.
3. Create several learning objectives for a community-service learning course that fits with your occupational therapy educational program's curriculum design.
4. Generate five researchable questions related to occupational therapy in community-based practice settings.
5. Develop a research proposal incorporating the principles of community-based participatory action research and mixed method designs.

REFERENCES

American Occupational Therapy Association. (2011). *Accreditation Council for Occupational Therapy Education (ACOTE) Standards and Interpretative Guide (effective July 31, 2013)*. Retrieved from http://aota.org/Educate/Accredit/Draft-Standards/50146.aspx?FT=.pdf

American Occupational Therapy Association. (2010). Telerehabilitation. *American Journal of Occupational Therapy, 64* (Suppl.), S92–S102. doi: 10.5014/ajot.2010.64S92-64S102

American Occupational Therapy Association. (2008). Occupational therapy practice framework: Domain and process (2nd ed.). *American Journal of Occupational Therapy, 62*, 625–683.

American Occupational Therapy Association. (2006). *AOTA's centennial vision*. Retrieved from http://aota.org/News/Centennial/Background/36516.aspx?FT=.pdf

American Telemedicine Association. (2011). *Resolving barriers to licensure portability for telerehabilitation professionals*. Retrieved from http://americantelemed.org/files/public/MemberGroups/Rehabilitation/RERC_TR_0107_11_03b.pdf

Barker, J. A. (1992). *Future edge: Discovering the new paradigms of success*. New York: William Morrow.

Baugher, E., & Pyne, K. (2012). Family minded: Supporting families with children with autism. *OT Practice, (17)*2, 15–19.

Baum, C., & Law, M. (1998). Community health: A responsibility, an opportunity and a fit for occupational therapy. *American Journal of Occupational Therapy, 52*(1), 7–10.

Blakeney, A. B., & Marshall, A. (2009). Water quality, health and human occupations. *American Journal of Occupational Therapy, 63,* 46–57.

Bockhoven, J. S. (1968). Challenge of the new clinical approaches. *American Journal of Occupational Therapy, 22,* 23–25.

Cahill, S., Daniel, D., Nelson-Stitt, M., Brager, S., Dostal, A., Hirter, S. (2009). Creating partnership to promote health and fitness in children. *OT Practice, 14*(6), 10–13.

Capra, F., and Steindl-Rast, D. (1991). *Belonging to the universe: Explorations on the frontiers of science and spirituality.* San Francisco: HarperCollins.

Cason, J. (2012). An introduction to telehealth as a service delivery model within occupational therapy. *OT Practice, 17*(7), CE-1–CE-7.

Cason, J. (2011). Molly asks. *OT Practice, 16*(1), 44.

Chase, C., Roche, S. (2011). Caroline Bartlett Crane Everyman's House: Historical home design and home modification today. *OT Practice, 16*(17), 14–17.

Christiansen, C. H., & Matuska, K. M. (2010). Health promotion research in occupational therapy. In M. Scaffa, S. M. Reitz, & M. Pizzi (Eds.), *Occupational therapy in the promotion of health and wellness* (pp. 528–540). Philadelphia: F.A. Davis Company.

Clark, F., Reingold, F. S., & Salles-Jordan, K. (2007). Obesity and occupational therapy (Position paper). *American Journal of Occupational Therapy, 61*(6), 701–703.

Conrad, D., and Hedin, D. (1991). School-based community service: What we know from research and theory. *Phi Delta Kappan, 72,* 743–749.

Cornish, E. (1980). Toward a philosophy of futurism. *Health Education, 11,* 10–12.

Crabtree, L. (2011). Autism is lifelong: Community integration of adults on the autism spectrum. *OT Practice (16)*12, 8–12.

Fagan, L. A., & Sabata, D. (2011). Home modifications and occupational therapy. AOTA Factsheet. Retrieved from http://aota.org/Consumers/Professionals/WhatIsOT/PA.Facts/39470.aspx

Fagan, L. A., Van Oss, T., Cabrera, C., Olivas De La O T., & Vance, K. (2008). Implementing the centennial vision in home and community health. *AOTA Home and Community Health Special Interest Quarterly, 15*(1), 1–4.

Fidler, G. S. (2000). Beyond the therapy model: Building our future. *American Journal of Occupational Therapy, 54*(1), 99–101.

Finn, G. L. (1972). The occupational therapist in prevention programs. *American Journal of Occupational Therapy, 26,* 59–66.

Freudenberg, N., Eng, E., Flay, B., Parcel, G., Rogers, T., and Wallerstein, N. (1995). Strengthening individual and community capacity to prevent disease and promote health: In search of relevant theories and principles. *Health Education Quarterly, 22*(3), 290–306.

Giles, D. E., and Eyler, J. (1994). The impact of a college community service laboratory on students' personal, social and cognitive outcomes. *Journal of Adolescence, 17,* 327–339.

Health Resources and Services Administration. (n.d.). *Telehealth.* Retrieved from http://hrsa.gov/ruralhealth/about/telehealth/

Horowitz, B. P. (2012). Service learning and occupational therapy education: Preparing students for community practice. *Special Interest Section Quarterly: Education, 22* (2), 1–4.

Kielhofner, G. (2005). Scholarship and practice: Bridging the divide. *American Journal of Occupational Therapy, 59,* 231–239.

Koestler, A. (1978). *Janus.* London: Hutchinson.

Kotler, P. D., & Koenig, P. K. (2012). Authentic partnerships with adults with autism: Sifting the focus to strengths. *OT Practice, (17)*2, 6–9.

Kugel, J. (2010). Combating childhood obesity through community practice. *OT Practice, 15*(15), 17–18.

Lau, C. (2011). Preventing childhood obesity through occupational therapy. *OT Practice, 16*(6), 11–17.

Letts, L. (2003). Occupational therapy and participatory research: A partnership worth pursuing. *American Journal of Occupational Therapy, 57,* 77–87.

Markus, G. B., Howard, J. P., & King, D. C. (1993). Integrating community service and classroom instruction enhances learning: Results from an experiment. *Educational Evaluation and Policy Analysis, 15,* 410–419.

McColl, M. A. (1998). What do we need to know to practice occupational therapy in the community? *American Journal of Occupational Therapy, 52*(1), 11–18.

McKenna, T. (2011). Roadside assistance: Occupational therapy's ethical obligation to older drivers and society. *OT Practice, 16*(2), 11–12.

Morris, A. L. (2009). Collaboration for accessibility and aging in place. *OT Practice, (14)*6, 14–17.

Mosley, L. J., Jedlika, J. S., Lequieu, E., & Taylor, F. D. (2008). Obesity and occupational therapy practice: Present and potential practice trends. *OT Practice, 13*(7), 8–16.

National Service Learning Clearinghouse. (2012). *What is service learning?* Retrieved from http://servicelearning.org/what-service-learning

Odgen, C. L., Carroll, M. D., Kit, B. K., & Flegal, K. M. (2012). *Prevalence of obesity in the U.S., 2009–2010. NCHS data brief, no. 82,* 2–8. Hyattsville, MD: National Center for Health Statistics.

Office of Behavioral and Social Sciences Research, National Institutes of Health. (2011). *Best practices for mixed methods research in the health sciences.* Retrieved from http://obssr.od.nih.gov/mixed_methods_research

Orentlicher, M. L., & Dougan, C. (2011). Person-centered planning: An innovative approach for transition planning. *OT Practice, (16)*1, CE-1–CE-8.

Rogers, E. M. (1995). *Diffusion of innovations* (4th ed.). New York, NY: The Free Press.

Rushdie, S. (1999). *The ground beneath her feet*. New York, NY: Henry Holt.

Sankaran, G., Cinelli, B., McConatha, D., and Carson, L. (1995). Voluntarism: An investment in preparing health professionals for the future. *Journal of Health Education, 26*(1), 58–60.

Scaffa, M. E., Van Slyke, N., & Brownson, C. A. (2008). Occupational therapy services in the promotion of health and prevention of disease and disability. *American Journal of Occupational Therapy, (62)*6, 694–703.

Shrestha, L. B., & Heisler, E. J. (2011). *The changing demographic profile of the United States*. A Congressional Research Service Report to Congress. Retrieved from http://fas.org/sgp/crs/misc/RL32701.pdf

Southwest Autism Research and Resource Center. (2012). *Programs: Vocational/ Life Skills Training*. Retrieved from http://autismcenter.org/Vocational.aspx

Stadnyk, R. L., Townsend, E. A., & Wilcock, A. A. (2010). Occupational justice. In C. Christiansen & E. Townsend (Eds.), *Introduction to occupation: The art and science of living, 2nd ed.* (pp. 329–358). Upper Saddle River, NJ: Pearson.

Stern, E., Prudencio, T., & Sadler, E. (2011). Shifting gears: Helping service members return to the road. *OT Practice, 16*(2), 6–7, 19.

Strzelecki, M. V. (2011). Green light go: Helping teens with disabilities take the wheel. *OT Practice, 16*(2), 8–10, 19.

Taylor, R. R., Braveman, B., & Hammel, J. (2004). Developing and evaluating community-based services through participatory action research: Two case examples, *American Journal of Occupational Therapy, 58*, 73–82.

U.S. Department of Education. (2006). *Part II Department of Education 34 CFR Parts 300 and 301*. Retrieved from http://idea.ed.gov/download/finalregulations.pdf

U.S. Department of Health and Human Services. (n.d.). *What are the reimbursement issues for telehealth*. Retrieved from http://hrsa.gov/healthit/toolbox/RuralHealthITtoolbox/Telehealth/whatarethereimbursement.html

Waite, A. (2011). Home teams: Practitioners work with contractors for home modifications. *OT Practice, 16*(17), 9–13.

Weissert, C., Knott, J., & Steiber, B. (1993). *Health professions education reform: Understanding and explaining states' policy options*. Michigan State University: The Department of Political Science and the Institute for Public Policy and Social Research.

Wilcock, A. (1998). *An occupational perspective on health*. Thorofare, NJ: SLACK.

Young, D. (2011). Assembling the team: Occupational therapy and the building profession. *OT Practice, (16)*17, 11.

Index

Page numbers followed by "f" denote figures, "t" denotes tables, and "b" denotes boxes